IFMBE Proceedings

Volume 86

The IFMBE Proceedings Book Series is an official publication of *the International Federation for Medical and Biological Engineering* (IFMBE). The series gathers the proceedings of various international conferences, which are either organized or endorsed by the Federation. Books published in this series report on cutting-edge findings and provide an informative survey on the most challenging topics and advances in the fields of medicine, biology, clinical engineering, and biophysics.

The series aims at disseminating high quality scientific information, encouraging both basic and applied research, and promoting world-wide collaboration between researchers and practitioners in the field of Medical and Biological Engineering.

Topics include, but are not limited to:

- Diagnostic Imaging, Image Processing, Biomedical Signal Processing
- Modeling and Simulation, Biomechanics
- Biomaterials, Cellular and Tissue Engineering
- Information and Communication in Medicine, Telemedicine and e-Health
- Instrumentation and Clinical Engineering
- Surgery, Minimal Invasive Interventions, Endoscopy and Image Guided Therapy
- Audiology, Ophthalmology, Emergency and Dental Medicine Applications
- Radiology, Radiation Oncology and Biological Effects of Radiation

IFMBE proceedings are indexed by by SCOPUS, EI Compendex, Japanese Science and Technology Agency (JST), SCImago.

Proposals can be submitted by contacting the Springer responsible editor shown on the series webpage (see "Contacts"), or by getting in touch with the series editor Ratko Magjarevic.

More information about this series at https://link.springer.com/bookseries/7403

Juliana Usman · Yih Miin Liew ·
Mohd Yazed Ahmad · Fatimah Ibrahim
Editors

6th Kuala Lumpur International Conference on Biomedical Engineering 2021

Proceedings of BioMed2021, July 28–29, 2021

Springer

Editors
Juliana Usman
Department of Biomedical Engineering
Faculty of Engineering
Universiti Malaya
Kuala Lumpur, Malaysia

Yih Miin Liew
Department of Biomedical Engineering
Faculty of Engineering
Universiti Malaya
Kuala Lumpur, Malaysia

Mohd Yazed Ahmad
Department of Biomedical Engineering
Faculty of Engineering
Universiti Malaya
Kuala Lumpur, Malaysia

Fatimah Ibrahim
Department of Biomedical Engineering
Faculty of Engineering
Universiti Malaya
Kuala Lumpur, Malaysia

ISSN 1680-0737 ISSN 1433-9277 (electronic)
IFMBE Proceedings
ISBN 978-3-030-90723-5 ISBN 978-3-030-90724-2 (eBook)
https://doi.org/10.1007/978-3-030-90724-2

This Springer imprint is published by the registered company Springer Nature Switzerland AG
The registered company address is: Gewerbestrasse 11, 6330 Cham, Switzerland

Conference Organization

Name

The 6th Kuala Lumpur International Conference on Biomedical Engineering 2021

Short Name

BioMed2021

Venue

July 28 and 29, 2021
Virtual Conference

Proceedings Editors

Juliana Usman
Liew Yih Miin
Mohd Yazed Bin Ahmad
Fatimah Ibrahim

Organized by

Department of Biomedical Engineering, Universiti Malaya, Malaysia

In Cooperation with

International Federation for Medical and Biological Engineering (IFMBE)

Endorsed by

Malaysia's Society of Medical and Biological Engineering (MSMBE)

Collaborators

Centre for Innovation in Medical Engineering (CIME)
Centre for Applied Biomechanics (CAB)

Organizing Committee

Advisors

Noor Azuan Abu Osman
Fatimah Ibrahim
Wan Abu Bakar Wan Abas

Chairman

Juliana Usman

Conference Director

Nasrul Anuar Abd Razak

Secretary

Farina Muhamad

Assistant Secretary

Hanie Nadia Shasmin

Treasurer

Mas Sahidayana Mohktar

Assistant Treasurer

Liyana Abu

Program Scientific and Technical

Mohd Yazed Ahmad
Hua-Nong Ting
Einly Lim
Nahrizul Adib Kadri
Nur Azah Hamzaid
Ahmad Khairi Abdul Wahab
Siew-Cheok Ng
Wan Safwani Wan Kamarul Zaman

Secretariat Committee

Nooranida Arifin
Khairunnisa Hasikin
Salmah Karman
Norita Mohd Zain
Norhafizal Ahmad

Azuan Othman
Razalee Rahimi Abd Manaf
Yuslialif Mohd Yusup
Mohd Khairul Amran
Muhairizam Manan
Mohamad Zaki Jaafar
Ahmad Ali-Emran
Ku Mohd Haziq Ku Yusof
Mohamad Ramadan Ramlee
Sainah Che Umar

Publications

Juliana Usman
Yih Miin Liew
Fatimah Ibrahim
Fairuz Hanum

Program Website

Chow-Khuen Chan
Mohd Yazed Ahmad

Public and Industry Relations

Khin-Wee Lai
Hamidreza Mohafez
Nahrizul Adib Kadri
Mas Sahidayana Mohktar
Wan Safwani Wan Kamarul Zaman
Adhli Iskandar Putera Hamzah
Abd Halim Mohamed

Preface

On behalf of the organizing committee, we are honored and delighted to welcome you to the 6th Kuala Lumpur International Conference on Biomedical Engineering (BioMed2021) after a decade-long hiatus. We are proud to be able to host this virtual conference amidst the global outbreak of the COVID-19 pandemic.

The BioMed2021 virtual conference aims to promote the latest research and developments related to the integration of engineering technologies in the fields of medical and life sciences. The virtual conference brings together leading academic icons, researchers, and industrial representatives to exchange and share their knowledge and research results in the latest innovations, research trends and concerns, challenges, and adopted solutions in the field of biomedical engineering.

The BioMed2021 virtual conference is organized by the Department of Biomedical Engineering, Universiti Malaya, in cooperation with the International Federation for Medical and Biological Engineering (IFMBE) and the endorsement from Malaysia's Society of Medical and Biological Engineering (MSMBE). The virtual conference also received support from the Centre for Applied Biomechanics (CAB) and the Centre for Innovation in Medical Engineering (CIME). Special thanks go to our sponsors Abex Medical System Sdn Bhd, Malaysia, BioApps Sdn Bhd, Malaysia, and to Springer for supporting the publication of the conference proceedings.

My highest appreciation goes to all the honorable plenary speakers, the forum panels, and the expert talk speakers for making this conference a globally recognized event. I take this opportunity to extend my heartfelt gratitude to the BioMed2021 organizing committee members for their enthusiasm, commitments, dedications, and hard work and the distinguished International Advisory Committee members for their invaluable support and assistance. Last but not least, I would like to thank all the authors, the reviewers, session chairs, and the delegates for their contributions and participation. The conference will not be a success without your expertise and active participation.

To all participants of BioMed2021, we hope that this conference will foster the exchange of new ideas and networking among researchers along with the joyful academic experience of BioMed2021.

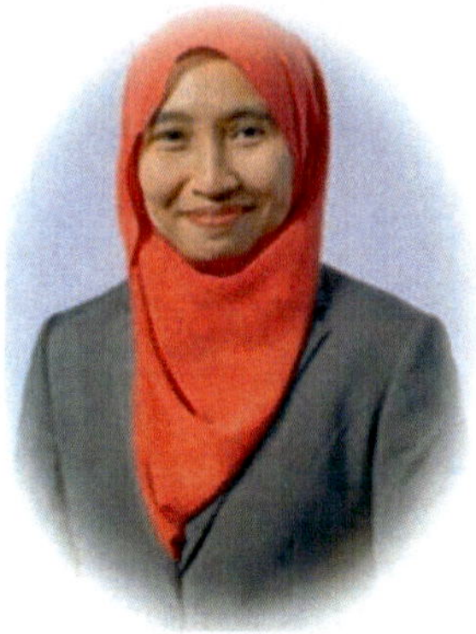

Kuala Lumpur, Malaysia

Dr. Juliana Usman
Conference Chair BioMed2021

Contents

AI and Computational Modeling

Formulation of Sensor Ranking Associated in Categorical Perception: A Pilot Study Using Machine Learning 3
Abdul Rauf A. Bakar, Khin Wee Lai, and Nur Azah Hamzaid

Analysis of Carotid Artery Ultrasound Images Using Gabor Filter, Maximally Stable Extremal Regions and Convolutional Neural Network 15
Soumyajyoti Dutta, Viththal Khandelwal, Rohan Sood, Samiappan Dhanalakshmi, and S. Latha

A Combinational Approach to Generate Nonlinear Foot Trajectories for Robotic Prothesis with Elementary Clinical Results 27
Mouaz Al Kouzbary, Hamza Al Kouzbary, Lai Kuan Tham, Jinjing Liu, Hanie Nadia Shasmin, Nooranida Arifin, and Noor Azuan Abu Osman

Eye-Controlled Wheelchair Improves Quality-of-Life on Paraplegic Patients in Home-Care Setting: A Case Study 37
Kamala Krishnan, Tan Lee Fan, and Danny Ng Wee Kiat

Fusion of Deep Features for Classification of Breast Cancer Using Multi-Deep CNNs 49
S. R. Sannasi Chakravarthy, N. Bharanidharan, and Harikumar Rajaguru

Improved Bald Eagle Search Optimization for Enhancing the Performance of Supervised Classifiers in Dementia Diagnosis 59
N. Bharanidharan, S. R. Sannasi Chakravarthy, and Harikumar Rajaguru

Classification of Walking Speed Based on Bidirectional LSTM 67
Wan Shi Low, Chow Khuen Chan, Joon Huang Chuah, Khairunnisa Hasikin, and Khin Wee Lai

Automated Segmentation of Metal and BVS Stent Struts from OCT Images Using U-Net 75
Yu Shi Lau, Li Kuo Tan, Chow Khuen Chan, Kok Han Chee, and Yih Miin Liew

Comparison of Blood Rheological Models in Patient-Specific Left Coronary Arteries with Varying Degrees of Stenosis 85
Noushin Anan, Nusrat S. Khan, Samreen T. Mahmud, Tahura Hossain, and M. Tarik Arafat

Wall Stress Analysis of Patient-Specific Left Ventricular Hypertrophy Models 93
Wei Jan Goh, Bee Ting Chan, Wan Naimah Wan Ab Naim, Shoon Hui Chuah, Einly Lim, and Yih Miin Liew

Computational Analysis of Newtonian and Non-Newtonian Rheological Models for Patient-Specific Intracranial Aneurysm 103
Farhan Muhib and M. Tarik Arafat

Electro-Mechanical Finite Element Model of Left Ventricular Hypertrophy 113
Zhi Chin Hew, Bee Ting Chan, Wan Naimah Wan Ab Naim, Socrates Dokos, Wah Yen Tey, and Yih Miin Liew

Modified Spotted Hyena Optimizer Based Leukemia Microscopic Images Classification 123
S. Aswath, N. Bharanidharan, R. S. Valarmathi, and Harikumar Rajaguru

A Strategic Corrective Maintenance Prioritization Assessment for Medical Equipment 133
Aizat Hilmi Zamzam, Ayman Khallel Ibrahim Al-Ani, Khairunnisa Hasikin, and Ahmad Khairi Abdul Wahab

Detection of Knee Osteoarthritis and Prediction of Its Severity Using X-ray Image Analysis and Patients Assessment Data: A Hybrid Design 143
Hamidreza Mohafez, Hamza Sayed, Maryam Hadizadeh, Lai Khin Wee, and Siti Anom Ahmad

Depression Detection Using Natural Language Processing on Bahasa Malaysia Non-clinical Text 153
Nur Aiman Mohd Fuad and Nik Nur Wahidah Nik Hashim

A Preliminary Study of IVOCT-Based Atherosclerosis Plaque Classification Technique 163
Sanjiv Rajkumar, Muhammad Safwan Soaib, Yih Miin Liew, Kok Han Chee, Ho Kin Tang, Kanendra Naidu, Nooranida Arifin, and Chow Khuen Chan

Biomechanics, Rehabilitation, and Education

The Effects of Prosthetic Knee Joints During Walking on Different Types of Surfaces: A Preliminary Study ... 173
Nur Amira Adlan, Nooranida Arifin, Noor Azuan Abu Osman, Hasif Rafidee Hasbollah, Saari Mohamad Yatim, Yusniza Mohd Yusof, and Chan Chow Khuen

Ground Reaction Force of Trilateral Amputee During Walking With and Without Upper Limb Prosthesis: Case Report ... 187
Nur Afiqah Hashim, Nasrul Anuar Abd Razak, and Noor Azuan Abu Osman

A Low-Cost Human Gait Analysis System ... 197
Siow Cheng Chan, Yu T'ng Chan, and Yu Zheng Chong

Qualitative Study of Prosthetic Liner Materials on Transtibial Amputees' Satisfaction in Term of Positional Pain and Discomfort ... 205
M. A. Mohamed Nizam, N. A. Abd Razak, N. A. Abu Osman, and R. A. Mohd Jaladin

Restoration of Gait Spatio-temporals After Anterior Cruciate Ligament Reconstruction ... 217
Maryam Hadizadeh, Hamidreza Mohafez, Khin Wee Lai, and Saidon Bin Amri

Surface Electromyography: A New Indicator of Fatigue Level ... 225
Fauzani Jamaluddin, Fatimah Ibrahim, and Siti Anom Ahmad

Relationship Between Handedness and Cognition Performance of University Undergraduates ... 233
Yin Qing Tan, Si Yun Tee, and Hong Kiat Ooi

Parents Involvement in Young STEM Learners and Talent Development: A Pilot Study ... 243
Nur Azah Hamzaid, Juliana Usman, Jegalakshimi Jewaratnam, Chan Chow Khuen, Suzieleez Syrene Abdul Rahim, and Mohd Faiz Azmi

Practice Analysis: The Service Delivery and Domains of Prosthetic and Orthotic Practitioners in Malaysia ... 251
Hasif Rafidee Hasbollah and Nooranida Arifin

A Conceptual Design and Control of a Novel Powered Ankle–Foot Prosthesis (RoMicP™) for Heavy Amputees ... 259
Jingjing Liu, Noor Azuan Abu Osman, Mouaz Al Kouzbary, Hamza Al Kouzbary, Nasrul Anuar Abd Razak, Hanie Nadia Shasmin, and Nooranida Arifin

The Treatment Impact of Partial Body Weight Supported Treadmill (PBWST) on Cerebral Palsy Kid Using Physio-Treadmill (*PhyMill*): A Case Study 269
Rabiatul Aisyah Ariffin, Mohd Azrul Hisham Mohd Adib, Nurul Shahida Mohd Shalahim, Narimah Daud, and Nur Hazreen Mohd Husni

Design and Testing of an Interim Transtibial Prosthetic Leg for Amputees Living in Rural Areas: A Case Study 277
Nur Azah Hamzaid, Mohamad Hasmizan Halim, and Chung Tze Yang

Immediate Effect of Flexing the Toes During Performing Salat on Hemodynamic Status 285
Fatimah Ibrahim, Mas Sahidayana Mokhtar, Nur Fara Ateeka Jaafar, and Nurul Fauzani Jamaluddin

Automatic Physio-Walker (*PhyWalk*) as a Rehabilitation Therapy for Children with Lower Disability 295
Mohd Azrul Hisham Mohd Adib, Mohd Hanafi Abdul Rahim, Rabiatul Aisyah Ariffin, Idris Mat Sahat, Mohd Hafiz Hasan, Nurul Anati Basirah Sulaiman, Siti Nurfarhana Mohamad Wahid, Mohd Firdaus Mak Nayan, Mohammad Fitri Abdullah, Suraya Najiha Mohd Ishak, Nurul Shahida Mohd Shalahim, and Narimah Daud

A Preliminary Study of Ankle Muscular Strategy During Single Leg Stance 303
Nureen Shahirah Ahmad Zaghlul, Siew Li Goh, Rizal Razman, Salmah Karman, and Chow Khuen Chan

The Prevalence of Lower Limb Musculoskeletal Pain Symptoms During Stop and Go Driving 313
Navien Arul Raj, Juliana Usman, Saad Jawaid Khan, and Siew-Li Goh

The Effect of Physical Non-operative Modalities on Pain in Osteoarthritis of the Knee 319
Salma Mohamed Saad, Nor Hazwani Ibrahim, Anusha Nair, Norita Mohd Zain, and Juliana Usman

Biosensors, Biosignals, and Biomedical Imaging

Infant-Wrap (*InfaWrap*) Device as Pediatric Technology Tool: The Heart Rate and SpO^2 Monitoring for Neonates 331
Mohd Hanafi Abdul Rahim, Mohd Azrul Hisham Mohd Adib, Mohamad Zairi Baharom, and Nur Hazreen Mohd Hasni

Optimization and Performance Evaluation of Apodization Function for Fiber Bragg Grating as Vital Sign Sensor 341
Ramya Arumugam, Ramamoorthy Kumar, and Samiappan Dhanalakshmi

Analysis of Heart Rate and Heart Rate Variability for Stress Evaluation 351
Li Ann Lim, Jee Hou Ho, Jong Chern Lim, Einly Lim, and Bee Ting Chan

Fabrication of Carbon Nanofibers Using MEMS Technique for Future Electrochemical Biosensors 363
Elyana Kosri, Fatimah Ibrahim, and Marc Madou

The Study of Polarization Properties of Agarose Gel in Normal Line of Light Transmission 373
Siti Nurainie Tukimin, Salmah Binti Karman, Wan Safwani Wan Kamarul Zaman, and Mohd Yazed Ahmad

Design of Rectifier Circuit to Harvest the RF Energy for Wearable Medical Devices 381
Hussein Yahya Alkhalaf, Mohd Yazed Ahmad, and Harikrishnan Ramiah

Assessing Clinical Usefulness of Readmission Risk Prediction Model 389
Kareen Teo, Ching Wai Yong, Joon Huang Chuah, Khairunnisa Hasikin, Maheza Irna Mohd Salim, Yan Chai Hum, and Khin Wee Lai

Prediction of Spine Decompression Post-surgery Outcome Through Transcranial Motor Evoked Potential Using Linear Discriminant Analysis Algorithm 397
Mohd Redzuan Jamaludin, Saw Lim Beng, Joon Huang Chuah, Khairunnisa Hasikin, Maheza Irna Mohd Salim, Yan Chai Hum, and Khin Wee Lai

Restoring Lesions in Low-Dose Computed Tomography Images of COVID-19 Using Deep Learning 405
K. A. Saneera Hemantha Kulathilake, Nor Aniza Abdullah, Abhishek Shivanand Lachyan, A. M. Randitha Ravimal Bandara, Dhrumil Deveshkumar Patel, and Khin Wee Lai

Detection of COVID-19 on Chest X-Ray Using Neural Networks 415
Anis Shazia, Tan Zi Xuan, Joon Huang Chuah, Hamidreza Mohafez, and Khin Wee Lai

Assessment of LV Myocardial Function in Aortic Stenosis Using Personalized 3D+ Time Cardiac MRI Modelling 425
Shoon Hui Chuah, Wen Dee Thong, Nor Ashikin Md Sari, Li Kuo Tan, Khairunnisa Hasikin, and Yih Miin Liew

Development of Automated Segmentation of the Thigh Muscles from Dixon MRI for Fat Fraction Quantification 437
Ashrani Aizzuddin Abd. Rahni, Mohd Izuan Ibrahim, Devinder Kaur Ajit Singh, Noor Ibrahim Mohamed Sakian, and Suzana Shahar

Longitudinal Assessment of Optical Properties in Early Demineralization of Enamel Using pH Cycling Model 445
Fatin Najwa, Yih Miin Liew, Ngie Min Ung, and Prema Sukumaran

Investigate the Velocity Difference Between MRI Measurement and CFD Simulation on Patient-Specific Blood Flow Analysis 453
Sheh Hong Lim, Mohd Azrul Hisham Mohd Adib, Mohd Shafie Abdullah, Nur Hartini Mohd Taib, Radhiana Hassan, and Azian Abd Aziz

A Preliminary Assessment of Neuro-Salutogenic Landscape Stimuli in Neighbourhood Parks: Theory-Based Model for Stress Mitigation 461
Sharifah Khalizah Syed Othman Thani, Ng Siew Cheok, and Hazreena Hussein

Development of a Mobile Augmented Reality System for Radiotherapy Practitioner Training 471
Kinersh Gopalakrishnan, Nor Aniza Azmi, Rozilawati Ahmad, Wan Nordiana Wan Abdul Rahman, and Ashrani Aizzuddin Abd Rahni

Visual Directed Deep Breathing with Heart Rate Variability Measurement in Mobile Application 479
Poh Foong Lee, Ming Chien Ong, Wei Liang Soon, Chean Swee Ling, and Paul E. Croarkin

Feature Selection for Identification of Fake Profiles on Facebook 489
John Benyen Munga and Prabu Mohandas

Tissue Engineering and Clinical Management

Feasibility of Using Saliva Samples and Laser-Induced Breakdown Spectroscopy for Dental Screening During Pandemic 501
Syafriandi, Siti Norhayati Md Yassin, Siti Norbaieah Mohd Hashim, Maheza Irna Mohamad Salim, Rania Hussein AlAshwal, Asnida Abdul Wahab, Mariaulpa Sahalan, Hum Yan Chai, and Lai Khin Wee

Determination of Suitable Bioactive Glass-Polymer Film Conditioned Medium Extracts for Potential Applications in Tissue Regeneration: A Preliminary Study 511
Siti Fatimah Samsurrijal, Siti Noor Fazliah Mohd Noor, Mamun Khan Sujon, and Khirun Musa

Cellulose Isolation from Oil Palm Empty Fruit Bunch (OPEFB) via Alkaline Hydrogen Peroxide Treatment 519
Nurul Athirah Syafiqah Mohamad Zulkifli, Farina Muhamad, and Bee Chin Ang

Identifying Bioglass and Liquid Exfoliation of Graphite/MWCNT Mixtures Through UV–Vis Spectroscopy 529
Siti Fatimah Samsurrijal, Nik Syahirah Aliaa Nik Sharifulden, Nur Syazana Azizan, David Yi San Chau, and Siti Noor Fazliah Mohd Noor

Increasing the Bacterial Cellulose Yield by Supplementation of Static Culture Medium 541
Farhana Islam and M. Tarik Arafat

Novel Method of Producing Free-Standing SU8-Based Carbon Scaffold as Biomedical Engineering Application 551
Vieralynda Vitus, Fatimah Ibrahim, and Wan Safwani Wan Kamarul Zaman

The Effect of microRNA Targeting IL-17RA in the Regulation of RANKL and OPG Expressions in Stem Cells from Human Exfoliated Deciduous Teeth 561
Wan Khairunnisaa Wan Nor Aduni, Rashidi Dzul Keflee, See Too Wei Cun, and Asma Abdullah Nurul

Synthesis of Polycaprolactone Using Novel Crude Lipase: Parameter Optimization 571
Paveethra Thegarathah, Muhamad Harith bin Amran, Jegalakshimi Jewaratnam, and Khanom Simarani

Experimental Study Between TPU Flex and Silicon Materials Mechanical Properties as an Alternatives in Development of the *CardioVASS* Heart Model 577
Nur Afikah Khairi Rosli, Mohd Azrul Hisham Mohd Adib, Mok Chik Ming, Nurul Natasha Mohd Sukri, Idris Mat Sahat, and Nur Hazreen Mohd Hasni

Assessment of the Cardiac Response to Sleep Arousal 593
Sobhan Salari Shahrbabaki and Mathias Baumert

Achieving Carbon-Balanced Ecosystem: Case Study of Carbon Sequestration Analysis in Universiti Malaya 601
Nurshafira Hazim Chan, Ayman Khallel Ibrahim Al-Ani, Nahrizul Adib Kadri, Sarah Abdul Razak, Hanee Farzana Hizaddin, Mohd Istajib Mokhtar, Muhammad Mokhzaini Azizan, Khin Wee Lai, and Khairunnisa Hasikin

Surface Water Quality Assessment: A Case Study of Merbok River, Kuala Muda, Kedah 611
Wen Yee Wong, Ayman Khallel Ibrahim Al-Ani, Sarah Abdul Razak, Hanee Farzana Hizaddin, Mohd Istajib Mokhtar, Muhammad Mokhzaini Azizan, and Khairunnisa Hasikin

AI and Computational Modeling

Formulation of Sensor Ranking Associated in Categorical Perception: A Pilot Study Using Machine Learning

Abdul Rauf A. Bakar, Khin Wee Lai, and Nur Azah Hamzaid

Abstract The concept of categorical perception has been enormously investigated to digitalize the process of auditory processing when perceiving speech stimulus at higher brain neurological signal. Despite the nature non-stationary property of electroencephalography (EEG) during any task processing, scientists and clinicians find it to be not well fitted in the healthcare setting application without professional monitoring, and even worst, the hearing aid device functionality was also reported at a low success rate. In this study, we embraced machine learning technology and extracting contribution into our auditory research area. The present pilot work aims to create a robust computational framework to formulate the sensor ranking principle in auditory speech perception. The ranking for sensors could facilitate in identifying the minimal set sensor-of-interest (ROI) that are sufficient in specific auditory task processing using an optimally trained model. The trained Support Vector Machine (SVM) highest performance reported at random 2 training dataset with scoring of 92.3% using 70% triple-random training dataset. Based on the sensor ranking, the C_Z electrode outperformed the other electrodes with scoring of 96.74%, followed by P_Z and F_{PZ} for the 2nd and 3rd rank (95.66% and 95.34% respectively). Our pilot study anticipated that the sensor ranking formula able to underline more precise neural correlates based on current auditory categorical perception response. The excellence sensor ranking in delivering a minimal set of sensor-of-interest (SOI) drive the capability of the SVM model in classifying auditory brain response in high-performance prediction metrics and possible reliability in the healthcare setting application.

Keywords Electroencephalography (EEG) · Categorical perception · Machine learning · Cortical auditory evoked potential (CAEP) · Support vector machine (SVM)

A. R. A. Bakar · K. W. Lai (✉) · N. A. Hamzaid
Department of Biomedical Engineering, Faculty of Engineering, Universiti Malaya, 50603 Kuala Lumpur, Malaysia
e-mail: lai.khinwee@um.edu.my

J. Usman et al. (eds.), *6th Kuala Lumpur International Conference on Biomedical Engineering 2021*, IFMBE Proceedings 86,
https://doi.org/10.1007/978-3-030-90724-2_1

1 Introduction

The necessity of a structured and accurate auditory brain system when perceiving sound stimulus is highly determined by an organized speech perception. Categorical perception (CP) is inherent from speech perception property to underpin how the process of listening and discrimination were established in auditory neurological categorization into invariant format [1–4]. Initially, CP predicted as an "isolated mode" during speech listening process [5] but yet the philosophy changes when more recent researchers discovered wider manifestation of CP in perception of colors [6], musical chord studies [7] and further in speech vowel continuum processing [3]. The shifting of neurological response from desired auditory signal mapping evident in daily verbal conversation when the hearing loss population experiences constant processing disruption, even worst in a noisy environment [3, 8].

It has been well documented that the reliance on electrophysiological data recorded through electroencephalography (EEG) help to convey attributed information in hearing research, including development of high quality hearing aids [9, 10]. Cortical auditory evoked potential (CAEP) refers to the neuronal electrical activity emanated from the scalp after the onset of auditory stimulus that are measured continuously with highly specific time-locked characteristics. Many studies showed how the contribution of neural mechanism at different perceptual state, morphology, learning experience, and stimulus acoustical properties and familiarities have complicate the auditory evaluation process to certain extent [11–14]. For example, it was reported that the CAEP components experienced response alteration at different stage of age in life, as a measure of maturational process [14, 15].

Post market survey had concluded that the poor performance of advanced hearing aids in delivering desired speech sound based on the feedback collected from hearing aid wearers, and yet the device abandonment contributed as the next step taken as part of the devices ineffectiveness [16–18]. Significantly, the complexities and existing influential factors had lead into several challenges in affirming clinical decision at research setting and healthcare locality. To date, increasing interest has been on the verge of establishing machine learning computational into healthcare clinical decision [19, 20]. With the opportunity of future availability of electronic health data in healthcare sector, scientist have utilized practical application of machine learning which are commonly used in medical imaging into various sectors of clinical diagnostic, i.e. in epilepsy studies [21], multiple sclerosis disease [22], sleep study [23], therapeutic research [24], speech and language [25] and recently in the auditory assessment [26, 27]. Remarkable work done in 2019 has used CAEP response and machine learning to distinguish brain response among age-related hearing loss when processing speech information [27]. Extended work also utilized the same capacity to classify hearing capability test groups and speech clarity and it is proven to work more effectively at left hemisphere region [28, 29].

While prior studies have identified the contribution of machine learning in classification process, we offer a new analysis to formulate how the trained computation classifier support sensor ranking in obtaining high level speech perception performance. The proposed pilot work could assist in determining the minimal set sensor-of-interest (SOI) to recognize precise neural correlates of auditory response in terms of any deficits or abnormalities. We focused to train the classifier algorithm before using it as a predictive tool. This pilot work would help to shed light on the next data driven approach in anticipating the brain neuronal response processing among hearing impairment population. The minimal sensor set that is sufficient for optimal classification process would develop further avenue on robust framework that could translate data driven response in hearing research area and development of digital hearing aid.

2 Research Methodology

2.1 Participants

Eight adult male subjects (age: 20–45 years) participated in the present work. All the recruited subjects were healthy, right-handed, and having a normal level of auditory sensitivity for both ears (<20 dB Hearing Level (HL) between 250 and 8000 Hz based on audiometry test) [29, 30]. Their health condition was confirmed based on medical history, medical assessment, and Pure Tone Audiometry (PTA) test by Otorhinolaryngology (ENT) physicians at University Malaya Medical Centre (UMMC), Kuala Lumpur, Malaysia. A simple Mini-Mental State Examination (MMSE) was performed to provide an extended measure of the subject's behavioural, cognitive, and memory proficiency [8, 31, 32]. All the subjects were briefly explained about the study protocol and signed written consent was obtained from all participants before the experiment. The study setup was approved by Medical Ethics Committee, UMMC (Institutional Review Board (IRB) No.: 1045.22) and conducted in line with the Code of Ethics (Declaration of Helsinki) by the World Medical Association (WMA) for research involving human subjects. Figure 1 presented the audiogram behavioral response of both ears across all participants.

2.2 Stimulus Description and EEG Data Acquisition

Two consonants-vowel (CV) speech tokens /ba/ and /pa/ with phonemes phonological contrast in terms of their voicing property (/b/ is voiced, /p/ is voiceless) were applied as auditory stimuli delivered at 80 dB Sound Pressure Level (SPL). The speech tokens were digitized at 250 ms with 10 ms rise/fall time to minimize the spectral platter phenomenon. The oddball paradigm setup was implemented for each token using pseudorandomized manner with 80% probability for standard stimulus and 20% probability for deviant stimulus at an interstimulus interval of 800 $\pm$ 200 ms. The

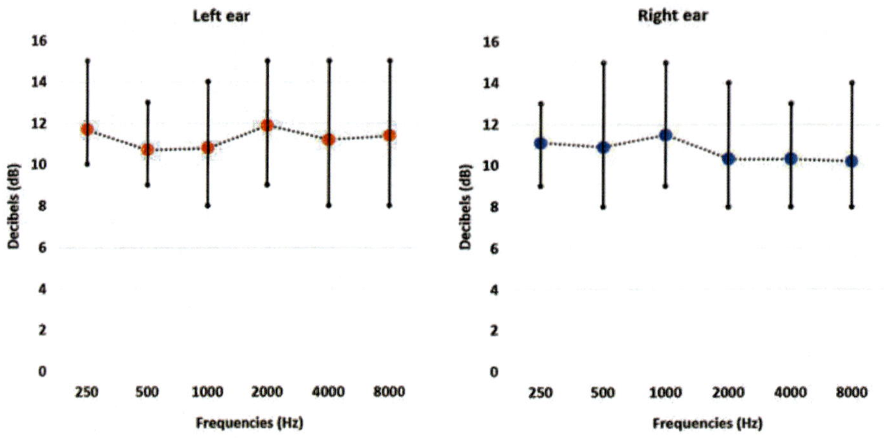

Fig. 1 The average (avg: centre point), maximum (max: top point) and minimum (min: bottom point) chart of both ears behavioral threshold for all recruited subjects using PTA test

speech token /ba/ was fixed as a deviant stimulus on every trial. To minimize the artifacts or noise from the surrounding, the experimental procedure was carried out passively in a soundproof chamber and auditory stimuli were presented binaurally using closed circumaural headphones HD 428 calibrated at ear level. To elevate the SNR (signal-to-noise ratio), a replication of two successful trials were applied with a total of 600 CVs were delivered in a clear condition with that of 480 responses from the standard stimulus and 120 responses from the deviant stimulus. All recruited subjects were allowed to have a short break between trials. All subjects were advised to stay awake and focused on the reading material supplied. The design of stimulus presentation is illustrated in Fig. 2.

Each speech token contained distinct voice fundamental frequency and specific formant frequencies (/ba/; F0: 217 Hz, F1: 740 Hz, F2: 1481 Hz, F3: 3228 Hz, F4: 4311 Hz; and /pa/; F0: 866 Hz, F1: 929 Hz, F2: 1523 Hz, F3: 3478 Hz, F4: 4438 Hz). The brain neural activity was recorded using a modified International 10–20 system of electrode placement via wireless EEG device Enobio 8 channels system

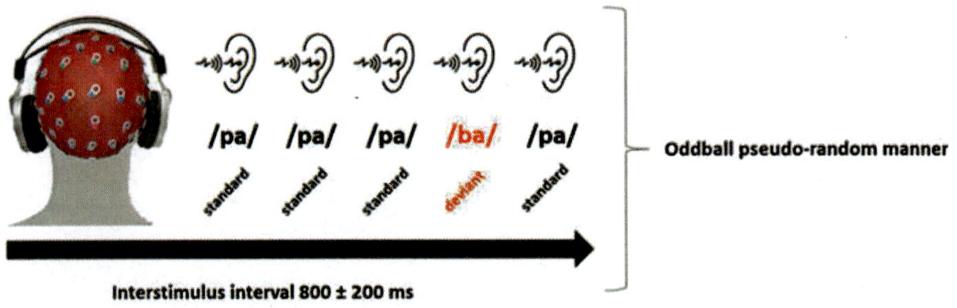

Fig. 2 Pseudorandomized design of speech stimulus presentation on both ears

(Neuroelectrics, Cambridge, MA, United States) at 500 Hz sampling frequency [8, 33, 34]. Silver-Silver Chloride (Ag/AgCl) electrodes were used on the EEG cap to continuously captured the EEG signal response from left hemisphere at specific positioning; F_{PZ}, F_Z, C_Z, P_Z, C_3, F_7, T_7, and P_7. Two additional electrodes were applied as reference (active Common Mode Sense (CMS)) and grounding at the right mastoid (passive Driven Right Leg (DRL)). A standard computer installed with Neuroelectrics NIC 1.3 software and MATLAB R2019a was used for the inter-software communication on stimulus delivery and presentation. The inter-electrodes impedance were maintained at below 5kΩ. All the recruited participants were brief to reduce any avoidable artifacts especially those from physiological and muscle origin [15, 35]. For instances, present research protocol adopted and developed from formerly established work on elicitation, acquisition and quantification of CAEP response in auditory passive listening mode [15, 28, 36].

2.3 CAEP Feature Analysis

The collected EEG signal responses were initially processed and analyzed using MATLAB R2019a software. The signal pre-processing technique eliminated the presence of ocular artifacts, power supply noise and baseline correction (at 100 ms pre-stimulus interval). The signals were bandpass filtered at 1–30 Hz. Any artifact-contaminated peak response emerged higher than $\pm 35\ \mu V$ were rejected upon analysis [37, 38]. The CAEP response were interpreted from these continuous EEG signal. Based on the two successful trials of EEG recording session, only the deviant CAEP response were averaged separately at each specific electrode positioning. The 800 ms time domain waveforms of the CAEP emanated after the deviant stimulus onset were constructed on each trials and were averaged between the trials to obtain the final individual CAEP waveform. Five components of CAEP amplitude were visually verified based on their standard windowing latencies namely as P1 (20–100 ms), N1 (60–160 ms), P2 (140–240 ms), N2 (160–300 ms) and P3 (280–470 ms) [15, 39–41] via automated CAEP components detection algorithm. It is documented that CAEP waveforms with low SNR were observed as a poor performance signal and excluded leaving about 95% of the signal data that was retained for further analysis.

2.4 Predictive Model Construction for Sensor Ranking

The machine learning model is a valuable tool in offering predictive measure based on the given training dataset to learn through adaptation, pattern learning and processing new future data with possible performance measure even in small data sizes [4, 42, 43]. In this pilot study, we trained SVM classifier to create a robust predictive model in ranking sensors performance at specific brain activity condition from CAEP. The SVM model learned the response function from the training dataset that represented in the time-domain waveform. The study randomly used 70% of the total data sizes as training dataset and another 30% as testing dataset. A five-fold cross-validation was iterated in order to fine-tuning on our sample data sizes and cater model overfitting [4, 44]. The randomized training dataset was repeated for three trials by evaluating classifier performance metrics, receiver operating characteristics (ROC) curve, area under the curve (AUC) and F1-score. Once all the triple-random SVM models learned the discriminant predictors, the 30% unseen data was submitted for automated prediction and were quantified separately. SVM classifier works by transforming non-linear data into higher-dimensional space predictors [45]. SVM developed a hyperplane having maximum margin to accurately separate the attributed class labels [43]. The accuracy performance of the trained SVM at each sensor position was calculated and ranked in comparison with the ground truth class labels.

3 Results and Discussion

The present work supplied the time-domain waveform as an input dataset to train the SVM classifier. We reported that there is no statistical significant difference between the trials across all subjects using paired sample t-test ($t = 1.14$, $p > 0.05$), thus the responses were averaged to be collectively known as specific individual response. Notably, the averaged time-domain waveform responses were used as ground truth labels in evaluating the model prediction performance. Figure 3 represented on the averaged CAEP multichannel waveforms across all recruited subjects measured in 800 ms window after deviant stimulus onset. The result showed that the trained

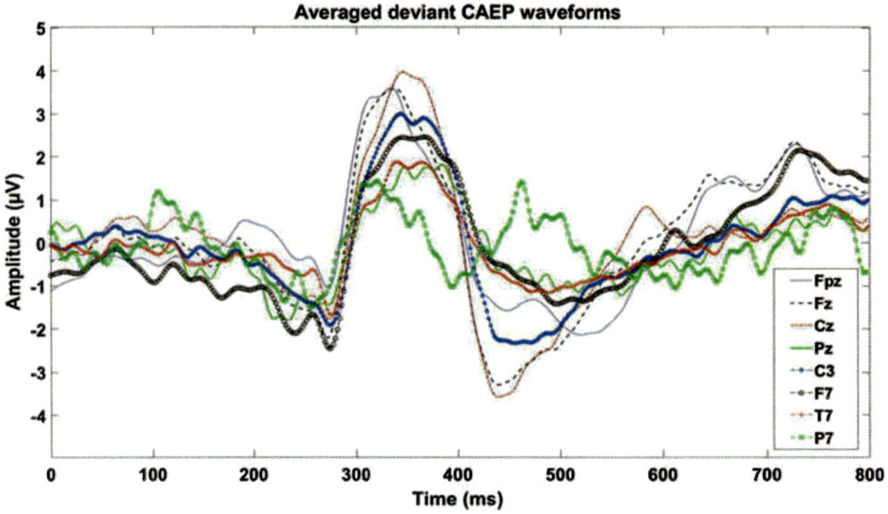

Fig. 3 Averaged CAEP waveform across all participants recorded on eight channel EEG electrodes

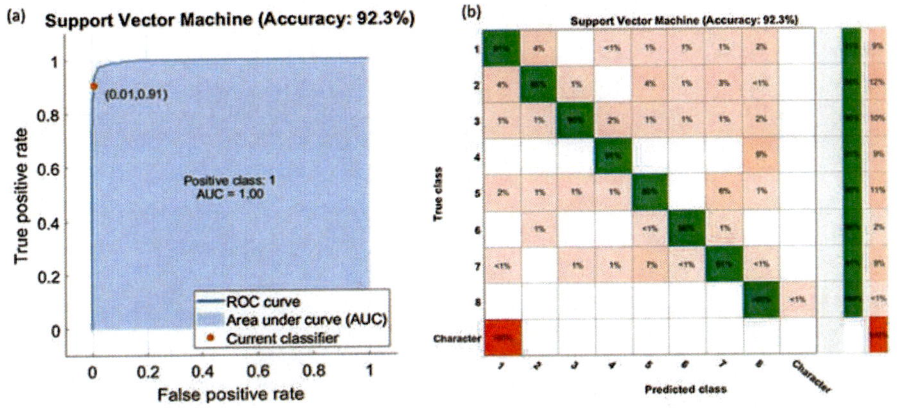

Fig. 4 Trained SVM with highest accuracy at 92.3%. Left **a** ROC curve plot. Right **b** confusion matrix plot using true positive rates false positive rates function (Predicted class label descriptions; class 1: F_{PZ}, class 2: F_Z, class 3: C_Z, class 4: P_Z, class 5: C_3, class 6: F_7, class 7: T_7, and class 8: P_7)

SVM achieved maximum tuning of 92.3% based on triple-random training dataset supplied using five-fold cross-validation. The ROC curve and confusion matrix table were displayed in Fig. 4.

Our findings proved that the training dataset was capable to develop a potentially good predictive SVM model with over 90% performance accuracy as recorded in all triple-random training dataset (Table 1). The mapping achievement corroborates with former investigations when the training accuracy percentage may reflect as an indicator on the capability of the model for next decoding label quantification [26, 46]. Therefore, triple-random training dataset have supported the SVM model to hold-out next testing dataset for the model validation and predictive measure.

We randomly used the 30% of the unseen data from overall hemispheric-specific data activity to test on the developed model. Figure 5 presented on the testing data accuracy on each sensor using triple-random trained SVM. As a whole, the fitted SVM model showed great potential to correctly predict the auditory response based on their class labels with capacity higher than 85% accuracy. The performance based on accuracies indexes underline the formulation of sensor ranking in highly specific auditory task response. Based on the sensor ranking prediction using triple-random

Table 1 Training performance of triple-random trained SVM model

Training data (K-Fold: 5)	Accuracy (%)	Prediction speed (observation/sec)	Training time (sec)	AUC (%)	F1 score (%)
Random 1	91.4	3500	28.03	98.42	98.00
Random 2	**92.3**	3500	28.18	**100.00**	**100.00**
Random 3	90.8	**3600**	**27.92**	98.13	98.00

The 'bold' represented on the top performer

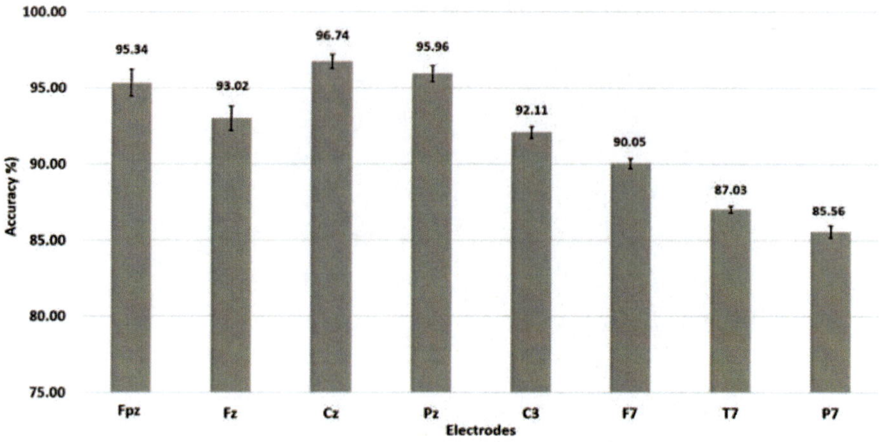

Fig. 5 Sensor ranking prediction using triple-random trained SVM model with error bars

trained classifier, C_Z, P_Z and F_{PZ} electrodes ranked at the highest top three among other SOI (96.47%, 95.66% and 95.34% respectively) and the lowest score situated for P7 electrodes (85.56%). The next 4th and 5th sensors ranking achieved by F_Z and C_3 electrodes with scoring of 93.02% and 92.11% respectively. The presented outperformed sensors resembled with the previous studies when C_Z and P_Z have shown clear indications of behavioral speech-in-noise perception involving children [47, 48], vowel sound susceptivity [49], and medium of benchmark on temporal and spatial processing deficits in auditory abnormalities affecting speech perception [4, 8, 50]. Here, we conveyed that SVM model could be a great classifier algorithm in learning the brain neurophysiological speech processing response. The successful of SVM model aligned with many studies which discussed about the achievement of SVM model in hearing research classification [27, 51, 52]. It has been further noted that C_Z, P_Z, F_{PZ}, F_Z, and C_3 fulfill the minimal set of SOI that potentially sufficient and capable to classify auditory brain response in high performance machine learning model.

4 Conclusion

In conclusion, the present pilot research built effective computational modelling that could identify the minimal sensor set through sensor ranking in delivering good machine learning performance. We demonstrated the capacity of the SVM model to be trained as a robust classifier. It is suggested that the formulation of sensor ranking using machine learning model development could equip us to focus on diversity manifestation of neurophysiological speech processing knowledge in a more precise SOI. However, the existing limited data size may contribute several challenges to automate the model at a greater scale, and given recommendation that the elevated number of data size would improve the model applicability. The future direction should look into how the development of robust multi-model assists in the classification of auditory speech signal processing at different perceptual states to distinguish response properties in the auditory process.

Acknowledgements This work was financially supported by the RU Geran, Universiti Malaya (ST005-2020) and Public Service Department of Malaysia (JPA). The authors declared no conflict of interest.

References

1. Zheng, H.-Y., Minett, J.W., Peng, G., Wang, W.S.Y.: The impact of tone systems on the categorical perception of lexical tones: an event-related potentials study. Lang. Cognit. Process. **27**(2), 184–209 (2012)
2. Bidelman, G.M., Lee, C.-C.: Effects of language experience and stimulus context on the neural organization and categorical perception of speech. Neuroimage **120**, 191–200 (2015)
3. Bidelman, G.M., Walker, B.S.: Attentional modulation and domain-specificity underlying the neural organization of auditory categorical perception. Eur. J. Neurosci. **45**(5), 690–699 (2017)
4. Mahmud, M.S., Ahmed, F., Yeasin, M., Bidelman, G.M.: Decoding categorical speech perception from evoked brain responses. In: 2020 IEEE Region 10 Symposium (TENSYMP), IEEE (2020)
5. Liberman, A.M., Mattingly, I.G.: A specialization for speech perception. Science **243**(4890), 489–494 (1989)
6. Franklin, A., Drivonikou, G.V., Clifford, A., Kay, P., Regier, T., Davies, I.R.: Lateralization of categorical perception of color changes with color term acquisition. Proc. Natl. Acad. Sci. **105**(47), 18221–18225 (2008)
7. Klein, M.E., Zatorre, R.J.: A role for the right superior temporal sulcus in categorical perception of musical chords. Neuropsychologia **49**(5), 878–887 (2011)
8. Ting, H.N., ABakar, A.R., Santhosh, J., Al-Zidi, M.G.: Effects of speech phonological features during passive perception on cortical auditory evoked potential in sensorineural hearing loss. Sains Malaysiana **46**(12), 2477–2488 (2017)
9. Van Yper, L.N., Dhooge, I.J., Vermeire, K., De Vel, E.F., Beynon, A.J.: The P300 auditory event-related potential as a method to assess the benefit of contralateral hearing aid use in bimodal listeners: a proof-of-concept. Int. J. Audiol. **59**(1), 73–80 (2020)
10. Engström, E., Kallioinen, P., von Mentzer, C.N., Lindgren, M., Ors, M., Sahlén, B., et al.: Computer-assisted reading intervention for children with sensorineural hearing loss using hearing aids: effects on auditory event-related potentials and mismatch negativity. Int. J. Pediatr. Otorhinolaryngol. **117**, 17–25 (2019)
11. Brown, A.D., Beemer, B.T., Greene, N.T., Argo IV, T., Meegan, G.D., Tollin, D.J.: Effects of active and passive hearing protection devices on sound source localization, speech recognition, and tone detection. PLoS One **10**(8) (2015)
12. Paulraj, M., Subramaniam, K., Yaccob, S.B., Adom, A.H.B., Hema, C.: Auditory evoked potential response and hearing loss: a review. Open Biomed. Eng. J. **9**, 17 (2015)
13. Durankaya, S.M., Mutlu, B., Isler, Y., Uzun, Y., Kırkım, G.: Comparison of cortical auditory evoked potential findings in presbycusis with low and high word-recognition score. J. Am. Acad. Audiol. (2020)
14. Silva, L.A.F., Magliaro, F.C.L., Carvalho, A., Matas, C.G.: Maturation of long latency auditory evoked potentials in hearing children: systematic review. CoDAS (2017)

15. Duncan, C.C., Barry, R.J., Connolly, J.F., Fischer, C., Michie, P.T., Näätänen, R., et al.: Event-related potentials in clinical research: guidelines for eliciting, recording, and quantifying mismatch negativity, P300, and N400. Clin. Neurophysiol. **120**(11), 1883–1908 (2009)
16. Jilla, A.M., Johnson, C.E., Danhauer, J.L., Anderson, M., Smith, J.N., Sullivan, J.C., et al.: Predictors of hearing aid use in the advanced digital era: an investigation of benefit, satisfaction, and self-efficacy. J. Am. Acad. Audiol. (2020)
17. Lerner, S.: Limitations of conventional hearing aids: examining common complaints and issues that can and cannot be remedied. Otolaryngol. Clin. North Am. **52**(2), 211–220 (2019)
18. Kozlowski, L., Ribas, A., Almeida, G., Luz, I.: Satisfaction of elderly hearing aid users. Int. Arch. Otorhinolaryngol. **21**(01), 92–96 (2017)
19. Wiens, J., Shenoy, E.S.: Machine learning for healthcare: on the verge of a major shift in healthcare epidemiology. Clin. Infect. Dis. **66**(1), 149–153 (2018)
20. Ghassemi, M., Naumann, T., Schulam, P., Beam, A.L., Ranganath, R.: Opportunities in machine learning for healthcare (2018). arXiv:1806.00388
21. Abbasi, B., Goldenholz, D.M.: Machine learning applications in epilepsy. Epilepsia **60**(10), 2037–2047 (2019)
22. Yperman, J., Becker, T., Valkenborg, D., Popescu, V., Hellings, N., Van Wijmeersch, B., et al.: Machine learning analysis of motor evoked potential time series to predict disability progression in multiple sclerosis. BioRxiv 772996 (2019)
23. Ravan, M.: A machine learning approach using EEG signals to measure sleep quality. AIMS Electron. Electr. Eng. **3**(4), 347 (2019)
24. Bălan, O., Moise, G., Moldoveanu, A., Leordeanu, M., Moldoveanu, F.: An investigation of various machine and deep learning techniques applied in automatic fear level detection and acrophobia virtual therapy. Sensors **20**(2), 496 (2020)
25. Baker, J.M., Chan, A.M., Marinkovic, K., Halgren, E., Cash, S.: Machine learning for learning how the brain recognizes speech and language. In: Statistical And Perceptual Audition 2010 (2010)
26. Xie, Z., Reetzke, R., Chandrasekaran, B.: Machine learning approaches to analyze speech-evoked neurophysiological responses. J. Speech Lang. Hear. Res. **62**(3), 587–601 (2019)
27. Mahmud, M.S., Ahmed, F., Al-Fahad, R., Moinuddin, K.A., Yeasin, M., Alain, C., et al.: Decoding age-related changes in the spatiotemporal neural processing of speech using machine learning. bioRxiv, 786566 (2019)
28. Mahmud, M.S., Ahmed, F., Al-Fahad, R., Moinuddin, K.A., Yeasin, M., Alain, C., et al.: Decoding hearing-related changes in older adults' spatiotemporal neural processing of speech using machine learning. Front. Neurosci. **14** (2020)
29. Mahmud, M.S., Ahmed, F., Yeasin, M., Alain, C., Bidelman, G.M.: Multivariate models for decoding hearing impairment using EEG gamma-band power spectral density. In: 2020 International Joint Conference on Neural Networks (IJCNN), IEEE (2020)
30. Mohammed, G., Al-Zidi, J.S., Siew-Cheok NG, Ibrahim Amer, I., Rauf, A., Bakar, A.: P2 and P3 as indicators of hearing aids performance in speech perception. Biomed. Eng./Biomedizinische Technik (2016)
31. Wang, R., Wang, J., Yu, H., Wei, X., Yang, C., Deng, B.: Power spectral density and coherence analysis of Alzheimer's EEG. Cogn. Neurodyn. **9**(3), 291–304 (2015)
32. Folstein, M.F., Folstein, S.E., McHugh, P.R.: Mini-mental state: a practical method for grading the cognitive state of patients for the clinician **12**(3), 189–198 (1975)
33. Ruffini, G., Dunne, S., Farrés, E., Cester, I., Watts, P.C., Ravi, S., et al.: ENOBIO dry electrophysiology electrode; first human trial plus wireless electrode system. In: Engineering in Medicine and Biology Society, 2007. EMBS 2007. 29th Annual International Conference of the IEEE, IEEE (2007)
34. Dubreuil-Vall, L., Ruffini, G., Camprodon, J.A.: Deep learning convolutional neural networks discriminate adult ADHD from healthy individuals on the basis of event-related spectral EEG. Front. Neurosci. **14**, 251 (2020)
35. Tandle, A., Jog, N., D'cunha, P., Chheta, M.: Classification of artefacts in EEG signal recordings and EOG artefact removal using EOG subtraction. Commun. Appl. Electron. **4**, 12–19 (2016)

36. Korczak, P.A., Stapells, D.R.: Effects of various articulatory features of speech on cortical event-related potentials and behavioral measures of speech-sound processing. Ear. Hear. **31**(4), 491–504 (2010)
37. Bidelman, G.M., Moreno, S., Alain, C.: Tracing the emergence of categorical speech perception in the human auditory system. Neuroimage **79**, 201–212 (2013)
38. Yi, H.G., Xie, Z., Reetzke, R., Dimakis, A.G., Chandrasekaran, B.: Vowel decoding from single-trial speech-evoked electrophysiological responses: a feature-based machine learning approach. Brain Beha. **7**(6), e00665 (2017)
39. Stapells, D.R.: Cortical event-related potentials to auditory stimuli. Handbook Clin. Audiol. **5**, 378–406 (2002)
40. Lightfoot, G.: Summary of the N1-P2 cortical auditory evoked potential to estimate the auditory threshold in adults. In: Seminars in Hearing. Thieme Medical Publishers (2016)
41. Steinhauer, K.: Event-related potentials (ERPs) in second language research: a brief introduction to the technique, a selected review, and an invitation to reconsider critical periods in L2. Appl. Linguist. amu028 (2014)
42. Papakostas, G.A., Diamantaras, K.I., Palmieri, F.A.: Emerging trends in machine learning for signal processing. Comput. Intell. Neurosci. **2017** (2017)
43. Hosseini, M.-P., Hosseini, A., Ahi, K.: A review on machine learning for EEG signal processing in bioengineering. IEEE Rev. Biomed. Eng. (2020)
44. McKearney, R.M., MacKinnon, R.C.: Objective auditory brainstem response classification using machine learning. Int. J. Audiol. **58**(4), 224–230 (2019)
45. Subasi, A., Gursoy, M.I.: EEG signal classification using PCA, ICA, LDA and support vector machines. Expert Syst. Appl. **37**(12), 8659–8666 (2010)
46. Ilyas, M., Naït-Ali, A.: Machine Learning Based Detection of Hearing Loss Using Auditory Perception Responses. In: 2019 15th International Conference on Signal-Image Technology and Internet-Based Systems (SITIS), IEEE (2019)
47. Benítez-Barrera, C.R., Key, A.P., Ricketts, T.A., Tharpe, A.M.: Central auditory system responses from children while listening to speech in noise. Hear. Res. **403**, 108165 (2021)
48. Mukari, S.Z.-M.S., Umat, C., Chan, S.C., Ali, A., Maamor, N., Zakaria, M.N.: Effects of age and type of stimulus on the cortical auditory evoked potential in healthy Malaysian children. J. Audiol. Otol. **24**(1), 35 (2020)
49. Silva, D.M., Rothe-Neves, R., Melges, D.B.: Long-latency event-related responses to vowels: N1–P2 decomposition by two-step principal component analysis. Int. J. Psychophysiol. **148**, 93–102 (2020)
50. Roque, L., Karawani, H., Gordon-Salant, S., Anderson, S.: Effects of age, cognition, and neural encoding on the perception of temporal speech cues. Front. Neurosci. **13**, 749 (2019)
51. Ibrahim, I.A., Ting, H.-N., Moghavvemi, M.: Formulation of a novel classification indices for classification of human hearing abilities according to cortical auditory event potential signals. Arab. J. Sci. Eng. **44**(8), 7133–7147 (2019)
52. Paulraj, M., Subramaniam, K., Yaccob, S.B., Adom, A.H.B., Hema. C.: A machine learning approach for distinguishing hearing perception level using auditory evoked potentials. In: 2014 IEEE Conference on Biomedical Engineering and Sciences (IECBES), IEEE (2014)

Analysis of Carotid Artery Ultrasound Images Using Gabor Filter, Maximally Stable Extremal Regions and Convolutional Neural Network

Soumyajyoti Dutta, Viththal Khandelwal, Rohan Sood, Samiappan Dhanalakshmi, and S. Latha

Abstract Stroke is considered as one of the leading reasons for death at present. The presence of plaque in the carotid artery (CA) is a factor that can be utilized to foresee the risk of diseases related to it (such as cerebral ischemia). Due to fat deposition or plaque formation in the wall of Carotid Artery, blood circulation system gets damaged resulting change in blood flow to brain. For a period of time, an increase in deposition can totally obstruct blood flow resulting reduced patency of the lumen. The purpose of this article is to provide a comprehensive overview of procedures used to investigate the carotid artery for the aim of detecting stroke, atherosclerosis, and other cardiovascular diseases which primarily suggests detection of wall thickening or plaque formation the lumen. For morphological evaluation of CA, ultrasound imaging has been the most clinically useful process. We go through the strategies for artery wall monitoring, intima–media segmentation, and lumen segmentation, which aids in determination of the magnitude of mentioned disease. The report images tend to contain speckle noise due to the photographic modality's properties, which degrades image clarity. For image denoising, the Anisotropic Diffusion Filter was used. Denoising techniques which prioritize edge preservation and have an edge seeking function as the diffusion coefficient is more accurate for the files to be examined for this study. A detailed parametric study of some filtering techniques is considered as the first step towards the approach. The second step of the process is feature extraction of the datasets. Two different approaches have been listed to round out this study. This includes maximally stable extremal regions (MSER), local binary pattern (LBP), image matrix study of region of interest (ROI) and application of Gabor Filter. The supporting argument regarding the recommended feature extraction process is strengthened by training a Convolutional Neural Network (CNN) model with the created database.

S. Dutta · V. Khandelwal · R. Sood · S. Dhanalakshmi (✉) · S. Latha
Department of Electronics and Communication Engineering, College of Engineering and Technology, SRM Institute of Science and Technology, SRM Nagar, Kancheepuram, Chengalpattu Dt., Tamil Nadu 603203, India
e-mail: dhanalas@srmist.edu.in

J. Usman et al. (eds.), *6th Kuala Lumpur International Conference on Biomedical Engineering 2021*, IFMBE Proceedings 86,
https://doi.org/10.1007/978-3-030-90724-2_2

Keywords Carotid artery · Atherosclerotic plaques · Anisotropic diffusion · LBP feature extraction · Image-matrix analysis · Gabor filter · CNN

1 Introduction

Using the North American symptomatic carotid endarterectomy trial process, the fear of stroke increases by 0.1–1.6% a year in asymptomatic persons with ICA stenosis of 75–80%. The risk increases to about 2–3% a year for people with higher degrees of stenosis [1, 2]. The detailed study of human anatomy [3] suggests that the state of CA is crucially important in this regard. Figure 1 shows a sample Carotid Artery ultrasound image.

To choose an effective pre-processing [4] and de-speckle filtering [5] framework detailed analysis of different filters is performed which includes edge preserving filter, Gaussian Filter [6, 7], Anisotropic Diffusion [8, 9] as mentioned in Sect. 2.1. These filters are extensively used for image processing in recent years. The definition of feature extraction [10–12] conveys the important shape and details found in a pattern, so that a systematic process may make the task of categorization and classification using the pattern easier. Analysis of two different approaches regarding the process is performed. One of them proposes conversion of image into a matrix and analyzing it in a systematic manner, while the other concentrates on the traditional methodology such as mathematical modelling [13] and implementation of transform algorithms as described in Sect. 2.2. Furthermore, the use of deep learning [14] algorithms on a database of extracted features opens up a lot of possibilities for automating CA stenosis risk prediction [15, 16]. The study and analysis regarding this are evident in recent times. So, far CNN models are yet to achieve the pinnacle of accuracy. To improve the existing methodologies, the application of deep learning algorithms regarding CA report analysis [17–20], characterization classification and segmentation [21, 22] is performed on the extracted data (from both normal and abnormal reports) via aforementioned process as depicted in Sect. 2.3.

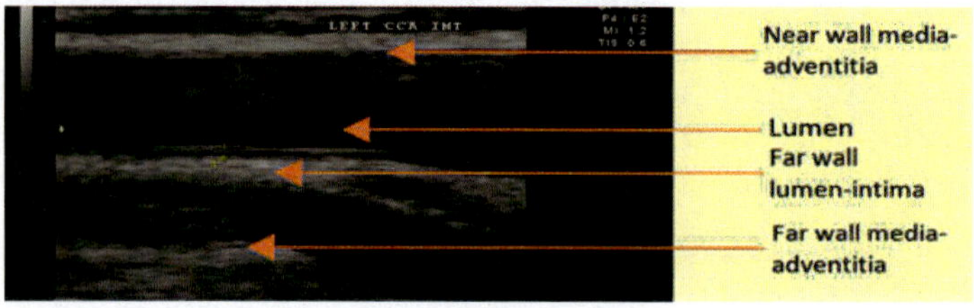

Fig. 1 Carotid artery ultrasound image

2 Proposed Methodology for Analysis of Carotid Artery Ultrasound Reports

The proposed methodology consists of various noise-reduction and image-improvement filters. Furthermore, the images are subjected to feature extraction method in order to acquire distinct and manageable segments for processing the important features for study and testing. Finally, a CNN model is trained with the processed data.

2.1 *Pre-Processing and Fundamental Analysis of Datasets*

Pre-processing of an image refers to the reduction of noise that degrades the image's quality. To eliminate the speckle noise, guided filter, Gaussian filter and anisotropic diffusion filter was used in this process. This research and technique entail examining the behaviour of these filters when applied to ultrasound images of the carotid artery. Mean squared error (MSE), peak signal-to-noise ratio (PSNR), and signal-to-noise ratio (SNR) are the chosen parameters used for the thorough analysis of the filters (Table 1), such as Anisotropic Diffusion Filter, Guided Filter, Gaussian Filter. The process flow of this study is mentioned in Fig. 2. In Gaussian blurring, the diffusion coefficient is constant. This is great for eliminating light, but it still blurs edges randomly. When the diffusion coefficient is used as an edge seeking function (such as Perona-Malik) the equations that emerge support diffusion within regions and prohibit it across strong edges. As a result, the image's edges will be retained when the noise is removed. The anisotropic diffusion filter works best with images that have been distorted by additive noise. The results (Table 1) clearly depict that in case of Gaussian Filter the MSE is very high (204.6272) which is drastically reduced (6.7085) when anisotropic diffusion filter is applied. Also, for the latter one the PSNR and SNR value is considerably higher than other filters.

Table 1 Performance of filters when applied to a normal report—right common carotid artery bulb

Filter type	Mean-squared error between reference image and filtered one (MSE)	Peak signal to noise ratio (PSNR)	Signal to noise ratio (SNR)
Anisotropic diffusion	**6.7085**	**39.8645**	**25.9748**
Guided filter	16.0771	36.0687	22.1790
Gaussian filter	204.6272	11.1314	11.1314

Bold values prove the improved performance of the aforementioned filter compared to the Guided and Gaussian filter

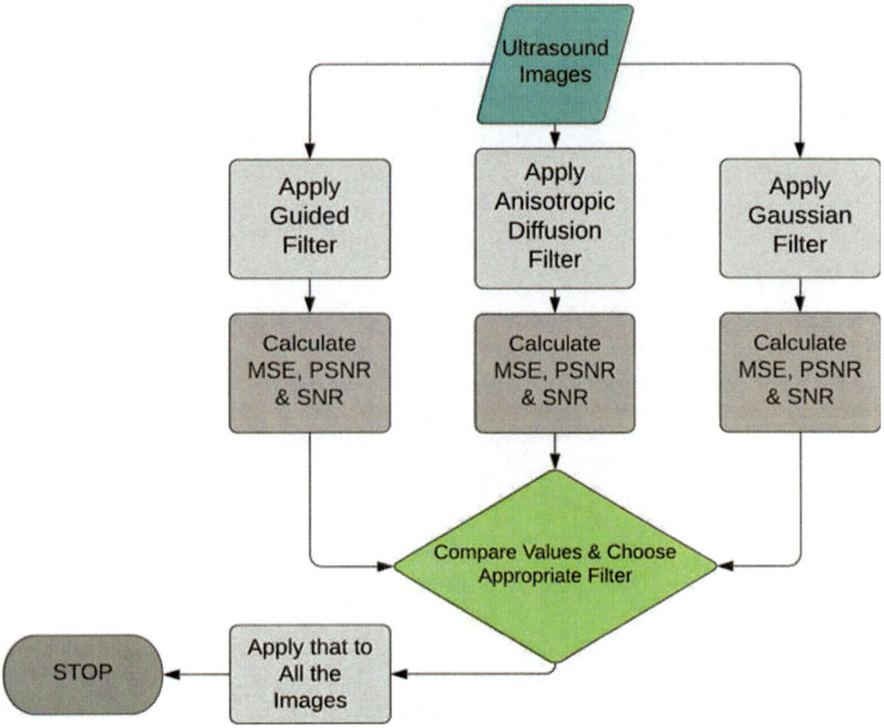

Fig. 2 Filter application and analysis process

2.2 Feature Extraction of the Pre-Processed Ultrasound Images

Feature extraction is described as a method that reduces a large collection of raw data into discrete and manageable segments for processing which preserves the important features for the study and analysis. This phase of study involves analysis of two different approaches mentioned in the following portion.

Approach 1: Analysis of LBP Feature Extraction and Plotting MSER Features

The feature extraction in this case is achieved using the linear binary pattern (LBP) feature extraction process (The process flow of this approach is depicted in Fig. 3). Initially, the feature extraction process is performed by applying Gabor filter (includes specification of optimum phase, bandwidth, wavelength, aspect ratio and orientation. For this purpose, phase value of 90 is recommended) followed by LBP feature extraction.

In addition, as a secondary procedure MSER (Maximally Stable Extremal Regions) features can also be plotted which is a key factor of approach 2 mentioned in the next section (Fig. 4a, b). This method clearly distinguishes between the

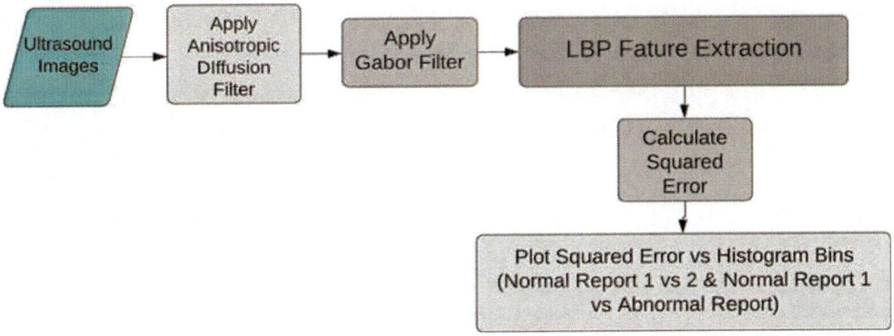

Fig. 3 Feature extraction process 1

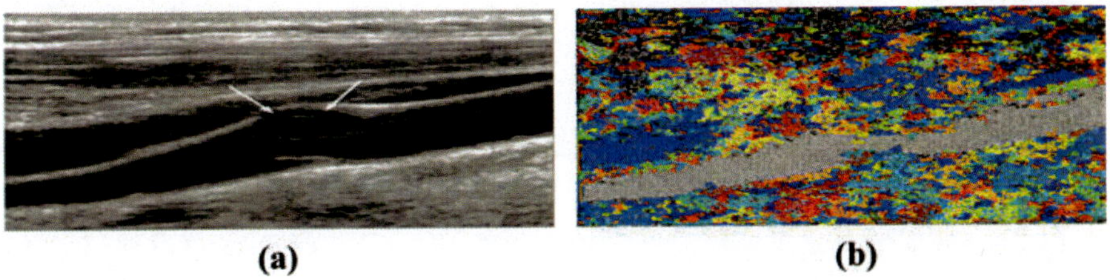

Fig 4 **a** Original ultrasound image, **b** outcome of plotting MSER features on Gabor filter output of the image

artery wall and the lumen, allowing for better data visualization through computer vision. The data is registered and squared error between two normal images is plotted vs. histogram bins (Fig. 5). In a similar way, the squared error between a normal and abnormal picture is measured and for ease of comparison, the data was recorded as a table. Finally, they are compared to one another (Fig. 5).

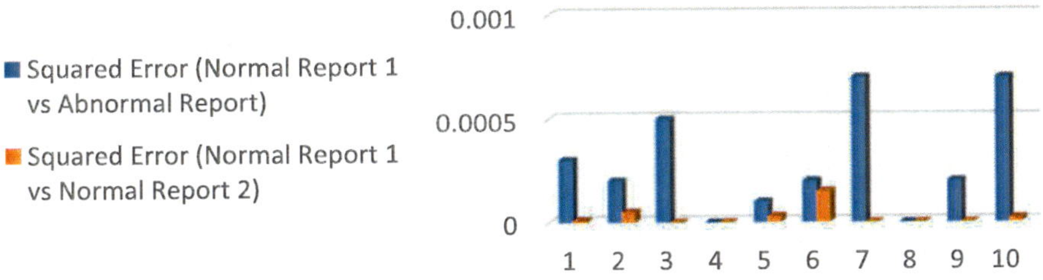

Fig. 5 Comparison of squared error (y axis) after LBP feature extraction w.r.t histogram bins (x axis)

Approach 2: Image-matrix Analysis for Feature Extraction

As mentioned in the complete process flow (Fig. 6), this method begins with application of Gabor filter and filtering ultrasound report image using an anisotropic diffusion filter. In the next step the MSER regions are plotted and the plotted image is converted into greyscale again. The ".jpg" file is converted into ".mat" file. This process is performed to represent the image as a matrix of pixel values. The region of interest (Fig. 7a, b) is now labelled, and the x and y coordinate values are saved. After this the boundary condition is applied to the image matrix and a secondary matrix is prepared containing only the pixel values of that region is created. Now, the mean for the row elements is calculated, and a M $\times$ 1 matrix (Table 2b) is created. The

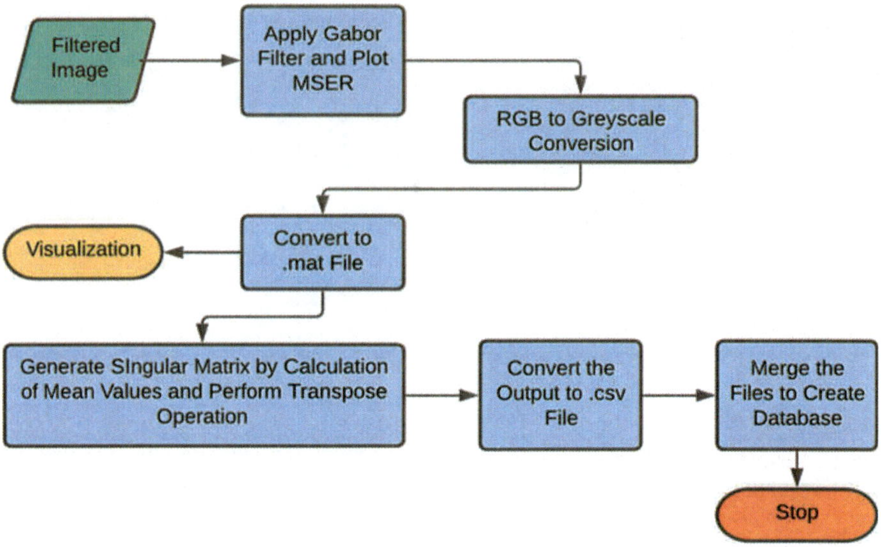

Fig. 6 Feature extraction process 2

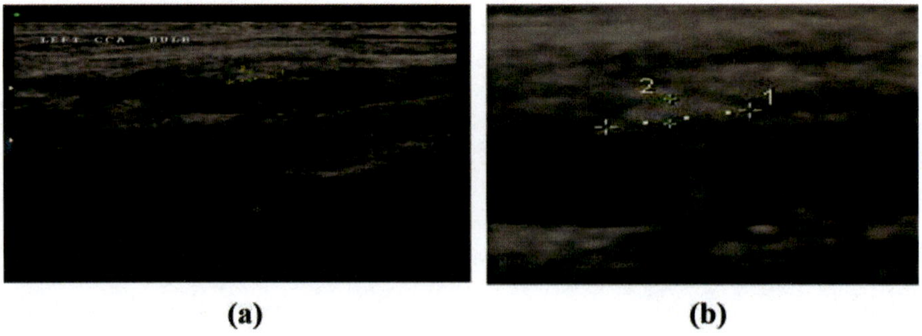

Fig. 7 **a** Original ultrasound image, **b** zoomed view of atherosclerotic plaque

Table 2 **a** Complete matrix representation of mentioned atherosclerotic plaque (left), **b** Matrix representation after generation of average values

12	11	3	6	5	4	3	3	3	4	3	3	3	3	3	3	2	2	2	4	5	7	8	8	7	7	6	5	4	1	2	2
5	5	2	2	2	0	0	1	3	4	3	3	3	3	3	3	1	1	1	3	4	6	8	9	8	8	7	5	5	2	2	3
3	3	2	2	1	1	1	2	3	3	3	2	4	7	7	6	4	6	5	4	3	3	3	5	7	6	6	5	4	4	3	3
3	2	2	1	1	2	2	3	3	3	5	7	10	10	8	7	5	4	3	2	2	2	2	3	3	2	2	1	1	3	3	2
3	2	2	2	2	2	3	3	4	4	6	8	10	10	9	8	5	5	4	3	3	3	2	1	1	0	0	0	0	3	3	2
3	2	2	2	2	3	3	4	4	4	5	6	7	7	7	7	6	7	7	7	6	5	3	1	1	1	1	2	2	3	3	2
3	2	2	3	3	3	3	4	4	5	4	4	4	5	5	6	7	8	9	9	8	6	3	1	2	2	2	3	3	3	3	2
3	2	2	3	3	3	4	5	5	5	4	4	4	4	5	7	6	7	8	9	7	5	3	1	1	2	2	3	3	3	3	2
3	2	1	2	2	2	3	4	4	4	4	4	3	3	3	4	4	4	5	5	4	3	2	1	1	2	2	3	3	4	4	2
2	2	1	1	1	1	2	3	3	3	4	4	3	3	2	2	2	2	2	2	2	2	1	0	1	2	2	3	4	5	4	3
2	2	1	1	1	1	2	3	3	3	4	4	3	3	2	2	1	1	1	1	1	1	1	0	1	1	3	4	5	5	5	3
2	1	1	1	1	1	2	3	3	3	4	4	3	3	2	2	0	0	0	0	0	0	0	0	0	1	3	4	5	5	4	4
1	1	1	1	1	1	2	3	3	3	4	4	3	3	2	2	0	0	0	0	0	0	0	1	2	2	2	3	3	3	3	2
1	1	1	1	1	1	2	3	3	3	4	4	3	3	2	2	1	1	1	1	1	1	2	3	2	2	2	1	1	0	1	1
1	1	1	1	1	1	2	3	3	3	4	4	3	3	2	2	1	1	1	1	1	1	2	4	3	2	2	0	0	0	0	0
1	1	1	1	1	1	1	1	1	1	2	2	2	2	2	2	1	1	1	1	1	1	1	2	2	2	2	2	2	1	1	1
1	1	1	1	1	1	1	1	1	1	2	2	2	2	2	2	1	1	1	1	1	1	1	2	2	2	2	2	2	1	1	1
1	1	1	1	1	1	1	1	1	1	1	1	1	1	1	1	1	1	1	1	1	1	1	1	1	1	1	1	1	1	1	1
1	1	1	1	1	1	1	1	1	1	1	1	1	1	1	1	1	1	1	1	1	1	1	1	1	1	1	1	1	1	1	1
1	1	1	1	1	1	1	1	1	1	0	0	0	0	0	0	1	1	1	1	1	1	1	0	0	0	0	0	0	1	1	1
1	1	1	1	1	1	1	1	1	1	0	0	0	0	0	0	1	1	1	1	1	1	1	0	0	0	0	0	0	1	1	1
1	1	2	1	1	1	1	1	1	1	1	1	1	1	1	1	1	1	1	1	1	1	1	0	0	0	0	0	0	2	2	2
1	1	2	1	1	1	1	1	1	1	1	1	1	1	1	1	1	1	1	1	1	1	1	1	1	1	1	1	1	2	2	3
1	1	2	1	1	1	1	1	1	1	1	0	0	0	0	0	0	0	0	0	0	0	1	2	2	2	2	2	2	1	3	5
2	2	2	1	1	1	1	1	1	1	2	2	2	1	1	0	1	1	1	1	1	1	1	1	1	2	2	3	3	3	6	11
2	2	1	1	1	1	1	1	1	2	5	4	3	2	2	1	3	3	3	3	3	3	2	1	2	3	3	5	5	7	11	17

(a)

4.6875
3.5938
3.7813
3.4063
3.5313
3.9063
4.0938
4
3.0313
2.3125
2.2188
1.9375
1.75
1.75
1.6875
1.375
1.375
1
1
0.625
0.625
0.9375
1.1563
1.0625
1.875
3.25

(b)

Fig. 8 QR code of atherosclerotic plaque for detailed matrix

latter method avoids handling large amounts of data and greatly simplifies the QR code generation process. The derived matrix value (Table 2a) is used to create the quick response (QR) code for easier data storage (Fig. 8). This makes data storage effective and reduces ambiguity.

Huge number text data can lead to mismanagement and increases the possibilities of inaccurate final outcome. QR codes are simple to create and if stored with proper file nomenclature a simple decoder can readily return the required numerical data.

2.3 *Model Training*

The data derived via feature extraction is trained with help of Convolutional Neural Networks. Convolutional Networks (convolutional neural networks, or CNNs) are a type of neural network that specialises in data processing with a known grid-like topology. (Such as time-series data, 1-D grid taking samples at regular intervals and image-data, that can be described as a 2-D grid of pixels). The term "CNN" refers to the network's use of the convolutional mathematical operation Convolution is a special kind of linear operation. Convolutional networks are essentially neural networks with at least one layer that uses convolution (1) (2) (A specialised Linear Operation) instead of general matrix multiplication.

$$s(t) = \int x(a)w(t-a)da \tag{1}$$

$$s(t) = (x^{*}w)(t) \tag{2}$$

At first, database is properly optimized for the model training purpose. Next phase is inclusion of library (TensorFlow, Numpy, Pandas, Keras are imported) and then complete data is read, described and converted into float 32 value. Now, the data is shaped properly with training and testing data is differentiated (training and testing of more than 550 data). Then, Activation and dropout are specified and added (Relu and Sigmoid). Optimizer is 'sgd' and loss is 'binary cross entropy'. The complete procedure followed regarding the training purpose is mentioned in Fig. 9 and the performance metrics of the training model is depicted in Fig. 10. The essential parameters for model training are plaque height and breadth. The plaque's 2D coordinates are recorded as a ROI, and the pixel values are evaluated. The model's operation can be summarized as the matching of plaque pixel values retrieved from abnormal reports with lumen region pixel values acquired from the report under investigation.

According to the Table 3 the performance metrics of the CNN model depicts a 97.45% validation accuracy and a final validation loss of 0.1235. The accuracy

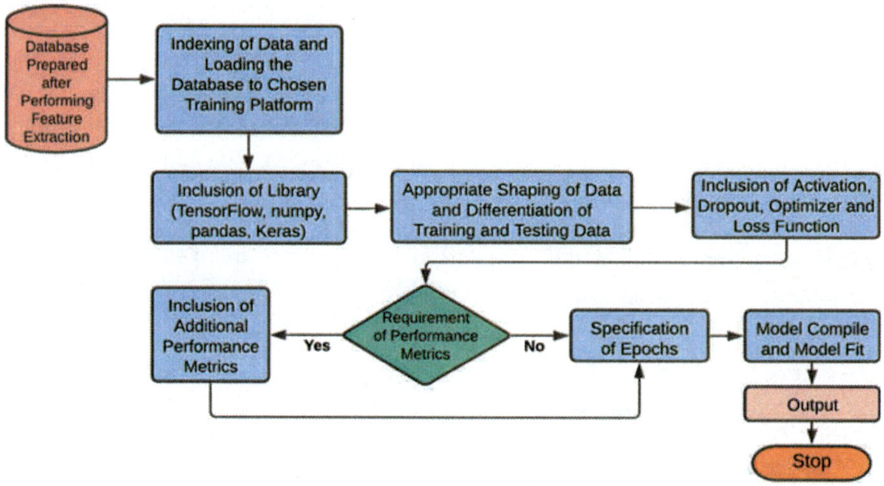

Fig. 9 Summarized flow-chart of the complete process including model training

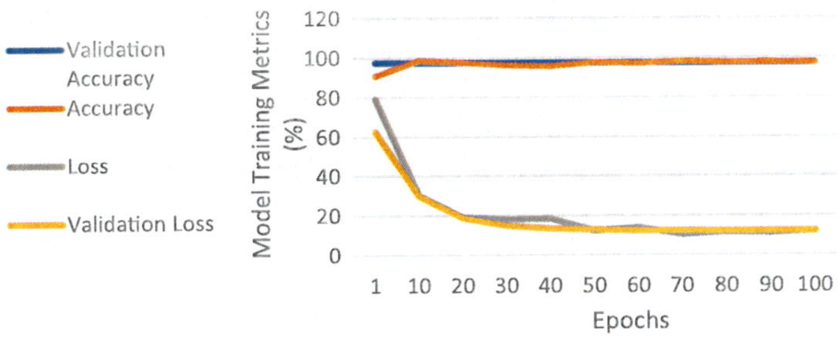

Fig. 10 Graphical representation of model training metrics

Table 3 Model training metrics

S. No	Value type	Accuracy (%)	Epoch	Loss	Epoch	Validation loss	Epoch
1	Minimum	95.10	12	0.0809	94	0.1199	100
2	Maximum	**98.64**	94	0.7907	1	0.6250	1
3	Average	97.25	–	**0.1189**	–	**0.1235**	–
4	Validation	**97.45**	1–100	N/A	N/A	N/A	N/A

ranges between 95.10% and 98.64% while the same for loss is 0.0809 (epoch 94) to 0.7907 (epoch 1). The range of validation loss lies between 0.1199 (epoch 100) and 0.6250 (epoch 1). The average accuracy and average loss are recorded as 97.25% and 0.1189. The same for validation loss is 0.1235.

3 Results and Discussion

The first phase of the research demonstrates how different filters perform when applied to ultrasound images. The calculated mean squared error between the original image and filtered image for the anisotropic diffusion filter is 9.3801, as shown in Table 1. The value for Guided Filter is 18.9699, while the value for Gaussian Filter is 220.2986. Anisotropic diffusion filters are clearly very effective in this regard. The PSNR and SNR values calculated also support the claim (i.e., Both PSNR and SNR values are greater for Anisotropic Diffusion Filters). The second phase consists of two different feature extraction approaches. Approach 1 encourages the use of existing methodologies and the development of a framework by combining them in logical order so that data visualization and extraction are simple to carry out and depict. Approach 2 is more detail-oriented. Every pixel value in the ROI (region of interest) is analysed, and the image matrix is converted into a QR code, resulting in a modern and sophisticated result. This makes data retrieval easier than ever before. If more information is required, a simple QR code scanner will return the matrix's raw value. In this way the pixel values can be analysed manually also if needed. Before the preparation of image matrices, the plotting of MSER on filtered images clearly separates the wall and lumen portion. If the data is visualized it can be easily inferred that only lumen region gets excluded from the MSER plot. A CNN model can be trained if there is a large enough database of ultrasound images.

After 100 epochs, a validation accuracy of 97.45% is achieved. It is apparent that using the proposed feature extraction approach during pre-processing has enhanced accuracy and validation accuracy (Fig. 11) compared to reference articles that only claim 50–60% validation accuracy using CNN model training and 95% via Transfer Learning. The minimum loss is recorded as 8.09% and the average loss is 11.89%. After running 100 epochs the final validation loss is obtained as 11.99% (Table 3). Validation loss is useful because it indicates how much the predictions deviate from what they ought to be before they are passed through the threshold. If we can obtain further reports and train them using our proposed method, the accuracy would be considerably higher than it has been so far. As a result, we will be able to achieve near-perfect automation. As the epoch is increased to 200 or higher, the loss steadily decreases.

$$\text{F1 Score} = (2 \times \text{Precision} \times \text{Recall})/(\text{Precision} + \text{Recall}) \tag{3}$$

```
Epoch 79/100
16/16 [==============================] - 0s 6ms/step - loss: 0.1675 - accuracy: 0.9597 - val_loss: 0.1219 - val_accuracy: 0.9745
Epoch 80/100
16/16 [==============================] - 0s 6ms/step - loss: 0.1148 - accuracy: 0.9767 - val_loss: 0.1217 - val_accuracy: 0.9745
Epoch 81/100
16/16 [==============================] - 0s 6ms/step - loss: 0.1282 - accuracy: 0.9724 - val_loss: 0.1216 - val_accuracy: 0.9745
Epoch 82/100
16/16 [==============================] - 0s 6ms/step - loss: 0.1368 - accuracy: 0.9692 - val_loss: 0.1214 - val_accuracy: 0.9745
Epoch 83/100
16/16 [==============================] - 0s 6ms/step - loss: 0.1325 - accuracy: 0.9715 - val_loss: 0.1213 - val_accuracy: 0.9745
Epoch 84/100
16/16 [==============================] - 0s 6ms/step - loss: 0.1240 - accuracy: 0.9733 - val_loss: 0.1212 - val_accuracy: 0.9745
Epoch 85/100
16/16 [==============================] - 0s 7ms/step - loss: 0.1024 - accuracy: 0.9803 - val_loss: 0.1210 - val_accuracy: 0.9745
Epoch 86/100
16/16 [==============================] - 0s 6ms/step - loss: 0.0976 - accuracy: 0.9819 - val_loss: 0.1209 - val_accuracy: 0.9745
Epoch 87/100
16/16 [==============================] - 0s 6ms/step - loss: 0.1161 - accuracy: 0.9761 - val_loss: 0.1208 - val_accuracy: 0.9745
Epoch 88/100
16/16 [==============================] - 0s 6ms/step - loss: 0.1468 - accuracy: 0.9671 - val_loss: 0.1207 - val_accuracy: 0.9745
Epoch 89/100
16/16 [==============================] - 0s 5ms/step - loss: 0.1480 - accuracy: 0.9665 - val_loss: 0.1206 - val_accuracy: 0.9745
Epoch 90/100
16/16 [==============================] - 0s 5ms/step - loss: 0.1152 - accuracy: 0.9754 - val_loss: 0.1205 - val_accuracy: 0.9745
Epoch 91/100
16/16 [==============================] - 0s 7ms/step - loss: 0.1092 - accuracy: 0.9786 - val_loss: 0.1205 - val_accuracy: 0.9745
Epoch 92/100
16/16 [==============================] - 0s 6ms/step - loss: 0.0963 - accuracy: 0.9819 - val_loss: 0.1204 - val_accuracy: 0.9745
Epoch 93/100
16/16 [==============================] - 0s 5ms/step - loss: 0.1344 - accuracy: 0.9698 - val_loss: 0.1203 - val_accuracy: 0.9745
Epoch 94/100
16/16 [==============================] - 0s 6ms/step - loss: 0.0809 - accuracy: 0.9864 - val_loss: 0.1202 - val_accuracy: 0.9745
Epoch 95/100
16/16 [==============================] - 0s 6ms/step - loss: 0.1316 - accuracy: 0.9709 - val_loss: 0.1202 - val_accuracy: 0.9745
Epoch 96/100
16/16 [==============================] - 0s 5ms/step - loss: 0.1302 - accuracy: 0.9728 - val_loss: 0.1201 - val_accuracy: 0.9745
Epoch 97/100
16/16 [==============================] - 0s 6ms/step - loss: 0.0835 - accuracy: 0.9861 - val_loss: 0.1200 - val_accuracy: 0.9745
Epoch 98/100
16/16 [==============================] - 0s 5ms/step - loss: 0.1117 - accuracy: 0.9768 - val_loss: 0.1200 - val_accuracy: 0.9745
Epoch 99/100
16/16 [==============================] - 0s 6ms/step - loss: 0.1010 - accuracy: 0.9804 - val_loss: 0.1199 - val_accuracy: 0.9745
Epoch 100/100
16/16 [==============================] - 0s 6ms/step - loss: 0.1421 - accuracy: 0.9689 - val_loss: 0.1199 - val_accuracy: 0.9745
<tensorflow.python.keras.callbacks.History at 0x7f79eb0c8310>
```

Fig. 11 Model training epoch results (after recommended feature extraction process)

The study is concluded by calculation pf F1 score or Sørensen–Dice Coefficient (3) and a 0.9425429471429471 F1 score suggests better precision and recall compared to the existing methodologies.

4 Conclusion

This section provides a detailed and conclusive review of methods used to examine the carotid artery in order to diagnose stroke, atherosclerosis, and other coronary disorders, with an emphasis on lumen wall thickening or plaque formation. The methods have been divided into phases. During phase one of the analysis, it was discovered that Anisotropic Diffusion filter outputs have less than half the mean squared error of Guided Filter outputs. Furthermore, they have a PSNR value of 8–12% higher. The Anisotropic Diffusion filter methodology is clearly superior regarding the aforementioned purpose. There are two processes in feature extraction stage. In approach 1 LBP Feature Extraction and histogram analysis is performed, which quickly provides the squared error between two images. These values are simple to plot, but yields lesser accuracy when used for CNN model training (i.e., 50–60%). The advantage of approach 2 is the level of detailing and ease of access. This method also allows for the examination of both the entire image and a specific ROI. The ability to mark ROI through computer vision adds a customized examination process to ultrasound reports. Furthermore, this format of final data (i.e., pixel value of MSER plotted images saved as.csv file) is easier to use as a database for deep learning algorithms that can predict the occurrence of stenosis or decrease in patency. The results shown in the previous sections strengthens the fact that the accuracy has significantly increased compared to the existing methods (97.45%). Also, average loss and validation loss (11.99% in the 100th epoch) has reduced significantly.

References

1. Kyriacou, E.C., Petroudi, S., Pattichis, C.S., Pattichis, M.S., Griffin, M., Kakkos, S., Nicolaides, A.: Prediction of high—risk asymptomatic carotid plaques based on ultrasonic image features. IEEE Trans. Inf Technol. Biomed. **16**(5), 966–973 (2012)
2. Arko, C., Jishnu, R.N., Taritro, G,S., Dhanalakshmi, L.S.: Diagnosis of atherosclerotic plaques in carotid artery using transfer learning. In: Fifth international conference on communication and electronics systems (ICCES 2020) IEEE conference record # 48766, IEEE Xplore ISBN (2020)
3. Romanes, G.J.: Cunningham's manual of practical anatomy (15th edn). Oxford University Press. ISBN 978-0-19-922908-6
4. Varma, S., Dhanalakshmi, S., Latha, S.: Performance evaluation of unpreprocessed and preprocessed ultrasound images of carotid artery using CNN algorithm. In: IOP Conference Series: Materials Science and Engineering, vol. 912 (2020)

5. Loizou, C.P., Pattichis, C.S., Christodoulou, C.I., Istepanian, R.S.H., Pantziaris, M., Nicolaides, A.: Comparative evaluation of despeckle filtering in ultrasound imaging of the carotid artery. IEEE Trans. Ultrason. Ferroelectr. Freq. Control **52**(10), 1653–1669 (2005)
6. Gedraite, E.S., Hadad, M.: Investigation on the effect of a Gaussian blur in image filtering and segmentation, IEEE Xplore ISSN: 1334–2630 (2011)
7. Deng, G., Cahill, L.W.: An adaptive Gaussian filter for noise reduction and edge detection. In: IEEE Conference Record Nuclear Science Symposium and Medical Imaging Conference (1993)
8. Choi, H., Jeong, J.: Despeckling images using a preprocessing filter and discrete wavelet transform-based noise reduction techniques. IEEE Sens. J. **18**(8), 3131–3139 (2018)
9. Sa-ing, V., Vorasayan, P., Suwanwela, N.C., Auethavekiat, S., Chinrungrueng, C.: Multiscale adaptive regularisation Savitzky–Golay method for speckle noise reduction in ultrasound images. IET J. IET Image Process. **12**(1), 105–112 (2017)
10. Kumar, G., Bhatia, P.K.: A detailed review of feature extraction in image processing systems. In: Fourth International Conference on Advanced Computing and Communication Technologies (2014)
11. Salau, A.O., Jain, S.: Feature extraction: a survey of the types, techniques, applications. IEEE 978-1-5386-9436-7 (2019)
12. Porebski, A., Vandenbroucke, N., Macaire, L.: Haralick feature extraction from LBP images for color texture classification. IEEE 978-1-4244-3321 (2008)
13. Dhanalakshmi, S., Venkatesh, C.: Nonlinear structure tensor based spatial fuzzy clustering for ultrasound carotid artery image segmentation with texture and IMT extraction using hilbert huang transform. Eur. J. Sci. Res. ISSN **80**(3), 1450–2216 (2012)
14. Goodfellow, I., Bengio, Y., Courville, A.: Deep Learning. MIT Press, ISBN 9780262035613 (2017)
15. Farook, M., Dhanalakshmi, S., Manikandan, V., Venkatesh, C.: Optimal feature selection for carotid artery image segmentation using evolutionary computation. Appl. Mech. Mater. Trans Tech Publ. 626 (2014)
16. Samiappan, D., Chakrapani, V.: Classification of carotid artery abnormalities in ultrasound images using an artificial neural classifier. Int. Arab J. Inf. Technol. **13**(6A), 756–762 (2016)
17. Lekadir, K., Galimzianova, A., Betriu, A., del Mar Vila, M., Igual, L., Rubin, D.L., Napel, S.: A convolutional neural network for automatic characterization of plaque composition in carotid ultrasound. IEEE J. Biomed. Health Inform. **21**(1), 48–55 (2017)
18. Menchón-Lara, R.-M., Sancho-Gómez, J.-L., Bueno-Crespo, A.: Early-stage atherosclerosis detection using deep learning over carotid ultrasound images. Appl. Soft Comput. Elsevier **49**, 616–628 (2016)
19. Abolmaesumi, P., Sirouspour, M.R., Salcudean, S.E.: Real-time extraction of carotid artery contours from ultrasound images. In: Proceedings 13th IEEE Symposium on Computer-Based Medical Systems, CBMS (2000)
20. Luijten, B., Cohen, R., De Bruijn, F.J., Schmeitz, H.A.W., Mischi, M., Eldar, Y.C., Van Sloun.: Adaptive ultrasound beamforming using deep learning. IEEE Trans. Med. Imaging 1–1 (2020)
21. Delsanto, S., Molinari, F., Giustetto, P., Liboni, W., Badalamenti, S., Suri, J.S.: Characterization of a completely user-independent algorithm for carotid artery segmentation in 2-D ultrasound images. IEEE Trans. Instrum. Meas. **56** (2007)
22. Samiappan, D., Chakrapani, V.: Classification of ultrasound carotid artery images using texture features. Int. Rev. Comput. Softw. **8**(4), 933–940 (2013)

A Combinational Approach to Generate Nonlinear Foot Trajectories for Robotic Prothesis with Elementary Clinical Results

Mouaz Al Kouzbary, Hamza Al Kouzbary, Lai Kuan Tham, Jinjing Liu, Hanie Nadia Shasmin, Nooranida Arifin, and Noor Azuan Abu Osman

Abstract One problem in the field of robotic prostheses' control is the generation of dynamic trajectories to be tracked by a low-level control system. In this work we are suggesting a combinational approach to estimate the foot trajectory for a robotic below-knee prostheses. The two-stage estimation is to identify foot angular speed based on tibia angular speed and acceleration using cascade neural network (CNN). Then, the foot angular position will be estimated from the first stage estimation using nonlinear autoregressive network with exogenous inputs (NARX). In this paper we are presenting the elementary results from a clinical trial for long distance treadmill walking. The two-stage method shows an average correlation of 0.986 in three walking speeds. Moreover, the average of root mean square errors (RMSEs) and mean absolute errors (MAEs) are 0.0517 and 0.0403 (rad), respectively. The result only shows the performance of the estimation method for one healthy participant. However, more analysis is required on the method ability to provide generalized subject-independent trajectories.

Keywords Robotic protheses · Powered ankle–foot · High-level control system · ANN · Nonlinear dynamic trajectory

1 Introduction

In the last decade, the number of lower-limb robotic prostheses started increasing [1]. The task of developing a universal control system proved to be challenging [2], where the safety measure is the priority. Two main roles that control system must fulfil are smooth motion and stable transition between terrains, and robust behavior against mechanical perturbations [3]. The most commonly used is the hierarchical control structure [2, 4]. However, the hierarchical control system still needs more

M. Al Kouzbary · H. Al Kouzbary · L. K. Tham · J. Liu · H. N. Shasmin · N. Arifin · N. A. Abu Osman (✉)
Center for Applied Biomechanics, Department of Biomedical Engineering, Faculty of Engineering, Universiti Malaya, Kuala Lumpur, Malaysia
e-mail: azuan@um.edu.my

J. Usman et al. (eds.), *6th Kuala Lumpur International Conference on Biomedical Engineering 2021*, IFMBE Proceedings 86,
https://doi.org/10.1007/978-3-030-90724-2_3

theoretical approach to guarantee control system stability recent works try to achieve the stability in [5–7]. One of the difficulties still facing the hierarchical control structure is the dynamic and user-independent high-level controller. One approach proposed in the literature is based on emulating the nonlinear central biological signals for transfemoral prosthesis [8]. Authors implemented an artificial recurrent neural network called central pattern generator (CPG), which is widely used in the field of bipedal robots. However, designing a specific CPG neural network based on the height, weight and age is required for each amputee. Moreover, the process of calibrating CPG's parameters is quite sophisticated.

In [9, 10], the authors designed a recurrent long short-term memory neural network (LSTM RNN) for estimating the ankle angle of the amputated leg on the basis of the kinematics of the intact limb. A problem with this neural network is that it necessitates a number of sensors attached to the subject, which increases the computation load and adds to the cost of the device. In this work we are presenting elementary result for an AI-based pattern generator for active prosthetic devices.

2 Method

In this section we are presenting the experiment design, sensors and statistical analysis methods used to study the elementary. The result shown is a part of a wider clinical study include seven healthy subjects. The participants were to walk on treadmill for three walking speeds (self-selected speed $\pm 2\%$) for 12 min, here we show the result of using the combination method on the data of one subject only. This study was granted approval from the Medical Research and Ethics Committee's (MREC) (Reference Number: KKM/NIHSEC/P19-2206(11)). All subjects agreed on participating in the study by signing a consent form. In previous study we show the ability of NARX (with 3–1 neurons structure) to estimate the angular position of body segments using the angular speed [11]. Independently we show an NARX (with structure 3-15-1 neurons) to be used as a pattern generator in three-level hieratical system [12], where the neural network was used to estimate the angular position of foot based on the angular speed of tibia. The use of NARX in both studies was required as an integration procedure requires a recurrent neural network structure. In order to enhance the estimation error of the pattern generator given in [12], we are suggesting two estimation steps. First, estimating the foot angular speed using tibia angular speed. Second, calculating the foot angular position using the estimated angular speed in step one. Figure 1 shows the block diagram of the suggested method. Where, ${}^{N}\upsilon_t$ and ${}^{N}\upsilon_t$ are the normalized tibia angular speed and acceleration, respectively. Neural networks weights and biases are donated by **w** and **b** (note we used superscript ^{2} to differentiate the NARX's wights and biases).

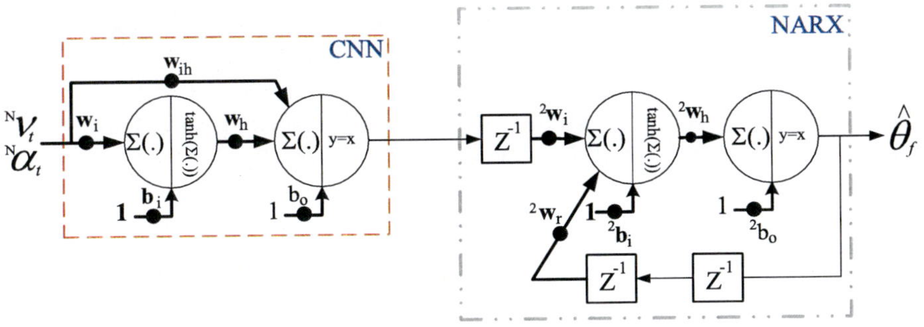

Fig. 1 Two-stage estimation technique to generate foot nonlinear trajectory.

2.1 Sensors and Experiment Setup

Four OPAL wearable devices (https://apdm.com/wearable-sensors/) were placed on the lower body segments as shown in Fig. 2. Each OPAL is equipped with 9 degree of freedom (DoF) with ability to stream data online with frequency up to 128 Hz. The subject (with 67 kg and 177 cm) was asked to stand still at the end of the trail to record data for sensors' alignment to a global coordinate system. The subject was

Fig. 2 Sensors location as shown placed on one participant in the clinical trial.

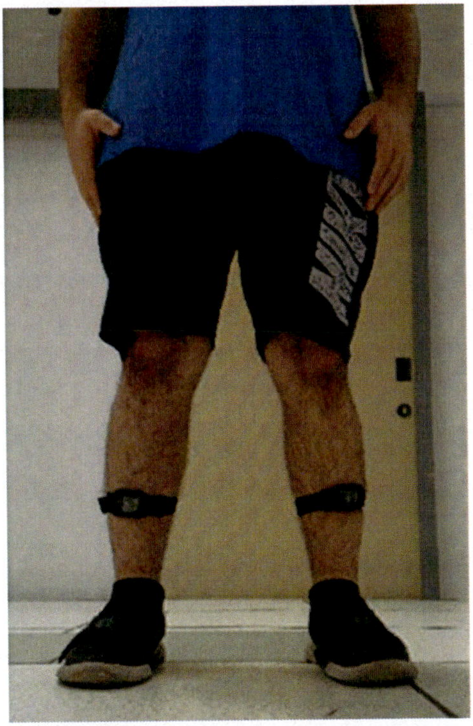

asked to walk at the three different speeds (3.6, 4.0 and 4.4 for slow, normal and fast respectively) The raw data of all sensors was analyzed in MATLAB® (2019a).

The gyroscopes' data passed through a second order low-pass filter with 24 [rad/s] cut-off frequency and critical damping ($\xi = 1$). The data processed only in the sagittal plane. Accelerometers' data were used to find the orientation using the complementary filter (CF) approach [13]. The estimated value of foot orientation is compared to the measured value using CF.

2.2 Neural Networks Design and Role

In this study we utilized two conventional neural networks (i.e., CNN and NARX). The CNN main role is to map the tibia angular speed (ν_t) and acceleration (α_t) to foot angular speed (ν_f). As shown in Fig. 3a the functional relationship between the CNN inputs (ν_t and α_t) and the target. Whereas the NARX main task is to numerically integrate the estimated foot angular speed (ν_f) and cancel the gyroscopic drift. As shown in [11] one can represent the role of the NARX algebraically as demonstrated in Eq. (1). Moreover, based on Eq. (1) we were able to select the inputs and the number of delay units required in the NARX structure. Where y[k] is the NARX's output, u[k] is the input, ω_n is the filter cut-off frequency, and T_s is the sampling time. Figure 3b illustrates the relation between foot angular position (θ_f) and speed (ν_f).

$$y[k] = \frac{(2 + \omega_n \cdot T_s) \cdot y[k-1]}{1 + \omega_n \cdot T_s} - \frac{y[k-2]}{1 + \omega_n \cdot T_s} + \frac{T_s \cdot (u[k] - u[k-1])}{1 + \omega_n \cdot T_s} \tag{1}$$

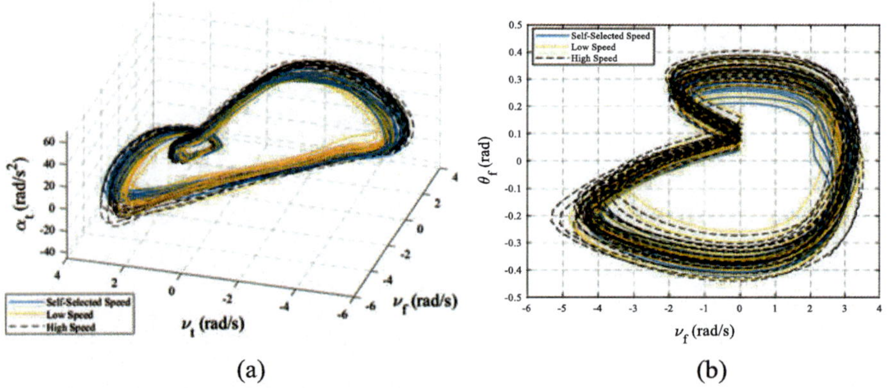

Fig. 3 Neural networks inputs-outputs relationship. In **a** the inputs-output relation which the CNN is required to map, and in **b** the input–output relation to be mapped by NARX. Self-selected, low, and high speeds are shown in solid blue line, yellow dots, and detached black line, respectively.

Table 1 The hyperparameters for BR training algorithm

Parameters	Value
Maximum number of epochs to train	75,000
Performance goal	0
Marquardt adjustment parameter	0.005
Decrease factor for mu	0.4
Increase factor for mu	10
Maximum value for mu	1e10
Maximum validation failures	inf
Minimum performance gradient	1e-18

Note The training of the NARX is done as shown in [11]

A series of 6 gait cycles (8.44 s) is used to train the CNN with single hidden layer and 12 neurons which can distinguish between 4 different manifolds, the selected training algorithm is Bayesian Regularization (BR) to avoid overfitting [14]. The training algorithm's hyperparameters are shown in Table 1.

2.3 *Statistical Analysis Tools*

In order to assess the result of the suggested method a number of statistical tools will be utilized. The estimated result will be compared to the measured values for CNN the measured value can be obtained directly from the foot gyroscope output in the global reference frame. However, the NARX output is compared to the fusion of the gyroscope and accelerometer using CF. We used the root mean square error (RMSE) and MAE to measure the method precision and accuracy, respectively. To identify signals' synchronization and similarity using normalized cross-correlation, the r-value should be greater than 0.75 to assume that estimations are acceptable. The t-test was used to identify the nature of the error signals (difference between the measurements and estimation of the two-level structure) where the estimation error should be a white noise (gaussian distribution). Finally, the model probabilistic consistency the measured and estimated signals histogram distribution will be analyzed based on the extreme value distribution.

Note: the statistical analysis is done for all the data set of the three trails ($5.52e^{05}$ samples).

3 Result and Discussion

In this section we are going to present the result, statistical assessment, and discussion of the networks' performance. Both neural networks and CF was built in MATLAB all algorithms run using Euler's discrete time solver. Figures 4 and 5 show the CNN and NARX performance, respectively. The average of the last 50 gait cycles is illustrated as solid lines, where the standard deviation is shown as a shadow around the average value. Table 2 summaries the performance of CNN throughout 12 min trial for three different speeds best performance is achieved for self-selected speed. The accuracy and precision dropped during high speed.

Table 3 shows the NARX performance based on the statistical analysis tools where again the best performance appeared for self-selected speed. However, the bias increased at low speed. The t-test shows that the NARX error is free of any drift all the noise is white whit high degree of certainty.

Finally, Fig. 6 illustrates the histograms of the NARX compared with CF the result show that the combined method is able to cancel the steady state error appeared in the performance of the NARX solely [12].

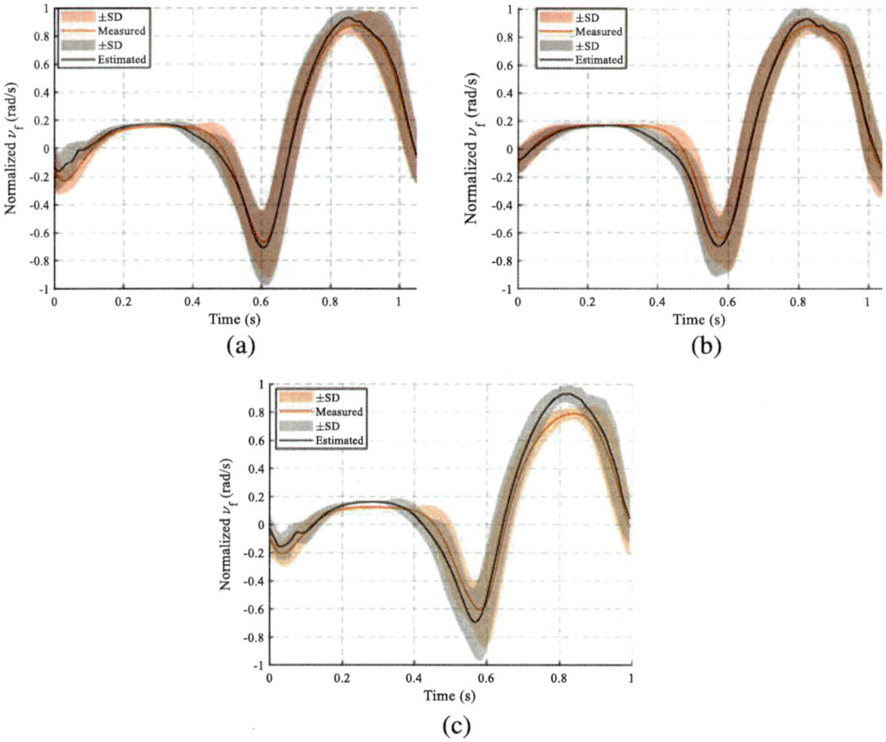

Fig. 4 The average value of foot angular speed and standard deviation of 50 consecutive gait cycles in three different walking speeds. The mean value and standard deviation of the estimated gait cycles are shown as a black line and gray shadow, respectively. The mean value and standard deviation of measured gait cycles are shown in a red line and pink shadow, respectively

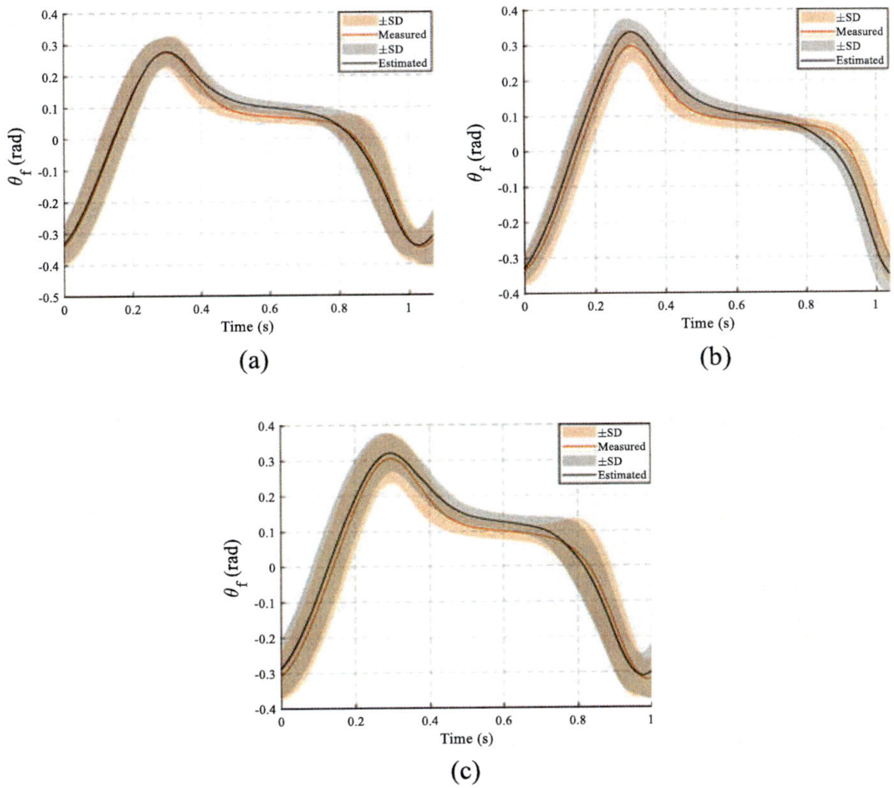

Fig. 5 The average value of foot angular position and standard deviation of 50 consecutive gait cycles in three different walking speeds. The mean value and standard deviation of the estimated gait cycles are shown as a black line and gray shadow, respectively. The mean value and standard deviation of measured gait cycles are shown in a red line and pink shadow, respectively

Table 2 Statistical evaluation of CNN performance

Speed	Cross-correlation	RMSE (rad/s)	MAE (rad/s)	t-test
Low	0.9856	0.3407	0.2424	h = 0 p = 0.9176
Self-selected	0.9869	0.3155	0.2203	h = 0 p = 1
High	0.9854	0.4192	0.3222	h = 0 p = 0.9056

4 Conclusion

In this paper we presented a method to generate foot pattern based on tibia angular speed, the suggested method was inspired by two previous work where NARX were

Table 3 Statistical parameters for NARX evaluation of foot angular position in sagittal plane.

Speed	Cross-correlation	RMSE (rad)	MAE (rad)	t-test
Low	0.9654	0.0636	0.0521	h = 0 p = 0.9621
Self-selected	0.9771	0.0420	0.030	h = 0 p = 0.8896
High	0.9748	0.0495	0.0388	h = 0 p = 1

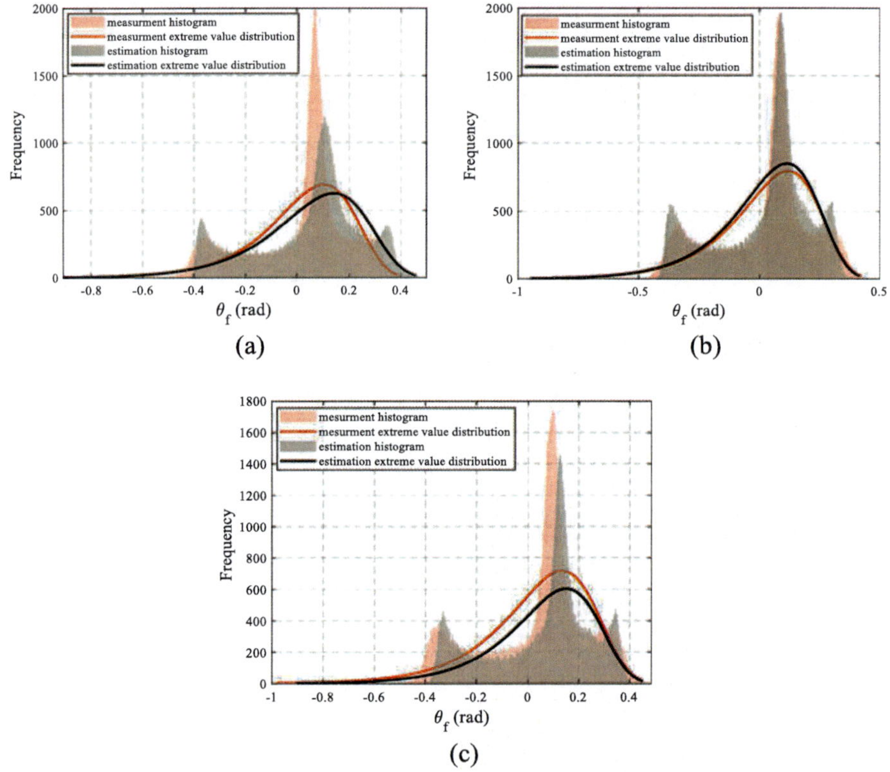

Fig. 6 NARX and CF histograms in gray and pink (for the three walking speeds), respectively. Along with the fitted extreme value distribution

used as pattern generator [12] and orientation estimator [11] The new method shows a promising result by canceling a static error which reported in [12]. The limitation of this study is that the CNN was trained using a 6 s window from the subject data more test and assessment of the method as a user independent technique. Furthermore, the method performance should be evaluated for walking with terrain/ speed changes.

References

1. Liu, J., Abu Osman, N.A., Al Kouzbary, M., et al.: Classification and comparison of mechanical design of powered ankle–foot prostheses for transtibial amputees developed in the 21st century: a systematic review. J. Med. Devices **15**(1), 010801 (2021)
2. Tucker, M.R., Olivier, J., Pagel, A., et al.: Control strategies for active lower extremity prosthetics and orthotics: a review. J. Neuroeng. Rehabil. **12**(1), 1–30 (2015)
3. Ahn, J., Hogan, N.: Walking is not like reaching: evidence from periodic mechanical perturbations. PloS One **7**(3), e31767 (2012)
4. Mouaz, A.K.: Robotic assistive ankle-foot prosthesis based on sensorless fuzzy logic control system/Mouaz Al Kouzbary. University of Malaya (2019)
5. Ames, A.D., Galloway, K., Sreenath, K., et al.: Rapidly exponentially stabilizing control lyapunov functions and hybrid zero dynamics. IEEE Trans. Autom. Control **59**(4), 876–891 (2014)
6. Alan, A., Taylor, A.J., He, C.R., et al.: Safe controller synthesis with tunable input-to-state safe control barrier functions (2021). arXiv:210308041
7. Ames, A.D., Coogan, S., Egerstedt, M., et al. (eds.): Control barrier functions: theory and applications. In: 2019 18th European Control Conference (ECC), IEEE (2019)
8. Nandi, G.C., Ijspeert, A., Nandi, A. (eds.): Biologically inspired CPG based above knee active prosthesis. In: 2008 IEEE/RSJ International Conference on Intelligent Robots and Systems, IEEE (2008)
9. Rai, V., Sharma, A., Rombokas, E. (eds.): Mode-free control of prosthetic lower limbs. In: 2019 International Symposium on Medical Robotics (ISMR), IEEE (2019)
10. Rai, V., Rombokas, E. (eds.): A framework for mode-free prosthetic control for unstructured terrains. In: 2019 IEEE 16th International Conference on Rehabilitation Robotics (ICORR), IEEE (2019)
11. Tham, L.K., Osman, N.A.A., Al Kouzbary, M., et al.: Biomechanical ambulatory assessment of 3D knee angle using novel inertial sensor-based technique. IEEE Access **9**, 36559–36570 (2021)
12. Al Kouzbary, H., Al Kouzbary, M., Tham, L.K., et al.: Generating an adaptive and robust walking pattern for a prosthetic ankle-foot by utilizing a nonlinear autoregressive network with exogenous inputs. IEEE Trans. Neural Netw. Learn. Syste. (2021)
13. Gui, P., Tang, L., Mukhopadhyay, S. (eds.): MEMS based IMU for tilting measurement: comparison of complementary and kalman filter based data fusion. In: 2015 IEEE 10th Conference on Industrial Electronics and Applications (ICIEA), IEEE (2015)
14. Foresee, F.D., Hagan, M.T. (eds.): Gauss-Newton approximation to Bayesian learning. In: Proceedings of International Conference on Neural Networks (ICNN'97), IEEE (1997)

Eye-Controlled Wheelchair Improves Quality-of-Life on Paraplegic Patients in Home-Care Setting: A Case Study

Kamala Krishnan, Tan Lee Fan, and Danny Ng Wee Kiat

Abstract A powered wheelchair is usually controlled with a joystick, but there are other input devices that can be used if the user lacks either coordination or the use of their hands or fingers. This study purposed to evaluate the impact after using the eye-controlled wheelchair in short term. Two elderly female subjects who suffer from stroke and spinal cord injury were recruited from a local old folks home-care. Both of them were manual wheelchair bounded and needs the assistance of their caregivers to wheel them around their home-care. Subjects' QoL after the eye-controlled usage was assessed using a self-designed questionnaire. The data were collected and analyzed descriptively. The collected data was interpreted as such to show the subjects' QoL progress during the 8 weeks of data collection. As in the fourth week, the QoL scores were: subject A (21/32) and subject B (22/32). In contrast, the QoL score increased from the 4th week to the 8th week. In the 8th week, the scores were: subject A (30/32) and subject B (29/32). Interpretation: The final week scores denoted that the subject's QoL has increased as in contrast to Week 1 scores with Subject A with 9 scores difference and Subject B with 7 scores difference. There was visible QoL score improvement in both subjects comparatively. In conclusion, this study achieved the study aim which is to evaluate the impact after using the eye-controlled wheelchair in short term.

Keywords Eye-controlled wheelchair · Paraplegic · Home-care

K. Krishnan (✉)
Faculty of Medicine and Health Science, Universiti Tunku Abdul Rahman, 43000 Kajang, Selangor, Malaysia

T. L. Fan · D. N. W. Kiat
Lee Kong Chian Faculty Engineering and Science, Universiti Tunku Abdul Rahman, 43000 Kajang, Selangor, Malaysia

J. Usman et al. (eds.), *6th Kuala Lumpur International Conference on Biomedical Engineering 2021*, IFMBE Proceedings 86,
https://doi.org/10.1007/978-3-030-90724-2_4

1 Introduction

1.1 Research Background

A wheelchair equipped with an electric motor is known as a powered wheelchair. This wheelchair is usually controlled with a joystick, but other input devices can be used if the user lacks either coordination or the use of their hands or fingers [1]. This wheelchair eliminates most of the muscle power usage which is basic in a manual wheelchair, whereby, the steering mechanism still requires an upright posture and some upper-body mobility and strength [2].

However, the upper limb strength is necessary to control a powered wheelchair but it is not applicable for patients who suffer from paraplegia. A neurological disorder can be simply defined as any disease which disturbs the physiology of both the central nervous system and peripheral nervous system will result in the neurological disorder [3]. In this study, two paraplegic neurological disorders were focused which are stroke and spinal cord injury.

American Heart Association (AHA) or American Stroke Association (ASA) had come with an updated definition of stroke, whereby stroke can be included in both silent hemorrhages and silent infarction (inclusive of retinal, spinal, and cerebral) [4]. Whether chronic, relapsing, or remitting, psychological stressors induce harm in stroke survivors owing to associated stroke recurrence, mortality, disability, reductions in quality of life (QOL), and cognitive impairment [5–8].

WHO defined spinal cord injury (SCI) as the damage that occurs at the spinal cord due to trauma (e.g. motor vehicle accident, falls) or due to degeneration/disease (e.g. malignancies). Secondary impairments of SCI can limit one's independent functionality as well as negatively impact the quality of life (QoL) [9–12].

In contemporary terms, any subjective improvement criteria can be simply recognized as QoL considerations [13]. Measurement of QoL assistive devices such as wheelchairs provides a meaningful way to determine the impact of health care when cure is not possible before their muscles deteriorate to more severe conditions.

Since there is no study found measuring the QoL in an eye-controlled wheelchair and the available studies [14–16] were only studied on studies the QoL in either manual or powered wheelchair users. Therefore, this study purposes to evaluate the impact after using the eye-controlled wheelchair in short term.

2 Method and Material

2.1 Study Design

This is a qualitative design study as the eye-controlled wheelchairs' were customized according to subjects' needs.

2.2 Procedure

The experiment began with the subject sat in the wheelchair (refer to Fig. 1). The Tobii 4C eye tracker is fixed with the laptop and the laptop screen was closely aligned in a range of 30–50 cm from the subject's eye level [17]. The Tobii Eye Tracking v2.9.0 software is installed on the laptop and the built-in "Gaze Trace" option gives the visual feedback of the user's focus point.

Prior to the experiment, verbal instructions were given regarding the procedure of eye-controlled wheelchair navigation and control. During the instruction, subjects could raise their questions and concerns regarding eye-controlled wheelchair usage. All queries raised were explained accordingly and once again the verbal consent is obtained to confirm their participation in this study.

Few trial sessions were allowed for the subjects to familiarize themselves with the eye-controlled wheelchair system with the presence of the researcher. Once the trials over, the subjects were allowed to control and navigate the eye-controlled wheelchair with minimal company by the researcher. This is to ensure an unbiased effect on the outcome measure with the presence of the researcher. The wheelchair navigation duration is solely based on the subject's will to move around and they are free to stop whenever they want. A minimum of 3 days/sessions per week was attempted by each subject.

The subjects were instructed to select their desired direction just by looking at the direction boxes displayed on the laptop screen. Each of the boxes represents a direction in terms of forward, right turn, left turn, and stop which aids in the eye-controlled wheelchair navigation and control.

Once a selection made, the wheelchair will drive accordingly. A wheelchair session was considered valid if the subject moves around the home-care upon selection using the eye-gaze for at least several minutes. During the wheelchair session, the subjects were given the freedom to move around the home-care and speak to their friends, staff, and visitors.

Each subject was accompanied by the researcher for the first 5 sessions, it is expected that the subjects will be familiarized and developed an ability to navigate and control the wheelchair by then. This reason lies in safety concerns and as an effort to encourage the subjects to use the eye-controlled wheelchair as both subjects have only experienced using the manual wheelchair. To add to the users' safety, the wheelchair speed was set at 0.2 m/s.

2.3 Participants

Two elderly female subjects were recruited from a local old folks home-care. The subjects are denoted as Subject A, 64 years old is suffering from spinal cord injury, and, Subject B, 75 years old is suffering from stroke. Both subjects had weak upper limbs and manual wheelchair bounded and required assistance from their caregivers

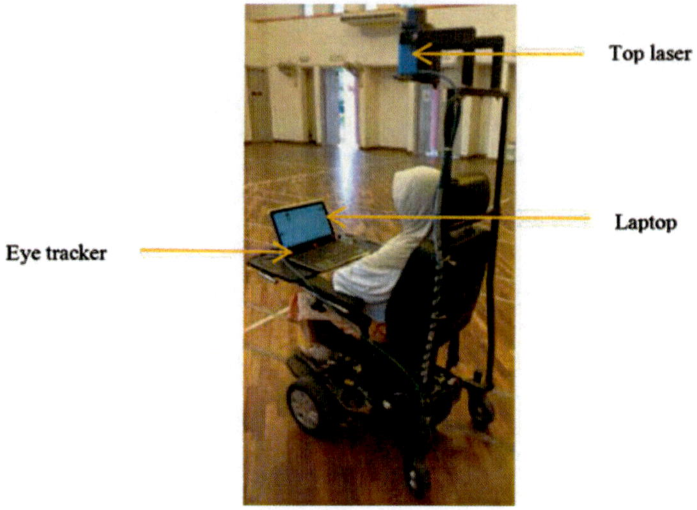

Fig. 1 The subject is looking at the direction box on displaced on the laptop screen to navigate the wheelchair

to wheel them around. Prior to the recruitment, ethical approval was obtained from the institute and old folk's home-care. Informed consent was obtained from the voluntary subjects who were pre-screened according to the inclusion criteria. The inclusion criteria of the subjects were: (1) mentally stable paraplegic patient and (2) manual wheelchair-bound. Exclusion criteria were any subjects who had experienced using with eye-controlled or brain-computer interface wheelchair.

2.4 *Measurement Tools*

Baseline assessments were conducted based on the inclusion criteria in order to follow the pre-designed standard by the university (UTAR) in conducting the research.

The data collection was performed by the same researcher throughout the 2 months. Since the researcher is also the data collector, therefore, few measures were strictly followed by the researcher to prevent bias. The measures are: (1) verbal information was given to the participants that their feedback will never affect their involvement in this study, (2) to read the questions in the same tone to both the participants and (3) record subjects' responses as it is.

The details on the QoL questionnaire as detailed below in ***Quality-of-Life (QoL) Questionnaire***.

Quality-of-Life (QoL) Questionnaire. Subjects' QoL after the eye-controlled usage was assessed using a self-designed questionnaire, Quality-of-Life in Relation with Wheelchair Questionnaire (QOLRW). QOLRW consists of 16 items and 5 domains, which are general feeling (4 items), self-esteem (2 items), social interaction/independence (2 items), user-friendly (4 items), and general health (4 items). A 5-point Likert scale ranging from 2 = Strongly Agree, 1 = Agree, 0 = Neutral, −1 = Disagree and −2 = Strongly Disagree was used in this questionnaire. In order to ease the subjects' response, a visual analog scale (VAS) was inserted along in the questionnaire to ease the scoring. Scoring was done by simply summing all and rate it as better, unchanged, or worse compared to the previous session. The total score is 32.

Questionnaire Administration. QOLRW was administered on weekly basis after the eye-controlled wheelchair navigation and control, however, the data will be interpreted as once a month. This is similar to a previous study that measures the QoL once a month [18]. The data collection duration is 2 months.

The researcher read out this questionnaire to the subjects individually and manually selected the subject's verbal answer by clicking to the pre-set Google Form on the smartphone. The raw data were auto-stored in the Google Drive.

3 Results

The Quality-of-Life (QoL) was measured using a self-designed questionnaire, Quality-of-Life in Relation with Wheelchair Navigation (QOLRW). Table 1 shows there is a progressively increase in the subjects' QoL over the period of study. Overall, the results revealed a positive impact with the wheelchair navigation on all domains which are general feeling, self-esteem, social interaction/independence, user-friendly, and general health as both the subject's steady QoL increased in comparison to the 4th week to the subsequent weeks until the 8th week. The results of QOLRW by domains for Subject A rated most items by domains as agree and strongly agree for general feeling, self-esteem, social interaction/independence, user-friendly, and general health domains. Similarly, for Subject B, she rated most items by domains as agree and strongly agree for general feeling, self-esteem, social interaction/independence, user-friendly, and general health domains during the first assessment. The result interpretation by subjects is as briefed in the next paragraph.

The collected data was interpreted as such to show the subjects' QoL progress during the 8 weeks of data collection. As in the fourth week, the QoL scores were: subject A (score: 21/32) and subject B (score: 22/32). Interpretation: Both subjects' scores were almost similar. In contrast, the QoL score increased from the 4th week to the 8th week. In the 8th week, the QoL scores were: subject A (score: 30/32) and subject B (score: 29/32). Interpretation: The final week scores denoted that the subject's QoL has increased as in contrast to Week 1 scores with Subject A with 9 scores difference and Subject B with 7 scores difference. There was visible QoL score improvement in both subjects comparatively.

Next, the differences between week 4 and week 8. The differences were simply calculated by deducting the week 8 score with week 4 by domains. Score difference

Table 1 QoL score after wheelchair usage

Subject	Domain	Week 4 Score	Week 8 Score	Score difference[1]	Total score by domain[2]	*Improvement in each domain (%)	Effect Size**
A	General feeling	5	7	2	8	25	Small
	Self-esteem	2	4	2	4	50	Small
	Social Interaction/independence	2	4	2	4	50	Small
	User-friendly	7	7	0	8	0	N/A
	General health	5	8	3	8	38	Small
	Total score	**21**	**30**	**9**	**32**	–	–
B	General feeling	4	6	2	8	25	Small
	Self-esteem	2	4	2	4	50	Small
	Social Interaction/independence	2	4	2	4	50	Small
	User-friendly	7	8	1	8	13	Small
	General health	7	7	0	8	0	N/A
	Total score	**22**	**29**	**7**	**32**	–	–

*Improvement in each domain (%) = $\frac{\text{Score difference}}{\text{Total score in the domain}} \times 100$

**Cohen's d, Small = 0.2, Medium = 0.5, and Large = 0.8 [18] obtained by Subject A: general feeling (score: 2), self-esteem (score: 2), social interaction/independence (score: 2), user-friendly (score: 0), and, general health (score: 3). Followed by the score difference obtained by Subject B: general feeling (score: 2), self-esteem (score: 2), social interaction/independence (score: 2), user-friendly (score: 1), and, general health (score: 0).

The total score by domains was as: general feeling (score: 8), self-esteem (score: 4), social interaction/independence (score: 4), user-friendly (score: 8), and, general health (score: 8).

Finally, the improvement of score in each domain (%) was calculated using this formula:

$$\text{Improvement in each domain (\%)} = \frac{\text{Score difference}}{\text{Total score in the domain}} \times 100$$

The percentage of improvement of each domain was calculated in order to find out the improvements of the QoL score differences in comparison to week 4 and week 8. Improvement of each domain by percentage Subject A: general feeling (25%), self-esteem (50%), social interaction/independence (50%), user-friendly (0%), and, general health (38%). While for Subject B: general feeling (25%), self-esteem (50%), social interaction/independence (50%), user-friendly (13%), and, general health (0%).

Next, the effect size was mentioned according to the improvement of each domain. Effect size is a statistical concept that measures the strength of the relationship between two variables on a numeric scale [23]. The effect size for Subject A is small for the stated domains: general feeling, self-esteem, social interaction/independence, and general health, and, for the user-friendly domain it is not applicable. While the effect size for Subject B is, also, small for the stated domains: general feeling, self-esteem, social interaction/independence, and user-friendly, and, general health domain it is not applicable. The small effect size shows that there is least difference is found between the week 4 and week 8 scores for each domain.

4 Discussion

This study purposed to evaluate the impact after using the eye-controlled wheelchair in short term. Two paraplegic patients were recruited and given the eye-controlled wheelchair for them to navigate and control to their desired direction in this study for 2 months duration.

In order to measure the QoL after the eye-controlled wheelchair usage, a questionnaire is used. Since the available questionnaires are either general health-related or specific disease-related. General health-related such as Short Form-36 (*SF-36*), Sickness Impact Profile (*SIP*), EuroQol Quality of Life Scale (*EQ-5D*), and McGill Quality of Life Questionnaire (*MQOL*) [19–21]. While, the existing disease-specific questionnaires are such as Stroke Specific Quality of Life (*SSQOL*)

[22], Spinal Cord Injury Quality-of-Life (*SCIQL-23*) [23], Quality of Life in Neurological Disorders (*Neuro-QoL*) [24], and Amyotrophic Lateral Sclerosis-Specific QOL Instrument-Revised (ALSSQOL-R) [25].

However, after reading through these questionnaires. It is found that some of these questionnaire domains did match with our key domains, however, there are still lacking to apt for our study purpose, which is to evaluate the impact after using the eye-controlled wheelchair in short term. Therefore, QOLRW, a self-designed questionnaire was developed and both face and content validated in accordance with the aim of the present study. Visual Analogue Scale (VAS) was used along with this QOLRW and the emoticons had eased the subjects to answer the questionnaires verbally.

Throughout the study, mobility from one place to another had resulted in a positive impact on the subjects' QoL, specifically in the domains of self-esteem, social interaction/ independence, user-friendly, and general health, and a negative impact on the domain of general feeling. Initially, Subject A stated that "it's quite difficult to get familiarize with the system" while, Subject B stated "it a new type of wheelchair to get to know", however, over time they both managed to get a good sense of control over the wheelchair. This has been expressed by themselves that the wheelchair made them feel "free and happy to move around" and to "socialize with others while sightseeing", as previously, they depended on their caregivers or friends' assistance to wheel them around their home-care.

In day-to-day life, both subjects enjoy going around the home-care and chat with the other folks, however, their interest was not being able to be fulfilled many of the times as they need someone to wheelchair them around. This is solely due to the limited presence of caregivers with more wheelchair dependents in their residing home-care. In specific, the reduction of QoL is found in terms of independence and social interaction. This statement is similar to a preliminary study, which studied the relationship between SCI manual wheelchair users' satisfaction and QoL and concluded that social circle and transportation usage were more related to QoL than to wheelchair users' satisfaction [15].

In this study, both subjects were taken care of by their caregivers who assist their activities of daily living (ADL) which include bathing, dressing, wheeling from one place to another, and so forth. Even though both subjects do have minimal hand function but they were still limited to control the manual or electric wheelchair due to their deteriorating health condition.

The functional limitation and quality of life are related to stroke-related impairments. This statement is supported in a recent article whereby this study result found that quite a number of stroke and spinal code injury (SCI) (type of neurological disorder) survivors had not fully regained their functional mobility and independence in performing their activity of daily life (ADL) [26, 27]. This fact is applicable for post-stroke patients for more than 2 years [26]. Furthermore, reduction of outdoor activities will lead to limited social participation as it decreases the subject's chances to meet and greet their friends within the home-care. In the worst case, limited social participation will lead to depression [26]. Mobility-affected stroke and SCI patients will be wheelchair dependent in nature, mostly mainly manual and powered wheelchair.

In contrary to the manual wheelchair, the eye-controlled wheelchair users need only minimal assistance during the wheelchair setup and later during the system shutting down at the end of usage. Subject A and Subject B have forwarded their wish to use the eye-controlled wheelchair almost every day, if possible. However, due to their disease progression, physiotherapy sessions and hospital visits made them take a break in between, but, this never stopped their will to use this eye-controlled wheelchair, whenever possible. Similarly, in a recent study, the QoL was measured with an independent eye-controlled home system usage [28] and mind-controlled brain painting application at the subject's home [29]. Both case studies had demonstrated improvement in QoL of paraplegic patients over a period of use of the devices.

5 Conclusion

Even though the subjects have minimal hand function, however, due to their disease progression, it may deteriorate their health which may reduce their ability to control and navigate a powered wheelchair via the usual method. Therefore, an eye-controlled wheelchair may serve as an alternative innovative method to control and navigate a powered wheelchair. In conclusion, this study achieved the study aim which is to evaluate the impact after using the eye-controlled wheelchair in short term. Despite the research were conducted for 2 months duration (short term), however, there is a positive impact found in both subjects' QoL where their improvements were able to be quantified.

Acknowledgements We would like to convey our appreciation to Dato' Prof. Dr. Goh Sing Yau, Universiti Tunku Abdul Rahman, Malaysia, for his guidance, the research subjects, and those who helped us both directly and indirectly.

Funding This work was supported by the Universiti Tunku Abdul Rahman Research (Malaysia) Fund 2018 Cycle 2, IPSR/RMC/UTARRF/2018-C2/T01.

Conflicts of Interest None

Ethical Approval and Consent to Participate This study was supported by Universiti Tunku Abdul Rahman Scientific and Ethical Review Committee (Ref: U/SERC/99/2018) and the Department of Social Welfare Malaysia (Ref: JKMM 100/12/5/2: 2018 / 326).

References

1. Tuisku, O., Bates, R., Štěpánková, O., Fejtová, M., Novák, P., Istance, H.: A survey of existing 'de-facto' standards and systems of gaze based mobility control. (Deliverable D2. 6, communication by gaze interaction (COGAIN), Project IST-2003–511598). In: Retrieved from the COGAIN Association website (2008). http://www.cogain.org/wiki/COGAIN_Reports
2. Simpson, R.C.: Smart wheelchairs: a literature review. J. Rehabil. Res. Dev. **42**(4) (2005)
3. Brodal, P.: The Central Nervous System: Structure and Function. Oxford University Press (2004)
4. Sacco, R.L., Kasner, S.E., Broderick, J.P., Caplan, L.R., Connors, J.J., Culebras, A., Elkind, M.S. et al.: An updated definition of stroke for the 21st century: a statement for healthcare professionals from the American Heart Association/American Stroke Association. Stroke **44**(7), 2064–2089 (2013)
5. Graf, R., LeLaurin, J., Schmitzberger , M., Freytes, I.M., Orozco, T., Dang, S., Uphold, C.R.: The stroke caregiving trajectory in relation to caregiver depressive symptoms, burden, and intervention outcomes. Topics in sTroke rehabilitation **24**(7), 488–495 (2017)
6. Ayerbe, L., Ayis, S., Crichton, S., Wolfe, C.D.A., Rudd, A.G.: The long-term outcomes of depression up to 10 years after stroke; the South London Stroke Register. J Neurol Neurosurg. Psychiatry **85**(5) (2014): 514–521
7. Nordin, N.A.M., Abd Aziz, N.A., Aziz, A.F.A., Singh, D.K.A., Othman, N.A.O., Sulong, S., Aljunid, S.M.: Exploring views on long term rehabilitation for people with stroke in a developing country: findings from focus group discussions. BMC Health Serv. Res. **14**(1), 1–10 (2014)
8. Samsiah, M., Das, S., Chee, S.Y., Rashidah, R., Siti, H., Ruth, P., Hamidah, H., Ho, S.E., Santhna, L.: The ideal measurement of the quality of life in post stroke patients: an urban study. Clin. Ter. **162**(3), 209–215 (2011)
9. Hachem, L.D., Ahuja, C.S., Fehlings, M.G.: Assessment and management of acute spinal cord injury: from point of injury to rehabilitation. J. Spinal Cord Med. **40**(6), 665–675 (2017)
10. Tulsky, D.S., Kisala, P.A., Victorson, D., Tate, D.G., Heinemann, A.W., Charlifue, S., Kirshblum, S.C., et al.: Overview of the spinal cord injury–quality of life (SCI-QOL) measurement system. J. Spinal Cord Med. **38**(3), 257–269 (2015)
11. Liu, C.W., Attar, K.H., Gall, A., Shah, J., Craggs, M.: The relationship between bladder management and health-related quality of life in patients with spinal cord injury in the UK. Spinal Cord **48**(4), 319–324 (2010)
12. Brown-Triolo, D.L., Roach, M.J., Nelson, K., Triolo, R.J.: Consumer perspectives on mobility: implications for neuroprosthesis design. J. Rehabil. Res. Dev. **39**(6), 659–670 (2002)
13. Aaronson, N.K.: Quantitative issues in health-related quality of life assessment. Health Policy **10**(3), 217–230 (1988)
14. Hosseini, S.M., Oyster, M.L., Kirby, R.L., Harrington, A.L., Boninger, M.L.: Manual wheelchair skills capacity predicts quality of life and community integration in persons with spinal cord injury. Arch. Phys. Med. Rehabil. **93**(12), 2237–2243 (2012)
15. Chan, S.C., Chan, A.P.: User satisfaction, community participation and quality of life among Chinese wheelchair users with spinal cord injury: a preliminary study. Occup. Ther. Int. **14**(3), 123–143 (2007)
16. Pettersson, I., Ahlström, G., Törnquist, K.: The value of an outdoor powered wheelchair with regard to the quality of life of persons with stroke: a follow-up study. Assist. Technol. **19**(3), 143–153 (2007)
17. Krishnan, K., Fan, T.L., Kiat, D.N.W., Yau, G.S.: Implementing a brain-computer interface wheelchair in home-care setting: preliminary result. In: Journal of Physics: Conference Series, vol. 1372, no. 1, p. 012020. IOP Publishing (2019)
18. Bartolucci, A.A., Tendera, M., Howard, G.: Meta-analysis of multiple primary prevention trials of cardiovascular events using aspirin. Am. J. Cardiol. **107**(12), 1796–1801 (2011)
19. Ferrucci, L., Koh, C., Bandinelli, S., Guralnik, J.M.: Disability, functional status, and activities of daily living. Encycl. Gerontol. 427–436 (2010)

20. McDowell, I.: Measuring Health: A Guide to Rating Scales and Questionnaires. Oxford University Press, USA (2006)
21. Robin Cohen, S., Mount, B.M., Bruera, E., Provost, M., Rowe, J., Tong, K.: Validity of the McGill quality of life questionnaire in the palliative care setting: a multi-centre Canadian study demonstrating the importance of the existential domain. Palliat. Med. **11**(1), 3–20 (1997)
22. Williams, L.S., Weinberger, M., Harris, L.E., Clark, D.O., Biller, J.: Development of a stroke-specific quality of life scale. Stroke **30**(7), 1362–1369 (1999)
23. Sullivan, G.M., Feinn, R.: Using effect size—or why the P value is not enough. J. Grad. Med. Educ. **4**(3), 279–282 (2012)
24. Gershon, R.C., Lai, J.S., Bode, R., Choi, S., Moy, C., Bleck, T., Miller, D., Peterman. A., Cella, D.: Neuro-QOL: quality of life item banks for adults with neurological disorders: item development and calibrations based upon clinical and general population testing. Qual. Life Res. **21**(3), 475–486 (2012)
25. Felgoise, S.H., Walsh, S.M., Stephens, H.E., Brothers, A., Simmons, Z.: The ALS specific quality of life-revised (ALSSQOL-R) user's guide. version 1.0. 2011 [Online].[cited 2011 Jan 15]
26. Azlin, N., Aziz, N.A., Saperi, B.S., Aljunid, S.M.: Functional limitation and health-related quality of life, and associated factors among long term stroke survivors in a Malaysian community. Med. J. Malaysia **71**(6), 313–321 (2016)
27. Tsang, W.W.N., Gao, K.L., Chan, K.M., Purves, S., Macfarlane, D.J., Fong, S.S.M.: Sitting tai chi improves the balance control and muscle strength of community-dwelling persons with spinal cord injuries: a pilot study. In: Evidence-Based Complementary and Alternative Medicine 2015 (2015)
28. Wolpaw, J.R., Bedlack, R.S., Reda. D.J., Ringer, R.J., Banks. P.G., Vaughan, T.M., Heckman, S.M. et al.: Independent home use of a brain-computer interface by people with amyotrophic lateral sclerosis. Neurology **91**(3), e258–e267 (2018)
29. Holz, E.M., Botrel, L., Kaufmann, T., Kübler, A.: Long-term independent brain-computer interface home use improves quality of life of a patient in the locked-in state: a case study. Arch. Phys. Med. Rehabil. **96**(3), S16–S26 (2015)

Fusion of Deep Features for Classification of Breast Cancer Using Multi-Deep CNNs

S. R. Sannasi Chakravarthy, N. Bharanidharan, and Harikumar Rajaguru

Abstract Breast cancer remains a deadly disease that frightens women in several parts of the world. At the same time, deep learning becomes the widely used and fast-growing area of traditional machine learning. The work experiments a newer computer-aided diagnosis (CAD) tool that comprises of feature extrication and classification through deep learning for assisting radiologists in breast cancer classification in mammogram images. And this is done by three different experimentations for determining the optimum way of robust classification. Herein, the first one makes use of pretrained Deep CNNs namely AlexNet, GoogleNet, Res-Net50, and DenseNet121. The second one is based on the experimentation of extracting features using the Deep CNNs and applied to a support vector machine (SVM) model. The last one is based on fusing the deep features for designing a robust classification framework. All these experimentations are evaluated using MIAS database. And finally, the results reveal that the fusing of deep features enhanced the classification performance of SVM, i.e., this deep feature fusion (feature set_3) with SVM provides a maximum classification accuracy of 96.739% than other approach.

Keywords Convolution neural networks · Support vector machine · Deep learning · Transfer learning · Gaussian · Breast cancer · Mammograms

1 Introduction

Globally, breast cancer is becoming a deadly and high frightening disease in women's health. Additionally, this type of cancer is globally witnessed as one of the most persistent cancer type among women [1]. Thus, earlier detection and diagnosis of this cancer type is significant to reduce mortality and successful treatment.

S. R. Sannasi Chakravarthy (✉) · H. Rajaguru
Department of ECE, Bannari Amman Institute of Technology, Sathyamangalam, India

N. Bharanidharan
Department of CSE, Dayananda Sagar University, Bangalore, India

J. Usman et al. (eds.), *6th Kuala Lumpur International Conference on Biomedical Engineering 2021*, IFMBE Proceedings 86,
https://doi.org/10.1007/978-3-030-90724-2_5

Medical imaging and analysis are the most efficient approach for the cancer diagnosis. For breast cancer, there are several distinct image modalities available such as digital mammographic procedure, magnetic resonance imaging (MRI), ultrasound (US), thermography, x-ray imaging and fine needle aspiration (FNA). But for the purpose of earlier detection, mammogram is the widely used procedure for breast cancer [2]. The mammographic procedure gives us high quality digital mammograms for visualizing the breast anatomy. Herein, several indicators are provided by mammograms for breast cancer diagnosis, they are: microcalcification, masses, and architectural distortions. In this, the crucial indicators are masses and microcalcifications which provide information of tumors in the primary stages whereas the last indicator is lesser significant as concern with the other two indicators [3]. Radiologist and clinical people could not provide us the precise evaluation of mammogram images due to several misconceptions among them during screening. Thus, a CAD tool is needed to assist them for better diagnosis and successful treatment. This will enhance the accuracy of diagnostic procedure and so considered as a secondary opinion for clinical people [4].

The aim of the work lies in designing an efficient CAD tool for breast cancer classification using deep learning techniques. The novelty lies in achieving the maximum classification performance by fusion of deep features. In literature, several works have been proposed [5–7] using fusion of deep features with different DCNNs, but the appropriate fusion of deep features extracted from distinct DCNNs is analysed in the paper. The work evaluated on Mammographic Image Analysis Society dataset, and the overall proposed workflow of the paper is given in Fig. 1.

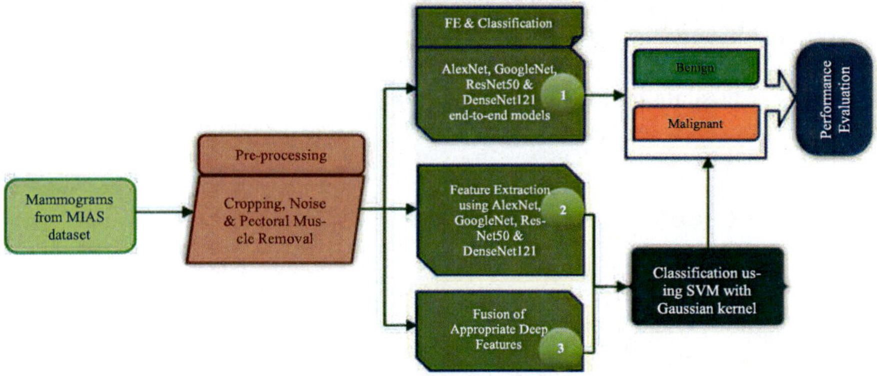

Fig. 1 Overall proposed workflow for breast cancer classification

2 Methodology

2.1 Dataset, Pre-Processing, and Augmentation

The effectiveness of the proposed work is examined using the mammograms of Mammographic Image Analysis Society (MIAS) database, a standard benchmark dataset for classification of microcalcification. The dataset is publicly available [8] and was developed by a group of United Kingdom (UK) research people. It consists of 322 mammograms where the work considers benign (64) and malignant (51) cases for severity classification problem. And all these mammograms were acquired at mediolateral oblique (MLO) views. The pre-processing of mammograms is essential to provide better classification and precise diagnosis of breast cancer.

The pre-processing steps of mammograms are graphically illustrated in Fig. 2 and summarised below:

- The dark areas or black part on either side of mammograms are cropped manually (Fig. 2b).
- The noise in mammograms is removed using adaptive median filtering [9] (Fig. 2b)
- The left MLO view mammograms in MIAS dataset are flipped uniformly so that all the mammograms will become right MLO view mammograms (Fig. 2c).
- For easy removal of pectoral muscles using pixel intensity, the mammograms are now enhanced using CLAHE – contrast limited adaptive histogram equalization [10] (Fig. 2d).
- Based on the pixel intensity and global thresholding [11], the pectoral muscles are removed as in (Fig. 2e).

The MIAS dataset is a powerful data corpus, but it is a smaller database due to limited volume of patients. So, image augmentation is performed to provide better

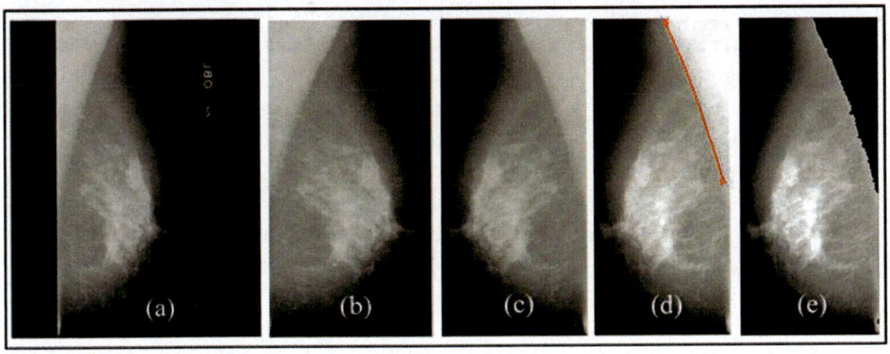

Fig. 2 Pre-processing of mammogram [*mias120.pgm*]

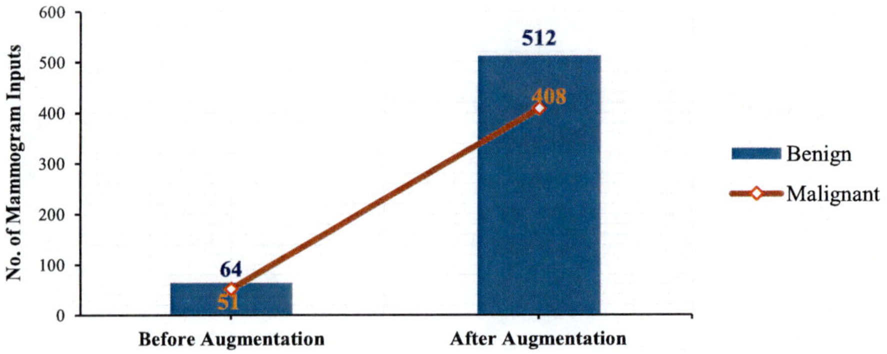

Fig. 3 Mammogram inputs used for evaluation of the work

results of classification using deep learning. After pre-processing step, the mammograms are then augmented i.e., new mammograms are generated based on the pre-processed one. This can be done by flipping and rotating the pre-processed mammograms by six distinct angles: 45°, 90°, 135°, 180°, 234°, 270°, and by horizontal and vertical flipping. Thus, the mammogram of benign and malignant cases is now $64 \times 8 = 512$ and $51 \times 8 = 408$. The number of cases in each severity before and after augmentation is illustrated in Fig. 3. After pre-processing, the size of mammogram input is reduced than the original and they are now cropped according to the deep CNN type.

2.2 *Feature Extraction and Transfer Learning*

In several machine learning applications, feature extraction is the challenging task; the emerging deep learning approaches have drawn more attention due to their higher classification performance and consistency [12]. The concept of transfer learning is used in the work for mammogram feature extraction where the deep CNNs are trained already with around 1.2 million image inputs (ImageNet dataset) with thousand output classes. The feature extraction is performed by replacing the final fully connected layer in deep CNNs with a newer layer for the severity classification of mammograms. Thus, the work utilizes the transfer learning technique to extract robust features for obtaining optimal representation of mammograms. The detailed description of deep CNNs used in the work is summarized in Table 1.

Table 1 Deep CNNs used in the classification of breast cancer

AlexNet	GoogleNet	ResNet50	DenseNet121
Input image (227 × 227 × 3)	Input image (224 × 224 × 3)	Input image (224 × 224 × 3)	Input image (224 × 224 × 3)
conv1 pool1 conv2 pool2 conv3 conv4 conv5 pool5	conv1 pool1 conv2 pool2 Inception (3a) Inception (3b) pool3 Inception (4a) Inception (4b) Inception (4c) Inception (4d) Inception (4e) pool4 Inception (5a) Inception (5b) average pooling	conv1 pool1 conv2_*x* conv3_*x* conv4_*x* conv5_*x* average pooling	conv1 pool1 Dense block1 Transition block1 Dense block2 Transition block2 Dense block3 Transition block3 Dense block4 average pooling
Fully connected (fc) (4096 × 2)	fully connected (fc) (1024 × 2)	Fully connected (fc) (2048 × 2)	Fully connected (fc) (1024 × 2)

2.3 *Feature Classification*

As shown in Fig. 1, in the experimentation (1), four distinct end-to-end deep CNNs are constructed (as shown in Table 1) using AlexNet, GoogleNet, ResNet50, and DenseNet121 architectures for classifying microcalcifications in mammograms. In experimentations (2) and (3), SVM algorithm with Gaussian kernel [13] is used for classification. The aim of the SVM algorithm is to classify the input features into targets using hyperplanes [14]. Herein, several hyperplanes are used for classifying 2 data points, but the one with maximum margin is the ideal one. The support vector is the vector that state the hyperplane [14].

3 Results and Discussion

All the experimentations in the work is done using a system with Intel Core i7 and having GPU of NVIDIA GeForce 940MX, 8 GB RAM on Windows 10 (×64) with MATLAB R2018b. The standard performance metrics [9] considered for the problem are sensitivity, accuracy, specificity, precision, and for validating, Cohen's kappa (κ) metric [15] is used. All the above metrics are derived from the parameters of confusion matrix obtained. The splitting of input subject for experimentation (1) is standard 70:30 training and testing ratio and followed 80:20 ratio for the remaining

Table 2 The performance of deep-CNNs for experimentation (1)

Deep-CNN	Accuracy (%)	Kappa score (κ)
AlexNet	60.145	0.211
GoogleNet	73.913	0.479
ResNet50	71.014	0.422
DenseNet121	**75.362**	**0.508**

The bold value in the table shows that the corresponding CNN architecture has provided the best value of classification accuracy

experimentations (2) and (3), because of using fivefold cross-validation. Moreover, the parameters of SVM are tuned using grid search method [16].

For experimentation (1), the five end-to-end deep-CNNs are retrained after fine tuning the fc layer, the primary learning rate and the iteration are chosen as 10^{-3} and 10^4 [17]. And the momentum and weight decay are chosen as 5×10^{-4} and 0.9 [17]. The mini-batch size and epochs are chosen as 4 and 20. In addition, the maximum iterations per epoch is chosen as the validation frequency for validating the results at each epoch. Other than these, all other parameters are set as default. The results obtained are tabulated in Table 2. As shown in Table 2, the kappa score of the Deep-CNNs is obtained in the range of 0.2–0.5 whereas the DenseNet121 model provides a maximum κ score of 0.508 with 75.362% accuracy.

In experimentation (2), the extraction of deep features is done and then fed to train and test the SVM algorithm with Gaussian kernel. The results obtained are given in Table 3. As in Table 3, the classification performance of SVM algorithm fed with deep features of Deep-CNNs has strengthened with the range of accuracy (77.1–94.022%). In this experiment also, the highest kappa score is obtained for DenseNet121–SVM algorithm as 0.879 with 94.175% of precision, which is due to its improved parameter efficiency and deep supervision nature of networks.

The third experimentation is done to determine the result if the deep features are fused for providing enhanced classification performance than others. For this, the work utilizes four different feature sets signifying distinct fusion of deep features. For generating these feature sets, the work makes use of the validated kappa score obtained in experimentation (1) which can be used for ranking the deep features

Table 3 The performance of deep-CNNs with SVM classifier for experimentation (2)

DCNN	Sensitivity (%)	Specificity (%)	Accuracy (%)	Precision (%)	Kappa (κ)
AlexNet	83.33	76.83	80.435	81.731	0.603
GoogleNet	79.41	74.39	77.174	79.412	0.538
ResNet50	94.12	91.46	92.935	93.204	0.857
DenseNet121	95.1	92.68	**94.022**	94.175	0.879

The bold value in the table shows that the corresponding CNN architecture has provided the best value of classification accuracy

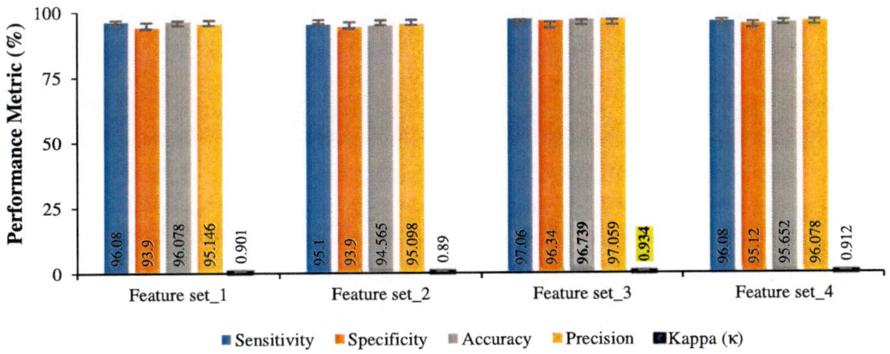

Fig. 4 Performance comparison of fused feature sets for experimentation (3)

of Deep-CNNs. Accordingly, the feature set_1 is the fusion of DenseNet121 and GoogleNet features, which have the maximum kappa score as compared with other models as shown in Table 2. Then the GoogleNet and ResNet50 features are fused due to their next highest kappa score (Table 2) to create the feature set_2. Now the deep features of DenseNet121 are added to feature set_2 to create the feature set_3. And finally, the feature set_4 is created by fusing the feature set_3 with the AlexNet features. The classification performance of these fused feature sets is compared and analyzed in Fig. 4, which reveals that the maximum of 96.739% accuracy is obtained for feature set_3 fed with SVM algorithm. And this was better than the accuracy of 94.022% attained using the DenseNet121 in experimentation (2). Furthermore, the precision and kappa score have increased to 97.059% and 0.934 respectively, which were better than the 94.175% of precision and 0.879 of validated κ score. Moreover, the next highest performance is achieved for feature set_4 which combines all the features of four Deep CNNs.

4 Conclusion, Limitations and Future Work

The precise and earlier breast cancer diagnosis is much needed for reducing the mortality and controlling the progression of tumor cells. Thus, the work focused to design a robust computer aided diagnostic tool for severity classification problem, where a novel CAD tool is proposed and explored different fusion of feature sets and chosen the one that provides the better classification performance. All these experimentations are carried out using digital mammograms taken from the MIAS dataset. The first experimentation was based on the classification using four fine-tuned end-to-end Deep-CNNs namely AlexNet, GoogleNet, ResNet50, and DenseNet121. To increase the performance, the second experimentation is done that used deep feature classification using SVM with Gaussian kernel. The results revealed that the classification performance obtained in experimentation (2) was better than that of experimentation (1). The third experimentation was done to investigate the fusion of appropriate deep features from different CNNs for further improvement where the performance of end-to-end Deep-CNNs was utilized for ranking the features. That is, fusion of GoogleNet, ResNet50, and DenseNet121 features (feature set_3) and fed with SVM provided a maximum accuracy of 96.739% with a validated kappa score of 0.934. Consequently, the work includes the analysis of above three experimentations for obtaining better classification performance for the problem. Thus, the results revealed that the proposed CAD model is competent of effectively classifying mammogram lesions. However, the study noted that the computational cost is increased when the deep features are combined for classification improvement of breast cancer. A feature reduction technique such as linear discriminant analysis (LDA) or principal component analysis (PCA) might be useful for getting rid of this increased computational cost. The future action of the work involves the experimentation on larger datasets such as Digital Database for Screening Mammography (DDSM) with different preprocessing techniques, with the consideration of feature reduction using LDA or PCA, and with different pretrained convolution neural network models.

References

1. Miller, K.D., Fidler-Benaoudia, M., Keegan, T.H., Hipp, H.S., Jemal, A., Siegel, R.L.: Cancer statistics for adolescents and young adults. CA: Cancer J. Clin. **70**(6), 443–459 (2020)
2. Duffy, S.W., Tabár, L., Yen, A.M.F., Dean, P.B., Smith, R.A., Jonsson, H., & Chen, T.H.H.: Mammography screening reduces rates of advanced and fatal breast cancers: results in 549,091 women. Cancer **126**(13), 2971–2979 (2020)
3. Dibden, A., Offman, J., Duffy, S.W., Gabe, R.: Worldwide review and meta-analysis of cohort studies measuring the effect of mammography screening programmes on incidence-based breast cancer mortality. Cancers **12**(4), 976 (2020)
4. Pisano, E.D.: AI shows promise for breast cancer screening. Nature **577**(7788), 35–36 (2020)
5. Jiang, F., Liu, H., Yu, S., Xie, Y.: Breast mass lesion classification in mammograms by transfer learning. In: Proceedings of the 5th International Conference on Bioinformatics and Computational Biology, pp. 59–62 (2017)
6. Ragab, D.A., Sharkas, M., Marshall, S., Ren, J.: Breast cancer detection using deep convolutional neural networks and support vector machines. Peer J, **7**, e6201 (2019)
7. Mendel, K., Li, H., Sheth, D., Giger, M.: Transfer learning from convolutional neural networks for computer-aided diagnosis: a comparison of digital breast tomosynthesis and full-field digital mammography. Acad. Radiol. **26**(6), 735–743 (2019)
8. Suckling J.P.: The mammographic image analysis society digital mammogram database. Digital Mammo, 375–386 (1994)
9. Chakravarthy, S.S., Rajaguru, H.: Automatic detection and classification of mammograms using improved extreme learning machine with deep learning. IRBM (2021). https://doi.org/10.1016/j.irbm.2020.12.004
10. Sahu, S., Singh, A.K., Ghrera, S.P., Elhoseny, M.: An approach for de-noising and contrast enhancement of retinal fundus image using CLAHE. Opt. Laser Technol. **110**, 87–98 (2019)
11. Sannasi Chakravarthy, S.R., Rajaguru, H.: Detection and classification of microcalcification from digital mammograms with firefly algorithm, extreme learning machine and non-linear

regression models: a comparison. Int. J. Imaging Syst. Technol. **30**(1), 126–146 (2020). https://doi.org/10.1002/ima.22364
12. Sannasi Chakravarthy, S.R., Rajaguru, H.: Deep-features with Bayesian optimized classifiers for the breast cancer diagnosis. Int. J. Imaging Syst. Technol. (2021). https://doi.org/10.1002/ima.22570
13. Xue, Y., Zhang, L., Wang, B., Zhang, Z., Li, F.: Nonlinear feature selection using Gaussian kernel SVM-RFE for fault diagnosis. Appl. Intell. **48**(10), 3306–3331 (2018)
14. Keerthi, S.S., Lin, C.J.: Asymptotic behaviors of support vector machines with Gaussian kernel. Neural Comput. **15**(7), 1667–1689 (2003)
15. Kraemer, H.C.: Kappa coefficient. Wiley StatsRef: Statistics Reference Online, 1–4 (2014)
16. Syarif, I., Prugel-Bennett, A., Wills, G.: SVM parameter optimization using grid search and genetic algorithm to improve classification performance. Telkomnika **14**(4), 1502 (2016)
17. Gao, F., Yoon, H., Wu, T., Chu, X.: A feature transfer enabled multi-task deep learning model on medical imaging. Expert Syst. Appl. **143**, 112957 (2020)

Improved Bald Eagle Search Optimization for Enhancing the Performance of Supervised Classifiers in Dementia Diagnosis

N. Bharanidharan, S. R. Sannasi Chakravarthy, and Harikumar Rajaguru

Abstract Evolutionary algorithms are widely used to improve the performance of machine learning techniques through various approaches. This paper focuses on increasing the accuracy of the machine learning techniques in diagnosing dementia through the usage of Improved Bald Eagle Search Optimization as a transformation technique. In the proposed Improved Bald Eagle Search Optimization, the control parameters are updated using the entropy-based gradient to reduce the error rate of the classification algorithm. Magnetic resonance images of 52 dementia and 52 non-dementia subjects obtained from the OASIS database are considered in this research work. Raw intensity values are taken as features and given as input to the transformation technique based on Improved Bald Eagle Search Optimization. Then the transformed values are classified through one of the three different supervised classifiers namely Naïve Bayes, Linear Discriminant Analysis, and Support Vector Machine. The accuracy of Support Vector Machine is 64% when no transformation technique is used and it is increased to 88% when Improved Bald Eagle Search Optimization is used for transforming the features.

Keywords Dementia · Machine learning · Improved bald eagle search optimization

1 Introduction

Various machine learning algorithms are developed in the last few decades to act as decision support systems in various fields [1]. Particularly in the medical field, computerized decision support systems will be very useful in diagnosing a disease. But in the medical field, the decision of machine learning algorithms should be accurate otherwise the ill-effects will be severe [2]. To improve the accuracy of

N. Bharanidharan (✉)
CSE Department, Dayananda Sagar University, Bangalore, India

S. R. Sannasi Chakravarthy · H. Rajaguru
ECE Department, Bannari Amman Institute of Science and Technology, Sathyamangalam, India

J. Usman et al. (eds.), *6th Kuala Lumpur International Conference on Biomedical Engineering 2021*, IFMBE Proceedings 86,
https://doi.org/10.1007/978-3-030-90724-2_6

machine learning algorithms various approaches are used such as feature selection, dimensionality reduction, transformation techniques, etc.

Dementia—a syndrome that affects memory, behavior, thinking, and the response of a human. Dementia is one of the common diseases in older people but still, it is not due to normal aging and so it is detected even in mid-aged people [3]. According to World Health Organization, more than fifty million humans are possessing dementia currently worldwide and around ten million humans are detected with dementia every year. Magnetic Resonance Imaging (MRI) of the brain region will be generally used in the diagnosis of dementia. Due to a large amount of data and the nature of complexity, a computerized decision support system with high accuracy will be very useful for dementia diagnosis [4].

Optimization algorithms are widely classified into gradient and non-gradient optimization algorithms [5] and they are extensively used in enhancing the accuracy of machine learning techniques in decision support systems. For example, gradient-based optimization algorithms namely Stochastic Gradient Descent, Adam optimizer are commonly used in training neural networks. On the other hand, non-gradient optimization algorithms are simple, possess derivation-free mechanisms, and belong to the meta-heuristic techniques category. Meta-heuristic algorithms comprise evolutionary algorithms, swarm-based algorithms, physics-based algorithms, bio-inspired algorithms, and nature-inspired algorithms [6]. Some of the meta-heuristic algorithms include genetic algorithm, Particle Swarm Optimization (PSO), harmony search, Tabu search, elephant herding optimization, cuckoo search, Bald Eagle Search (BES), etc.

Meta-heuristics are mostly used to enhance the performance of machine learning algorithms through feature selection and neural network training [7]. In some research works, meta-heuristics are used as a transformation technique to improve the accuracy of machine learning algorithms [8, 9]. To the best of our knowledge, BES is not reported as a transformation technique and so this research work focuses on implementation and improvisation of the BES as transform. Control parameters (weights) of BES are updated through an entropy-based gradient in the proposed Improved Bald Eagle Search (IBES) and this can be considered as the main novelty of this paper.

The remaining paper is structured as follows: the original BES algorithm is presented in the next section; dataset and methodology will be explained in the third section; implementation of BES and IBES algorithms will be dealt in fourth and fifth sections respectively; final results are discussed in the sixth section and conclusion is presented in the last section.

2 Bald Eagle Search

BES optimization algorithm is proposed through the inspiration from the hunting behavior of Bald Eagles [10]. During their hunting process, three stages can be witnessed: select space, search space, and swooping. During the select stage, the

Eagles will choose the best area for hunting and this mathematically modeled as:

$$p_{i,new} = p_{best} + \propto * r * (p_{mean} - p_i) \tag{1}$$

Here $p_{i,new}$ and p_i are new position and old position positions of ith Bald Eagle respectively; p_{best} refers to the search space currently chosen based on previous experiences and p_{mean} denotes the mean position of previous iterations; α is a control parameter that decides the position change and usually it will be varied from 1.5 to 2; r is a random value in the range [0,1].

During the search stage, Bald Eagles use spiral movement to search for prey in the selected search space and this is represented using the following equations:

$$p_{i,new} = p_i + y(i) * (p_i - p_{i+1}) + x(i) * (p_i - p_{mean}) \tag{2}$$

Here $x(i)$ and $y(i)$ present in Eq. (2) are given by,

$$x(i) = \frac{xr(i)}{\max(|xr|)} \tag{3}$$

$$y(i) = \frac{yr(i)}{\max(|yr|)} \tag{4}$$

$xr(i)$ and $yr(i)$ present in Eqs. (3) and (4) are given by,

$$xr(i) = r(i) * \sin(\theta(i)) \tag{5}$$

$$yr(i) = r(i) * \cos(\theta(i)) \tag{6}$$

$\theta(i)$ and $r(i)$ present in Eqs. (5) and (6) are given by,

$$\theta(i) = a * \pi * rand \tag{7}$$

$$r(i) = \theta(i) * R * rand \tag{8}$$

In the last stage of hunting, the bald eagles swoop towards the food from its best position and this is represented using the following equations:

$$p_{i,new} = rand * p_{best} + y1(i) * (p_i - c_2 * p_{best}) + x1(i) * (p_i - c_1 * p_{mean}) \tag{9}$$

Here $x1(i)$ and $y2(i)$ present in Eq. (9) are given by,

$$x1(i) = \frac{xr1(i)}{\max(|xr|)} \tag{10}$$

$$y1(i) = \frac{yr1(i)}{\max(|yr|)} \quad (11)$$

$xr1(i)$ and $yr1(i)$ present in Eqs. (10) and (11) are given by,

$$xr1(i) = r(i) * \sinh(\theta(i)) \quad (12)$$

$$yr1(i) = r(i) * \cosh(\theta(i)) \quad (13)$$

$\theta(i)$ and $r(i)$ present in Eqs. (12) and (13) are given by,

$$\theta(i) = a * \pi * rand \quad (14)$$

$$r(i) = \theta(i) \quad (15)$$

Here a and R are control parameters that decide the spiral motion and *rand* is the random number in the range [0,1].

3 Methodology

OASIS database contains dementia brain MRI images and 52 demented and non-demented subjects are considered in this study. Raw intensity values are considered as features in this research work and they are given as input to the IBES based transformation technique as shown in Fig. 1. Then the transformed values are given as input to any one of the supervised classifiers namely: Naïve Bayes Classifier (NBC) [11], Linear Discriminant Analysis (LDA) [12], and Support Vector Machine (SVM) [13]. Then the popular metrics namely Accuracy (ACC), Error Rate (ER), Sensitivity (SENS), Specificity (SPEC), False Positive Rate (FPR), and Precision (PREC) are used to quantify the classification performance [14].

During the implementation of supervised classifiers, 80% of MRI images are considered for training, and the remaining is considered for testing. Stratified sampling is used to split the dataset into training and testing sets. To avoid overfitting and better performance, tenfold cross-validation is used. To find the best control parameters for supervised classifiers, a randomized search is utilized.

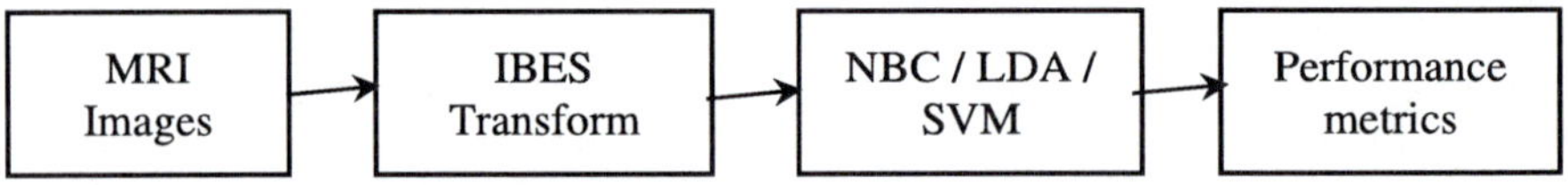

Fig. 1 Flowchart depicting the proposed methodology

4 BES Transform

To train neural networks and to solve feature selection/numerical optimization problems, the positions of Bald Eagles are initialized randomly. But to use BES as transform, the raw intensity values are assigned as positions of Bald Eagles initially. Then using Eqs. (1) to (15), the positions will be updated iteratively. The best position p_{best} is identified through fitness function. The inverse of Euclidean distance between the target and current position of Bald Eagle is considered as the fitness function.

Through experiments, it is found that the ideal value for the target is equal to 300. BES possess three control parameters namely α, *a* and R. Through experiments [10], the ranges of these control parameters are stated as below: α – [1.5, 2]; *a* – [5, 10]; R – [0.5, 2]. The ideal value for these control parameters can be found using the trial and error method. But before finding the ideal values for control parameters, the ideal value for the maximum number of iterations will be found as shown in Fig. 2. During this process, the control parameter values are fixed with their median value according to the range mentioned above. Through a similar process, ideal values for control parameters α, *a* and R can be found as depicted in Figs. 3 and 4. The ideal values are: maximum number of iterations = 10, α = 1.9, *a* = 6 and R = 1.7.

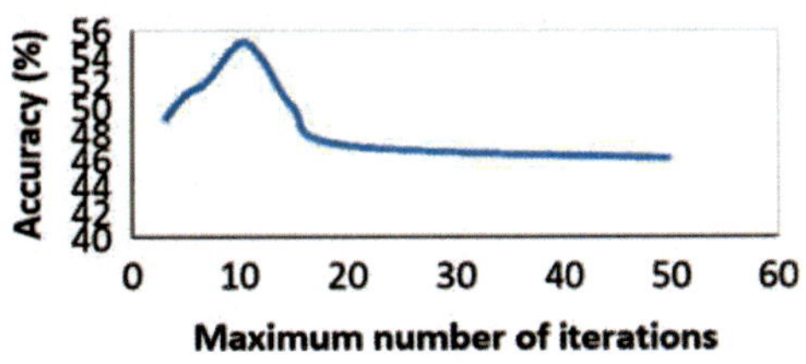

Fig. 2 Searching the ideal value for maximum number of iterations

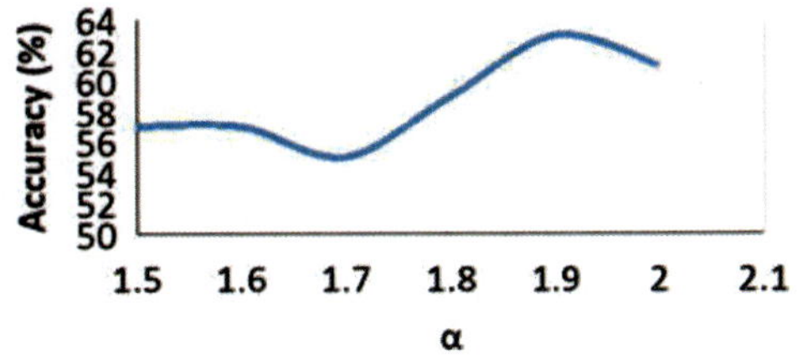

Fig. 3 Searching the ideal value for control parameter 'α'

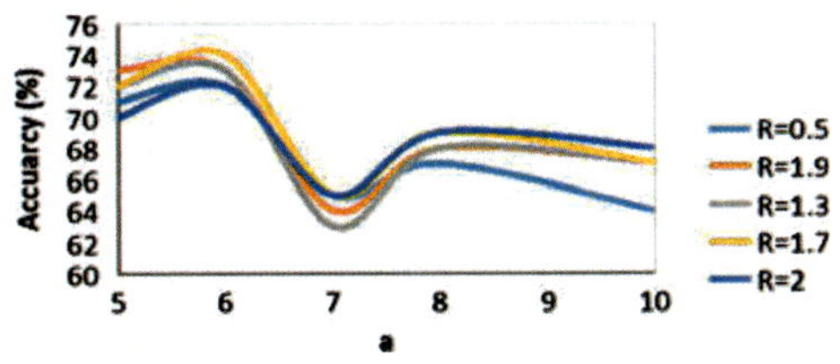

Fig. 4 Searching the ideal value for control parameters 'a' and 'R'

5 IBES Transform

Through Figs. 3 and 4, the importance of the control parameters can be witnessed i.e., sometimes even a small change in control parameter has a huge effect on accuracy. In the BES transform, the ideal values for the three control parameters are found using the trial and error method. Then these values are fixed for all iterations. It will be more beneficial to change the control parameters value in each iteration in an appropriate manner. Hence this research paper proposes the usage of gradient-based control parameter change in each iteration as shown in Eq. (16).

$$w_{t+1} = w_t + \varepsilon * \frac{\partial L}{\partial w_t} \tag{16}$$

Here w_{t+1} and w_t are the new and old control parameters and ε is the learning rate. $\frac{\partial L}{\partial w_t}$ is the loss function with respect to change in control parameter value and in the proposed method it is found using Eq. (17).

$$\frac{\partial L}{\partial w_t} = \frac{E(t) - E(t-1)}{w(t) - w(t-1)} \tag{17}$$

In Eq. (17), E represents the entropy, w represents the control parameter and t represents the iteration number. In each iteration, a change in entropy with respect to change in control parameter is calculated and this value is used to update the value of the control parameter in the next iteration.

6 Results and Discussion

The six popular classification metrics mentioned in the third section are calculated for all the three classifiers without any transform and those results are mentioned as NB, LDA and SVM in Table 1. Then BES and IBES are used as a transform for all the three classifiers using the methodology mentioned in sections four and five respectively. To justify the performance of BES and IBES, another popular meta-heuristic technique, PSO [15] is used as transform. The accuracy of various classifiers and transforms are plotted in Fig. 5. From Fig. 5, the efficiency of the proposed IBES based transform can be witnessed clearly. When the SVM classifier is considered, the IBES transform usage provides the highest accuracy of 88% while the BES transform usage provides the accuracy of 78% and when no transform is used, the accuracy of the SVM classifier is 64% only. It should be also noted the proposed transform has produced a significant increase in accuracy for both NB and LDA. This improvement is primarily due to the change of control parameter iteratively using the entropy-based gradient technique. On the other hand, PSO and IPSO based transform failed to provide any significant performance enhancement for the supervised classifiers; it is just providing some slight accuracy increment.

Table 1 Performance metrics of various techniques used

	ACC	ER	SENS	SPEC	FPR	PREC
NB	62	38	62	62	38	56
LDA	62	38	69	57	43	56
SVM	64	36	63	65	35	59
BES-NB	74	26	79	69	31	67
BES-LDA	72	28	77	68	32	66
BES-SVM	78	22	79	77	23	73
IBES-NB	78	22	83	74	26	72
IBES-LDA	79	21	83	77	23	74
IBES-SVM	88	12	90	86	14	84
PSO-NB	59	41	60	58	42	53
PSO-LDA	63	37	69	58	42	57
PSO-SVM	61	39	52	68	32	56
IPSO-NB	62	38	67	58	42	56
IPSO-LDA	64	36	69	60	40	58
IPSO-SVM	65	35	54	74	26	62

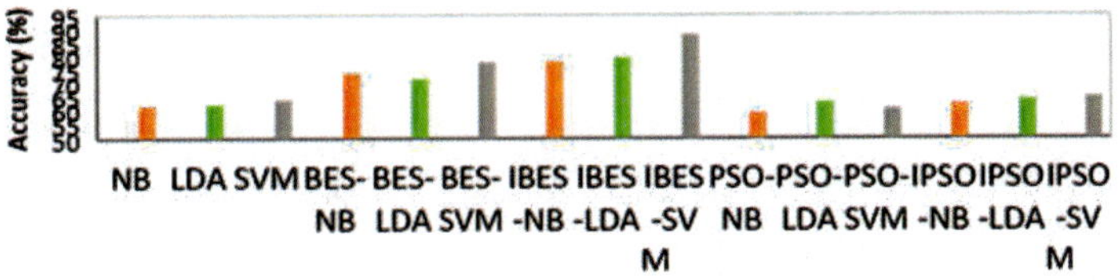

Fig. 5 Accuracy comparison of various techniques

7 Conclusion

This research paper mainly concentrated on the implementation of BES and IBES transform to improve the accuracy of three supervised classifiers namely NB, LDA, and SVM in diagnosing dementia. In IBES, the entropy-based gradient method is proposed to update the control parameters iteratively since the ideal value for the control parameters is found using the trial and error method in BES and notably, these values are fixed for all iterations in BES. In classifying the dementia images, IBES transform has improved the accuracy of NB, LDA and SVM classifiers significantly when compared to BES, PSO and IPSO transforms. Remarkably 88% accuracy is attained for the SVM classifier when IBES transform is used. Our future work will be in the direction of using different statistical measures instead of entropy for calculating the appropriate control parameter in each iteration.

References

1. Osisanwo, F.Y., Akinsola, J.E.T., Awodele, O., Hinmikaiye, J.O., Olakanmi, O., Akinjobi, J.: Supervised machine learning algorithms: classification and comparison. Int. J. Comput. Trends Technol. **48**(3), 128–138 (2017)
2. Riddhi, S.K., Dr. Salankar, S.S., Babar, M.: Literature survey on detection of brain tumor from MRI images. IOSR J. Electron. Commun. Eng. (IOSR-JECE) **10**(1), 80–86 (2015)
3. International statistical classification of diseases and related health problems. In: 10th Revision. Geneva, World Health Organization (1992)
4. Paraskevaidi, M., Martin-Hirsch, P.L., Martin, F.L.: Progress and challenges in the diagnosis of dementia: a critical review. ACS Chem. Neurosci. **9**(3) (2018)
5. Mirjalili, S., Mirjalili, S.M., Lewis, A.L.: Grey wolf optimizer. Adv. Eng. Softw. **69**, 46–61 (2014)
6. Dhiman, G., Kumar, V.: Spotted hyena optimizer: a novel bio-inspired based metaheuristic technique for engineering applications. Adv. Eng. Softw. **114**, 48–70 (2017)
7. Koumi, F., Aldasht, M., Tamimi, H.: Efficient feature selection using particle swarm optimization: a hybrid filters-wrapper approach. In: 10th International Conference on Information and Communication Systems (ICICS), Irbid, Jordan (2019)
8. Bharanidharan, N., Rajaguru, H.: Dementia MRI image classification using transformation technique based on elephant herding optimization with Randomized Adam method for updating the hyper-parameters. Int. J. Imaging Syst. Technol. 1–25 (2020). https://doi.org/10.1002/ima.22522
9. Bharanidharan, N., Harikumar, R.: Modified grey wolf randomized optimization in dementia classification using MRI images. IETE J. Res. (2019). https://doi.org/10.1080/03772063.2020.1715852
10. Alsattar, H.A., Zaidan, A.A., Zaidan, B.B.: Novel meta-heuristic bald eagle search optimisation algorithm. Artif. Intell. Rev. **53**, 2237–2264 (2020)
11. Sanchis, A., Juan, A.: A word-based naïve Bayes classifier for confidence estimation in speech recognition. IEEE Trans. Audio Speech Lang. Process. **20**(2), 564–565 (2012)
12. Tharwat, A., Gaber, T., Ibrahim, A., Hassanien, A.E.: Linear discriminant analysis: a detailed tutorial. AI Commun. **30**(2), 169–190 (2017)
13. Magnin, B., Mesrob, L., Kinkingnéhun, S., Pélégrini-Issac, M.: Support vector machine-based classification of Alzheimer's disease from whole-brain anatomical MRI. Neuroradiology **51**(2), 73–83 (2008)
14. Fielding, A.H.: Cluster and Classification Techniques for the Biosciences. Cambridge University Press, Cambridge (2006)
15. Kennedy, J., Eberhart, R.: Particle swarm optimization. IEEE International Conference on Neural Networks, Australia **4**, 1942–1948 (1995)

Classification of Walking Speed Based on Bidirectional LSTM

Wan Shi Low, Chow Khuen Chan, Joon Huang Chuah, Khairunnisa Hasikin, and Khin Wee Lai

Abstract Walking speed is a powerful predictor of health events which are related to musculoskeletal disorder and mental disease. One of the established computerized technique which employed to perform the gait analysis is motion analysis system. This system allows researchers to perform quantification or estimation on human pose and body shape from multiple camera with or without markers. However, it was reported that the high degree of variability within the data representation of gait has resulted important patterns to be undetectable. Through this study, we have developed a stacked bidirectional LSTM (Bi-LSTM) to interpret human walking speed based on kinematic data. A Bi-LSTM has higher training capability compared to a unidirectional LSTM, whereby it enables additional training by traversing the data forward and backward. We employed this model to classify the gait patterns of different walking speeds from 27 sets of gait data with total of 453 gait cycles collected from the walking trial, captured via via Vicon Motion System (Vicon MX, Oxford Metrics, UK). Kinematic parameters of the gait cycles were employed as the input layer of the Bi-LSTM deep learning architecture. Our proposed framework has achieved a prediction accuracy of 77% to classify different speed (slow, normal and fast) conditions. It was also observed that with the prediction accuracy is improved with an increased number of stacked Bi-LSTM layers.

Keywords Walking speed · Motion analysis system · Bidirectional LSTM

W. S. Low · C. K. Chan · K. Hasikin · K. W. Lai (✉)
Department of Biomedical Engineering, Faculty of Engineering, Universiti Malaya, Kuala Lumpur, Malaysia
e-mail: lai.khinwee@um.edu.my

J. H. Chuah
Department of Electrical Engineering, Faculty of Engineering, Universiti Malaya, Kuala Lumpur, Malaysia

J. Usman et al. (eds.), *6th Kuala Lumpur International Conference on Biomedical Engineering 2021*, IFMBE Proceedings 86,
https://doi.org/10.1007/978-3-030-90724-2_7

1 Introduction

The correlation between walking speed with functional decline has made it a widely used predictor for various health issue. Generally, higher risk of disability, cognitive impairments [1], falls, mortality [2], cardiovascular disease [3] and dementia [4] are found among individuals with slower gait speeds. Previous studies has concluded that the ability to maintain maximum walking speed was found to be reduced with age [5]. Such a condition can be resulted from numerous physiological factors, including joint problems [2], muscle weakness [6], reduction in hip flexor flexibility and neurological diseases [1]. Furthermore, results from some recent research have shown that the proximal redistribution of joint work found at elderly became more apparent with faster walking speed. In light of that, exploration on the impact of gait speed on biomechanical variables is critical for clinicians who frequently depend on the outcomes of gait analysis to predict functional conditions and optimize patient care.

Over the last decades, the technological advancements have given rise to the invention of computerized measurement method in gait analysis. These methods enable accurate quantification of whole-body pose thus provide clinicians with a comprehensive understanding of underlying condition which affect patient's mobility. One of the established technique of computerized gait analysis is motion capture system. It acquires the spatio-temporal data of a moving human via sensors and processes the acquired data by using mathematical model [7]. Generally, a motion capture system can be categorized into 2 groups which are optoelectronic system and markerless motion capture system. An optoelectronic system employs the emission or detection of infrared light to deduce a 3D position [8]. The system used in conjunction with retro-reflective markers whereby these markers are mounted upon the area of interest according to marker placement protocols. Multicamera setups will localize markers in a predefined 3-dimensional volume, allowing relative markers' position to be identified using output coordinate frame for individual body segments [9]. A marker-based technology is typically utilized by biomechanical and clinical studies for adapting the analysis techniques to the complexity necessary of an underlying research question. On the contrary, a markerless method estimates the pose and body shape of a person from multiple camera views without markers [10]. To achieve highly robust motion capture in unconstrained video, the predefined articulated model will be matched against multiple image sequence and iteratively refined to determine the best fit model of the data. Its major application area includes smart surveillance, human identification, and character animation. Despite the fact that motion analysis has been proven to be therapeutically beneficial, the routine clinical use of gait analysis is found with limited growth. Various variables, such as the variability of human's body appearance, the nonlinear and non-rigid nature of human motion, and self-occlusion [11], cast doubt on its therapeutic use. As a result of these circumstances, data representations of gait tend to be vast and contain a high degree of variability, rendering potentially important patterns within the data to be unrecognizable. To filter these data, it is crucial to develop a data-driven method which can extract the intrinsic and distinguishable gait patterns from camera or sensor measurement. A deep learning method which equipped with the attribute to learn and uncover the underlying distribution of data, are well suited for achieving this objective.

Machine learning, is a paradigm that focus on devising analytical models, which built on the foundation of human faculties of learning, adapting, memorizing and recognising [12]. It allows the computer system to automatically learn from data and make predictions based on the past experiences rules and observation. A machine learning has proved its important in gait-phase detection. In this case, using a learning system to understand and classify human physical activities such as sitting, walking, running and others [13, 14], enable clinician to assess the biomechanical and physiological variables of a patient on long-term basis. Furthermore, the learning algorithms can reveal hidden relationships between sensor data and biomechanical variable, in particular time series model of human motion [14]. For example, Luo et al. employed a support vector machines (SVM) algorithm to automatically produce a set of rules that identify normal and abnormal gait based on the sequence of detected gait phases [15]. Begg and Kamruzzaman applied SVM for the automatically identification of young-old gait types from their respective gait parameters which recorded using PEAK 3D motion analysis system and force platform [16]. Despite its higher classification accuracies, SVMs require high computational cost, which strongly discourages its usage when facing large-scale and real-time gait classification problems. To combat this issue, convolutional neural networks (CNNs), whose attributes include local feature extraction, weight sharing, and pooling, are employed [17]. In literature, researches has applied CNN methods using kinematics and kinetic features to forecast other kinetic parameters, but also infer additional gait kinematics. It is widely applied on data which was collected via wearable sensors to estimate the reference joint angle [18]. For instance, Gholami et al. used CNN as a regression model to evaluate the performance of single shoe-mounted accelerometer in monitoring the lower extremity running kinematics in the sagittal plane [19]. Zhao and Zhou proposed a CNN model for gait labelling and authentication [20]. However, CNNs has presented some challenges when deal with the temporal information of input data It is because CNN can only learn the short-term motion features between the adjacent frames rather than the periodic motion cue of gait sequence. As human gait is highly individual, CNN based algorithm might not be able to generalize when the threshold values are needed to be adapted to each user individually [20]. In this case, a recurrent neural network (RNN) which has achieved promising results in automatic speech recognition and machine translation, is reported to be dominant in gait sequence modelling tasks. Recently, a research team from University Carlos III of Madrid employed RNN as feature extraction algorithm on the smartphone scenario [21]. In their study, the gait data were fragments into gait cycles, and transformed into feature vectors by mean of RNN. It was found that an error rate for the tested algorithm would be lower (EER = 7.55%) when more users were added into the tested database. Noteworthy, for standard RNNs models, the range of contextual information that can be approached is limited as it can only catch time dependency in rather short sequences of data. Consequently, the earlier layers will learn very little for a longer input sequences. This issue is referred to as varnishing gradient. To address this problem, a modified version of RNN has been invented: long short-term memory (LSTM). These networks are distinguished by the presence of a memory space controlled by various gates, which allows for the modelling of temporal dependencies in sequential data [22]. The effectiveness of these methods for gait event detection was also proven, using a LSTM network to categorise gait events in children [23]. Feng et al. trained a LSTM model on human joints data to characterize the gait sequence representation, which can be used for gait recognition [24]. Liu et al. used a one-layer LSTM to learn the inherent spatial–temporal correlations of gait characteristics and detect the aberrant knee joint trajectories based on other joint [25]. Notably, a hidden state of LSTM takes information from the past without any prior knowledge about the future. A bidirectional LSTM model can take into account of any arbitrary amount of context on both sides of the sequences and eliminate the problem of limited context [26].

The aim of this work is to develop learning algorithm in advancing automatic analysis of human gait and interpreting human walking speed using kinematic data. For this purpose, we propose a bidirectional LSTM model for supervised classification whereby the model is trained to capture the temporal dependencies and characteristics of human gait data for classification of walking speed.

2 Methods

2.1 Data Labelling

There were 27 sets of gait data with a total of 453 gait cycles collected from the walking trial using Vicon Nexus. It consisted of kinematic parameters, which included the ankle, hip and knee angles from sagittal, frontal and transverse planes. These parameters were employed as cores to differentiate the gait speed in our proposed neural network training. To train the machine learning model, data labelling were performed on each set of gait cycle. The sequential data of our studied walking speed were re-labelled such that "Slow" = 0, "Normal" = 1, and "Fast" = 2 (Table 1).

Table 1 Gait cycles for various walking speed

Categories	Numerical representative	Amount of gait cycle
Slow	0	151
Normal	1	155
Fast	2	147

2.2 Deep Learning Framework Development and Validation

In this study, the neural networks were trained using Keras and TensorFlow as its backend, with Google Colab on free Tesla K80 GPU. The Bi-LSTM network was used as classifier to capture the sequential relationship in the acquired kinematic data. The proposed model consisted of an input layer, 3Bi-LSTM layers, a softmax layer and a classification layer. It has the ability to learn forward and backward temporal dependencies by characterizing the probable correlation within the data sequence. Due to the presence of repetitive action within the individual gait, the proposed network can extract the common temporal characteristic from periodic gait patterns. For sequential gaits, the network can learn the dependencies associated with the gait's sequence. In this case, the transition between the two distinct gait patterns is crucial for reinforcing the inter-connections among the cells on Bi-LSTM layers. The network employed a batch size of 500 with the Adam optimizer to run for 2500 epochs. A learning rate of 0.0001 was set as the default parameter. A dropout of 0.2 was applied to all BiLSTM layers to prevent the data from overfitting. The rectified linear unit (ReLU) was adopted in the densely connected layer as non-linear activation function to improve the learning algorithm of the model. In the output layer, a softmax activation function was used to calculate the probabilities of each walking speed over the studied speed classes. The developed model was validated by evaluating the prediction accuracy of different gait speeds from testing data of 20%. The impact of the number of stacked Bi-LSTM layers will too be discussed in the study.

3 Result and Discussion

3.1 Classification Performance of the Proposed 3 Layers Bi-LSTM Deep Learning Framework

As showed in the Figs. 1 and 2, the training epochs for training and test data are represented by blue and orange lines respectively. Both plots show good convergence of the model across epochs with regard to loss and classification accuracy. From Fig. 1, the accuracy is found to be increased drastically at around 350th epochs and the increment is slowing down after this point. At 1000th epochs, the percentage for both training and test increases to 79.7% and 77.2% respectively, and does not show an increase in accuracy with higher iterations. Therefore, 1000 epochs are considered as the ideal value for the training epochs of this model. The plot of test loss decreases to a point of stability and has a small gap with the training loss. Therefore, it can be deduced that a good fit is achieved in our model. Both test and training loss stops at 1000th epochs respectively.

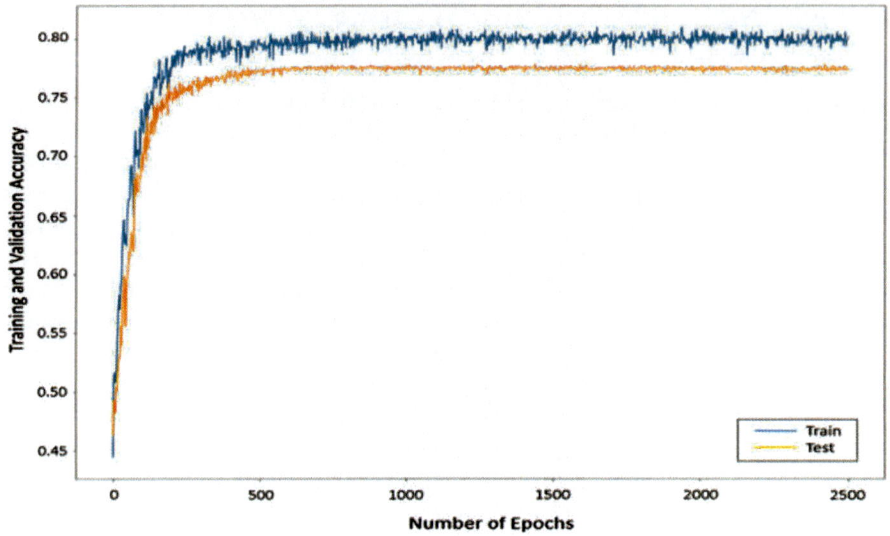

Fig. 1 Training and validation accuracy of proposed Bi-LSTM model

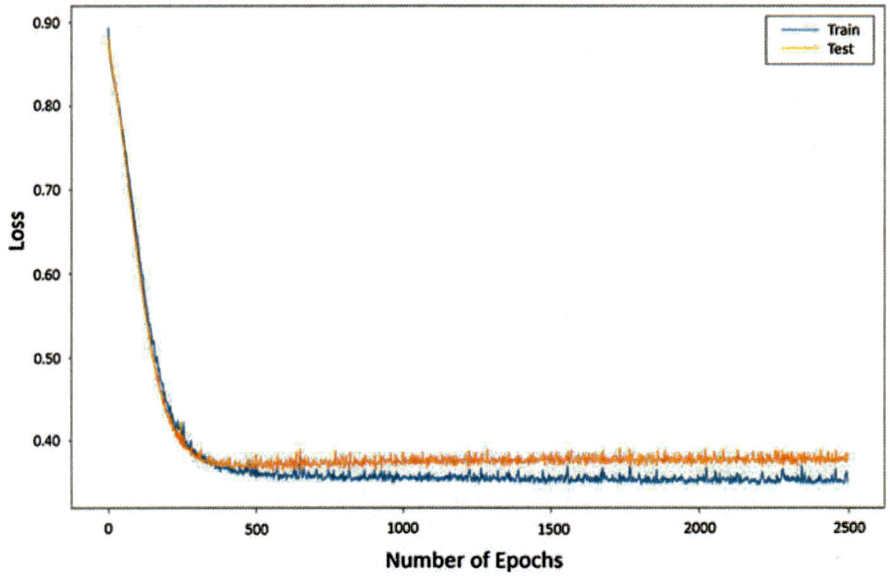

Fig. 2 Average loss of proposed Bi-LSTM model

Table 2 Table captions should be placed above the tables

No. of stacked Bi-LSTM layers	Loss	Accuracy (%)
1	0.39873	69.9
2	0.33423	72.3
3	0.28904	77.2

3.2 Impact of the Number of Stacked Bi-LSTM Layers

Table 2 depicts the prediction accuracy and loss values when the maximum prediction accuracy values of 1, 2, and 3 layers, respectively, are attained. With the addition of more stacked Bi-LSTM layers, the prediction accuracy improves while the prediction loss decreased. The capacities of the network increase when stacking more layers as it can help to extract more features. However, it should be noted that there is a tradeoff between the number of layers and the computational complexity to achieve a boost in accuracy with feasible network training time.

4 Conclusion

This paper presented the supervised classification of various walking speed by extracting features based on kinematic data. Preliminary result obtained using BiLSTM networks are capable of accounting for the temporal backward and forward correlations within the sequences of the gait data. The training and testing accuracy of our proposed model were 70.7% and 77.2%, respectively. In future, we will further investigate the effectiveness of BiLSTM model with kinetic data. Different network architectures and component will be studied for better modelling and improving the learning capacity of current model.

Acknowledgements This work was supported by RU Geran – Fakulti Program, Universiti Malaya (GPF008A-2018).

References

1. Carcreff, L., et al.: Walking speed of children and adolescents with cerebral palsy: laboratory versus daily life. Front. Bioeng. Biotechnol. **8**, 812 (2020)
2. Middleton, A., Fritz, S.L., Lusardi, M.: Walking speed: the functional vital sign. J. Aging Phys. Act. **23**(2), 314–322 (2015)
3. Shih, Y.-L., Shih, C.-C., Chen, J.-Y.: The association between walking speed and risk of cardiovascular disease in middle-aged and elderly people in Taiwan, a community-based, cross-sectional study. PLoS ONE **15**(7), e0235277–e0235277 (2020)
4. Grande, G., et al.: Measuring gait speed to better identify prodromal dementia. Exp. Gerontol. **124**, 110625 (2019)

5. Buddhadev, H.H., Smiley, A.L., Martin, P.E.: Effects of age, speed, and step length on lower extremity net joint moments and powers during walking. Hum. Mov. Sci. **71**, 102611 (2020)
6. Jordan, K., Challis, J.H., Newell, K.M.: Walking speed influences on gait cycle variability. Gait Posture **26**(1), 128–134 (2007)
7. Nakano, N., et al.: Evaluation of 3D markerless motion capture accuracy using OpenPose with multiple video cameras. Front. Sports Act. Living **2**, 50 (2020)
8. Akhtaruzzaman, M.D., Shafie, A.A., Khan, M.R.: Gait Analysis: systems, technologies, and importance. J. Mech. Med. Biol. **16**(07), 1630003 (2016)
9. Zago, M., et al.: 3D tracking of human motion using visual Skeletonization and Stereoscopic vision. Front. Bioeng. Biotechnol. **8**(181) (2020)
10. Corazza, S., et al.: A markerless motion capture system to study musculoskeletal biomechanics: visual hull and simulated annealing approach. Ann. Biomed. Eng. **34**(6), 1019–1029 (2006)
11. Colyer, S.L., et al.: A review of the evolution of vision-based motion analysis and the integration of advanced computer vision methods towards developing a markerless system. Sports Med. Open **4**(1), 24 (2018)
12. Khera, P., Kumar, N.: Role of machine learning in gait analysis: a review. J. Med. Eng. Technol. **44**(8), 441–467 (2020)
13. Mannini, A., Sabatini, A.M.: Machine learning methods for classifying human physical activity from on-body accelerometers. Sensors (Basel) **10**(2), 1154–1175 (2010)
14. Halilaj, E., et al.: Machine learning in human movement biomechanics: best practices, common pitfalls, and new opportunities. J. Biomech. **81**, 1–11 (2018)
15. Luo, J., Tang, J., Xiao, X.: Abnormal gait behavior detection for elderly based on enhanced wigner-ville analysis and cloud incremental SVM learning. J. Sensors **2016**, 5869238 (2016)
16. Begg, R., Kamruzzaman, J.: A comparison of neural networks and support vector machines for recognizing young-old gait patterns. In: TENCON 2003. Conference on Convergent Technologies for Asia-Pacific Region, pp. 354–358 (2003)
17. Dorschky, E., et al.: CNN-based estimation of sagittal plane walking and running biomechanics from measured and simulated inertial sensor data. Front. Bioeng. Biotechnol. **8**, 604 (2020)
18. Zhang, Y., et al.: A comprehensive study on gait biometrics using a joint CNN-based method. Pattern Recogn. **93**, 228–236 (2019)
19. Gholami, M., Napier, C., Menon, C.: Estimating lower extremity running gait kinematics with a single accelerometer: a deep learning approach. Sensors (Basel) **20**(10) (2020)
20. Zhao, Y., Zhou, S.: Wearable device-based gait recognition using angle embedded gait dynamic images and a convolutional neural network. Sensors (Basel) **17**(3) (2017)
21. Fernandez-Lopez, P., et al.: Recurrent neural network for inertial gait user recognition in smartphones. Sensors (Basel) **19**(18) (2019)
22. Donahue, J., et al.: Long-term recurrent convolutional networks for visual recognition and description. IEEE Trans. Pattern Anal. Mach. Intell. **39**(4), 1939–3539 (2017)
23. Kidzinski, L., Delp, S., Schwartz, M.: Automatic real-time gait event detection in children using deep neural networks. PLoS One **14**(1), e0211466 (2019)
24. Feng, Y., Li, Y., Luo, J.: Learning effective Gait features using LSTM, pp. 325–330 (2016)
25. Liu, D., et al.: Deep rehabilitation gait learning for modeling knee joints of lower-limb exoskeleton. In: 2016 IEEE International Conference on Robotics and Biomimetics (ROBIO), Qingdao, China (2016)
26. Aljarrah, A.A., Ali, A.H.: Human Activity Recognition using PCA and BiLSTM Recurrent Neural Networks, 156–160 (2019)

Automated Segmentation of Metal and BVS Stent Struts from OCT Images Using U-Net

Yu Shi Lau, Li Kuo Tan, Chow Khuen Chan, Kok Han Chee, and Yih Miin Liew

Abstract Percutaneous Coronary Intervention (PCI) is an effective treatment for coronary artery diseases. PCI treatment is usually carried out with stent implantation to provide structural support to balloon dilated blood vessel, reducing risk of re-narrowing. Intravascular Optical Coherence Tomography (OCT) can provide a series of cross-section images depicting the internal structure of the artery and residing stent during PCI treatment. Stent struts segmentation for OCT images is necessary to provide quantitative data regarding quality of stent deployment during PCI and severity of restenosis during follow-up examination. Manual segmentation of stent struts is not efficient and infeasible due to large number of stent struts presented in each pullback of OCT images. Thus, automated stent struts segmentation is necessary to help clinicians in getting quantified data from OCT images within intraoperative time frame. In this paper, an automated stent strut segmentation algorithm was developed, utilizing 3D information of stent structure and state-of-the-art U-Net. The implementation of the algorithm preserves the spatial resolution of the full-size OCT images without down-sampling. The algorithm was trained and tested on both Bioresorbable Vascular Scaffold (BVS) and metal stent images. It achieved Dice's coefficient of 0.82 for BVS images, precision of 0.90 and recall of 0.85 for metal stent images. This algorithm works for both BVS and metal stents OCT images and adapts to different stent conditions.

Keywords Stent strut segmentation · Optical coherence tomography · U-Net · Deep learning · Percutaneous coronary intervention

Y. S. Lau · C. K. Chan · Y. M. Liew (✉)
Faculty of Engineering, Department of Biomedical Engineering, Universiti Malaya, Kuala Lumpur, Malaysia
e-mail: liewym@um.edu.my

L. K. Tan
Faculty of Medicine, Department of Biomedical Imaging, Universiti Malaya, Kuala Lumpur, Malaysia
e-mail: lktan@um.edu.my

K. H. Chee
Faculty of Medicine, Department of Medicine, Universiti Malaya, Kuala Lumpur, Malaysia

J. Usman et al. (eds.), *6th Kuala Lumpur International Conference on Biomedical Engineering 2021*, IFMBE Proceedings 86,
https://doi.org/10.1007/978-3-030-90724-2_8

1 Introduction

According to the report from American Heart Association in 2018, heart diseases are the main killer of humans in the United States. Among the heart diseases, coronary artery disease contributed to the highest percentage (43.8%) of death annually [1]. Percutaneous Coronary Intervention (PCI) is one of the common methods for the treatment of the coronary artery disease, in which stent implantation is used to expand the narrowed vessel. Restenosis is the possible complication of PCI treatment, which is the recurrence of vessel blockage. Current clinical assessment of stent deployment and restenosis through an imaging modality, known as intravascular Optical Coherence Tomography (OCT), is by visual inspection. This assessment is subjective and suffers from high inter-observer variability. On the other hand, manual assessment is very tedious and time consuming, which is infeasible to complete within intraoperative time frame. Automated stent struts segmentation in OCT images can help to resolve these problems.

2 Literature Review

Previous research utilized the special signature of metal stent struts, i.e. each individual strut has a trailing shadow, to perform stent struts detection in OCT images. The intensity profile of polar OCT images was used to determine the position of stent struts. Afterwards, different researchers introduced different methods for false positive removal, for instance, to remove guide wire that can appear similar to metal stent struts with shadow using common guidewire's properties [2], bagged decision trees [3], Bayesian network and 3D information of stent [4], and artificial neural network [5]. Some research teams focused on metal stent struts covered by neointimal tissue, whereby metal stent struts have unusually low intensity and no trailing shadow. Xu et al. [6] used ridge detector based on Hessian matrix to segment this kind of stent struts. This team sought for approximation of stent area rather than localization of each strut. Thus, an ellipse was fitted on the stent struts segmented by ridge detector. Tsantis et al. [7], on the other hand, used strut scale-space signatures derived from local maxima of Laplacian of Gaussian responses across consecutive scales for metal stent struts detection. Probabilistic neural network was further utilized for feature extraction and classification to optimize the detection of stent strut position. Recently, researchers adapted machine learning technique to overcome the variabilities in the appearance of metal stent struts in the OCT images. 'You Only Look Once' version 3 (YOLOv3), Region-based Fully Convolutional Network (R-FCN) [8] and U-Net [9] were example of machine learning techniques adapted for metal stent struts detection.

Apart from metal stent, Bioresorbable Vascular Scaffold (BVS) is implemented and used for implantation during PCI. It has the advantage in terms of better biocompatibility than metal stent. Despite having similar functionality in PCI treatment, BVS struts appear very different from metal stent struts in OCT images. Thus, different efforts are needed to implement BVS struts detection in OCT images. Wang et al. [10] used intensity profile and gradient profile to differentiate BVS struts from background while Bologna et al. [11] used intensity thresholding for segmentation. Other groups of researchers adopted machine learning technique for BVS struts detection, for example, cascade classifier trained by AdaBoost algorithm with dynamic programming [12], U-Net [13], and convolutional neural network with weakly supervised localization [14].

Most of the studies had worked on segmenting one type of stents solely. In this paper, we aim for a deep learning algorithm, which can work on both metal and BVS stents. The algorithm adopted in this work is modified from U-Net framework. To preserve resolution of the original image, the OCT images were not resized, but were cropped into subimages before feeding into the neural network for training and testing. 3D information of stent in the form of neighboring images was provided to improve correctness of stent struts segmentation.

3 Research Methodology

3.1 IVOCT Data Preparation

A total of 26 pullbacks (each consisting of $\approx$370 images) from 16 patients were pre-labelled manually to prepare the ground truth data. These pullbacks consisted of either metal stents or BVS stents. These images were acquired from the University of Malaya Medical Center (UMMC) catheterization laboratory using Illumien Optis IVOCT Systems (St. Jude Medical) and the study were approved by University of Malaya Medical Ethics Committee (Ref: 20, 158–1554). These data were randomly divided into training and testing sets, which meant 20 pullbacks for training and 6 pullbacks for testing. Labelling was performed using ImageJ software. A contour was drawn manually on each stent strut in the OCT images under the supervision of a clinical expert. These contours were then converted into binary masks.

3.2 Training and Testing Implementation

While using the binary masks as labels of the stent struts, it is challenging for the deep learning training as the size of stent struts is very small compared to the size of the whole OCT image. The imbalance between the area of white (stent struts) and black (non-stent pixels) in binary masks is high. This may lead to bias in the learning of the neural network as it might always deliver output of a background label regardless of the input, as the overall accuracy metric will be dominated by large quantity of background pixels. To avoid this problem, rather than feeding the whole OCT image as the input into the neural network, the 3D OCT images were cropped into subimages

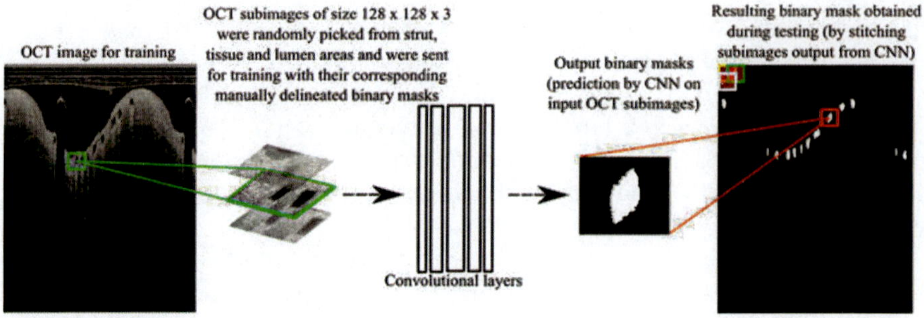

Fig. 1 Overview of algorithm for automated stent strut segmentation

of size 128 × 128 × 3 (Fig. 1). Cropping of images can resolve problem of imbalance data, at the same times, preserve the spatial information. However, cropping resulted in the loss of the full-view information of the images that can be originally learned by the neural network. Nevertheless, this loss of information is offset by including 3D information of stent (i.e. including both subimages before and after the slice of interest) for network training based on the property of stent wire continuity along the longitudinal direction of the OCT images.

The subimages for training were thereafter randomly cropped from struts, tissue and dark lumen areas in proportion of 5:4:1, in order to force the neural network to learn the variation in areas with rich texture rather than the textureless area of dark lumen. Manually delineated binary masks were provided as reference for the neural network to learn and to predict the stent struts.

During the testing phase, the testing images were cropped into subimages of the same size as the training subimages using a sliding window (128 × 128 × 3) before passing into the neural network. The stride size was set to half of the window size. The neural network outputs predicted masks of size 128 × 128 × 1, which were then stitched back to produce the full-size image (Fig. 1).

3.3 Convolutional Neural Network Architecture

The architecture of deep learning neural network (U-Net) used for the segmentation of stent struts is presented in Table 1.

U-Net is a fully convolutional neural network that is commonly applied for biomedical image segmentation. In this study, the input of the neural network was 3-channel grayscale image of size, 128 × 128 × 3 while the output was a binary image of size, 128 × 128 × 1. The kernel size was 3 × 3 for convolutional layers, 2 × 2 for deconvolutional layers and 1 × 1 for the last convolutional layer. The number of filters in the convolutional or deconvolutional layers were increased or decreased by a multiple of 16 starting from 64 across the convolutional neural network. The activation function for all convolutional or deconvolutional layers was Rectified Linear

Table 1 Convolutional neural network (CNN) architecture for stent strut segmentation of each OCT subimages of size, 128 × 128 × 3. The final output of this CNN is a binary mask of stent struts of size, 128 × 128 × 1

Encoding	Repeat	Output size	Decoding	Repeat	Output size
Input	No	128 × 128 × 3	DeConv1	No	32 × 32 × 256
Conv1	Yes	128 × 128 × 64	ConCat1	No	32 × 32 × 512
MaxPool1	No	64 × 64 × 64	Conv5	Yes	32 × 32 × 256
Conv2	Yes	64 × 64 × 128	DeConv2	No	64 × 64 × 128
MaxPool2	No	32 × 32 × 128	ConCat2	No	64 × 64 × 256
Conv3	Yes	32 × 32 × 256	Conv6	Yes	64 × 64 × 128
MaxPool3	No	16 × 16 × 256	DeConv3	No	128 × 128 × 64
Conv4	Yes	16 × 16 × 512	ConCat3	No	128 × 128 × 128
			Conv7	Yes	128 × 128 × 64
			Output	No	128 × 128 × 1

Units (ReLU) except that for last layer with usage of a sigmoid function. Zero padding was applied for all layers. To down-sample the images to half of their size, the size of max pooling window was set to 2 × 2. During up-sampling process, skip connection was performed via concatenation to retain information from earlier layers. Output from each deconvolutional layer (in decoding path) was concatenated with output from convolutional layers (in encoding path) of the same matrix size. Dropout was performed at the rate of 0.5 after each convolution process to reduce overfitting during training.

The loss function used for this neural network was weighted binary cross entropy. A higher weight was placed on the minority class (in this case, the stent pixels). This is another effort to resolve the problem of imbalanced data in the binary masks. Adam optimization algorithm was used to optimize the output of neural network to be as close as possible to the ground truth binary masks provided to it. The optimization was performed based on the loss calculated from the weighted binary cross entropy function. The learning rate was set to be 0.001.

3.4 Validation

The accuracy of the deep learning neural network for automated stent struts segmentation was evaluated against manually delineated ground truth stent struts in the testing sets. Consistent with the published works in literature review [4, 12], for a fair assessment, the performance of the segmentation algorithm in segmenting the two types of stents (i.e. metal stents and BVS stents) were assessed using two different metrics. The performance on BVS stents were assessed using Dice's coefficient, which measures the amount of overlap between ground truth struts and the predicted struts. Dice's coefficient is more suitable to be used for BVS stent struts as it has larger cross-section in OCT images, i.e. 10 times greater than the metal stent strut. Dice's coefficient was computed using Eq. (1)

$$\text{Dice} = (2 \times \text{TP})/((\text{TP} + \text{FP}) + (\text{TP} + \text{FN})) \tag{1}$$

whereby TP, FP and FN correspond to true positive, false positive and false negative pixels, respectively.

For metal stents, precision and recall were used to access the accuracy. They were calculated using TP, FP and FN as well, as shown by Eqs. (2) and (3), except that TP was defined differently. Centroids of the metal stent struts were extracted from the predicted and ground truth mask and the Euclidean distance between their centroids was calculated. A Euclidean distance of less than or equal to 50 μm [5] was used as a threshold to decide on the TP strut. A predicted strut with centroid outside this tolerance with any ground truth strut was considered a FP, whereas a ground truth strut with centroid outside this tolerance with any predicted strut was considered a FN. Since metal stents constitute a rather small cross-section in the OCT image, this point-based assessment is a better choice.

$$\text{Precision} = \text{TP}/(\text{TP} + \text{FP}) \tag{2}$$

$$\text{Recall} = \text{TP}/(\text{TP} + \text{FN}) \tag{3}$$

4 Results and Discussion

4.1 Results

Figure 2 shows the sample polar OCT images with segmented BVS and metal stent struts. The BVS stent struts were freshly implanted whereas the metal stent struts were covered by a layer of neointimal tissue signifying restenosis. The predicted stent struts were shown to match well with the gold standard stent struts. Both images show the feasibility of the proposed implementation of U-Net framework to segment both BVS and metal stent strut without specific customization for either one as in previous publications [2, 4, 6, 10, 12, 13].

Table 2 shows the overall accuracy of the proposed segmentation framework on the testing images. Overall Dice's coefficient, for all 3 pullbacks of testing OCT images with BVS was 0.82. Overall precision and recall for all 3 pullbacks of testing OCT images with metal stent struts were 0.90 and 0.85 respectively.

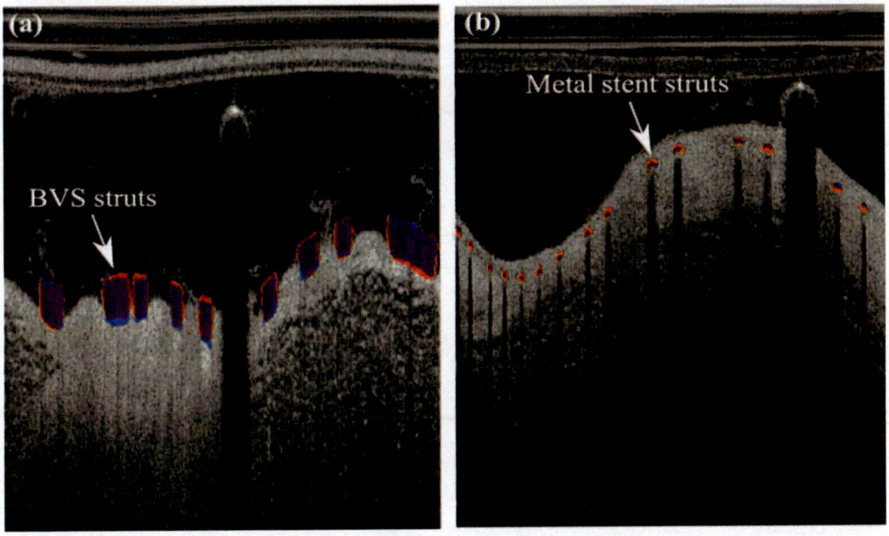

Fig. 2 OCT images with, **a** BVS struts and **b** metal stent struts, overlaid with predicted segmentation (red) and gold standard segmentation (blue)

Table 2 Accuracy of U-Net on stent strut segmentation

Type of stents	Dice's coefficient	Precision	Recall
Metal	–	0.90	0.85
BVS	0.82	–	–

4.2 Discussion

In this paper, the automated stent strut segmentation algorithm used binary masks as labels because binary masks would not be restricted by the types, numbers and locations of stent struts in OCT images during segmentation. The algorithm was modified from U-Net, which is a fully-convolutional network originally developed for biomedical image segmentation purposes. It suits our stent struts segmentation as it can input images (OCT images) and output images (binary masks). Functions like dropout regularization and skip connection introduced to further enhance the basic U-Net can prevent overfitting and improve training efficiency.

Although U-Net is appropriate for biomedical images, we may need to consider different conditions in our case of segmentation. Our targets of segmentation, i.e. stent struts, are small features in OCT images. Thus, we decided to crop the OCT images into subimages to reduce the proportional difference in size. Meanwhile, this kept us from needing to resize the images, retaining full resolution of OCT images. Neighboring 3D information of stent structure was provided to the neural network to compensate for the loss of full view information.

The automated algorithm achieved high accuracy for stent strut segmentation. Compared to published methods [2–14] that required selective application based on stent type, the proposed technique is proven to work on OCT images irrespective of the stent types (metal stent or BVS) residing in the images. Besides, this algorithm can segment stents of different levels of apposition, i.e. malapposed, freshly implanted and embedded. This increased the clinical usability of the algorithm compared to other studies as it has less restriction, for example, Cao et al. [12] only proved their works over baseline data or team Wang et al. [10] needed prior knowledge of data as baseline or follow-up. Thus, this algorithm provides a means for accessing stent deployment and restenosis accordingly.

5 Conclusion

In conclusion, this paper presented a deep learning algorithm for automated stent struts segmentation in OCT images. It aimed for segmenting both metal stents and BVS. The results show the algorithm working for different stent types and different levels of stent apposition, it is thus more applicable to clinical implementation. In future, the generality of the neural network can be improved by involving larger amounts of training data.

Acknowledgements This research was funded by the Malaysia Ministry of Higher Education Fundamental Research Grant Scheme (FRGS/1/2018/SKK03/UM/02/1) and Faculty Research Grant GPF (GPF026A-2019).

References

1. Benjamin, E.J., Virani, S.S., Callaway, C.W., Chamberlain, A.M., Chang, A.R., Cheng, S., Chiuve, S.E., Cushman, M., Delling, F.N., Deo, R.: Heart disease and stroke statistics-2018 update: a report from the American Heart Association. Circulation **137**(12), e67 (2018)
2. Wang, A., Eggermont, J., Dekker, N., Garcia-Garcia, H.M., Pawar, R., Reiber, J.H., Dijkstra, J.: Automatic stent strut detection in intravascular optical coherence tomographic pullback runs. Int. J. Cardiovasc. Imaging **29**(1), 29–38 (2013)
3. Lu, H., Gargesha, M., Wang, Z., Chamie, D., Attizzani, G.F., Kanaya, T., Ray, S., Costa, M.A., Rollins, A.M., Bezerra, H.G., Wilson, D.L.: Automatic stent detection in intravascular OCT images using bagged decision trees. Biomed. Opt. Express **3**(11), 2809–2824 (2012). https://doi.org/10.1364/BOE.3.002809
4. Wang, Z., Jenkins, M.W., Linderman, G.C., Bezerra, H.G., Fujino, Y., Costa, M.A., Wilson, D.L., Rollins, A.M.: 3-D stent detection in intravascular OCT using a Bayesian network and graph search. IEEE Trans. Med. Imaging **34**(7), 1549–1561 (2015)
5. Nam, H.S., Kim, C.S., Lee, J.J., Song, J.W., Kim, J.W., Yoo, H.: Automated detection of vessel lumen and stent struts in intravascular optical coherence tomography to evaluate stent apposition and neointimal coverage. Med. Phys. **43**(4), 1662–1675 (2016)

6. Xu, C., Schmitt, J.M., Akasaka, T., Kubo, T., Huang, K.: Automatic detection of stent struts with thick neointimal growth in intravascular optical coherence tomography image sequences. Phys. Med. Biol. **56**(20), 6665 (2011)
7. Tsantis, S., Kagadis, G.C., Katsanos, K., Karnabatidis, D., Bourantas, G., Nikiforidis, G.C.: Automatic vessel lumen segmentation and stent strut detection in intravascular optical coherence tomography. Med. Phys. **39**(1), 503–513 (2012)
8. Jiang, X., Zeng, Y., Xiao, S., He, S., Ye, C., Qi, Y., Zhao, J., Wei, D., Hu, M., Chen, F.: Automatic detection of coronary metallic stent struts based on YOLOv3 and R-FCN. Comput. Math. Methods Med. 2020 (2020)
9. Wu, P., Gutiérrez-Chico, J.L., Tauzin, H., Yang, W., Li, Y., Yu, W., Chu, M., Guillon, B., Bai, J., Meneveau, N.: Automatic stent reconstruction in optical coherence tomography based on a deep convolutional model. Biomed. Opt. Express **11**(6), 3374–3394 (2020)
10. Wang, A., Nakatani, S., Eggermont, J., Onuma, Y., Garcia-Garcia, H.M., Serruys, P.W., Reiber, J.H., Dijkstra, J.: Automatic detection of bioresorbable vascular scaffold struts in intravascular optical coherence tomography pullback runs. Biomed. Opt. Express **5**(10), 3589–3602 (2014)
11. Bologna, M., Migliori, S., Montin, E., Rampat, R., Dubini, G., Migliavacca, F., Mainardi, L., Chiastra, C.: Automatic segmentation of optical coherence tomography pullbacks of coronary arteries treated with bioresorbable vascular scaffolds: application to hemodynamics modeling. PloS One **14**(3), e0213603 (2019)
12. Cao, Y., Jin, Q., Lu, Y., Jing, J., Chen, Y., Yin, Q., Qin, X., Li, J., Zhu, R., Zhao, W.: Automatic analysis of bioresorbable vascular scaffolds in intravascular optical coherence tomography images. Biomed. Opt. Express **9**(6), 2495–2510 (2018)
13. Zhou, W., Chen, F., Zong, Y., Zhao, D., Jie, B., Wang, Z., Huang, C., Ng, E.Y.: automatic detection approach for bioresorbable vascular scaffolds using a u-shaped convolutional neural network. IEEE Access **7**, 94424–94430 (2019)
14. Gessert, N., Latus, S., Abdelwahed, Y.S., Leistner, D.M., Lutz, M., Schlaefer, A.: Bioresorbable scaffold visualization in IVOCT images using CNNs and weakly supervised localization. In: Medical Imaging 2019: Image Processing, p. 109492C. International Society for Optics and Photonics (2019)

Comparison of Blood Rheological Models in Patient-Specific Left Coronary Arteries with Varying Degrees of Stenosis

Noushin Anan, Nusrat S. Khan, Samreen T. Mahmud, Tahura Hossain, and M. Tarik Arafat

Abstract For computational analysis, it is essential to select a suitable blood model to depict the blood flow of healthy and atherosclerotic arteries uniquely as they tend to differ. In this study, four different blood models—Carreau, Casson, Herschel-Bulkley, and non-Newtonian power law have been compared by performing computational fluid dynamics (CFD) simulations in healthy and atherosclerotic patient-specific arteries. Hemodynamic parameters—wall shear stress (WSS), relative residence time (RRT), and global non-Newtonian importance factor (I_G factor) were analyzed for evaluating the blood models. All the blood models exhibited noticeable changes in the hemodynamic parameters with an increasing degree of stenosis. WSS had a similar distribution over a cardiac cycle for all models but showed different magnitudes. Casson and non-Newtonian power law model exhibited risk-identifying RRT range for high and low stenosis degrees. Analysis of the I_G factor revealed that the Carreau model represented blood viscosity more appropriately by exhibiting both Newtonian and non-Newtonian behavior of blood in both healthy and diseased arteries. Extensive analysis of the concerned parameters demonstrated that Carreau and Herschel-Bulkley models could predict the variation of blood flow in healthy and diseased arteries more precisely than Casson and non-Newtonian power law models, which either overestimated or underestimated the values of these parameters at different degrees of stenosis.

Keywords Blood rheological models · Hemodynamic parameters · Patient-specific geometries

---

N. Anan · N. S. Khan · T. Hossain
Department of Biomedical Engineering, Military Institute of Science and Technology (MIST), Dhaka 1216, Bangladesh

S. T. Mahmud · M. T. Arafat (✉)
Department of Biomedical Engineering, Bangladesh University of Engineering and Technology (BUET), Dhaka 1205, Bangladesh
e-mail: tarikarafat@bme.buet.ac.bd

J. Usman et al. (eds.), *6th Kuala Lumpur International Conference on Biomedical Engineering 2021*, IFMBE Proceedings 86,
https://doi.org/10.1007/978-3-030-90724-2_9

1 Introduction

The pathophysiology of atherosclerosis is highly influenced by blood flow dynamics, as dysfunctions of the blood vessels tend to occur in oscillatory and low wall shear stress (WSS) regions [1]. Therefore, hemodynamic parameters: WSS and other WSS-based descriptors significantly impact the onset and distribution of atherosclerosis. Computational fluid dynamics (CFD) is a non-invasive, low-cost, and efficient tool to predict plaque initiation and progression by investigating the local hemodynamics of the blood vessels [1, 2]. However, the performance of CFD models depends on the precise depiction of blood rheology since the blood viscosity fluctuates with the flow shear rate [3, 4]. For instance, blood flow within larger and straight arteries has a higher shear rate with Newtonian properties compared to bifurcated or stenosed arteries where shear rate decreases due to downstream flow, demonstrating altered rheological properties [1, 5]. Thus, different rheological blood models can be numerically simulated in CFD to investigate which model renders the most realistic hemodynamics to effectively predict atherosclerosis progression.

In the past, very few studies have considered diseased coronary arteries to study the effects of different blood rheological models using CFD. To illustrate, a research study investigated the hemodynamics only in healthy right coronary artery models using nine non-Newtonian models and stated that the Newtonian model is valid at a medium shear rate [6]. Moreover, in most studies, atherosclerotic patients with varying degrees of stenosis were not considered while studying the behavior of blood models. This is significant as the local hemodynamics are largely impacted by stenosis severity, which is the basis of most clinical decisions [7]. Although a recent study has evaluated the effects of some non-Newtonian models on the patient-specific stenosed left anterior descending (LAD) branch of the left coronary artery (LCA) with different stenosis severities, they have not considered the influence of bifurcation which is vital for analyzing any branch of the LCA [8]. To date, no study has been carried in both healthy and atherosclerotic patient-specific left coronary arteries with varying degrees of stenosis to assess the outcomes of different blood models corresponding to the patient-specific artery geometry.

The goal of our present study was to compare the four blood rheological models-Carreau, Casson, Herschel-Bulkley, and non-Newtonian power law, on both healthy and diseased patient-specific bifurcating branches of the left coronary artery and assess which blood model gives the most accurate result for different degrees of stenosis. For this regard, we numerically investigated the effect of each rheological model on the hemodynamic descriptors—WSS, relative residence time (RRT), and global non-Newtonian importance factor (I_G factor).

2 Materials and Methods

2.1 3D Reconstruction and Mesh Generation

Two patient-specific geometries, one having 0% stenosis (healthy) and the other having 30% stenosis in LAD and 80% stenosis in left circumflex (LCx) were generated from CT angiogram images using 3D reconstruction software MIMICS (Materialise Inc., Belgium). The 3D reconstructed geometries had approximate measurements of 9.2 mm along left main stem (LMS), 11.97 mm along LAD, and 9.72 mm along LCx [9]. The models were discretized by tetrahedral meshes after performing the mesh independence test with pressure drop (ΔP) and wall shear stress (WSS) at the artery wall as the control parameters. Element sizes were varied between 0.5 and 0.1 mm and by analyzing the trend of control parameters, fine meshes were generated considering the appropriate element size. Additionally, an inflation of about 1/10th of the inlet diameter of the models was generated.

2.2 Blood Models and Boundary Conditions

The blood was modeled as a laminar and incompressible fluid with four different non-Newtonian viscosity models as summarized in Table 1 with a density of 1060 kg/m^3. As the inlet boundary condition, a pulsatile velocity waveform was applied at the inlet of LCA, whereas for the outlet boundary condition, a pulsatile pressure waveform was imposed at the outlets of the LAD and LCx [12, 13].

Table 1 Different blood viscosity models [6, 10, 11]

Blood model	Effective viscosity, μ	Parameter values
Carreau model	$\mu = \mu_\infty + (\mu_0 - \mu_\infty)\left[1 + (\lambda\dot{\gamma})^2\right]^{\frac{n-1}{2}}$	$\lambda = 3.313$ s $n = 0.3568$ $\mu_0 = 0.056$ Pa.s $\mu_\infty = 0.0035$ Pa.s
Casson model	$\mu = \frac{\mu_\infty^2}{\dot{\gamma}} + \frac{2\mu_\infty N_\infty}{\sqrt{\dot{\gamma}}} + N_\infty^2$ $N_\infty = \sqrt{\mu_p (1 - HCT)^{-0.25}}$ $\mu_\infty = \sqrt{0.625\ HCT}$	$\mu_\infty = 0.00145$ Pa.s $HCT = 0.4$
Herschel-Bulkley model	$\mu = k\dot{\gamma}^{\eta-1} + \left(\frac{\tau_0}{\dot{\gamma}}\right))$	$\tau_o = 0.0175$ Pa $\eta = 0.8601$ $k = 8.9721 \times 10^{-3}$ kg s^{n-1} m^{-1}
Non-Newtonian power law model	$\mu = k\dot{\gamma}^{\eta-1}$	$\eta = 0.7$ $k = 0.00622$ kg s^{n-2} m^{-1}

2.3 Numerical Methods

The continuity and Navier–Stokes equations governing the fluid motion into the left coronary artery were numerically solved using Ansys Fluent (Ansys Inc., USA). A first-order central-difference scheme was used to discretize the diffusion term of the Navier–Stokes equation. Pressure velocity coupling was performed by implementing the semi-implicit method for pressure linked (SIMPLE) algorithm and hybrid initialization was applied. CFD simulations were performed with 64 steps having a step size of 0.0125 s and 100 iterations per time step. In each patient-specific LCA model, the result was converged to a residual target of less than 1×10^{-5} per time-step.

3 Result and Discussion

The diseased patient had plaques located at the LAD and LCx regions proximal to the bifurcation. Thus, for both the patients, WSS was measured taking a definite point at the proximal regions of the LAD and LCx. In the LAD region for 30% stenosed artery, WSS was observed to decrease in comparison with the healthy artery for all the blood models, as shown in Fig. 1. The formation of plaque creates backflows decreasing the velocity at that region, resulting in decreased WSS [1, 14]. Carreau, Herschel-Bulkley, non-Newtonian power law models showed 60%, 58%, and 61%

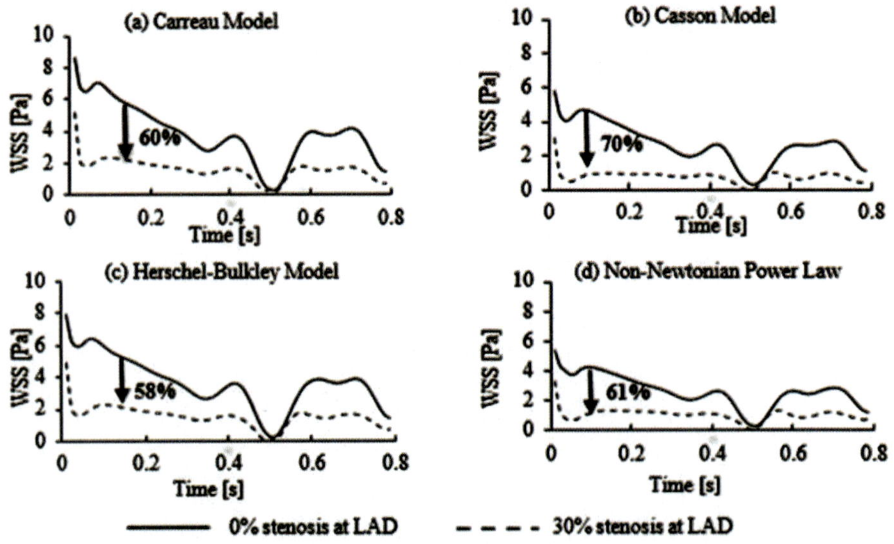

Fig. 1 WSS distribution for 0% (healthy) and 30% (diseased) stenosis at proximal LAD regions using different blood models: **a** Carreau model, **b** Casson model, **c** Herschel-Bulkley model and **d** non-Newtonian power law models

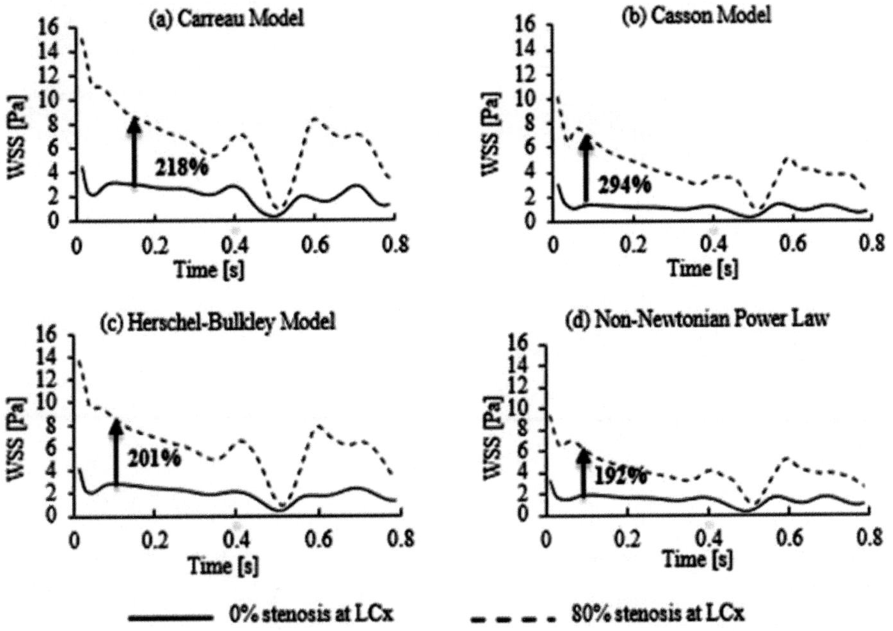

Fig. 2 WSS distribution for 0% (healthy) and 80% (diseased) stenosis at proximal LCx regions using different blood models: **a** Carreau model, **b** Casson model, **c** Herschel-Bulkley model and **d** non-Newtonian power law models

average decrease of WSS at 30% stenosis, respectively. However, the Casson model showed a 10% higher variation in WSS values from the other blood models exhibiting a 70% decrease in WSS. In Fig. 2, the comparison of WSS at the proximal LCx regions of a healthy artery and an 80% stenosed artery exhibited an increasing pattern in the case of the stenosed artery for all the blood models. At a higher degree of stenosis the velocity of flow increases owing to the severe decrease in lumen diameter, inhibiting backflow and increasing the value of WSS [15]. Carreau and Herschel-Bulkley models exhibited a 218% and 201% average decrease in WSS, respectively.

Casson model overestimated the WSS with the maximum average increase of 294%, whereas the non-Newtonian power law model underestimated it with the minimum average increase of 192%. Thus, at a lower degree of stenosis, Casson and non-Newtonian power law were observed to be more suitable for performing simulations, whereas at a higher degree of stenosis Carreau and Herschel-Bulkley models would give better results.

Region of high RRT reflects the intimal accumulation of lipids due to oscillation and flow recirculation, causing progression of atherosclerosis and areas having greater than 8 Pa^{-1} of RRT are prone to plaque formation [2]. These risk zones and the benign range within 0–8 Pa^{-1} have been focused on in Fig. 3. In the healthy artery, higher RRT was observed in the bifurcation region due to abrupt change in geometry. However, in the atherosclerotic artery, bifurcation and the LCx region

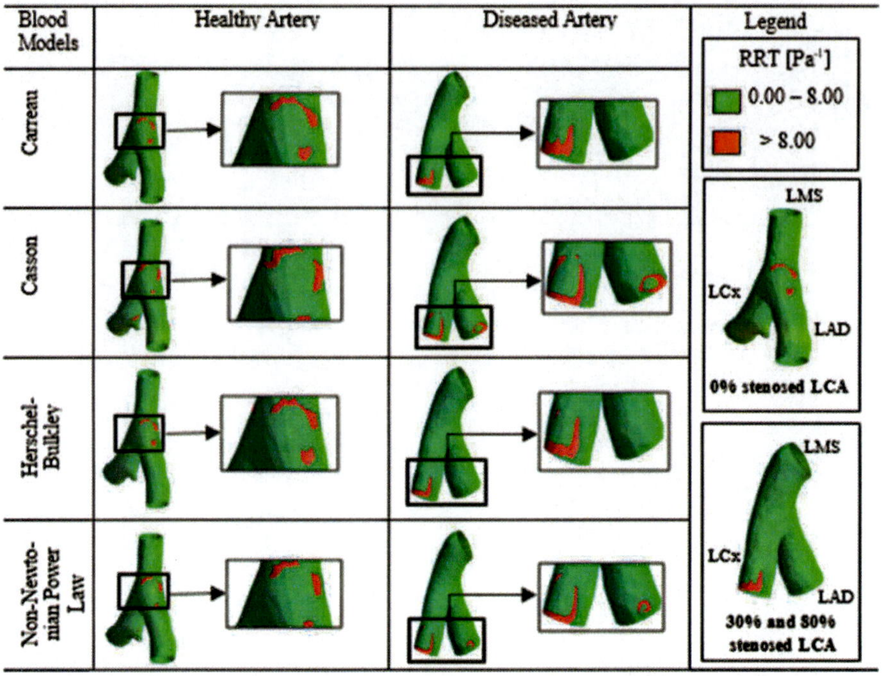

Fig. 3 RRT contour plots for each patient-specific geometry at cardiac cycle, t = 0.79 s

with severe stenosis of 80% had higher RRT where the lumen size decreased due to stenosis. In this case, the Carreau model was capable of showing values closer to the threshold of 8 Pa^{-1} (between 15 and 22 Pa^{-1}) comparing to the values found in the other three models (22–84 Pa^{-1}). In the case of LAD (30% stenosis), Casson and non-Newtonian power law blood models identified the post stenotic region as the risk-prone region for plaque progression. However, this region was captured as low-risk prone region (1.6–3.2 Pa^{-1}) by Carreau and Hershel-Bulkley blood models.

For distinct boundary condition and LCA geometry global non- Newtonian importance factor I_G is defined in Eq. (1), where N = total number of nodes on the artery wall, i = grid node index combining the cells on the arterial wall, μ = actual dynamic blood viscosity and μ_∞ = Newtonian blood viscosity, 0.00345 Pa.s [6].

$$I_G = \frac{1}{N} \frac{\left[\sum_{i=1}^{N} (\mu - \mu_\infty)^2\right]^{\frac{1}{2}}}{\mu_\infty} \tag{1}$$

Table 2 represents the I_G factors for the blood models at 0.3 and 0.6 m/s inlet velocities. Non-Newtonian blood properties influence the stress on artery walls, which can promote the onset and progression of lesions and its effects become important at low velocities of blood flow [16]. Previous studies anticipated that at the low velocity

Table 2 Global non-Newtonian importance factor I_G at inlet velocities 0.3 m/s and 0.6 m/s for healthy and diseased patient

Inlet velocity (m/s)	Patient	Carreau	Casson	Herschel-Bulkley	Non-Newtonian power law
0.3 (systole)	Healthy	0.20	0.21	0.13	0.30
	Diseased	0.26	0.41	0.13	0.44
0.6 (diastole)	Healthy	0.18	0.24	0.11	0.25
	Diseased	0.19	0.32	0.16	0.23

the I_G value is high whereas at high velocity it is low [1]. Low I_G values point to the Newtonian behavior of blood. A scheme similar to Johnston et al. study was applied, to decide the cut-off I_G 0.2 and 0.25 above which blood flow was considered to be non-Newtonian for the healthy and diseased artery, respectively [6, 11]. In the case of the healthy patient, among the four blood models studied, the Carreau model depicted the non-Newtonian and Newtonian behavior of blood. Casson and non-Newtonian power law blood models were more sensitive to the non-Newtonian fluid nature as they showed higher values of I_G. Hershel-Bulkley showed I_G values less than 0.2, representing more sensitivity to Newtonian property. I_G value decreased with the increase of velocity for Carreau, Hershel-Bulkley, and non-Newtonian power law models. However, in the case of the Casson blood model, there was a slight increase in I_G. This might be due to the applied boundary condition and the artery geometry corresponding to a specific patient. In the case of the diseased patient, the three blood models except Casson showed a reduction in I_G during diastole, thus approached the Newtonian model. During systole, these models showed an increase in I_G, and hence, exhibited the importance of Newtonian behavior.

4 Conclusion

Our study aimed at analyzing the outcome of four different blood models, Carreau, Casson, Herschel-Bulkley, and non-Newtonian power law in imitating blood flow through healthy and atherosclerotic arteries and elucidating how the use of a specific blood model differentiates the flow profile of an atherosclerotic artery from a healthy one. Analysis of the hemodynamic parameters showed that the Carreau model was able to portrait differences between the healthy and atherosclerotic arteries more vividly than the remaining three models. Next to the Carreau model, the Herschel-Bulkley model presented better outcomes though the values were slightly lower than the Carreau model. On the other hand, Casson and non-Newtonian power law models gave much-deviated results, where the values of the parameters were either underestimated or overestimated. Overall, it can be concluded that Carreau and Herschel-Bulkley models were able to depict the changes in a flow profile better than the other two models.

References

1. Skiadopoulos, A., Neofytou, P., Housiadas, C.: Comparison of blood rheological models in patient specific cardiovascular system simulations. J. Hydrodyn. **29**(2), 293–304 (2017)
2. Zhang, J.-M., et al.: Hemodynamic analysis of patient-specific coronary artery tree. Int. J. Numer. Methods Biomed. Eng. **31**(4), e02708 (2015)
3. Yilmaz, F., Yasar Gundogdu, M.: A critical review on blood flow in large arteries; relevance to blood rheology, viscosity models, and physiologic conditions. **20**, 197–211 (2008)
4. Bodnár, T., Sequeira, A., Prosi, M.: On the shear-thinning and viscoelastic effects of blood flow under various flow rates. Appl. Math. Comput. **217**(11), 5055–5067 (2011)
5. Mehri, R., Mavriplis, C., Fenech, M.: Red blood cell aggregates and their effect on non-Newtonian blood viscosity at low hematocrit in a two-fluid low shear rate microfluidic system. PloS One **13**(7) (2018)
6. Johnston, B.M., et al.: Non-Newtonian blood flow in human right coronary arteries: steady state simulations. J. Biomech. **37**(5), 709–720 (2004)
7. Shaw, L.J., et al.: Optimal medical therapy with or without percutaneous coronary intervention to reduce ischemic burden. Circulation **117**(10), 1283–1291 (2008)
8. Abbasian, M., et al.: Effect of non-Newtonian blood flow on coronary artery hemodynamics in a cohort of patients with stenosed artery. In: ASME 2018 5th joint US-European fluids engineering division summer meeting. American Society of Mechanical Engineers (2018)
9. Gholipour, A., Ghayesh, M.H., Zander, A.: Nonlinear biomechanics of bifurcated atherosclerotic coronary arteries. Int. J. Eng. Sci. **133**, 60–83 (2018)
10. Caballero, A.D., Laín, S.: Numerical simulation of non-Newtonian blood flow dynamics in human thoracic aorta. Comput. Methods Biomech. Biomed. Engin. **18**(11), 1200–1216 (2015)
11. Razavi, A., Shirani, E., Sadeghi, M.R.: Numerical simulation of blood pulsatile flow in a stenosed carotid artery using different rheological models. J. Biomech. **44**(11), 2021–2030 (2011)
12. Liu, B., et al.: Influence of model boundary conditions on blood flow patterns in a patient specific stenotic right coronary artery. Biomed. Eng. Online **14**(1), S6 (2015)
13. Mahalingam, A., et al.: Numerical analysis of the effect of turbulence transition on the hemodynamic parameters in human coronary arteries. Cardiovasc. Diagn. Therapy **6**(3), 208 (2016)
14. Chaichana, T., Sun, Z., Jewkes, J.: Haemodynamic analysis of the effect of different types of plaques in the left coronary artery. Comput. Med. Imaging Graph. **37**(3), 197–206 (2013)
15. Al-allaq, A.A., Mahmoud, N.S.: Numerical study of the efects of aneurysm and stenosis in the left coronary artery on the human blood stream. Eng. Technol. J. **35**(1 Part (A) Engineering), 29–40 (2017)
16. Jahangiri, M., Saghafian, M., Sadeghi, M.R.: Effect of six non-Newtonian viscosity models on hemodynamic parameters of pulsatile blood flow in stenosed artery. J. Comput. Appl. Res. Mech. Eng. (JCARME) **7**(2), 199–207 (2018)

Wall Stress Analysis of Patient-Specific Left Ventricular Hypertrophy Models

Wei Jan Goh, Bee Ting Chan, Wan Naimah Wan Ab Naim, Shoon Hui Chuah, Einly Lim, and Yih Miin Liew

Abstract Left ventricular hypertrophy (LVH) is a complex heart disease characterised by abnormal heart wall. A wall stress analysis may provide insight on ventricular wall mechanics, and it should be conducted with patient-specific geometry for accurate assessment. This study aims to investigate the distribution of stress on the left ventricular (LV) wall of LVH patients in diastolic filling phase using the finite element method. The patient-specific LV geometries of two LVH patients were compared with two healthy subjects. The effect of individual factors in contributing to wall stress was also studied by adapting the model settings for investigation. Our results showed that the excessive wall stress observed in LVH patients ($\sigma_{\_c}$: 6068 ± 342 Pa, $\sigma_{\_z}$: 3785 ± 161 Pa, $\sigma_{\_r}$: 384 ± 649 Pa), when compared to healthy subjects ($\sigma_{\_c}$: 2662 ± 82 Pa, $\sigma_{\_z}$: 1486 ± 239 Pa, $\sigma_{\_r}$: 0.1 ± 47 Pa), were mainly contributed by the elevated filling pressure. Besides, an abnormal stress variation was also observed in LVH patients, especially near the region with wall thickening and distinct local wall curvature. A high convexity area was observed to have high circumferential stress and low longitudinal stress, while the opposite was noted at the local high concavity area. These findings indicate the importance of patient-specific models in wall stress assessment of LVH patients.

Keywords Patient-specific · Hypertrophy · Wall stress

W. J. Goh · B. T. Chan (✉)
Department of Mechanical, Materials and Manufacturing Engineering, Faculty of Science and Engineering, University of Nottingham, Selangor, Malaysia
e-mail: BeeTing.Chan@nottingham.edu.my

W. N. W. Ab Naim
Faculty of Mechanical and Automotive Engineering Technology, Universiti Malaysia Pahang, Pahang, Malaysia

S. H. Chuah · E. Lim · Y. M. Liew
Department of Biomedical Engineering, Faculty of Engineering, Universiti Malaya, Kuala Lumpur, Malaysia

J. Usman et al. (eds.), *6th Kuala Lumpur International Conference on Biomedical Engineering 2021*, IFMBE Proceedings 86,
https://doi.org/10.1007/978-3-030-90724-2_10

1 Introduction

Left ventricular hypertrophy (LVH) is an abnormal increase in left ventricular (LV) mass due to thickening and enlargement of the heart wall [1], and it has been proven to be a strong predictor of cardiovascular disease complications [2]. One of the main causes of LVH is the continuous pressure overload on the LV wall of the heart, which triggers a compensatory response of increasing thickness in the heart tissue to cope with the condition. As the wall thickens, the heart will lose its elasticity and efficiency in pumping blood throughout the body, leading to congestive heart failure and irregular rhythms. This pressure overload is typically caused by aortic stenosis, aortic coarctation or systemic hypertension [3–5]. LVH is more common in people who have high blood pressure and treating the disease may ease the symptoms and reverse the hypertrophy. However, cardiovascular patients with LVH in the early stages may not even be aware of their condition because it develops gradually. Measuring the ejection fraction (EF) is not a good predictor of LVH development [5, 6] since the percentage of blood pumped out by the diseased heart could still be maintained despite the LV wall thickening [7].

The wall stress analysis may be used as a potential indicator to predict the occurrence of LVH. Using the Laplace analysis, LV wall stress has been quantified based on the assessment of the heart wall geometry. But the method involves geometry assumption and is not able to present the varying stress on the wall [8]. Although the influence of LV wall thickness and curvature on wall stress has been studied [9], the wall features are assumed to be uniformly distributed in the geometry, even though the wall thickness of LVH patients is heterogenous and local curvatures are present [10]. An accurate assessment of LV wall stress is only feasible with patient-specific modelling [11]. Recent studies developed personalised 3D models to evaluate the wall mechanics of LVH patients by utilising the information from magnetic resonance imaging [1, 10]. However, the information of wall mechanics relies on the temporal and spatial resolution of the imaging modality. To overcome this limitation, a patient-specific finite element model has emerged as a useful assessment tool. Existing finite element LV models were predominantly focused on other heart diseases, such as myocardial infarction and aortic diseases [12–14], while development of LVH patient-specific model using finite element method is limited.

The present study aims to develop patient-specific finite element models of LVH patients to investigate wall stress distribution. The finite element models of healthy subjects are also constructed to serve as a baseline comparison. It is hypothesized that abnormal wall stress may occur in LVH patients and a patient-specific model is required to accurately determine the stress variation.

Table 1 List of parameter values for healthy (control) and LVH conditions

LV models	Ejection fraction (%)	Early diastolic volume (ml)	End diastolic volume (ml)	α	μ (Pa)
Control 1	67.8	33.8	105.0	9.7	230
Control 2	72.2	34.1	122.6	9.7	200
Patient 1	35.1	211.4	325.9	20	1720
Patient 2	31.4	184.3	268.7	20	2400

2 Methodology

2.1 Patient-Specific Geometries

Four cases (two LVH patients and two healthy subjects) were simulated using the finite element method to investigate the stress distribution on the LV wall. The healthy subjects served as the baseline control. The LV geometry of two control subjects and two LVH patients at early diastole were reconstructed from previous work [1]. The LV volume and EF of all subjects were obtained from the motion corrected LV models as stated in Table 1 [15].

2.2 Material Properties

The LV wall was modelled with hyperelastic behaviour material using first-order Ogden constitutive equation as stated in (Eq. 1),

$$W = \frac{u}{\alpha}\left(\overline{\lambda_1}^{\alpha} + \overline{\lambda_2}^{\alpha} + \overline{\lambda_3}^{\alpha} - 3\right) + K/2(J-1)^2 \tag{1}$$

where $\overline{\lambda_p}(p = 1, 2, 3)$ are the principal stretches, μ and α are material constants, J is the volume ratio and K is the bulk modulus of 28 kPa [16]. Table 1 also recorded the material constants (α and μ) for each subject. These material constants were selected so that the specific-end diastolic volume was achieved with predefined filling pressure, i.e. 8 mmHg for the controls [17] and 24 mmHg for LVH patients [18]. The wall stiffness was assumed to be constant throughout the model.

2.3 Discretisation and Implementation

The initial state of the LV model was at early diastole, which was assumed to have zero or minimal residual stress. To simulate diastolic filling phase, a uniform pressure

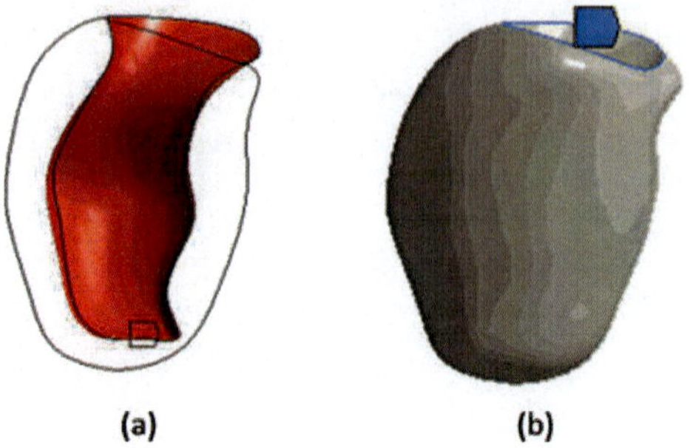

Fig. 1 Implementation of boundary conditions on patient-specific LV model: **a** filling pressure applied on endocardium (red surface), **b** fixed constraint on wall basal edge (blue line)

was applied onto the endocardial surface to inflate the LV cavity. To prevent rigid body motion, the degree of freedom of the LV basal edge was suppressed in all directions. The implementation of boundary conditions was illustrated in Fig. 1.

The LV wall of each model was discretised using 10-node tetrahedral quadratic elements. Mesh independence study was performed on each model, and the final meshes (33–40 K elements) were chosen with an acceptance criterion of less than five percent change in radial stress. The finite element models were solved using ANSYS Mechanical R2020 and simulations were conducted on an Intel i5 7th Gen processor with 8 GB RAM.

2.4 *Effects of Individual Contributing Factors on Wall Stress*

In this study, the patient models demonstrated a combined effect of increased filling pressure and enhanced wall stiffness. As such, the impact of individual factors on wall stress was examined. The abnormal conditions (increased filling pressure and wall material parameters) were implemented on *Control 1* whilst normal conditions were applied on *Patient 1* (Table 2). The stress results of these adapted models were analysed by comparing to the patient-specific models from Table 1. The effects of wall thickening and local curvature of LVH patients were studied by assessing the models under same settings (i.e. *Control 1* vs. *Patient 1_normal pressure and stiffness; Patient 1* vs. *Control 1_abnormal pressure and stiffness*).

Table 2 Adapted models of *Control 1* and *Patient 1*

Adapted model	Pressure (mmHg)	α	μ (Pa)
Control 1_abnormal pressure and stiffness	24	20	1720
Control 1_abnormal pressure	24	9.7	230
Patient 1_normal pressure and stiffness	8	9.7	230
Patient 1_normal pressure	8	20	1720

3 Results and Discussion

This study presents the discrepancy of wall stress between controls and LVH patients using patient-specific finite element models. The patient-specific conditions of two healthy and two LVH patients were simulated, and their LV wall stress were examined in circumferential, longitudinal, and radial directions.

Figure 2 illustrates the distribution of wall thickness in each model. The end-diastolic wall thickness varied among the patient-specific geometries. The controls showed a normal wall thickness with more uniform distribution (<9 mm) while the LVH patients exhibited localised wall hypertrophy (>9 mm) [1]. Particularly, *Patient 1* (Fig. 2c) had thicker LV wall at the basal and mid regions, while a greater wall thickness was observed at the mid and apical regions of *Patient 2* (Fig. 2d). The maximal wall thickness of LVH patients (12.5 ± 0.5 mm) was substantially larger than the controls (8 ± 1.2 mm) at end diastole.

Due to the complex LV geometric curvature and inconsistent wall thickness in LV geometries, the accuracy of Laplace analysis was often compromised [11]. Hence, patient-specific models with sufficient spatial resolution would be useful in obtaining the variations of wall stress. Figure 3 shows the distribution of longitudinal, circumferential and radial stress across the LV wall of a control and LVH patient. In the control, the circumferential wall stress varied transmurally, with the greatest stress observed at the endocardium and the lowest at the epicardium, whereas it was vice versa for radial stress. However, this result trend was not always observed in LVH patients, particularly near the region with wall thickening (short-axis base level of *Patient 1*). From the results of longitudinal stress distribution, both control and patient groups showed remarkably high stress at region with high concavity, whereas the high convexity area demonstrated low stress.

The average wall stress at the short-axis basal, mid, and apical levels of all subjects are depicted in Table 3. Overall, the average wall stress in LVH patients ($\sigma_{\_c}$: 6068 ± 342 Pa, $\sigma_{\_z}$: 3785 ± 161 Pa, $\sigma_{\_r}$: 384 ± 649 Pa) were substantially greater than controls ($\sigma_{\_c}$: 2662±82 Pa, $\sigma_{\_z}$: 1486±239 Pa, $\sigma_{\_r}$: 0.1±47 Pa). The circumferential stress was highest in all subjects, followed by longitudinal stress and radial stress. The circumferential stress had the most significant role in counteracting elevated chamber pressure in these patients. Although the implementation of filling pressure and wall stiffness were comparable in each group, there was a discrepancy in average wall stress due to the anatomical features of individual LV geometry.

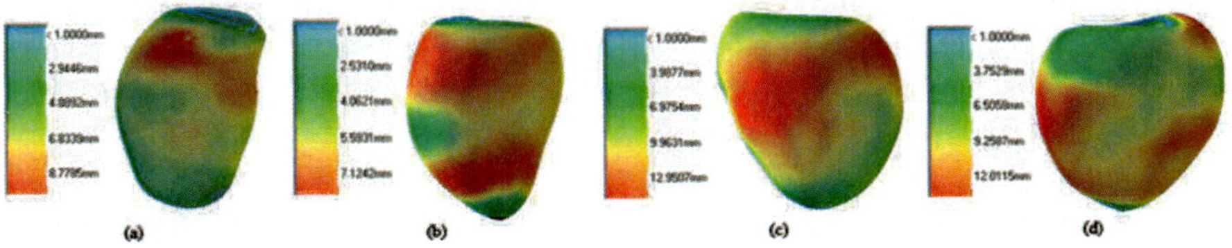

Fig. 2 End-diastolic wall thickness in controls (**a**, **b**) and LVH patients (**c**, **d**). The colour bar indicates wall thickness in mm

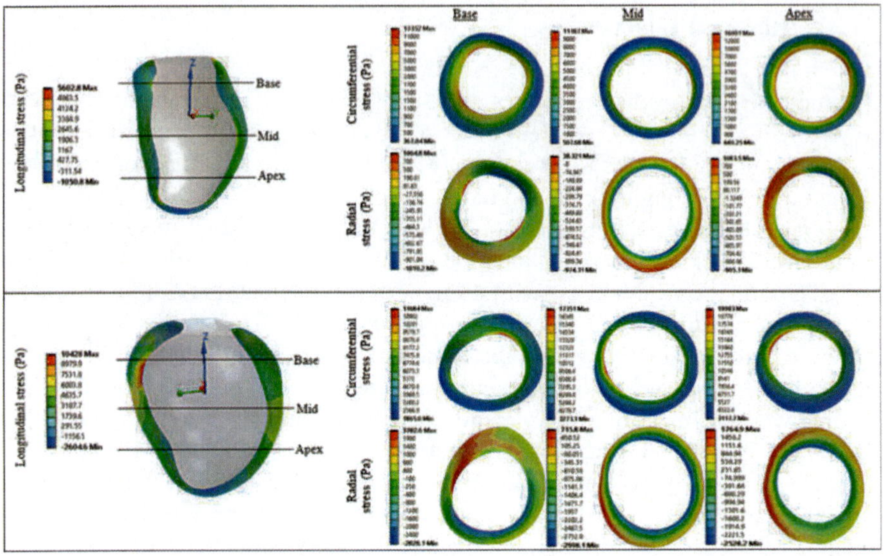

Fig. 3 Contour plots of longitudinal stress (long-axis), circumferential and radial stresses (short-axis) at end-diastole for *Control 1* (top) and *Patient 1* (bottom)

Table 3 Average end-diastolic circumferential, longitudinal and radial stresses at the short-axis basal, mid, and apical levels of each model

Model	Circumferential stress, σ_c (Pa)			Longitudinal stress, σ_z (Pa)			Radial stress, σ_r (Pa)		
	Base	Mid	Apex	Base	Mid	Apex	Base	Mid	Apex
Control 1	1932.1	2467.3	3411.3	933.5	1570.6	1448	−4.6	−233.9	138.3
Control 2	1953.8	3302.1	2903.1	1803.5	2017.4	1143.5	−82.0	−151.1	333.9
Patient 1	4450.6	7066.7	7412	3440.2	4527.0	3047.5	391.0	−918.0	301.7
Patient 2	4127.6	6639.4	6711.8	4514.2	4986.6	2197.1	2620.6	−875.6	782.8

Figure 4 shows the circumferential stress of *Control 1, Patient 1* and adapted models in long-axis view. From the results, an analogous circumferential stress distribution was observed between the models with different filling pressure (i.e. *Control 1* vs. *Control 1_abnormal pressure*; *Patient 1* vs. *Patient 1_normal pressure*). However, the stress magnitude was elevated in models with abnormal high pressure. The same happened for longitudinal and radial stress. Compared with different wall stiffness *(Control 1_abnormal pressure* vs. *Control 1_abnormal pressure and stiffness; Patient 1_normal pressure* vs. *Patient 1_normal pressure and stiffness),* the models with more compliant wall showed greater wall stress because the LV wall had to withstand a larger filling volume. Irrespective of the difference in filling pressure and wall stiffness, the maximal circumferential stress was noticed in both control and LVH patients at the endocardial region with high convexity. This indicated that

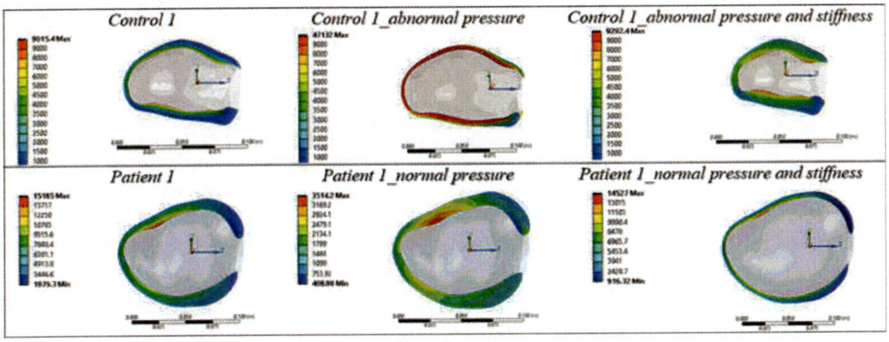

Fig. 4 Circumferential stress of *Control 1, Patient 1,* and the adapted models in long-axis view. The colour bar represents stress magnitude in Pa

wall stress variation was dependent on geometrical shape, and this distinct feature was characterized by the patient-specific LV geometry. The local convexity was even more significant in LVH patients with hypertrophic cardiomyopathy [19].

Figure 5 summarizes the effects of individual factors on wall stress. In both *Control 1* and *Patient 1,* the radial stress (σ_r) changed three-fold to act against the same pressure change. The impact of wall stiffness was less significant than the filling pressure in diastolic filling. With three-fold higher filling pressure, the maximal longitudinal (σ_z) and circumferential stress (σ_c) in *Control 1* had substantially increased about five times. Interestingly, *Patient 1* only showed three to four times (instead of five) increase in the two wall stress when subjected to three-fold filling pressure change. This could be due to the LV wall thickening in *Patient 1,* which caused the stress to be distributed transmurally across wall. The local wall curvatures of the patient might also contribute to this observation. A previous study had reported the correlation of wall thickness and curvatures with wall stress in the left atrium,

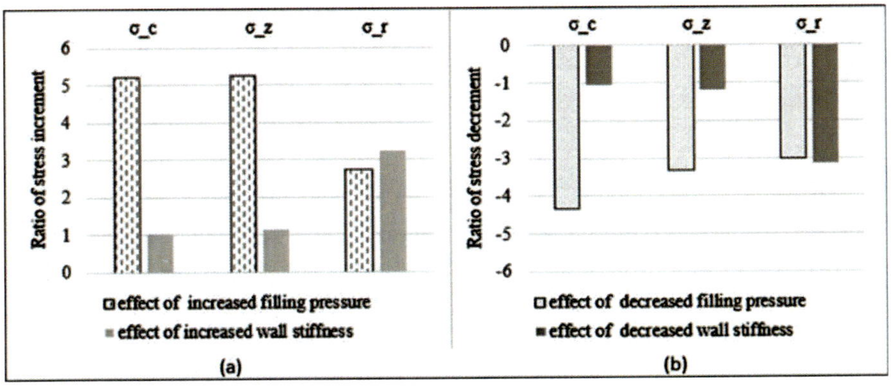

Fig. 5 Comparison of filling pressure and wall stiffness effects on maximal wall stresses for **a** *Control 1* and **b** *Patient 1*

where the thickness had a predominant role than curvatures [20]. More detailed investigations into this correlation would be required in LVH patients with regard to its relevance to LV remodelling.

One of the limitations of this preliminary study was the non-inclusion of myocardial fibre orientation in the finite element model. An isotropic wall expansion was assumed, thus the LV wall untwisting motion was not considered. Therefore, all the types of wall stress were studied in cylindrical coordinate, but not along the fibre direction. Furthermore, the model implementation was restricted to diastolic filling phase with constant pressure. The LVH patients in this study appeared to have the phenotype of hypertensive heart disease, with both systolic and diastolic dysfunction. Future work could consider improving the patient-specific model with inclusion of diastolic transient filling, systolic simulation and myocardial fibre incorporation for more realistic wall movement. More subjects and patients with varying degrees of disease severity and phenotypes should also be included for better result validity.

4 Conclusion

This study investigated the end-diastolic wall stress distribution in LVH patients using a patient-specific finite element model. Excessive wall stress experienced by LVH patients in this study was mainly due to elevated filling pressure during diastole. In addition, an abnormal diastolic wall stress variation was also observed due to LV wall thickening and distinct local geometrical curvatures in LVH patients. This highlights the importance of using a patient-specific model in wall stress assessment of LVH patients. Further investigations would be required to correlate the local geometrical features with regional wall stress and remodelling in LVH patients.

Acknowledgements This study was supported by the University of Nottingham Malaysia Pump Priming Grant 2020 and Universiti Malaya Faculty Research Grant (GPF053B-2020).

References

1. Chuah, S.H., et al.: Phenotyping of hypertensive heart disease and hypertrophic cardiomyopathy using personalized 3D modelling and cardiac cine MRI. Phys. Medica **78**(May), 137–149 (2020). https://doi.org/10.1016/j.ejmp.2020.08.022
2. Paoletti, E., et al.: The worsening of left ventricular hypertrophy is the strongest predictor of sudden cardiac death in haemodialysis patients: a 10 year survey. Nephrol. Dial. Transplant. **19**(7), 1829–1834 (2004). https://doi.org/10.1093/ndt/gfh288
3. Alkema, M., Spitzer, E., Soliman, O.I.I., Loewe, C.: Multimodality imaging for left ventricular hypertrophy severity grading: a methodological review. J. Cardiovasc. Ultrasound **24**(4), 257–267 (2016). https://doi.org/10.4250/jcu.2016.24.4.257
4. Katholi, R.E., Couri, D.M.: Left ventricular hypertrophy: major risk factor in patients with hypertension: update and practical clinical applications. Int. J. Hypertens. **2011** (2011). https://doi.org/10.4061/2011/495349

5. Loncaric, F., et al.: Pathophysiology and treatment of hypertensive left ventricular hypertrophy. Facta Univ. Ser. Med. Biol. **39**(3), 137–149 (2018). https://doi.org/10.1007/s11906-014-0428-x
6. Curtis, J.P., et al.: The association of left ventricular ejection fraction, mortality, and cause of death in stable outpatients with heart failure. J. Am. Coll. Cardiol. (2003). https://doi.org/10.1016/S0735-1097(03)00789-7
7. Smiseth, O.A., Torp, H., Opdahl, A., Haugaa, K.H., Urheim, S.: Myocardial strain imaging: how useful is it in clinical decision making? Eur. Heart J. **37**(15), 1196–1207b (2016). https://doi.org/10.1093/eurheartj/ehv529
8. Zhong, L., Ghista, D.N., Tan, R.S.: Left ventricular wall stress compendium. Comput. Methods Biomech. Biomed. Engin. **15**(10), 1015–1041 (2012). https://doi.org/10.1080/10255842.2011.569885
9. Choi, H.F., D'hooge, J., Rademakers, F.E., Claus, P.: Influence of left-ventricular shape on passive filling properties and end-diastolic fiber stress and strain. J. Biomech. **43**(9), 1745–1753 (2010). https://doi.org/10.1016/j.jbiomech.2010.02.022
10. Zhao, X., et al.: Left ventricular wall stress is sensitive marker of hypertrophic cardiomyopathy with preserved ejection fraction. Front. Physiol. **9**(MAR), 1–14 (2018). https://doi.org/10.3389/fphys.2018.00250
11. Gsell, M.A.F., et al.: Assessment of wall stresses and mechanical heart power in the left ventricle: finite element modeling versus Laplace analysis. Int. J. Numer. Method. Biomed. Eng. **34**(12), 1–18 (2018). https://doi.org/10.1002/cnm.3147
12. Leong, C.N., et al.: The role of end-diastolic myocardial fibre stretch on infarct extension. Int. J. Numer. Method. Biomed. Eng. **36**(1), 1–17 (2020). https://doi.org/10.1002/cnm.3291
13. Wenk, J.F., et al.: Regional left ventricular myocardial contractility and stress in a finite element model of posterobasal myocardial infarction. J. Biomech. Eng. **133**(4), 44501 (2011)
14. Wollmuth, J.R., et al.: Left ventricular wall stress in patients with severe aortic insufficiency with finite element analysis. Ann. Thorac. Surg. **82**(3), 840–846 (2006). https://doi.org/10.1016/j.athoracsur.2006.03.100
15. Liew, Y.M., et al.: Motion corrected LV quantification based on 3D modelling for improved functional assessment in cardiac MRI. Phys. Med. Biol. **60**, 2715 (2015)
16. Bettendorff-Bakman, D.E., Schmid, P., Lunkenheimer, P.P., Niederer, P.: A finite element study relating to the rapid filling phase of the human ventricles. J. Theor. Biol. (2006). https://doi.org/10.1016/j.jtbi.2005.05.009
17. Peverill, R.E.: Understanding preload and preload reserve within the conceptual framework of a limited range of possible left ventricular end-diastolic volumes. Adv. Physiol. Educ. **44**(3), 414–422 (2020). https://doi.org/10.1152/ADVAN.00043.2020
18. Zile, M.R., et al.: Heart failure with a normal ejection fraction: Is measurement of diastolic function necessary to make the diagnosis of diastolic heart failure? Circulation **104**(7), 779–782 (2001). https://doi.org/10.1161/hc3201.094226
19. Tarkiainen, M. et al.: Left ventricular septal convexity in differentiating hypertrophic cardiomyopathy from hypertensive heart disease—cardiac MRI study. Eur. Heart J. **41**(Supplement_2), 2020 (2020). https://doi.org/10.1093/ehjci/ehaa946.0210
20. Augustin, C.M., et al.: The impact of wall thickness and curvature on wall stress in patient-specific electromechanical models of the left atrium. Biomech. Model. Mechanobiol. **19**(3), 1015–1034 (2020). https://doi.org/10.1007/s10237-019-01268-5

Computational Analysis of Newtonian and Non-Newtonian Rheological Models for Patient-Specific Intracranial Aneurysm

Farhan Muhib and M. Tarik Arafat

Abstract This computational study is conducted to compare different blood models using a patient-specific intracranial aneurysm. A proper blood rheological model with varying viscosity gives different analytical results than assuming blood to be of constant characteristic. Computational analysis is done on a patient-specific intracranial aneurysm model to compare the results of the Newtonian model with the non-Newtonian power-law model (NNPL) and Herschel-Bulkley (HB) model. The results are presented in terms of wall shear stress (WSS), oscillatory shear index (OSI), dynamic viscosity, and strain rate. The peak WSS inside the aneurysm for the Newtonian model is 65.84% higher than the peak value obtained for the non-Newtonian power-law model. Moreover, the area percentage of the aneurysm covered with low WSS (less than 5 Pa) for the HB model is 6.28% lower than that of the Newtonian model. On the contrary, 6.55% of the aneurysm shows OSI values higher than 0.45 for the HB model, and the area percentage is 6.72% for the Newtonian model. Three different viscous models showed that viscous models influence the outcome of computational analyses to a great extent, and an appropriate viscous model must be identified, which can be used to simulate proper blood behavior during computational analysis.

Keywords Intracranial aneurysm · Non-Newtonian blood models · Patient-specific

1 Introduction

An intracranial aneurysm is a pathological outgrowth of the vascular wall in a cerebral blood vessel. Intracranial aneurysms are relatively common compared to the occurrence of an aneurysm in other vasculatures. According to a study conducted in China, rupture of these aneurysms may result in hemorrhagic stroke, which causes death in 46% of the cases [1]. Patients, who survive the stroke, often suffer from

F. Muhib · M. Tarik Arafat (✉)
Department of Biomedical Engineering, Bangladesh University of Engineering and Technology (BUET), Dhaka 1205, Bangladesh
e-mail: tarikarafat@bme.buet.ac.bd

J. Usman et al. (eds.), *6th Kuala Lumpur International Conference on Biomedical Engineering 2021*, IFMBE Proceedings 86,
https://doi.org/10.1007/978-3-030-90724-2_11

paralysis and 50% of those become permanently disabled [2]. However, the conventional medical imaging modalities do not provide much information regarding the rupture risk of aneurysms. To predict aneurysm rupture risk, physicians are considering using image-based computational fluid dynamics (CFD), which is supposed to go through a lot of developments within the next few years.

One of the most important factors while developing CFD models of biological organs is mimicking the properties of blood. Characteristics of blood flow depend on several rheological properties like viscoelasticity, deformation rate, and shear stress. However, a common issue in previous works was that researchers modeled blood as a Newtonian fluid [3]. In reality, blood is a shear-thinning, Bingham plastic fluid because of the disaggregation of the stacks of red blood cells and the orienting of individual red blood cells. The assumption of the blood being a Newtonian fluid is often impractical and only correct for limited scenarios like flow through a narrow channels. As mentioned in previous studies, blood flowing through vessels has an erythrocyte-free peripheral plasma layer, a Newtonian fluid, and the core region of suspension of all erythrocytes, which is non-Newtonian fluid [4]. This suggests that it is appropriate to model blood during simulation that has two-fluid nature, where its property will change depending on the inlet velocity condition and strain rate.

A recent study challenged the commonly used assumption of neglecting non-Newtonian effects in CFD simulations of intracranial blood flow and concluded that the Newtonian assumption might be inappropriate to mimic blood flow [5]. However, the discrepancies among viscous models were not shown through any computational simulation in the study. With this in mind, we designed our current study to find a proper rheological model that can mimic the non-Newtonian behavior of blood flow. The non-Newtonian models considered in our study are the non-Newtonian power-law model (NNPL) and Herschel-Bulkley (HB) model, as previous studies used these models to compare blood behavior in the coronary artery [6]. Simulations are done on a patient-specific model of anterior communicating artery aneurysm for different phases of a cardiac cycle. A comparative analysis is done among different hemodynamic parameters to identify the extent to which the hemodynamic parameters depend on viscous models used while conducting computational analyses.

2 Methodology

2.1 Three-Dimensional Model Generation

CT scan images of an aneurysm at the anterior communicating artery were used to create a three-dimensional vasculature model (see Fig. 1). A three-dimensional model of the intracranial aneurysm was generated from the DICOM images using MIMICS Medical software (see Fig. 1).

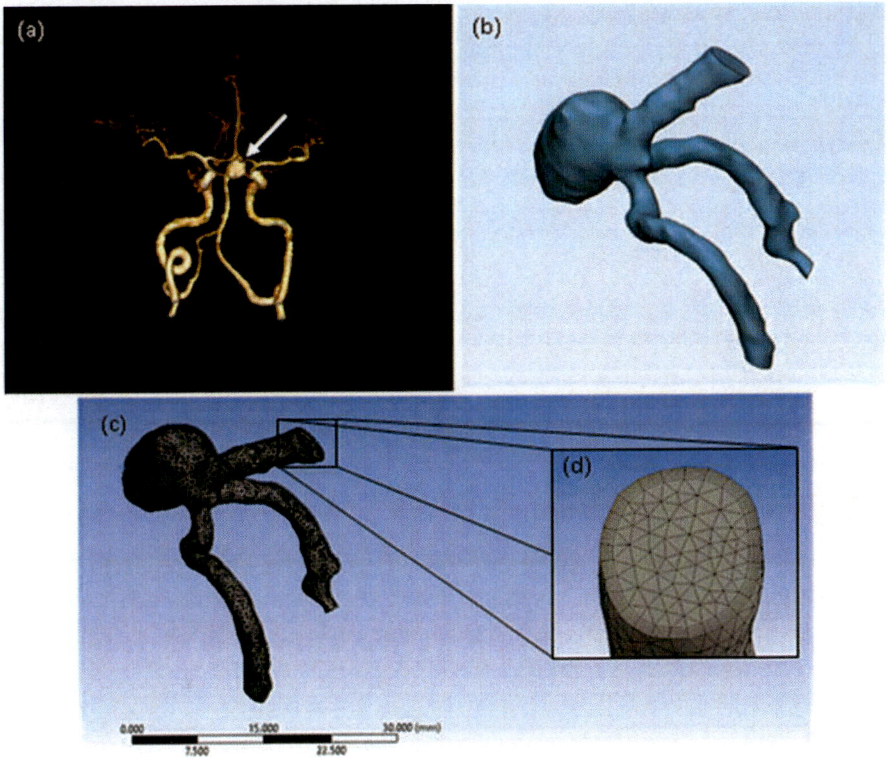

Fig. 1 **a** CT-DSA of an anterior communicating artery aneurysm (white arrow); **b** processed 3D model of the aneurysm; **c** meshing of the aneurysmal artery; and **d** inflation on the artery wall

2.2 Meshing

ANSYS meshing tools were used for the finite-volume meshing of the three-dimensional geometry (see Fig. 1). A mesh independence study was conducted to determine the optimum meshing parameters. The minimum size of mesh was set to a mesh setting with 0.07 mm, and five layers of inflation were implemented at the walls of the geometry with a total thickness of 0.2 mm and 1.2 growth rate for accurate calculation of WSS and other parameters. The meshing was completed with 1,597,153 elements. The skewness of 90% of the elements less than 0.75 and orthogonal quality of all elements above 0.1 with this setting indicates a good mesh quality.

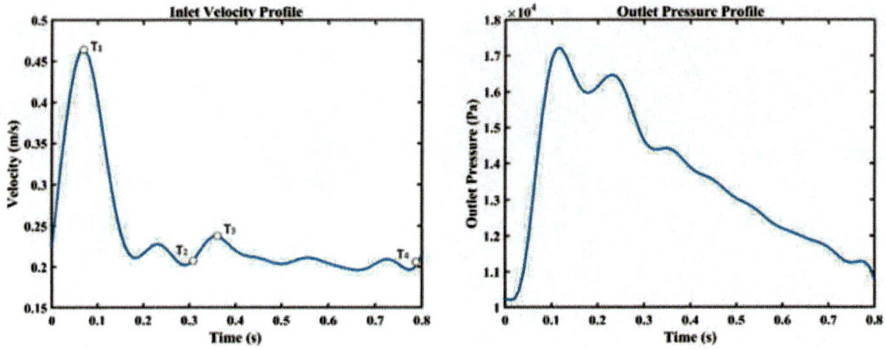

Fig. 2 Velocity waveform profile at the inlet (left) and pressure waveform profile at the outlets (right)

2.3 Boundary Conditions and Material Properties

The density of blood was assumed to be 1060 kg m^{-3}. The mass flow profile through the artery should be similar to anatomical flow in the carotid artery, which is pulsatile and changes with different phases of the cardiac cycle. The velocity profile for the anterior communicating artery was adopted from Ku et al. [7].

A pulsatile pressure waveform was imposed at the outlets, which was adopted from the works of Lee et al. [8]. Assuming the patient had a normal blood pressure condition, the outlet pressure range was approximately 80–130 mmHg, where the maximum pressure was during peak systole, and it decreased through the diastolic part (see Fig. 2). The vessel walls were assumed to be rigid, and a no-slip condition was applied to the walls.

2.4 Non-Newtonian Blood Models

To compare different rheological models of blood, computational analyses were performed using Newtonian, non-Newtonian power-law, and Herschel-Bulkley models. Previous research works determined the input parameters for these models based on theoretical studies and by parameter fitting to experimental viscosity data obtained under steady-state and at certain shear rates [9]. Those parameters were used in this experiment to create the rheological models and run the numerical analyses. The characteristic equations and the input parameters used are shown in Table 1.

Table 1 Blood viscosity models with input parameters

Model name	Equations and input parameters
Newtonian model	$\mu = 0.0035$ Pa s
Herschel-Bulkley model	$\mu = \kappa \dot{\gamma}^{n-1} + \left(\frac{\tau_o}{\dot{\gamma}}\right)$ Where, consistency index, $\kappa = 8.9721 \times 10^{-3}$ kg s^{n-2} m^{-1}, $n = 0.8601$, yield stress, $\tau_o = 0.0175$ Pa
Non-Newtonian power-law model	$\mu = \kappa \dot{\gamma}^{n-1}$ Where, $\kappa = 0.012171$ kg s^{n-2} m^{-1}, $n = 0.7991$

The values of variables used to model blood using the equations were obtained by theoretical knowledge and experimental analyses. It appears that viscosity is denoted by μ (Pa-s), shear rate is denote by $\dot{\gamma}$ (s^{-1})

2.5 Simulation Setup

ANSYS FLUENT was used to numerically solve the 3D incompressible Navier–Stokes equation and rheological model equations. The 'SIMPLE' solution method was used in the CFD solver with second-order accuracy to solve the flow-governing Navier–Stokes equation. The second-order upwind differencing scheme was applied for solving the momentum equations. The absolute convergence criteria for residuals were 10^{-4}. A total simulation of 1.6 s was performed for two cardiac cycles with a time step size of 0.01 s.

3 Results and Discussions

3.1 Viscosity and Strain Rate

Blood, being a Bingham fluid, shows different viscosity values depending on strain rate. At a lower strain rate, the viscosity is higher, and the viscosity is lower at a higher strain rate. Figure 3 shows the change of strain rate and viscosity at a point on the most burgeoned region of the aneurysm changing with time. This figure clearly shows that the strain rate is highest during the systolic period of the cardiac cycle ($t = 0.07$ s), and at that time, the viscosity is lowest for NNPL and HB models. NNPL model shows a relatively lower viscosity value compared to the HB model throughout the cardiac cycle, which becomes 20.36% lower during systole. However, the viscosity of blood should not be much less than 0.0035 Pa-s, and based on that, the NNPL model does not perform as a viable choice for modeling blood.

Figure 4 shows the viscosity distribution contour along the aneurysmal wall for three rheological models. The Newtonian model shows constant viscosity at every region, where the viscosity value for the NNPL and HB models varies at different regions of the aneurysm depending on varying strain rates.

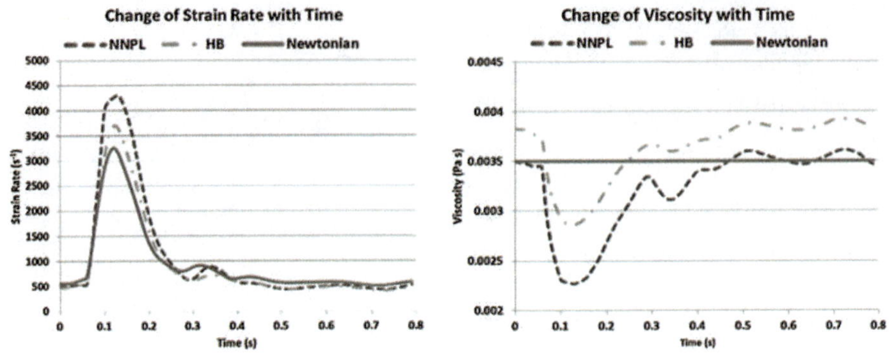

Fig. 3 Change of strain rate (left) and viscosity (right) value with time at an arbitrary point inside the aneurysm

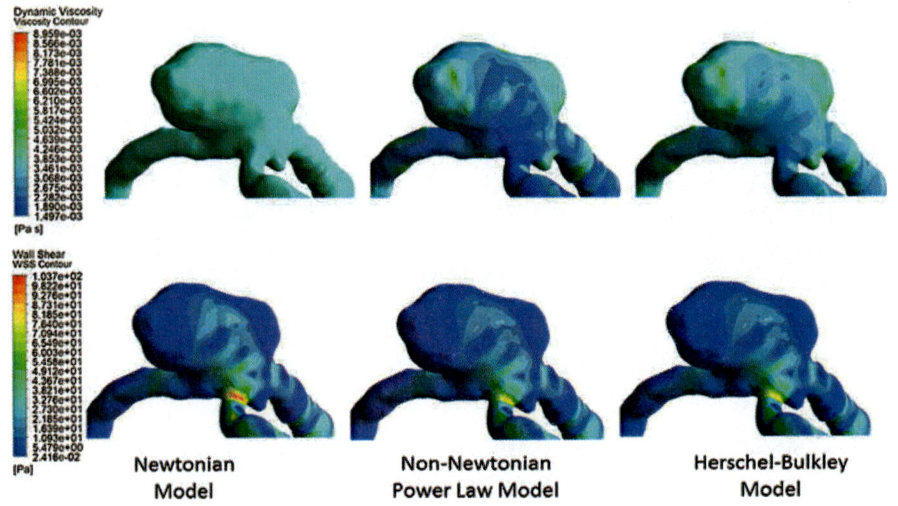

Fig. 4 Contour plots of the viscosity (top) and WSS distribution (below) during peak systole for three different rheological models

3.2 *Wall Shear Stress Distribution*

Wall shear stress (WSS) is one of the most important hemodynamic parameters in assessing the risk of rupture of aneurysms. Many previous studies proved that lower WSS regions inside the aneurysms indicate vulnerability, and the value can be as low as 0.01 Pa in the growing regions during systole [10, 11]. Figure 4 shows the WSS distribution inside the aneurysm for different models during peak systole. WSS value for the Newtonian model ranges from 0.06 to 85.4 Pa inside aneurysm (see Fig. 5(i)). The maximum WSS for the NNPL model is around 51 Pa which is about

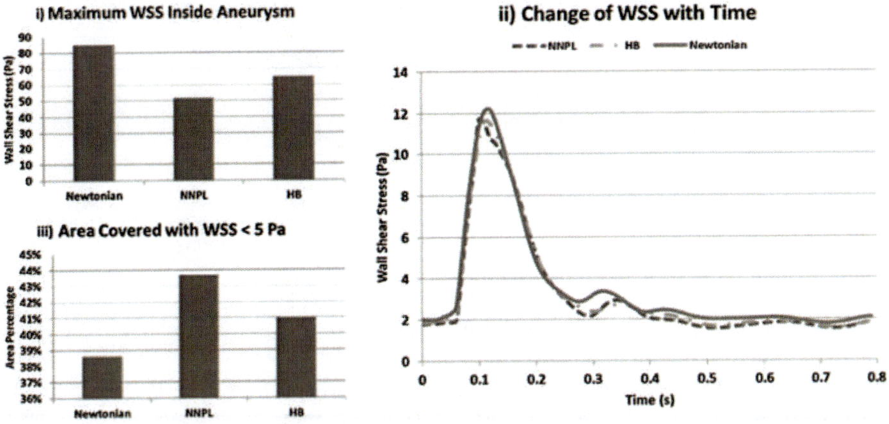

Fig. 5 **i** The bar chart shows the maximum value of WSS inside the aneurysm, **ii** WSS value at an arbitrary point inside the aneurysm for three different viscosity models, **iii** area percentage of aneurysm covered with low WSS

20.8% lower than that of the HB model. This is the result of underestimating the blood viscosity of the NNPL model observed in Sect. 3.1.

The discrepancy among the three viscosity models is more cogent from the graph shown in Fig. 5(ii), where the change of WSS value with time is displayed. To generate the graph, an arbitrary point was selected at the most burgeoned region of the aneurysm. From the graph, we can see that the value of WSS for the Newtonian model is higher than the other two models for most of the parts of a cardiac cycle. The other two models, the non-Newtonian power-law and the Herschel-Bulkley models, show almost the same value throughout the cardiac cycle. However, the second bar chart in Fig. 5(iii) shows that for the Newtonian model, the lowest percentage of area, 38%, is covered with a lower than 5 Pa WSS value during peak systole, which agrees with the previous observations. On the contrary, 43.7% and 41% of the area is covered with WSS values less than 5 Pa for NNPL and HB models, respectively. The values of the WSS distribution of the HB model are more acceptable compared to the NNPL model as it shows viscous behavior similar to the actual viscous property of blood.

3.3 *Oscillatory Shear Index*

Oscillatory shear index (OSI) is another important hemodynamic parameter used for assessing aneurysm rupture risk. The areas inside the aneurysm with a higher value of OSI indicate the reverse flow of blood in those regions, and according to previous studies, these regions have a higher risk of rupture in the future [12]. Figure 6 shows the area percentage of the aneurysm and its branches during peak systole covered

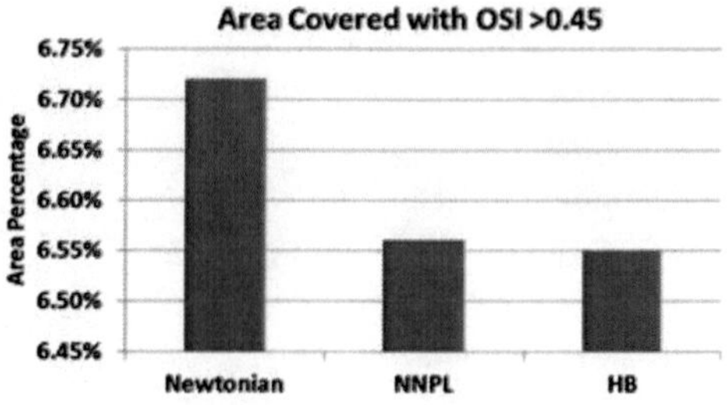

Fig. 6 Area percentage of aneurysm covered with high OSI

with a higher value of OSI, regions more susceptible to rupture. More than 6.7% of the aneurysm is covered with a high OSI value for the Newtonian model. The other two models show almost similar results, which are about 2.4% less than that of the Newtonian model (see Fig. 6). The higher viscosity values during systole compared to the other two rheological models is the main reason behind the higher value of OSI inside the aneurysm for the Newtonian model. Fluid with the higher viscous property during systole created vortices and reversed flow within the aneurysm, which may lead to damage of the internal layer of the artery and stimulate the growth of the aneurysm. NNPL and HB models showed lower viscosity during systole, which led to a lower amount of areas with reverse flow.

4 Conclusion

In this study, we identified clear distinctions between Newtonian, non-Newtonian power-law, Herschel-Bulkley viscosity models in terms of wall shear stress, oscillatory shear index, and strain rate. Whereas most of the previous studies focused solely on a specific stage of the cardiac cycle, we showed the effect of using different viscous models throughout a complete cardiac cycle. The values of these parameters can be assessed for any point of a cardiac cycle from the graphs. Based on the results discussed above, we can conclude that the HB model showed more similarity to the actual characteristic of blood compared to the other two rheological models and can be used to model blood in future computational studies. However, this study, too, had some flaws. Using more aneurysm models and using patient-specific boundary conditions would provide more accurate and reliable results. Further studies should address this issue and conduct a more expanded study to find the proper viscosity model to simulate the model in a computational setting.

Acknowledgements The project is funded by the ICT Ministry, Bangladesh under grant no. 56.00.0000.028.20.004.20-340.

References

1. Souza, S.D.: Aneurysmal Subarachnoid Hemorrhage. J. Neurosurg. Anesth. **27**, 21–23 (2015). https://doi.org/10.1097/ANA.0000000000000130
2. Wallace, M.C.: Outcome and Cost of Aneurysmal Subarachnoid Hemorrhage. https://doi.org/10.1016/j.nec.2009.10.014
3. Sun, H.T., Sze, K.Y., Tang, A.Y.S., et al.: Effects of aspect ratio, wall thickness and hypertension in the patient-specific computational modeling of cerebral aneurysms using fluid-structure interaction analysis. Eng. Appl. Comput. Fluid Mech. **13**, 229–244 (2019). https://doi.org/10.1080/19942060.2019.1572540
4. Sankar, D.S., Lee, U.: Two-fluid Herschel-Bulkley model for blood flow in catheterized arteries. J. Mech. Sci. Technol. **22**, 1008–1018 (2008). https://doi.org/10.1007/s12206-008-0123-4
5. Saqr, K.M., Mansour, O., Tupin, S., et al.: Evidence for non-Newtonian behavior of intracranial blood flow from Doppler ultrasonography measurements. Med. Biol. Eng. Comput. **57**, 1029–1036 (2019). https://doi.org/10.1007/s11517-018-1926-9
6. Soulis, J.V., Giannoglou, G.D., Chatzizisis, Y.S., et al.: Non-Newtonian models for molecular viscosity and wall shear stress in a 3D reconstructed human left coronary artery. Med. Eng. Phys. **30**, 9–19 (2008). https://doi.org/10.1016/j.medengphy.2007.02.001
7. Ku, J.P., Elkins, C.J., Taylor, C.A.: Comparison of CFD and MRI flow and velocities in an in vitro large artery bypass graft model. Ann. Biomed. Eng. **33**, 257–269 (2005). https://doi.org/10.1007/s10439-005-1729-7
8. Lee, C.J., Zhang, Y., Takao, H., et al.: A fluid-structure interaction study using patient-specific ruptured and unruptured aneurysm: the effect of aneurysm morphology, hypertension and elasticity. J. Biomech. **46**, 2402–2410 (2013). https://doi.org/10.1016/j.jbiomech.2013.07.016
9. Laboni, F.S., Rabbi, M.F., Arafat, M.T., et al.: Computational analysis of left coronary bifurcating artery using different blood rheological models. AIP Conf. Proc. **2121**, 100002-(1-8) (2019). https://doi.org/10.1063/1.5115933
10. Jiang, P., Liu, Q., Wu, J., et al.: Hemodynamic findings associated with intraoperative appearances of intracranial aneurysms. Neurosurg. Rev. (2018). https://doi.org/10.1007/s10143-018-1027-0
11. Wang, Y., Leng, X., Zhou, X., et al.: Hemodynamics in a middle cerebral artery aneurysm before its growth and fatal rupture: case study and review of the literature. World Neurosurg. **119**, e395–e402 (2018). https://doi.org/10.1016/j.wneu.2018.07.174
12. Liang, L., Steinman, D.A., Brina, O., et al.: Towards the clinical utility of CFD for assessment of intracranial aneurysm rupture—a systematic review and novel parameter-ranking tool. J. Neurointerv. Surg. **11**, 153–158 (2019). https://doi.org/10.1136/neurintsurg-2018-014246

Electro-Mechanical Finite Element Model of Left Ventricular Hypertrophy

Zhi Chin Hew, Bee Ting Chan, Wan Naimah Wan Ab Naim, Socrates Dokos, Wah Yen Tey, and Yih Miin Liew

Abstract Left ventricular hypertrophy (LVH) is one of the common heart diseases that contribute to global morbidity and mortality. LVH can be further classified into concentric LVH (cLVH), eccentric LVH (eLVH) and concentric left ventricular remodeling (cLVR) based on the changes in wall structure and cardiac function. This study simulated LVH cases by using an electro-mechanical left ventricular (LV) model. The simulation was performed on three LVH cases, with a healthy model used for baseline reference. The pressure–volume loops, LV wall thickening index (*TI*), shortening strain (*SS*) and thickening strain (*TS*) were evaluated. Although all LV models had a preserved ejection fraction, differences in *TI, SS* and *TS* were noted. The cLVH (*TI*: 24.4%, *SS*: −20.2%, *TS*: −52.5%) and eLVH (*TI*: 10.3%, *SS*: −81.2%, *TS*: 9.4%) models showed remarkable difference compared to the healthy model, whereas less significant discrepancy was noted in cLVR (*TI*: 5.1%, *SS*: −0.6%, *TS*: −7.3%). Distinct geometric features of increased wall thickness and chamber enlargement

Z. C. Hew · W. Y. Tey
Department of Mechanical Engineering, Faculty of Engineering, UCSI University, Kuala Lumpur, Malaysia

B. T. Chan (✉)
Department of Mechanical, Materials and Manufacturing Engineering, Faculty of Science and Engineering, University of Nottingham Malaysia, Selangor, Malaysia
e-mail: BeeTing.Chan@nottingham.edu.my

W. N. Wan Ab Naim
Faculty of Mechanical and Automotive Engineering Technology, Universiti Malaysia Pahang, Pahang, Malaysia

S. Dokos
Graduate School of Biomedical Engineering, UNSW Sydney, Sydney, Australia

W. Y. Tey
Malaysia-Japan International Institute of Technology, University Teknologi Malaysia, Skudai, Malaysia

Y. M. Liew
Department of Biomedical Engineering, Faculty of Engineering, Universiti Malaya, Kuala Lumpur, Malaysia

J. Usman et al. (eds.), *6th Kuala Lumpur International Conference on Biomedical Engineering 2021*, IFMBE Proceedings 86,
https://doi.org/10.1007/978-3-030-90724-2_12

were observed to affect the operative chamber stiffness in cLVH and eLVH. The *TI*, *SS* and *TS* results indicate wall mechanics impairment in cLVH and eLVH patients.

Keywords Hypertrophy · Strains · Wall thickening

1 Introduction

Left Ventricular Hypertrophy (LVH) is one of the common heart diseases that contribute to morbidity and mortality worldwide [1]. It is characterised by the appearance of abnormal left ventricular (LV) wall thickness and mass. LVH may be further classified into concentric LVH (cLVH), eccentric LVH (eLVH) and concentric LV remodeling (cLVR). cLVH occurs due to pressure overload, where the LV wall thickness and mass will increase to preserve heart function. In eLVH, there is decreased wall thickness in patients with deteriorating cardiac function due to volume overload [1]. Compared to a healthy heart, cLVR has no significant effect on LV wall structure, but there is notable increase in wall concentricity. Although LVH is usually reversible when the underlying cause is treated, the geometrical changes caused by the condition will affect cardiac performance and influence disease outcome.

Clinically, left ventricular ejection fraction (LVEF) is a standard assessment for heart function. Although LVEF is strongly associated with impaired heart function, studies have reported that it may not be a good outcome predictor for LVH patients [2], as an enlarged heart may still pump out a constant volume of blood. To overcome this limitation, myocardial wall mechanics have been developed as a potential tool to detect cardiac dysfunction. Imaging modalities, such as tissue doppler imaging and speckle tracking echocardiography, are widely used to assess myocardial deformation [3]. Nevertheless, the quantification of complete 3D deformation of the heart poses a challenge because the assessment is based on selected 2D chamber views, and the process is largely dependent on the observer's expertise. Although recent advanced imaging modalities are able to provide 3D assessment, but there is a trade-off in image quality due to limited frame rate and spatial resolution, besides taking a long acquisition time [3]. In addition, the high variability of patient characteristics also poses a challenge to determine the impact of individual risk factors on wall mechanics using imaging techniques.

On the other hand, computational modelling has emerged as a useful tool in understanding the mechanisms of cardiac disease and predicting the outcome. Computer models have been shown to be useful in studying the impact of individual risk factors in heart disease [4]. Numerous computational heart models have been developed to comprehend the pathophysiology of heart diseases, such as myocardial infarction [5], cardiomyopathy [6] and heart valve diseases [7]. However, there is a lack of attention in the development of LVH models through the investigation of myocardial wall mechanics and cardiac performance. This study aims to simulate various LVH models using the electro-mechanical finite element models adapted from fluid structure studies [4, 8]. The wall mechanics of LVH models are described as wall thickening index, shortening and thickening strains.

2 Methodology

2.1 LV Wall Geometry and Simulation Cases

The LV geometry was modelled as a 3D half prolate spheroid with height *h*, diameter *D* and wall thickness *t* as illustrated in Fig. 1 (left). Myocardial fibre varied continuously across the myocardium, oriented from +60° at the epicardium to −60° at the endocardium. The incorporation of myocardial fibre and its orientation in the LV wall was shown in Fig. 1 (right). The LV wall geometry was further divided into 17 segments according to the American Heart Association (AHA) model [9] for post-processing of results.

Three LVH models (cLVH, eLVH and cLVR) and a healthy counterpart were constructed based on measurements from published literature on the human heart [10–14]. The selected geometrical dimensions and characteristics of each LV model were listed in Table 1. The relative wall thickness was determined as two times of wall thickness *t* divided by the endocardial diameter *D* [9, 10]. These LV geometries were constructed at the original zero-stress configuration.

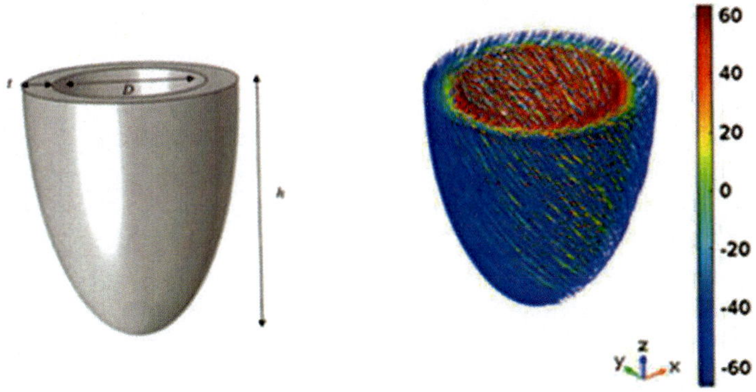

Fig. 1 3D left ventricular (LV) wall with labelled geometrical dimensions (left) and incorporation of fibre orientation (right) in an American Heart Association 17-segment heart model. Colour bar represents the fibre angle (degrees)

Table 1 Geometrical dimensions and characteristics of left ventricular hypertrophy (LVH) models

Model parameters	Healthy	cLVH	eLVH	cLVR
Height, *h* (mm)	70	68	70	70
Diameter, *D* (mm)	45	45	50	41
Wall thickness, *t* (mm)	9	15	9	10
Relative wall thickness	0.4	0.6	0.3	0.4

2.2 Boundary Conditions and Simulation Protocol

The simulation protocol was adapted from previous fluid–structure model studies [4, 8]. A pressure load was imposed on the endocardium of the LV geometry until the end diastolic volume (EDV) was achieved. Subsequently, the simulation starts at systole (isovolumetric contraction (IVC) and ejection), where an active stress induced by electrical impulses across the myocardium was coupled with the mechanical model to generate myocardial contraction during systole. This was followed by diastole (isovolumetric relaxation (IVR) and filling). The basal surface of the LV model was constrained in all directions to prevent rigid body motion. During IVC, LV volume was held constant while LV pressure, *Plv* (mmHg), was solved concomitantly. IVC phase would end when LV pressure reached 80 mmHg. In ejection phase, a three-element Windkessel model was used to compute the P_{lv} associated with the effect of blood ejection as stated in Eq. 1 and 2 [15].

$$P_{lv} = P_{sys} + Q_a R_a \quad (1)$$

$$C\frac{dP_{sys}}{dt} + \frac{P_{sys}}{R_{sys}} - Q_a = 0 \quad (2)$$

where P_{sys} (mmHg) denotes the systemic pressure and Q_a (mL·s^{-1}) represents the ejected flow rate or rate of LV volume change. The values of Windkessel parameters were set as follows: systemic impedance, $R_{sys} = 1.25$ mmHg·s·mL^{-1}, aortic impedance, $R_a = 0.06$ mmHg·s·mL^{-1} and peripheral capacitance, $C = 2.75$ mL·mmHg^{-1} [4]. The ejection phase stopped when P_{sys} is greater than P_{lv} and that indicates the aortic pressure is greater than the pressure in LV wall.

During IVR phase in diastole, the LV volume was held constant while P_{lv} was solved concurrently, which was the same as the implementation in IVC. IVR was terminated when LV pressure dropped to 0 mmHg and that indicates LV relaxation. In the final phase (i.e. filling), P_{lv} at the end of IVR phase had increased from zero to end diastolic pressure (EDP) as the load was imposed on the endocardium. The EDP was 12 mmHg in the healthy model and slightly increased at 13 mmHg in all LVH models with preserved LVEF.

2.3 Model Discretisation and Implementation

The 3D LV wall geometry was discretised into quadratic tetrahedral elements. Mesh convergence study was performed until the changes of LV pressure and volume were within five percent. A total of 5212 elements with an average element size of 6.9 mm were used in this study. The finite element analysis was performed using the COMSOL Multiphysics software (v5 COMSOL AB, Sweden). A PARDISO fully coupled solver was used to solve the equations with maximum time step of 20 ms in diastole and 10 ms in systole. All software calculations were carried out using an Intel(R) Core TM i5-5200 2.7 GHz processor with 12 GB RAM.

2.4 Assessments of Myocardial Wall Mechanics

The myocardial wall mechanics were evaluated using wall thickening index, longitudinal and radial strains. Wall thickening index (*TI*) was calculated as the amount of maximal changes in wall thickness from end systole (ES) to end diastole (ED) [16] using Eq. (3):

$$TI(mm) = \frac{1}{11}\sum_{i=7}^{17}\left[(t_{ES})_i - (t_{ED})_i\right] \tag{3}$$

The shortening strain (*SS*) that characterised the myocardial shortening of base-apex on the endocardial surface was calculated using Eq. (4).

$$SS(\%) = \frac{1}{11}\sum_{i=7}^{17}\left[\frac{(d\_\max_{ES})_i - (d\_\max_{ED})_i}{d\_\max_{EDi}} \times 100\%\right] \tag{4}$$

and thickening strain (*TS*), which represented the myocardial wall thickening or thinning, was calculated using Eq. (5).

$$TS(\%) = \frac{1}{11}\sum_{i=7}^{17}\left[\frac{(t\_\max_{ES})_i - (t\_\max_{ED})_i}{t\_\max_{EDi}} \times 100\%\right] \tag{5}$$

where i represents the number of segments, t represents an average wall thickness of the segment, *d*_max is the maximal base-apex distance, *t*_max is the maximal wall thickness, ES and ED represents end systole and end diastole, respectively.

The endocardium was used in *SS* calculation because the maximal global longitudinal strain occurred on this surface [17]. The basal segments (1–6) were excluded from calculations because the basal surface was constrained in this implementation to prevent a rigid body motion, while basal segments usually showed minimal contractility [16].

3 Results and Discussion

This study evaluated the *TI, SS* and *TS* of LVH models using the electro-mechanical finite element model. A healthy model was used as the baseline reference. Table 2 records the model conditions obtained from the implemented protocol. The concentricity was calculated as the ratio of LV mass to EDV [18], in which the LV mass was calculated as the product of the wall volume and myocardial tissue density (1.05 g/cm^3) [19]. All LV models showed a preserved LVEF (>50%), but the LVH models had larger LV mass and concentricity than the healthy model.

The model implementation was verified with the result of pressure–volume (PV) loops (Fig. 2). Compared to the healthy model, the PV loops of both cLVH and cLVR were skewed to the left, while the diastolic filling curves were raised slightly upwards. An increased LV pressure was also observed in cLVH throughout the systolic phase and in late systole for cLVR. On the contrary, the PV loop of eLVH was skewed to the right, and the diastolic filling curve and systolic pressure were slightly below the healthy model. The results of PV loops were in agreement with a study by Warriner et al. [20].

Myocardial tissues would shorten and lengthen throughout the cardiac cycle because of the contraction and relaxation of the heart muscle. Therefore, LV performance could be affected by the presence of wall abnormality. In this study, all LVH models had preserved LVEF, but the results of *TI, SS* and *TS* indicated that there was a heart abnormality, especially in cLVH and eLVH. The results of *TI, SS* and *TS* for each model are shown in Fig. 3.

A different trend was noted between *TI* and *TS*, although both results were calculated from wall thickness. *TI* characterised the overall score of myocardial contractility, whereas *TS* represents the deformation degree of the myocardial wall. Based on the healthy control, cLVH exhibited significant *TI* increment (24.4%) with a remarkable reduction in *TS* (−52.6%) and *SS* (−20.2%). Meanwhile, eLVH showed increments in *TI* (10.3%) and *TS* (9.4%), but *SS* was significantly impaired (−81.2%). The

Table 2 Model conditions obtained from the implemented protocol

	Healthy	cLVH	eLVH	cLVR
End systolic volume, ESV (mL)	45	40	54	36
End diastolic volume, EDV (mL)	112	107	123	94
LV ejection fraction, LVEF (%)	60	63	56	62
LV mass (g)	94	181	105	99
Concentricity	0.8	1.7	0.9	1.1

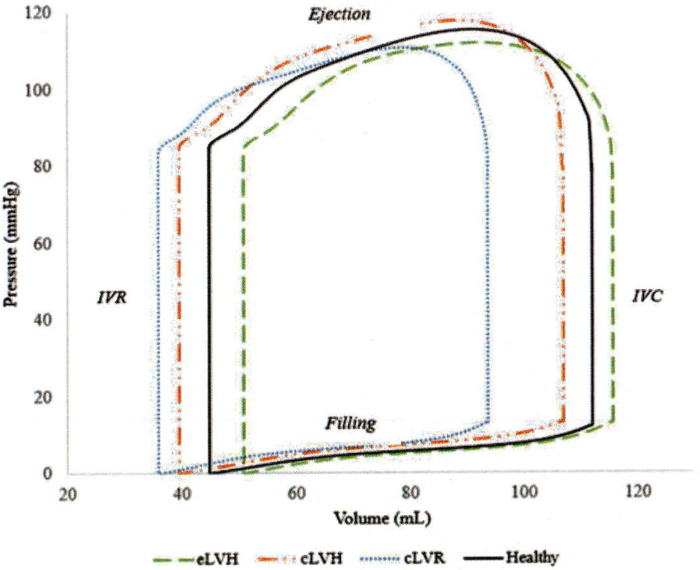

Fig. 2 Pressure–Volume (PV) loops retrieved from the LVH models and healthy control

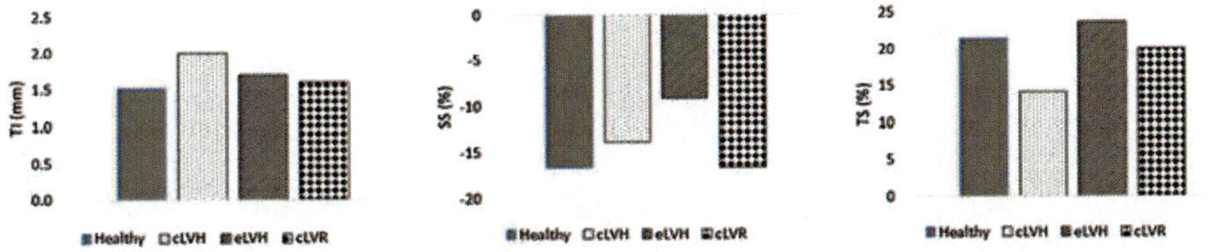

Fig. 3 Results of thickening index *(TI)*, shortening strain *(SS)* and thickening strain *(TS)* in healthy and LVH models. The negative value of *SS* represents myocardial shortening

result trends were in line with the previous study that reported wall strain impairment on LVH patients, while hypertrophic cardiomyopathy patients (cLVH) exhibited an excessive *TI* when compared to the healthy subjects [16]. An excessive *TI* occurred in cLVH due to increased wall thickness and LV mass, which was followed by eLVH. The *TS* calculation was normalised to ED wall thickness. Therefore, the eLVH with smallest ED wall thickness would show the greatest *TS*, while cLVH had the lowest *TS* when ED wall thickness was the highest. Meanwhile, the cLVR had the least difference from the healthy model in *TI* (5.1%), *SS* (−0.6%) and *TS* (−7.3%). Further investigations were required to identify the impact of these mechanics impairment.

Figure 4 indicates the regional wall deformation of LVH models at the short-axis taken from two-thirds of the LV height-level from base during ES and ED. From all the models, the sub-endocardial layer contributed greatly to the wall displacement as compared to the mid and subepicardial layer. This observation was in agreement with a previous study [21]. In terms of deformation degree, cLVH showed the largest

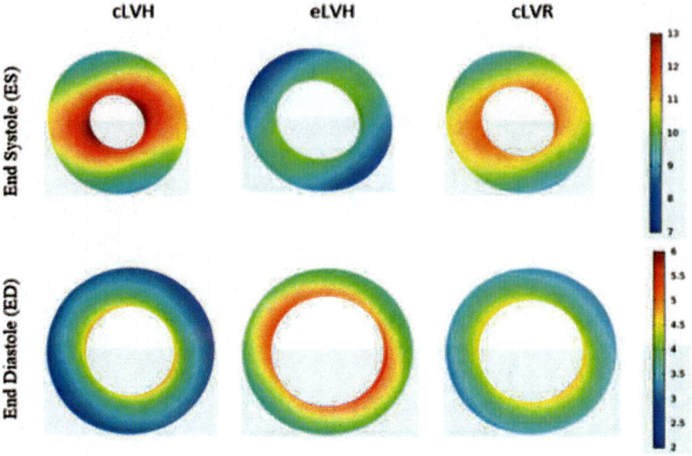

Fig. 4 Wall deformation at the apical region during ES (top) and ED (bottom). The colour bar represents total displacement (mm)

ES displacement, while the greatest ED displacement occurred in eLVH, and vice versa. This was because the increased LV mass (wall thickening) in cLVH would elevate the operative chamber stiffness during systolic contraction, but impair diastolic relaxation. The opposite happened in eLVH, which had a more compliant operative chamber stiffness due to chamber dilation. The regional deformation contours in Fig. 4 might imply that myocardial fibre orientation could play a role in wall deformation, which demanded further analysis on LV twisting and untwisting.

Study limitations. This study characterised LVH in simple geometries only with uniform wall thickness. The top basal surface of the LV model was fixed to prevent rigid body motion. This implementation would introduce high stress and thus, affect the strain on the wall near the constrained site. However, the result analysis was careful to exclude the affected area at basal regions. The LVH models were simulated for one full cardiac cycle only, and these could be improved by simulating for more cycles and using finer mesh sizes to compare the validity of result parameters (*TI*, *SS* and *TS*).

4 Conclusion

This study evaluated the wall mechanics in LVH geometries using the electromechanical finite element model. The models were validated based on the PV loops while intrinsic wall impairment of eLVH and cLVH were disclosed by the distinctive *TI*, *SS* and *TS*. The wall thickening of cLVH had elevated the operative chamber stiffness to enhance systolic contraction, but impair diastolic relaxation and vice versa in eLVH due to the chamber dilation. Future works would incorporate the patient specific LVH geometries, which had varying geometrical shape and non-uniform wall thickness.

Acknowledgements This study was supported by University of Nottingham Malaysia Pump Priming Grant 2020 and Universiti Malaya Faculty Research Grant (GPF053B-2020).

References

1. Aronow, W.S.: Hypertension and left ventricular hypertrophy. Ann. Transl. Med. **5**(1), 5–8 (2017)
2. Loncaric, F., Bijnens, B., Stiges, M.: Added value of cardiac deformation imaging in differential diagnosis of left ventricular hypertrophy. Glob. Cardiol. Sci. Pract. **3**, 2018 (2018)
3. Amzulescu, M.S., et al.: Myocardial strain imaging: review of general principles, validation, and sources of discrepancies. Eur. Hear. J. Cardiovasc. Imaging **20**(6), 605–619 (2019)
4. Chan, B.T., et al.: Impact of myocardial infarction on intraventricular vortex and flow energetics assessed using computational simulations. Int. J. Numer. Method. Biomed. Eng. **35**(6), 1–17 (2019)
5. Leong, C., et al.: Electromechanics Modeling of the Effects of Myocardial Infarction on Left Ventricular Function, pp. 5684–5687 (2015)
6. Sengupta, S., Ghosh. U., Sarkar. S., Das. S.: A Mathematical Approach to Characterize Left Ventricular Hypertrophy from ECG Diagrams, vol. 1, pp. 1–5 (2017)
7. Alkema, M., Spitzer. E., Soliman, O.I.I., Loewe. C.: Multimodality imaging for left ventricular hypertrophy severity grading: a methodological review. J. Cardiovasc. Ultrasound (2016)
8. Bakir, A.A., Al Abed, A., Stevens, M.C., Lovell, N.H., Dokos, S.: A multiphysics biventricular cardiac model: Simulations with a left-ventricular assist device. Front. Physiol. **9**(SEP), 1–25 (2018)
9. Jung, J., Kim, Y.H., Kim, N., Yang, D.H.: Patient-specific 17-segment myocardial modeling on a bull's-eye map. J. Appl. Clin. Med. Phys. **17**(5), 453–465 (2016)
10. Debry, N., et al.: Prognostic significance of left ventricular concentric remodelling in patients with aortic stenosis. Arch. Cardiovasc. Dis. **110**(1), 26–34 (2017)
11. Katz, D.H., Beussink, L., Sauer, A.J., Freed, B.H., Burke, M.A., Shah, S.J.: Prevalence, clinical characteristics, and outcomes associated with eccentric versus concentric left ventricular hypertrophy in heart failure with preserved ejection fraction. Am. J. Cardiol. **112**(8), 1158–1164 (2013)
12. Mizuguchi, Y., Oishi, Y., Miyoshi, H., Iuchi, A., Nagase, N., Oki, T.: Concentric left ventricular hypertrophy brings deterioration of systolic longitudinal, circumferential, and radial myocardial deformation in hypertensive patients with preserved left ventricular pump function. J. Cardiol. **55**(1), 23–33 (2010)
13. Rodrigues, J.C., et al.: The relationship between left ventricular wall thickness, myocardial shortening, and ejection fraction in hypertensive heart disease: insights from cardiac magnetic resonance imaging. J. Clin. Hypertens. **18**(11), 1119–1127 (2016)
14. Garg, S. et al.: Concentric hypertrophy and LV dilation. Circ. Hear. Fail. **10**(8), e003959 (2017)
15. Leong, C., et al.: The role of infarct transmural extent in infarct extension : a computational study. Int. J. Numer. Method. Biomed. Eng. **33**(2), e02794 (2017)
16. Chuah, S.H., et al.: Phenotyping of hypertensive heart disease and hypertrophic cardiomyopathy using personalized 3D modelling and cardiac cine MRI. Phys. Medica **78**(May), 137–149 (2020)
17. Nagata, Y., Wu, V.C.C., Otsuji, Y., Takeuchi, M.: Normal range of myocardial layer-specific strain using two-dimensional speckle tracking echocardiography. PLoS ONE **12**(6), 1–16 (2017)

18. Bang, C.N., et al.: Four-group classifcation of left ventricular hypertrophy based on ventricular concentricity and dilatation identifes a low-risk subset of eccentric hypertrophy in hypertensive patients. Circ. Cardiovasc. Imaging **7**(3), 422–429 (2014)
19. Devereux, R.B., et al.: Echocardiographic assessment of left ventricular hypertrophy: comparison to necropsy findings. Am. J. Cardiol. **57**(6), 450–458 (1986)
20. Warriner, D.R., et al.: Closing the loop: modelling of heart failure progression from health to end-stage using a meta-analysis of left ventricular pressure-volume loops. PLoS ONE **9**(12), 1–19 (2014)
21. Johnson, C., Kuyt, K., Oxborough, D., Stout, M.: Practical tips and tricks in measuring strain, strain rate and twist for the left and right ventricles. Echo Res. Pract. **6**(3), R87–R98 (2019)

Modified Spotted Hyena Optimizer Based Leukemia Microscopic Images Classification

S. Aswath, N. Bharanidharan, R. S. Valarmathi, and Harikumar Rajaguru

Abstract Applications of accurate machine learning techniques in medical field are increasing every day. This research paper proposes a novel Modified Spotted Hyena Optimizer as transformation technique to improve the performance of popular machine learning algorithms in classifying the Leukemia microscopic images. In the proposed transform, control parameter of Spotted Hyena Optimizer is found using Weightless Swarm Algorithm iteratively. Microscopic images of 26 leukemia and 26 normal subjects are obtained from C-NMC website and considered in this study. Statistical features namely mean, variance, skewness and kurtosis are extracted from microscopic images and given as input to the proposed transform. Then the transformed values are given as input to any one of the four supervised classifiers: K-Nearest Neighbor, Decision Trees, Random Forest, and Stochastic Gradient Descent. When the Modified Spotted Hyena Optimizer is for transforming the features in Stochastic Gradient Descent classifier, highest accuracy of 90% is achieved while the accuracy offered is only 65% when no transform is used.

Keywords Leukemia · Modified spotted hyena optimizer · Stochastic gradient descent

1 Introduction

Machine Learning can be used in various fields either to predict or to detect. Machine Learning is used as a prominent tool in data analytics, Natural Learning Processing, Computer vision, Speech Recognition, Medical Image analysis, etc. [1]. Many

S. Aswath (✉) · R. S. Valarmathi
Department of ECE, Vel Tech Rangarajan Dr. Sagunthala R&D Institute of Science and Technology, Chennai, India

N. Bharanidharan
Department of CSE, Dayananda Sagar University, Bangalore, India

H. Rajaguru
Department of ECE, Bannari Amman Institute of Technology, Sathyamangalam, India

J. Usman et al. (eds.), *6th Kuala Lumpur International Conference on Biomedical Engineering 2021*, IFMBE Proceedings 86,
https://doi.org/10.1007/978-3-030-90724-2_13

Machine Learning algorithms are available which can be used for the related application. Though the learning done by the computer has to be accessed periodically with testing, all models developed for any application will have both training as well as testing. Therefore, the performance of that particular model can be tweaked with some modifications to achieve the desired results. Nowadays in the medical field machine learning algorithms are been widely used for diagnosis purposes.

Acute Lymphoblastic Leukemia (ALL) is a malignant disorder in the bone marrow and different blood-forming organs producing elevated numbers of bizarre or immature leucocytes. These leucocytes suppress the manufacturing of regular blood cells, resulting in anemia and some other symptoms. It is very important to detect leukemia very early to save the patient's life. In the diagnosis of blood-related diseases and disorders, Microscopic images play a pivotal role [2]. Manually checking the blood samples is time-consuming and tedious work. Moreover it is also limited by the risk of human error. Therefore, to avoid these kinds of risks and cons, a computer-assisted detection system that can distinguish cancerous cells from normal cells is needed.

Metaheuristic techniques are mostly categorized as evolutionary-based, physics-based, and swarm-based. Apart from the other optimization techniques, Swarm Intelligence (SI) holds a very big advantage as they are nature-inspired optimization algorithms. These algorithms are designed with the base of the collective intelligence of the social behavior of the social creatures and it is the most preferred one due to its adaptability, non-derivative structure, and choosing the features carefully to avoid local optima [3]. To name a few SI algorithms: Ant Colony Optimization, Particle Swarm Optimization (PSO), Artificial Bee Colony, Bat algorithm (BA), Dragonfly algorithm (DA), Spotted Hyena Optimizer (SHO), etc. [4–6].

SI algorithms are mostly used to enhance the accuracy of supervised classifiers algorithms through feature selection and neural network training [7]. In some research works, SI algorithms are used as a transform to improve the performance of supervised classifiers [8, 9]. To the best of our knowledge, SHO is not reported as a transformation technique and so this research work focuses on implementation of SHO and Modified Spotted Hyena Optimizer (MSHO) as transformation techniques. Control parameters (weights) of SHO are updated through Weightless Swarm Optimization (WSO) in the proposed MSHO.

The remaining paper is structured as follows: the methodology used in this research work is presented in the next section; original SHO implementation will be explained in the third section; implementation of MSHO algorithm will be dealt in fourth section; results are discussed in the fifth section and conclusion is presented in the last section.

2 Methodology

A microscopic image dataset named C-NMC is collected from the cancer imaging archives website. The microscopic images of 26 cancer subjects and 26 normal subjects which comprises 2699 ALL images and 3389 normal B-lymphoid

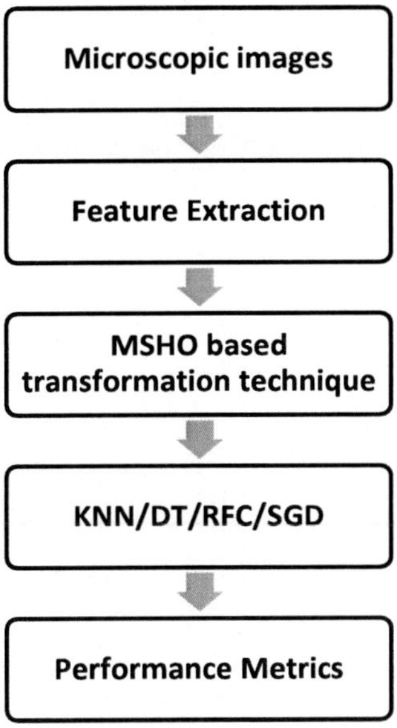

Fig. 1 Proposed methodology

precursor's images are considered in this analysis. The overall methodology followed in this work has been described in Fig. 1.

Each microscopic image is divided into 25 sub-divisions. Statistical features namely mean, variance, skewness and kurtosis are extracted from each sub-division. So the number of features obtained per microscopic image will be 100 (25 sub-divisions * 4 features). Since the SHO is a population-centered technique, the number of points of the feature under consideration should be large and for this purpose, the input image is divided into 25 sub-divisions. The ideal value for the number of sub-divisions in a single microscopic image is calculated through experiments and found as 25.

The extracted statistical features are given as input to the MSHO transform. After reaching the maximum number of iterations in MSHO, the transformed feature values will be given as input to any one of the four supervised classifiers: K-Nearest Neighbor (KNN), Decision Trees (DT), Random Forest Classifier (RFC), and Stochastic Gradient Descent (SGD). Finally the images will be categorized as either normal or leukemia and six performance metrics are calculated for comparison.

During the implementation of supervised classifiers, 80% of MRI images are considered for training, and the remaining is considered for testing. Stratified sampling is used to split the dataset into training and testing sets. To avoid overfitting and better performance, tenfold cross-validation is used. To find the best control parameters for supervised classifiers, a randomized search is utilized.

3 Spotted Hyena Optimizer

Based on the inspiration from social relationship and aggressive behavior of spotted hyena, SHO is developed [10]. The following equations represent that hunting behavior of the spotted hyena.

$$D_h = A \cdot L_h - L_k \tag{1}$$

$$L_k = L_h - E \cdot D_h \tag{2}$$

where D_h is the distance between the prey (target) and spotted hyena, L_k represents the position of all the other spotted hyenas except the first spotted hyena and L_h represents the location of the first spotted hyena, A and E are control parameters which can be represented as follows,

$$A = 2 \cdot rd_1 \tag{3}$$

$$E = 2h \cdot rd_2 - h \tag{4}$$

where

$$\mathrm{h} = 5 - (\mathrm{it} * (5/\mathrm{Maxit})) \tag{5}$$

Here "it" represents the number of iterations. Moreover the iteration value starts from 1 and goes on increasing to a limit when the closest match to the target is achieved. rd_1 and rd_2 are random vectors in [0,1]. The group of clusters with N number of optimal solutions is given by,

$$C_h = L_k + L_{k+1} + L_{k+2} + \ldots\ldots + L_{k+N} \tag{6}$$

Here N represents the total number of spotted Hyenas which can be calculated by using the below equation

$$\mathrm{N} = \mathrm{No.\ of\ count}(\mathrm{L_h}, \mathrm{L_{h+1}}, \mathrm{L_{h+2}}, \ldots\ldots, \mathrm{L_{h+M}}) \tag{7}$$

where M is a random vector in [0.5, 1]. Once the prey is located and all the hyenas are surrounded it then it can start attacking the prey. The mathematical formula to model that attack is given below

$$L(x + 1) = \frac{C_h}{N} \tag{8}$$

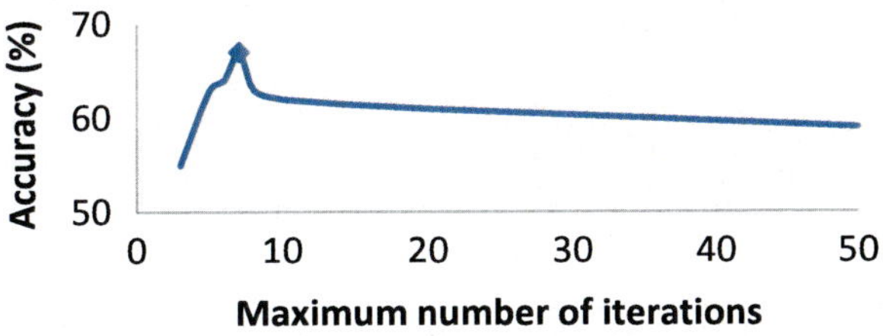

Fig. 2 Finding ideal value for maximum number of iterations

where L(x + 1) saves the best solution and updates the location of other search agents with respect to the location of the best search agent. Therefore, the SHO algorithm let all the search agents to update their position with respect to the position of the target and attack towards the target or prey.

4 SHO Based Transformation Technique

The positions of Spotted Hyenas are usually initialized randomly to train the neural networks and to solve feature selection problems. But to use SHO as transform, the statistical features are assigned as positions of Spotted Hyenas initially. Then using Eqs. (1)–(8), the positions will be updated iteratively. The best position p_{best} is identified through fitness function. The inverse of Euclidean distance between the target and current position of Spotted Hyena is considered as the fitness function.

Through experiments, it is found that the ideal value for the target is equal to 260. SHO possess two control parameters namely A and E and the values for these two control parameters are updated iteratively using Eqs. (3) and (4). Maximum number of iterations is used as termination criterion and ideal value for maximum number of iterations is found as 7 using trial and error method as shown in Fig. 2.

5 MSHO Based Transformation Technique

From Eq. (1), it is very evident that the control parameter A plays a significant role in finding the distance between the prey and the spotted hyena whereas the coefficient vector E is not needed there. Moreover, E depends upon the iteration number and A is independent of the number of iterations. So A is considered as more significant than E and the same is verified through experiments also. Hence the value of A is altered in the MSHO using Weightless Search Optimization (WSO) [11] as depicted in Fig. 3.

In WSO, 100 particles are initialized randomly and the position of those particles will be updated using equations of WSO and this will be repeated until maximum number of iterations are reached for WSO (maxit_WSO). Then mean of the 100 particles will be used to decide the value of weight, w and with respect to MSHO,

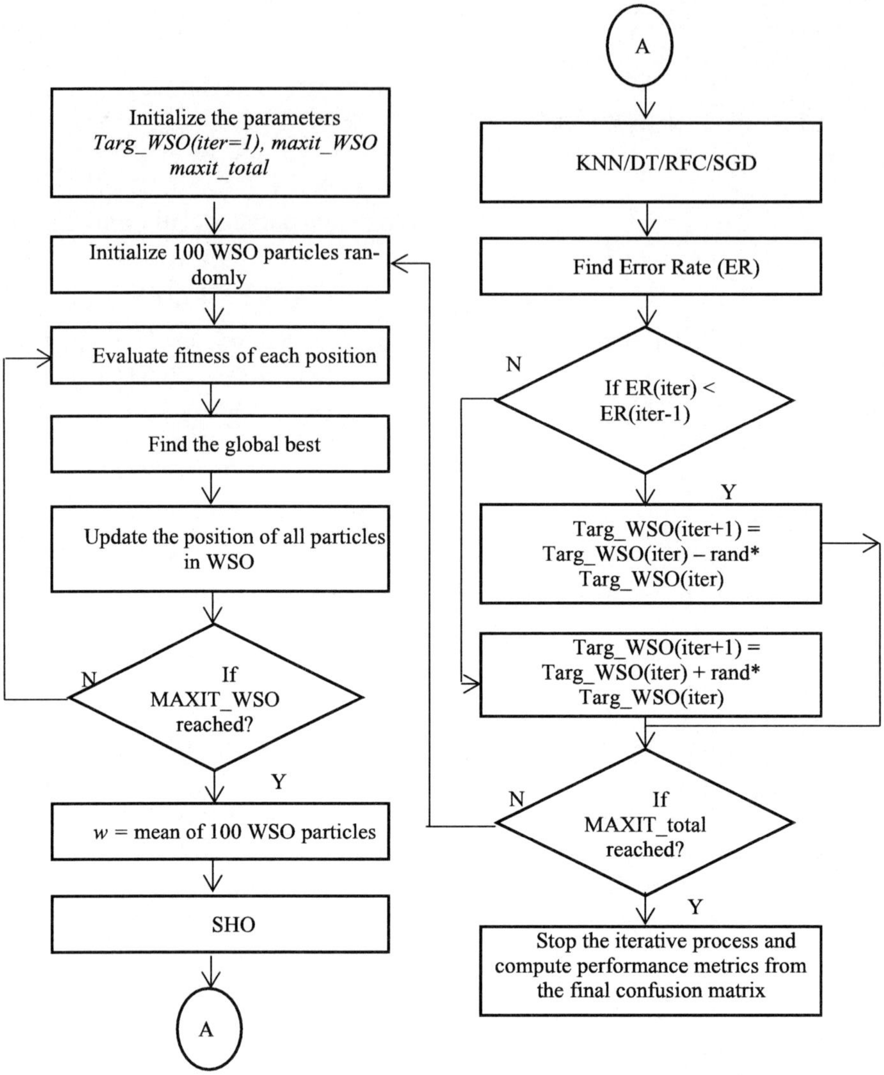

Fig. 3 Flowchart of proposed MSHO algorithm

control parameter A is considered as w. Using the new value of A, spotted hyenas positions will be updated and then the final transformed values are given as input to classifier. From the result of classifier, Error Rate (ER) will be computed and based on ER, the target of WSO (Targ_WSO) will be changed. This process will be repeated until maximum number of iterations for the total process (MAXIT_total) is met.

6 Results and Discussion

The performances of all the classifiers are quantized using the six different commonly used metrics namely Accuracy (ACC), F1 score, Mathews Correlation Coefficient (MCC), Error Rate (ER), Sensitivity (SENS) and Specificity (SPEC) [12]. These metrics are computed for all the four base classifiers without any transform and mentioned as KNN, DT, RFC and SGD in Table 1. To substantiate the results produced by SHO and MSHO, another popular SI technique, PSO is used as transform. The capacity of the proposed MSHO transform can be clearly seen in Fig. 4 through accuracy comparison. The highest accuracy of 90% is achieved when MSHO is used as transform for SGD while 83% and 65% accuracies are achieved for SGD in case of SHO transform and no transform usage respectively. It is also worthy to note that, the proposed MSHO enhances accuracy of all the four classifiers significantly.

Table 1 Simulation results

	ACC	F1	MCC	ER	SENS	SPEC
KNN	54	50	8	46	46	62
DT	60	57	19	40	54	65
RFC	63	63	27	37	62	65
SGD	65	63	31	35	58	73
PSO-KNN	58	56	15	42	54	62
PSO-DT	65	64	31	35	62	69
PSO-RFC	69	69	38	31	69	69
PSO-SGD	69	68	39	31	65	73
SHO-KNN	67	67	35	33	65	69
SHO-DT	75	75	50	25	73	77
SHO-RFC	77	77	54	23	77	77
SHO-SGD	83	83	65	17	85	81
MPSO-KNN	65	64	31	35	62	69
MPSO-DT	71	71	42	29	69	73
MPSO-RFC	75	75	50	25	77	73
MPSO-SGD	77	76	54	23	73	81
MSHO-KNN	79	78	58	21	77	81
MSHO-DT	85	85	69	15	85	85
MSHO-RFC	87	86	73	13	85	88
MSHO-SGD	90	91	81	10	92	88

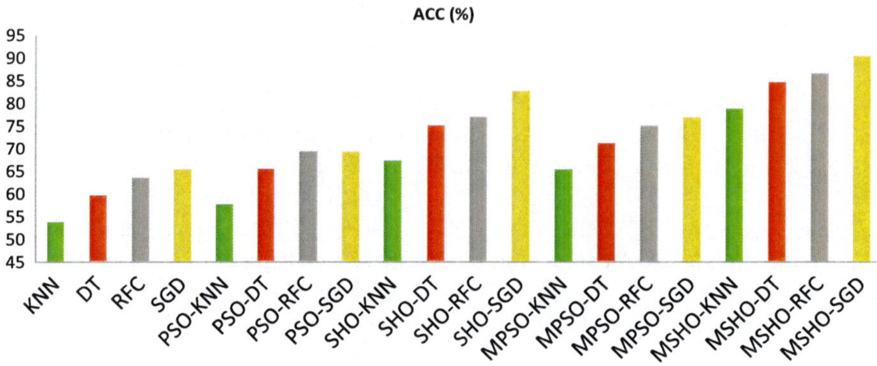

Fig. 4 Accuracy comparison

7 Conclusion

To classify the leukemia microscopic images, machine learning techniques are widely used. But the accuracy of the machine learning technique is a biggest issue and researchers are searching for the ways to improve it. This research work implements the MSHO algorithm as transform for increasing the performance of four machine learning techniques namely KNN, DT, RFC, and SGD in leukemia microscopic image classification. The control parameter of SHO namely A is updated using WSO in the proposed MSHO transform and it offers better results comparatively. Notably highest accuracy of 90% is attained for SGD when MSHO transform is used. Through Table 1, the capacity of MSHO to improve all the four classifiers' performance can be witnessed clearly. In future, other optimization algorithms need to be tested.

References

1. Vapnik, V.: Statistical Learning Theory. John Wiley & Sons (1998)
2. Xing, F., Yang, L.: Machine learning and its application in microscopic image analysis. In: The Elsevier and MICCAI Society Book Series, pp. 97–127 (2016)
3. Mirjalili, S., Mirjalili, S.M., Lewis, A.: Grey wolf optimizer. Adv. Eng. Soft. **69**, 46–61 (2014)
4. Sahab, M.G.: A review on traditional and modern structural optimization: problems and techniques. Metaheuristic Appl. Struct. Infrastruct. (2019). https://doi.org/10.1016/B978-0-12-398364-0.00002-4
5. Yang, X.-S.: Particle swarm optimization. Nat.-Inspired Optim. Algorithms **8**, 111–121 (2021)
6. Binitha, S., Siva Sathya, S.: A survey of bio inspired optimization algorithms. Int. J. Soft Comput. Eng. **2**(2),137–151 (2012)
7. Koumi, F., Aldasht, M., Tamimi, H.: Efficient feature selection using particle swarm optimization: a hybrid filters-wrapper approach. In: 10th International Conference on Information and Communication Systems (ICICS), Irbid, Jordan (2019)
8. Bharanidharan, N., Rajaguru, H.: Dementia MRI image classification using transformation technique based on elephant herding optimization with Randomized Adam method for updating

the hyper-parameters. Int. J. Imaging Syst. Technol. 1–25 (2020). https://doi.org/10.1002/ima.22522
9. Bharanidharan, N., Harikumar, R.: Modified grey wolf randomized optimization in dementia classification using MRI images. IETE J. Res. 1–10 (2019). https://doi.org/10.1080/03772063.2020.1715852
10. Dhiman. G., Kumar. V.: Spotted Hyena optimizer—a novel bio-inspired based metaheuristic technique for engineering applications. Adv. Eng. Softw. **114**, 48–70 (2017)
11. Ting, T.O., Man, K.L., Guan, S.-U., Nayel, M., Wan, K.: Weightless swarm algorithm (WSA) for dynamic optimization problems. Netw. Parallel Comput. 508–515 (2012)
12. Fielding, A.H.: Cluster and Classification Techniques for the Biosciences. Cambridge University Press, Cambridge (2006)

A Strategic Corrective Maintenance Prioritization Assessment for Medical Equipment

Aizat Hilmi Zamzam, Ayman Khallel Ibrahim Al-Ani, Khairunnisa Hasikin, and Ahmad Khairi Abdul Wahab

Abstract The utilization of effective medical equipment significantly contributes to the quality of healthcare services. Breakdown of medical equipment can jeopardize healthcare delivery, maintenance expenditure, and resources. The implementation of equipment assessment for corrective maintenance throughout the equipment life cycle during the maintenance phase may enhance the medical equipment reliability and availability. The study aims to develop the corrective maintenance prioritization assessment system in managing the rectification work of breakdown medical equipment. The proposed system was developed by considering nine medical equipment features, which involve 1028 equipment with 19 categories located in public health clinics. The assessment of medical equipment uses the machine learning of k-Means clustering technique to analyze the equipment database to generate priority levels. The assessment by applying the k-Means clustering algorithm classifies the medical equipment into three priority levels. The corrective maintenance prioritization assessment system can assist the clinical engineers in managing the rectification expenditure, reporting, preparation, workforce, and material. This prioritization system can be incorporated with a real-time asset management database system in healthcare institutions for continuous supervision.

Keywords Medical device · Unsupervised machine learning · Prioritization

1 Introduction

The efficacy of healthcare services significantly depends on the medical equipment [1]. Nowadays, the production of high technological medical equipment plays a more vital part in modern healthcare [2]. Furthermore, the achievement of healthcare

A. H. Zamzam · A. K. I. Al-Ani · K. Hasikin (✉) · A. K. A. Wahab
Department of Biomedical Engineering, Faculty of Engineering, Universiti Malaya, 50603 Kuala Lumpur, Malaysia
e-mail: khairunnisa@um.edu.my

A. H. Zamzam
Engineering Services Division, Ministry of Health Malaysia, 62590 Putrajaya, Malaysia

J. Usman et al. (eds.), *6th Kuala Lumpur International Conference on Biomedical Engineering 2021*, IFMBE Proceedings 86,
https://doi.org/10.1007/978-3-030-90724-2_15

institution cost-effectiveness and the quality of healthcare delivery hinge on the management of medical equipment maintenance effectiveness throughout the service life [3]. Hence, it is important to keep the equipment up, maintain safety, and mitigate the breakdown rate [4].

Lack of maintenance, preparation, and management are the common basis of medical equipment failure [5]. The breakdown of the equipment substantially jeopardizes the delivery of healthcare services to the community and affects the profitability of the healthcare institution. A strategic corrective maintenance program may assist the clinical engineers in rectifying the breakdown equipment in an effective way.

This paper aims to develop the corrective maintenance prioritization assessment system in managing the rectification work of breakdown medical equipment. The assessment of medical equipment applies the machine learning technique to analyze and measure the equipment database to generate priority levels. The application of machine learning can overcome the manual involvement in mathematical approaches in determining the criteria weightages. Besides, the proposed model in this study may assess various types of medical equipment utilized in healthcare institution.

This proposed model may assist the clinical engineers to prioritize the medical equipment corrective maintenance and strategize a better preparation on the rectification activities. Identification of priority degree in preparation process contributes to a better execution work planning [6].

2 Methods

The proposed model of the medical equipment corrective maintenance prioritization assessment system is presented in Fig. 1.

The model comprises several processes, which are dataset requirement, data preprocessing and organizing, feature extraction, data normalization, cluster analysis and prioritization clusters. To begin the process of achieving the corrective maintenance prioritization clusters, there are nine features of medical equipment involved. These nine features are associated with equipment in terms of purpose, maintenance history, and condition. The cluster analysis and measurement of corrective maintenance prioritization assessment system on these features use the k-Means clustering

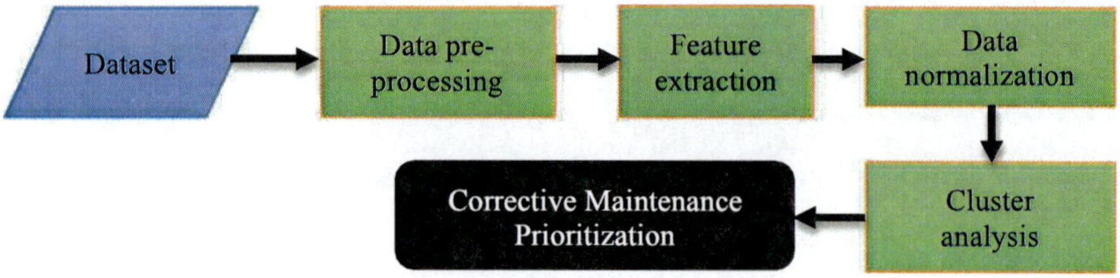

Fig. 1 Block diagram of the corrective maintenance prioritization assessment

technique [7]. This k-Means technique is an approach of separating and partitioning the specific dataset into pre-determined numbers. The selection of this clustering technique is done based on several related studies made and it is observed as a suitable partitioning method [8–10]. The development tools of corrective maintenance prioritization assessment model use MATLAB R2020b with several toolboxes, which are Statistics and Machine Learning Toolbox, Classification Learner Toolbox and Optimization Toolbox.

2.1 Dataset

The dataset of 1028 units with various types of medical equipment is the sample of this model development. The several medical equipment types comprised of emergency, laboratory, imaging, and physiology equipment were acquired from the asset management record of public health clinics in Malaysia. The records of 19 categories were taken from the year of 2015 to October 2020 as a cut-off period. Table 1 tabulates the category and quantity of medical equipment involved in this study.

Table 1 Category and quantity of medical equipment

Medical equipment	Quantity
Automated chemistry analyzer	4
Laboratory Bilirubinometer	59
Automatic external defibrillator	62
Manual external defibrillators	47
Densitometers	8
Infant incubators	7
Infusion pumps	2
Laryngoscopes	25
Physiologic monitoring systems	31
Nonheated nebulizers	158
Pulse oximeter	77
Phototherapy units	5
General Xray machine	37
Manual pulmonary resuscitator	38
Pharmacy weighing unit	3
Ultrasonic scanner	121
Sensitometers	7
Autoclave unit	321
Treadmills	16

Table 2 Medical equipment features and criteria

Features	Criteria
Function	Life support (5); therapeutic (4); diagnostic (3); analytic (2); miscellaneous (1)
Request to repair time (response time)	Time to respond to the breakdown equipment (average/day)
Maintenance complexity	Extensive maintenance (3); average maintenance (2); Visual inspection and basic check (1)
Repair time	Duration of the equipment repair (average/day)
Number of failures	Frequency of equipment failures (vary)
Asset status	Functioning (0); malfunctioning (1)
Backup or alternative unit	Yes (0); No (1)
Operations	Criticality (6–1)
Maintenance cost	Accumulation of repair expenses (vary)

* (5)—ranges of rating

The inputs of nine medical equipment features involve various criteria in light of the medical equipment descriptions. Table 2 shows the medical equipment features and criteria.

Function. Refers to the medical equipment service intention [3, 4], which consists of five criteria. Life support refers to highly essential equipment, which could harm the patient life and cause of death if the unit fails to operate properly. The remediation and treatment of a patient's illness refer to the therapeutic equipment, whereas detecting any possibility of diseases refers to diagnostic equipment. Any laboratory process of taking human samples for further analysis refers to the analytical equipment and any equipment used to assist the main medical activity refers to miscellaneous equipment.

Request to Repair Time. Time taken by the maintenance personnel to attend any equipment breakdown after receiving a report from the users [3]. The longer response time can cause a healthcare service disruption.

Maintenance Complexity. Comprises of extensive maintenance, average maintenance, and basic inspection [11, 12]. Extensive maintenance requires highly skilled workers to upkeep and troubleshoot the medical equipment. Checking and testing procedures, which involve safety and performance tests refer to average maintenance whereas visual examination, functional test, cleaning, and battery replacement are duties in basic maintenance.

Repair Time. Also known as Mean Time to Repair (MTTR). This feature is the duration of undertaking the equipment repair, recondition and overhaul works [3, 4]. The longer duration of repairs may disrupt the healthcare services to the patients.

Number of Failures. The number of failure events throughout the equipment service life [13, 14]. Require further attention for the higher number of failure events.

Asset Status. It consists of functioning and non-functioning status. The equipment is considered malfunctioning when it fails to operate as specified by the manufacturer.

Backup or Alternative Unit. Refers to temporary substitute equipment during the breakdown of main unit [15, 16]. The allocation of temporary substitute equipment is beneficial to avoid discontinue of medical services due to the failure of main equipment.

Operations. This segregation of this feature comprises six utilization levels and has been registered into asset management record.

Maintenance Cost. The maintenance cost refers to the rectification and overhaul expenses [17], which covers materials, workmanship, and administration.

2.2 *Corrective Maintenance Prioritization Assessment System*

The ultimate objective of this corrective maintenance prioritization assessment system is to assign the medical equipment into specified groups based on the features and criteria obtained. The groups are divided into three, which are high, medium, and low. The application of the k-Means clustering technique on the equipment dataset partitions the medical equipment into these three groups and turns the list of data to labelled dataset. From the labelled dataset, the priorities of corrective maintenance exercise can be recognized.

The data pre-processing involves the raw dataset conversion into the medical equipment features elements. At this process, only the equipment status of malfunctioning is considered. Then, the dataset requires a normalization process, where the values of every feature and criterion are significantly wide-ranging. The normalization of the dataset is important to ensure the distance of every feature value is weighted proportionately to avoid measurement domination and outlier creation. Therefore, the dataset is scaled with mean is equal to 0 and standard deviation is equal to 1, where the calculations are based on the following formulas:

$$z - score = \frac{\chi - \mu}{\sigma} \tag{1}$$

$$\sigma = \sqrt{\frac{1}{n-1}\sum_{i=1}^{n}(\chi i - \overline{\mathrm{X}})} \tag{2}$$

where χ is the equipment data, μ is mean, σ is standard deviation, and n is the number of equipment. The configuration of k-Means parameters has been fined-tune, where the distance metric is set to Squared Euclidean and replicate is set to 5 before proceeding to clustering analysis. The distance metric calculation is based on the following formulation:

$$d(x, c) = (x - c)(x - c)' \tag{3}$$

where d is the distance, x is the equipment feature value, and c is the centroid.

3 Results

The corrective maintenance prioritization assessment system results, which consists of three priority levels is tabulated in Table 3. The corrective maintenance prioritization assessment system involves eight features of medical equipment, which considers only breakdown equipment before normalization data and subsequently the process of clustering measurement. Thus, all functioning and good condition of the equipment have been omitted in this process. The total of 1028 units of medical equipment are segregated into three priority levels for the purpose of corrective maintenance prioritization and the numbers of unit at every level are presented in Table 3.

Table 4 summarizes the results of the clustering analysis on medical equipment for the corrective maintenance prioritization system. The system only considers malfunctioning medical equipment and thus, asset status at all priority level is malfunctioning. The low priority medical equipment of corrective maintenance prioritization demonstrates that the highest readings of response time are six days, the time taken to repair the equipment is 29 days, and the highest number of breakdowns is eight times. Furthermore, there is a substitute temporary equipment and the maximum accumulation of repair cost is MYR8k. The medium corrective maintenance prioritization level indicates that the longest response time and rectification time are 69 and 253 days, respectively. Besides, the equipment classified under this level requires performance and safety tests, or basic routine inspection. There is no temporary substitute unit and the highest rectification total cost is MYR10k. The high priority of equipment requires vital attention for corrective maintenance. In this priority level, the highest response time is 148 days, time to repair is 478 days, and the number of failures is up to 29 times throughout its service life. The high priority equipment

Table 3 Priority levels of medical equipment

	Level of priority		
	High	Medium	Low
No. of medical equipment	375	651	2

Table 4 Corrective maintenance prioritization system findings

Equipment features	Level		
	Low	Medium	High
Asset status response time (max. days)	Malfunctioning 6 days (average)	Malfunctioning 69 days (average)	Malfunctioning 148 days (average)
Maintenance complexity	–	1–2 (Basic check and average maintenance)	3 (Extensive maintenance)
Repair time (max. days)	29 days (average)	253 days (average)	478 days (average)
Number of failures (max.)	8 times	9 times	26 times
Backup and alternative unit	Yes	No	No
Maintenance cost	Highest cost: MYR8k	Highest cost: MYR10k	Highest cost: MYR86k

needs extensive technical work during maintenance activity. Moreover, no temporary substitute unit is provided and the most expensive repair work is MYR86k.

By considering eight medical equipment features and its criteria, it summarizes the total number of 1028 malfunctioning medical equipment are successfully prioritized by using the k-Means clustering method. Table 4 shows that the high priority level comprises of high characteristics of medical equipment compared to medium and low priority equipment. Furthermore, the low priority level significantly shows that the substantial indications of medical equipment fall under this category can be seen on its response time, repair time, backup and alternative units, and maintenance expenditure.

4 Discussion

The configuration of Squared Euclidean distance with replication number to 5 by applying the k-Means method is capable to develop a practical corrective maintenance prioritization assessment system of medical equipment. The priority levels generated from this system can assist clinical engineers who oversee and monitor the performance of medical equipment by prioritizing the corrective maintenance workload. Furthermore, the identification of medical equipment priority level in corrective maintenance is purely dependent on the database, where there is no user's involvement which requires great expertise and comprehensive knowledge. The analysis of patterns and trends in the medical equipment database determine the degree of priority. As a result, the outcomes of the system harmonize three aspects of management, clinical, and technical, and the priority level output can be generated rapidly and consistently.

The system could assist clinical engineers in understanding the actual failure of the equipment. This understanding leads the clinical engineers in preparing the appropriate report on corrective maintenance, which can cover scheduling, workforce and material to restore the malfunctioning equipment. Connecting and interacting among profession is difficult in the healthcare sector [18]. Through the effective report, this difficulty could be mitigated.

The application of this system could assist clinical engineers in managing the medical equipment corrective maintenance especially related to financial matters. The expenditures of replacement parts, third party service providers, materials, and tools can be managed from the indication of equipment priority level for corrective maintenance. In addition, the clinical engineers may control the regular and daily assignment by planning the effective program of corrective maintenance in accordance with the equipment priority level. The higher level may alert the clinical engineers to perform a thorough examination of the breakdown equipment in identifying the root-cause. Hence, the clinical engineers may devise a better corrective maintenance strategy for better equipment reliability and safety to use.

5 Conclusion

This study established the medical equipment corrective maintenance prioritization assessment system using the k-Means clustering technique. It can be a supportive tool during the maintenance phase of the equipment life cycle, which involves restoration, rectification and overhaul activities. This clustering method seems to be appropriate in prioritizing the medical equipment into three priority levels. This partitioning technique appears to be adequate in categorizing the medical equipment into three priority degrees. The system may avoid manual involvement in mathematical measurement, which need substantial expertise in clinical, technical and managerial aspects. Moreover, it can be applied in any kind of medical equipment stationed in the healthcare facility. This supportive tool can assist in terms of maintenance schedule, expenses control, resources handling, and reporting preparation. Thus, the reliability, availability and safety aspects of medical equipment can be achieved in delivering better healthcare services to the community. The corrective maintenance prioritization assessment system can be integrated with the existing real-time archive to provide a comprehensive function to the asset management system.

References

1. Badnjević, A., et al.: Measurement in medicine—past, present, future **50**(1), (2015)
2. Eliash, C., Lazar, I., Nissim, N.: SEC-C-U: the security of intensive care unit medical devices and their ecosystems. IEEE Access **8**, 64193–64224 (2020)

3. Hamdi, N., et al.: An intelligent healthcare management system: a new approach in work-order prioritization for medical equipment maintenance requests. J. Med. Syst. **36**(2), 557–567 (2012)
4. Jamshidi, A., et al.: A comprehensive fuzzy risk-based maintenance framework for prioritization of medical devices. Appl. Soft Comput. **32**, 322–334 (2015)
5. Wang, B., Rice, W.P.: JCAHO's equipment inclusion criteria revisited—application of statistical sampling technique. J. Clin. Eng. **28**(1), 37–48 (2003)
6. Santoso, L.W., et al.: Cluster analysis to determine the priority of operating room scheduling. In: AIP Conference Proceedings, pp. 020058. AIP Publishing LLC (2018)
7. Paluszek, M., Thomas, S.: MATLAB machine learning. Apress (2016)
8. Jayatilake, S.M.D.A.C., Ganegoda, G.U.: Involvement of machine learning tools in healthcare decision making. J. Healthcare Eng. **2021**, 6679512 (2021)
9. Wu, W., et al.: Decision-making support for the evaluation of clustering algorithms based on MCDM. Complexity **2020**, 9602526 (2020)
10. Koksal, A., Ozdemir, A., Ata, O.: RCAM based maintenance plan of the power transformers using k-means clustering algorithm. In: 2017 19th International Conference on Intelligent System Application to Power Systems (ISAP), pp. 1–6. (2017)
11. Ben Houria, Z., et al.: Quantitative techniques for medical equipment maintenance management. European J. Ind. Eng. **10**(6), 703–723 (2016)
12. Hutagalung, A.O., Hasibuan, S.: Determining the priority of medical equipment maintenance with analytical hierarchy process. Int. J. Online Biomed. Eng. **15**(10), 107–120 (2019)
13. Jarikji, Y., Hussein, B., H.-H. M.: A quantitative model for replacement of medical equipment based on technical and economic factors. Int. J. Artif. Organs **42**(8), 278–285 (2019)
14. Saleh, N., Balestra, G.: Comprehensive framework for preventive maintenance priority of medical equipment. In: 2015 37th Annual International Conference of the IEEE Engineering in Medicine and Biology Society. pp. 1227–1230 (2015)
15. Saleh, N., et al.: Preventive maintenance prioritization index of medical equipment using quality function deployment. IEEE J. Biomed. Health Inform. **19**(3), 1029–1035 (2015)
16. Taghipour, S., Banjevic, D., Jardine, A.K.S.: Prioritization of medical equipment for maintenance decisions. J. Oper. Res. Soc. **62**(9), 1666–1687 (2011)
17. Tawfik, B., Ouda, B.K., Abd El Samad, Y.M.: A fuzzy logic model for medical equipment risk classification. J. Clin. Eng. **38**(4), 185–190 (2013)
18. Curtis, K., Tzannes, A., Rudge, T.: How to talk to doctors—a guide for effective communication. Int. Nurs. Rev **58**(1), 13–20 (2011)

Detection of Knee Osteoarthritis and Prediction of Its Severity Using X-ray Image Analysis and Patients Assessment Data: A Hybrid Design

Hamidreza Mohafez, Hamza Sayed, Maryam Hadizadeh, Lai Khin Wee, and Siti Anom Ahmad

Abstract Knee osteoarthritis (KOA) is a degenerative disease associated with cartilage loss, causes limitations in the range of movement, and known to be one of the most disabling age-associated diseases around the world. It is vital to predict its presence and severity at early stage to tailor the interventions and treatments properly. Traditionally, X-ray Images are graded by radiologists to quantify KOA severity; however, this approach suffers from high levels of subjectivity due to the semi-quantitative nature of grading systems. Numerous attempts have been made to recruit automated X-ray image analysis to quantify KOA severity, but few studies have used pertinent assessment data such as symptoms and medications being used to establish accurate predictive model. So, we proposed a statistical model built on combination of features extracted from X-ray images and patients' data using ordinal regression analysis. The results revealed that the developed model based on combination of KOA X-ray key features and patient assessment data is able to predict the severity of KOA with high level of accuracy (89.2%) and acceptable level of inter-rater reliability with quadratic weighted Cohen's Kappa coefficient (QWK) of 0.8337. The study outcomes suggested that variables showing impaired knee functions are the best indicators to quantify knee OA presence and severity that may be used in conjunction with X-ray biomarkers for developing intervention and targeted treatment.

Keywords Knee osteoarthritis · X-ray image analysis · Kellgren-Lawrence · Model development · Early detection · Joint space width · Patient assessment data

H. Mohafez (✉) · H. Sayed · L. K. Wee
Department of Biomedical Engineering, Faculty of Engineering, Universiti Malaya, Jalan Universiti, 50603 Kuala Lumpur, Malaysia
e-mail: h.mohafez@um.edu.my

M. Hadizadeh
Centre for Sport and Exercise Sciences, Universiti Malaya, Jalan Universiti, 50603 Kuala Lumpur, Malaysia

S. A. Ahmad
Department of Electrical and Electronic Engineering, Faculty of Engineering, Universiti Putra Malaysia, Selangor, Malaysia

J. Usman et al. (eds.), *6th Kuala Lumpur International Conference on Biomedical Engineering 2021*, IFMBE Proceedings 86,
https://doi.org/10.1007/978-3-030-90724-2_16

1 Introduction

Knee osteoarthritis (KOA) is a rheumatic disorder that causes the degeneration of articular cartilage in the knee joint and is the most common type of OA as it affected 263 million people worldwide [1]. There is no specific cause of the disease, however, several factors such as obesity, age, joint trauma can increase the possibility of having KOA. Moreover, female gender seems to be associated with higher prevalence and severity of KOA than male gender Pain is the most prominent symptom of KOA which can ranges from hardly perceptible to agonizing and further immobilizing. Other symptoms include stiffness, restricted movement of the knee and impairment between the healthy knee and the diseased knee [2, 3]. KOA treatment strategies aim only to relive pain and restore mobility through using treatment plans usually include weight loss, exercise, injections of pain killers and anti-inflammatory medications, physical and occupational therapy and finally, surgeries such as arthroplasty, osteotomy or joint replacement [4]. There is a high demand to quantify the severity of KOA at early stages owing to its deniable impacts on disability and patient's economic status. Knowing the severity level of knee OA facilitates the determination of appropriate intervention to be taken and helps monitoring of its progression over time. In the state of art, the gold standard procedure for the diagnosis of KOA is a clinical examination followed by X-ray imaging analysis of the knee. Knee radiographs are evaluated by a trained radiologist to detect changes in the cartilage by evaluating joint space width (JSW), presence of changes in the bone structure such as the formation of osteophytes and subchondral sclerosis and grading the severity of the condition using widely used grading system, Kellgren and Lawrence (KL) [5]. However, KL grade system only provides a semi-quantitative scale, which causes ambiguity and uncertainty; and suffers from subjectivity leads to disagreement among raters [6]. In addition, the X-ray images are insensitive at early stage and in case that only acquired one time [7].

So, computer aided diagnosis has been used to overcome the subjectivity of KOA quantification through X-ray image analysis. Several attempts have been made to develop automated and semi-automated prediction of KOA severity using X-ray image analysis [7–9]. However, all these attempts could not manage to solve the subjectivity of KL grading system due to lack of patients' data being used in prediction of KOA severity [2]. As a result, developing a statistical model based on patients' data such as functional impairment, pain, symptoms, and whether being under medication may strengthen prediction ability by introducing variables that strongly contribute towards KOA prediction and offer additional advantages by reducing the cost of treatment and early-stage interventions. Moreover, fusion of patients' data and features extracted from X-ray images may diminish the subjectivity of available grading systems.

2 Materials and Methods

2.1 Data Collection

We used the Osteoarthritis Initiative (OAI) database collected from multi-center longitudinal and observational study of knee OA which is accessible at https://nda.nih.gov/oai/.

2.1.1 Database and Data Screening Procedure

The OAI dataset holds X-ray images (from both knees) of 4796 patients and their questionnaire data at baseline which contains 92 variables (binary, ordinal, and continuous) such as medication history, functional impairment, their vital signs, and symptoms of KOA such as pain. The database was manually inspected to select a subset of candidate predictors clinically relevant and formerly known as risk factors for KOA [3, 10]. Then, the completeness of the data in terms of missing values for each candidate features was checked and those with less than 10% missing values were kept for further analysis. Initial screening revealed that only 2951 individuals with the mean age of 60.5 ± 9.1 years, have sufficient questionnaire data on the 16 potential candidate features. To make the manual delineation of ROI by an experienced radiologist feasible, it's required to reduce the number of subjects to a manageable amount of X-ray images. The priori power analysis using G-power software was performed by setting effect size to medium ($f^2 = 0.15$), the significance level (α) to 0.05, the power ($(1 - \beta)$ to 0.8, and number of predictors to 16 (Number of clinically relevant candidate features from patient's characteristics) with the estimated required sample size of 143 (number of knees). So, 72 individuals from 5 patient groups (0–4 grades) were randomly selected with respect to their distribution in OAI database. Table 1 shows the distribution of KOA severity in OAI database and our experimental setup.

Two experts independently assessed, blinded to each other's rating, all images in OAI database using KL grading system; and disagreements between them were adjudged in a consensus session with the presence of a third reader. In case the ratings were not adjudged, a senior expert radiologist made the final decision.

Table 1 Distribution of KOA severity within OAI database and used dataset

Level of severity	OAI database	Used dataset
Level 0 (Normal)	1251	30
Level 1 (Doubtful)	520	13
Level 2 (Mild)	730	18
Level 3 (Moderate)	370	9
Level 4 (Severe)	80	2

2.1.2 Image Processing Chains

The OAI database includes bilateral posteroanterior (PA) fixed flexion view X-ray images acquired at an irradiation angle of 10° tilt in the caudal direction such that the anterior thigh contacted with the cassette, tips of the toes placed on the same plane as of the cassette, and the feet externally rotated 10°.

Joint space width (JSW) is mainly used as a determinant quantitative feature in monitoring extremity and progression of knee osteoarthritis [11, 12]. Although the segmentation of tibiofemoral joint as the region of interest (ROI) commonly was preformed manually through using hand drawn contours and cropping of the joint area, it's time consuming and tedious. So, lots of semi-automated and fully automated algorithms were proposed [8, 13, 14]. We designed a protocol for manual segmentation of tibiofemoral joint by developing a graphical user interface (GUI) in MATLAB which helped the radiologist to manually select the tibiofemoral joint and crop it from the pre-processed X-ray images using a hand-drawn rectangular contour, followed by delineating the femur and tibial edges and identifying the medial condyle and lateral condyle of tibial plateau. Then, the radiologist identified the minimum vertical distance between the tibial plateau and femur edge of medial and lateral sides to calculate the medial joint space width (JSW_M) and lateral joint space width (JSW_L), respectively (Fig. 1). In our experiment, an experienced radiologist applied the delineation protocol on 144 X-ray images repeatedly, 5 times with at

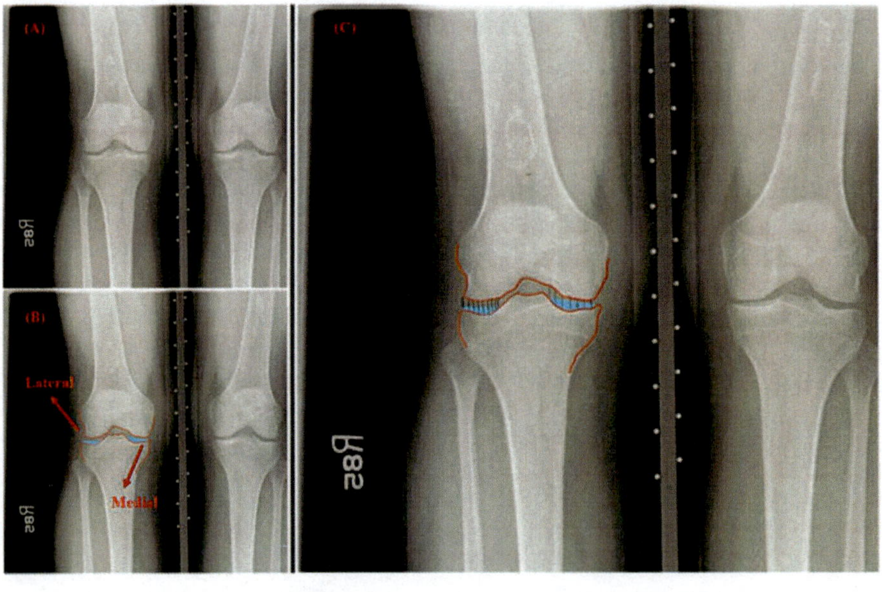

Fig. 1 Manual segmentation of tibiofemoral joint. **a** Pre-processed KOA X-ray bilateral images; **b** delineation of the femur and tibial edges and identification of the medial condyle and lateral condyle of tibial plateau; **c** The minimum vertical distance between the tibial plateau and femur edge of medial and lateral sides was identified by a radiologist and then calculated

least 20-min intervals between delineations to avoid learning. It's reported that the best repeatability will be achieved if a single clinician delineates all knee images, each one, if possible, several times [15]. The pre-processing chain and delineation protocol for manual segmentation of ROI can be found in supplementary material 1.

The estimated repeatability coefficient (RC) and Intra-class Correlation Coefficient (ICC) were used as a measure of intra-operator repeatability and intra-operator reliability, respectively. In other words, the consistency of single radiologist in segmentation of tibiofemoral joint for all 144 X-ray images (72 subjects) was evaluated through above mentioned parameters using SPSS for Windows, version 24.

2.2 Data Analysis

The research final goal was to develop a reproducible, accurate and objective method for prediction of knee osteoarthritis presence and severity through information obtained from X-ray images and patient's data. So, 3 statistical models were developed based on features extracted from X-ray images (JSW_M and JSW_L), from patients' data, and combination of these two types of information. We used K-fold cross validation approach to evaluate and compare the three developed models, and the same training and testing sets were used in all 3 models to have valid comparisons among them. Then, the error is averaged across all "K" trials. The details of model development and performance evaluation are as follows.

2.2.1 Model Development Based on X-ray Features, Patients' Questionnaire Data, and Their Combination

Although KL grade score suffers from subjectivity, it's required to build the statistical models based on KL grade score (ordinal scale 0–4) as there is no gold standard to predict KOA severity. Due to having an ordinal outcome, severity of KOA, the ordinal logistic regression analysis was used to build the predictive model. So, the ordinal logistic regression model was fitted on training data set and its prediction performance was tested on validation set. That is to say, the coefficients of two predictors, JSW_M and JSW_L, were estimated using training set, followed by performance evaluation of developed model using validation set.

The patient's questionnaire data at baseline contains 92 variables (binary, ordinal, and continuous) such as medication history, functional impairment, their vital signs, and symptoms of KOA such as pain. After manual inspection of questionnaire data, 16 clinically relevant candidate predictors were selected (supplementary material 2), followed by checking their possible multicollinearity to avoid information redundancy by using Pearson correlation, polychoric correlation, and polyserial correlations between continuous variables, between categorical predictors, and between continuous and categorical variables, respectively. Then, the ordinal logistic regression was fitted on the whole dataset (144 images) to determine which of independent variables (out of 16) have statistically significant effect on our outcome variable, KOA severity; and to identify how well our model was able to predict the outcome. Afterwards, the ordinal logistic regression model was fitted on training data set (coefficient estimation of candidate patients' questionnaire data) and its prediction performance was tested on validation set using the K-fold cross validation technique.

Finally, using patients' questionnaire data together with features extracted from X-ray images may lead to identify key variables with higher predictive performance, compensate the subjectivity of KL grading system, and be useful in monitoring the patients over time and designing early treatments. So, we combined the candidate predictors from patients' data, those had statistically significant effect on outcome variable, with JSW_M and JSW_L taken from X-ray images, followed by developing statistical model using ordinal logistic regression as detailed above.

The performance of the three developed models was validated and compared using three measures: accuracy (ACC), mean absolute error (MAE), mean and quadratic weighted Cohen's Kappa coefficient (QWK) [16, 17].

3 Results and Discussion

3.1 *Manual Segmentation of Tibiofemoral Joint Collection*

The estimated RC (i.e. measure of agreement between delineations made on the same image) was 0.062 ± 0.02 mm and 0.081 ± 0.03 for JSW_M and JSW_L, respectively meaning that difference between any two delineations of individual image by that individual operator was estimated to be no more than 0.062 mm and 0.081 mm (for JSW_M and JSW_L, respectively) on 95% of occasions and laid on the confidence interval 0.042–0.082 mm and 0.051–0.11 mm. Based on the rule of thumb proposed by Fayers and Machin [18], the ICC = 0.816 for JSW_M and ICC = 0.835 for JSW_L are considered high as a measure of intra-operator reliability of manual segmentation. This means 8.4 and 6.5% of variability in measurement of JSW_M and JSW_L, quality measure of manual delineation, were estimated due to the error of measurement process and the operator involved. So, the results indicated that the proposed protocol for manual segmentation of tibiofemoral joint can properly work in case of manageable number of X-ray images.

3.2 *Meaningful Predictors from Patient Assessment Data*

The deviance goodness-of-fit test indicated that the regression model fitted to the observed data, $\chi^2(364) = 182.723$, $p = 0.860$. We ran the GENLIN procedure to estimate the parameters of the model. Out of eight categorical candidate predictors, the following five had statistically significant effect on outcome variable, severity of KOA: Sex ($p = 0.023$), used medication for pain, aching or stiffness past 12 months ($p = 0.041$), having surgery on right knee ($p = 0.031$), having surgery on left knee ($p = 0.039$), and ever Dr. said patient has rheumatoid arthritis or other inflammatory arthritis ($p = 0.015$). In addition, the following continuous predictors had statistically significant on outcome variable: Right knee pain during walking ($p = 0.027$), left knee pain during walking ($p = 0.034$), left knee symptoms: knee catch or hang up when moving ($p = 0.038$), and right knee symptoms: knee catch or hang up when moving ($p = 0.026$). So, we managed to determine the patient assessment variables with the highest predictive ability of KOA (9 out of 16) which may help the clinicians to design and implement appropriate intervention at early stage. The results revealed that variables showing impaired knee functions are the best indicators to quantify knee OA presence and severity that may be used in conjunction with X-ray biomarkers for developing early intervention and targeted treatment which were in line with the findings of previous studies [3, 10].

3.3 *Model Evaluation and Comparison*

Table 2 illustrates the performance of three developed model using ordinal regression analysis on validation data set for different K values during K-fold cross validation. The results indicate that the highest accuracy of 89.2% and 88.7% belongs to model 3 which is built on combination of patient assessment predictors and X-ray features for K = 8 and K = 6, respectively. Similarly, model 3 performed the best among the three with QWK of 0.8837 for K = 8 and 0.8321 for K = 6. The mean average error (MAE) of model 3 was the least among all models with the value of 0.374 for K = 6, followed by model 2 with the value of 0.378 for K = 6. In summary, the model 3 that's built on combination of meaningful features extracted from X-ray images, JSW_M and JSW_L, and variables from patient assessment data that had the highest predictive ability had the best performance among three developed models.

Table 2 Comparison of ACC, MAE, and QWK among three developed models built on X-ray features, patients' questionnaire data, and their combination for different K values

	K = 4			K = 6			K = 8		
	ACC (%)	MAE	QWK	ACC (%)	MAE	QWK	ACC (%)	MAE	QWK
Model 1	82.7	0.451	0.7957	84.2	0.436	0.8018	83.8	0.418	0.8119
Model 2	83.1	0.396	0.8015	85.6	**0.378**	0.8116	84.3	0.385	0.8223
Model 3	88.4	0.382	0.8274	88.7	**0.374**	0.8321	**89.2**	0.380	**0.8337**

Model 1: Built on X-ray features; Model 2: Built on patient assessment data; and Model 3: Built on combination of X-ray features and patient assessment data
The bold values represents the key values for which the best performance occurred

Clinicians commonly use the X-ray images for assessment of KOA severity and functional impairment. It is expected that the X-ray image analysis provides objective and accurate impairment measure, while indeed not all impairments lead to knee anatomical transformation. So, prediction of KOA severity still relies on subjective perception of physician and patient side by side. Our aim was to find out whether statistical model based on combination of X-ray features and patient assessment data is capable to predict the KOA presence and severity, that was achieved with high level of accuracy (89.2%).

We also found that the performance of statistical model built on patient assessment data is comparable to the model built on the features extracted from X-ray images as highlighted in previous findings [2, 19, 20]. Using a single cohort database in building statistical models is one the potential limitations in our study that can be addressed by analyzing longitudinal cohort [17].

4 Conclusion

The study outcomes revealed that the patient assessment data is able to predict the KOA severity with high level of accuracy, and in particular when combined with KOA X-ray key features, joint space width. Additionally, they can be used to design effective intervention at early stage and to monitor the patient's improvement throughout the treatment. That is to say, we may identify the individuals currently using pain killers and experiencing limited knee functions in their daily activity by observing the variables with higher predictive ability; and develop early intervention. More importantly, we managed to address a potential limitation of any statistical model that is only developed based on assessing X-ray images through using KL grading system, by combining the X-ray features and patient assessment data as suggested by Abedin [2].

References

1. James, S.L., Abate, D., Abate, K.H., Abay, S.M., Abbafati, C., Abbasi, N., …, Abdelalim, A.: Global, regional, and national incidence, prevalence, and years lived with disability for 354 diseases and injuries for 195 countries and territories, 1990–2017: a systematic analysis for the global burden of disease study 2017. The Lancet **392**(10159), 1789-1858 (2018)
2. Abedin, J., Antony, J., McGuinness, K., Moran, K., O'Connor, N.E., Rebholz-Schuhmann, D., Newell, J.: Predicting knee osteoarthritis severity: comparative modeling based on patient's data and plain X-ray images. Sci. Rep. **9**(1), 1–11 (2019)
3. Heidari, B.: Knee osteoarthritis prevalence, risk factors, pathogenesis and features: part I. Caspian J. Intern. Med. **2**(2), 205 (2011)
4. Clausen, B., Holsgaard-Larsen, A., Søndergaard, J., Christensen, R., Andriacchi, T.P., Roos, E.M.: The effect on knee-joint load of instruction in analgesic use compared with neuromuscular exercise in patients with knee osteoarthritis: study protocol for a randomized, single-blind,

controlled trial (the EXERPHARMA trial). Trials **15**(1), 444 (2014). https://doi.org/10.1186/1745-6215-15-444
5. Kellgren, J., Lawrence, J.: Radiological assessment of osteo-arthrosis. Ann. Rheum. Dis. **16**(4), 494 (1957)
6. Abdelaziz, H., Balde, O.M., Citak, M., Gehrke, T., Magan, A., Haasper, C.: Kellgren-Lawrence scoring system underestimates cartilage damage when indicating TKA: preoperative radiograph versus intraoperative photograph. Arch. Orthop. Trauma Surg. **139**(9), 1287–1292 (2019)
7. Saleem, M., Farid, M.S., Saleem, S., Khan, M.H.: X-ray image analysis for automated knee osteoarthritis detection. SIViP **14**(6), 1079–1087 (2020). https://doi.org/10.1007/s11760-020-01645-z
8. Pandey, M.S., Rajitha, B., Agarwal, S.: Computer assisted automated detection of knee osteoarthritis using X-ray images. Sci. Technol. **1**(2), 74–79 (2015)
9. Stachowiak, G.W., Wolski, M., Woloszynski, T., Podsiadlo, P.: Detection and prediction of osteoarthritis in knee and hand joints based on the X-ray image analysis. Biosurf. Biotribol. **2**(4), 162–172 (2016)
10. Hunter, D.J., McDougall, J.J., Keefe, F.J.: The symptoms of osteoarthritis and the genesis of pain. Rheum. Dis. Clin. North Am. **34**(3), 623–643 (2008). https://doi.org/10.1016/j.rdc.2008.05.004
11. Altman, R., Alarcón, G., Appelrouth, D., Bloch, D., Borenstein, D., Brandt, K., …, Wolfe, F.: The American college of rheumatology criteria for the classification and reporting of osteoarthritis of the hip. Arthritis Rheum. **34**(5), 505–514 (1991).https://doi.org/10.1002/art.1780340502
12. Cicuttini, F., Ding, C., Wluka, A., Davis, S., Ebeling, P.R., Jones, G.: Association of cartilage defects with loss of knee cartilage in healthy, middle-age adults: a prospective study. Arthritis Rheum. **52**(7), 2033–2039 (2005). https://doi.org/10.1002/art.21148
13. Mengko, T.L., Wachjudi, R.G., Suksmono, A.B., Danudirdjo, D.: Automated detection of unimpaired joint space for knee osteoarthritis assessment. Paper presented at the Proceedings of 7th International Workshop on Enterprise networking and Computing in Healthcare Industry, 23–25 June 2005. HEALTHCOM (2005)
14. Schmidt, J.E., Amrami, K.K., Manduca, A., Kaufman, K.R.: Semi-automated digital image analysis of joint space width in knee radiographs. Skeletal Radiol. **34**(10), 639–643 (2005). https://doi.org/10.1007/s00256-005-0908-9
15. Jones, T.D., Plassmann, P. An active contour model for measuring the area of leg ulcers. IEEE Trans. Med. Imaging **19**(12), 1202–1210 (2000). https://doi.org/10.1109/42.897812
16. Amigó, E., Gonzalo, J., Mizzaro, S., Carrillo-de-Albornoz, J.: An effectiveness metric for ordinal classification: formal properties and experimental results (2020). https://doi.org/10.18653/v1/2020.acl-main.363
17. Yong, C.W., Teo, K., Murphy, B.P., Hum, Y.C., Tee, Y.K., Xia, K., Lai, K.W.: Knee osteoarthritis severity classification with ordinal regression module. Multi. Tools Appl. (2021). https://doi.org/10.1007/s11042-021-10557-0
18. Fayers, P.M., Machin, D.: Quality of Life: The Assessment, Analysis and Interpretation of Patient-Reported Outcomes. John Wiley & Sons (2013)
19. Antony, J., McGuinness, K., O'Connor, N.E., Moran, K.: Quantifying radiographic knee osteoarthritis severity using deep convolutional neural networks. In: 2016 23rd International Conference on Pattern Recognition (ICPR), pp. 1195–1200. IEEE (2016)
20. Tiulpin, A., Tevenot, J., Rahtu, E., Lehenkari, P., Saarakkala, S.: Automatic knee osteoarthritis diagnosis from plain radiographs: a deep learning-based approach. Sci. reports **8**, 1727 (2018)

Depression Detection Using Natural Language Processing on Bahasa Malaysia Non-clinical Text

Nur Aiman Mohd Fuad and Nik Nur Wahidah Nik Hashim

Abstract Depression is viewed as the largest cause of the world mental illness statistic, and it keeps increasing globally including Malaysia. Two main issues that prevent early diagnosis of depression in Malaysia are the limited number of psychologist ratios to patients and the stigma from the society that relates depression with insanity. In addition, research have shown that technology using bio-signals can be an alternative method that supports clinician's decision for early diagnosis of depression. The main objective of this study is to develop an automatic detection depression via the language usage in written text using Natural Language Processing (NLP). This work will be examining the text file of 51 subjects with depression and 53 non-depressed subjects. In the initial investigation, we identified the common and frequently used word used by each class. Subjects in the depressed group often use the word such as words "penat" and "bosan". These texts were then classified using common classifier models. Using Term Frequency-Inverse Document Frequency, Multinomial Naïve Bayes produces the best accuracy of 95%.

Keywords Detection depression · Natural Language Processing (NLP) · Text classification

1 Introduction

Depression is one of the types of mental health illness that deals with the feeling of anger, loneliness, sadness, despair, and hopelessness. These feelings will interfere with the patients' daily activities. Therefore, it is important to have a reliable method to detect depression. There is various type of assessment to detect depressive symptoms such as BDI-II, PHQ-9, and HAMD. These assessments are a bunch of question that will be asked to the potential patient, and they must complete it.

N. A. Mohd Fuad · N. N. W. N. Hashim (✉)
Department of Mechatronics, Faculty of Engineering, International Islamic University Malaysia, Kuala Lumpur, Malaysia
e-mail: niknurwahidah@iium.edu.my

J. Usman et al. (eds.), *6th Kuala Lumpur International Conference on Biomedical Engineering 2021*, IFMBE Proceedings 86,
https://doi.org/10.1007/978-3-030-90724-2_17

There are so many reasons why we are trying to develop an automatic depression detection. The first issue is there is a problem in early diagnosis due to the limited number of psychologist ratios to patients. This happens because the number of depressed patients increases year by year. In Malaysia, about thirty per cent of the netizens are diagnosed to suffer from depression. This percentage is expected to be increased significantly in 2020, due to a pandemic. Secondly, the stigma or the mindset of the patient. They do not want to be seen as "crazy" by society. Hence, they are more inclined to hide their depression until the end and suffering alone by themselves. Lastly, depression detection can be detected through technology. For example, using a bio signal. This can be proved due to the application electrocardiogram (ECG) and electroencephalogram (EEG) in detecting depression.

As the number of potential depression patients increases among Malaysian, the way or method to detect the depression needs to be improved. Instead of meeting a psychiatrist and performing several tests maybe there is another alternative method which can detect the depression accurately. This paper will focus on how to detect depression among Malaysian through the linguistic traces of depression in Bahasa Malaysia faster and efficiently.

2 Literature Review

2.1 Depression and Text

Text Classification for Early Depression Detection. First of all, the text classification by using Naïve Bayes for the EDD. This type of text classification is the most used algorithm. As opined by Nadeem [1], the Naïve Bayes classifier is one of the machine learning text classifications. Next, the Support Vector Machine (SVM). This is another machine learning text classification that is able to give an accurate result without too much training data [2].

Last of all, Deep Learning. This method is inspired by the neural networks of the humans, and it is divided into two types: The Convolutional Neural Networks (CNN) and the Recurrent Neural Networks (RNN) [2]. In their paper, Tadesse et al. [3] mentioned that by using CNN can increase the accuracy and the performance of text classification which contains the neurons.

Common Words Used by Depressed People. There are many common words used by depressed people as described by the reviewed literature and all of them show the symptom of depression. All the words are showing the symptoms of depression such as "loneliness", "feel alone", "worth" and "blame" whereas these examples of words show the signs of depression which are loneliness and hopelessness as highlighted by [4]. It should be noted that most texts or posts are written in the first-person pronouns like "I", "me" and "myself" instead of "we", "us" [5]. The depressed people also show their negative emotion more than positive emotion, as the result they tend to use negative words such as "hate", "ugly" and "unhappy". According to Oyong et al. [6], they found the same thing by analyzing the Indonesian Twitter posts. The Indonesian use the words that indicate their loneliness, anxiety, depressed and negative emotion. For example, "bimbang" (worry), "putus asa" (give up), "sunyi" (lonely), and "panik" (panic).

In Malaysia, the common words used by the depressed Malaysian are "memang", "kena", "mesti" [7]. In English, these words mean "have to", "must" and "should". As highlighted by Nadzirah, a clinical psychologist in IIUM Kuantan Hospital [7], these words are the common words used by the depressed patient in Malaysia that indicate they have a narrow mind. She also stated that many words that have been mentioned by the patient show their negative emotion, anxiety, and overthinking. Based on her experience in interviewing her depressed patients, the patients tend to filter out the positive emotion. The example of words that have always been used by them to indicate their negative feelings are "mati" and "kosong".

2.2 *Depression Text Corpus*

Based on the reviewed papers, certain researchers take the free-text clinical documents. This was done by Zhou et al. [8] which took the clinical documents of the 1200 patients' discharge summaries, used 600 of them for the training and the remaining as the testing data. Other researchers also collected about 1,800,000 clinical documents from 13,000 patients [9]. Lastly, Stasak et al. [10] used Black Dog Institute Affective Sentences (BDAS) corpus for their research. BDAS is an institute dealing with various types of mental health.

On the other hand, many researchers also obtained their depression text corpus via online platforms for such as Twitter and Reddit. Nadeem [1] and Oyong et al. [6] take the tweets as their text corpus. The text corpus needs to be corrected its text-spelling before it can be used. The study must include the lexicon symptom that contains the regional jargon and the slang used by social media users in Indonesia and English [6]. Meanwhile, in the paper of Wolohan et al. [11], they took about 12,106 Reddit users' posts which contain about 149,089,719 words to detect the depressed user.

Lastly, the customized or individualized depression text corpus which the corpus has to be obtained by collecting the data by ourselves.

2.3 *Performance of Text Automatic Depression Detection*

Free-Text Clinical Documents. Zhou et al. [8] database is based on the free-text clinical document of discharged ischemic heart disease patients who had been hospitalized between early year 2011 and the end of year 2013 at different hospitals in the United States. They choose 1200 patients' discharge summaries randomly and divide the documents into two datasets. Six hundred training datasets and six hundreds of documents that will be used for testing. The discharge summary contains the information regarding the hospital course, medication releases upon the discharge and care plan.

Reddit Post. According to Tadesse et al. [3], they train their model based on the dataset that had been built and it consists of the list of non-depressed users and depressed users. Based on these users, the data corpus is divided into two, depression indicative posts (1293) and the standard posts (548) which are written by the non-depressed users.

Using Social Media Post. Asad et al. [4] used two datasets containing user's SNS posts (Facebook and Twitter). The depression detection in the paper is based on the post of 100 Twitter users' tweets in one week and 50 Facebook users' last year posts.

3 Research Methodology

3.1 Database Collection

All procedures performed were in accordance with the ethical standards and has been approved by the IIUM Research Ethical Committee (IREC 2019-006). The database was divided based on gender and diagnostic groups of depressed and healthy. A total of 51 depressed and 53 healthy subjects were required to sign an informed consent and to be neither under the influence of alcohol, toxicity, nor experiencing respiratory problems.

Using online platform, subjects were also asked to report whether they have received a diagnosis of Major Depressive Disorder (MDD) by any hospital's psychiatrist and also required to fill in the Malay Beck Depression Inventory-II (Malay BDI-II) and Patient Health Questionnaire-9 (PHQ-9). One recording from each subject answering the question about what situation that usually causes them to feel stressed were gathered and transcribed.

3.2 Data Pre-processing

Test and Train Data. The obtained data will be divided into the training dataset and the testing dataset by using the ratios of 80:20 from each group of research subjects. 43 transcribed speech from depressed research subject and 40 transcribed speech from healthy are selected to be used as train dataset. Thus, 83 transcribed speeches will be used as a training dataset and the remaining data will be the testing dataset.

Noise Cleaning. The gathered data should be cleaned to remove the unwanted text through many rounds to avoid the inaccurate result. According to Ameisen [12], the good rule thumb is to look at the collected data first, then, clean it up so that you know what you should clean [12]. Zhao [13] stated that the commonly used cleaning steps for all the text data are:

1. Make each of the words lower case.
2. Eliminate the punctuation.
3. Get rid of the numerical values.
4. Take out certain words based on the listed stop words.
5. Deal with the typo.

Stop words. After dealing with noise cleaning or data cleaning, both the training data and testing data should be filtered and remove the stop words. Stop words is a list of frequently used words or vocabularies in any language. By removing the stop words, the accuracy of the classification model can be increased as there are only meaningful and valuable tokens left. And it also can reduce the size of the dataset and decrease the time taken for the training as well.

3.3 Feature Extraction

Tokenization. The assembled database is a text file that contains a series of words. Hence, this file needs to be converted into the numerical feature vector in order to run the machine learning algorithm [14]. This can be achieved through the process of tokenization. Tokenization is the process of replacing data with the generated number that will be decided by the algorithm, token.

Term Frequency, Inverse Document Frequency (TF-IDF). Without TF-IDF, there is some favouritism attached as the current tokenization [15]. In order to enhance the tokenization step and make the model focus more on meaningful words, TF-IDF has been introduced to the picture. TF-IDF give the weightage on words by how infrequent they are in the data set [12]. In other words, the worth of a worth rises proportionally to the count, however, the value of it inversely proportional to the frequency of the word in the text file [16]. With this, to separate and classify two groups become easier.

3.4 Classification Model

Five common classification models were implemented in this study on the extracted features from the texts. These classifiers are listed below.

1. **Extra Tree Classifier**. A classifier which sums up the results of multi cross-correlation decision trees collected in "forest" to give out the result of the the classification.
2. **AdaBoost Classifier**. A classifier which is a short form for Adaptive Boosting. This classifier combines multiple classifiers in order to increase the accuracy

by re-assign the weights to each instance with higher weight to categorize the instances incorrectly.

3. **Random Forest Classifier**. One of ensemble learning methods that build a collection of decision trees at the training time.
4. **Multinomial Naïve Bayes**. Naïve Bayes algorithm is suitable for large data sets. Its algorithm is the fittest one as it studies every feature separately, computes for each category its probability and then does the prediction about the category based on the highest probability.
5. **Logistic Regression**. According to Logistic Regression (LR) is the commonly preferred classifier to classify the data due to its adaptability, explainability, and it is very simple to train.

4 Result and Discussion

4.1 Data Processing

After the first round of data cleaning by eliminating the punctuation, making each of the words lower case and getting rid of the numerical values, and the feature of data is extracted using the feature of Bag of Words (BOW). One of the objectives of this paper is to analyze the common word used by the depressed subjects and their text pattern. Then, by using the BOW and the words frequency for each text file, we can obtain the common word used by depressed subjects. The common words can deliver by each of the research subjects regarding their feelings for the past of three days are represented in Word Cloud as shown in Figs. 1, 2, 3, and 4.

Based on the Word Cloud, certain observations can be made. Firstly, the majority of non-depressed female participants mention the word "stress" in their transcribed speeches compared to the other research subjects and this shows that the frequency of word "stress" in the text file is not related to depression. Next, it can be observed that the non-depressed participants are likely to mention how happy they are; however, the depressed participants tend to talk about dark emotions such as sadness, worry,

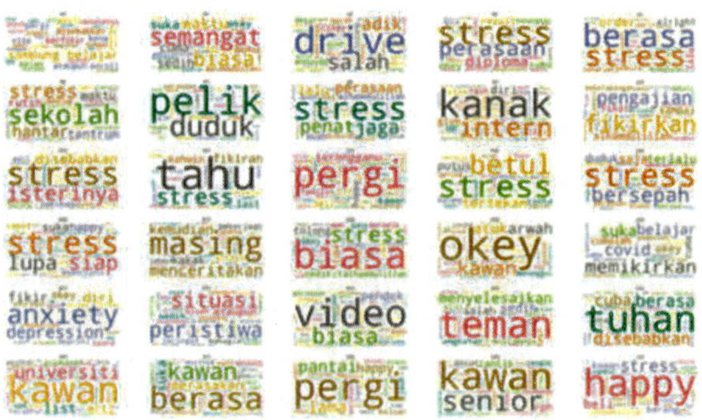

Fig. 1 Word Cloud of non-depressed female subjects

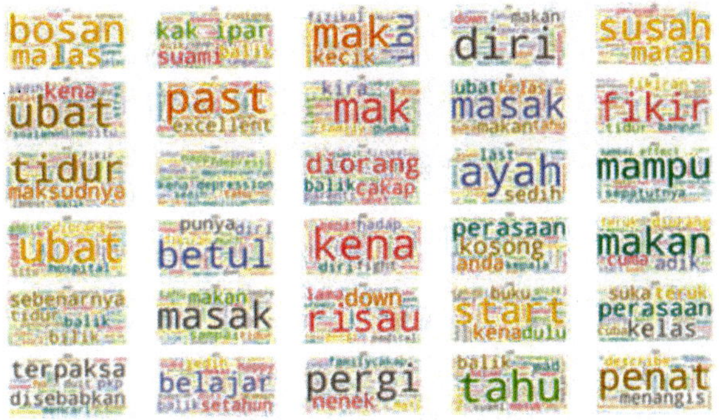

Fig. 2 Word Cloud of depressed female subjects

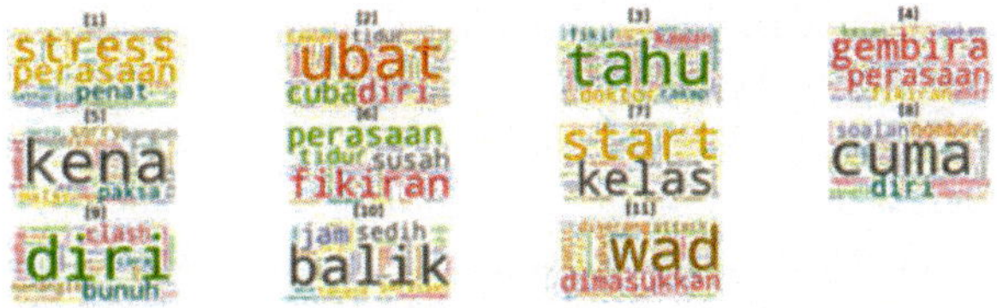

Fig. 3 Word Cloud of depressed male subjects

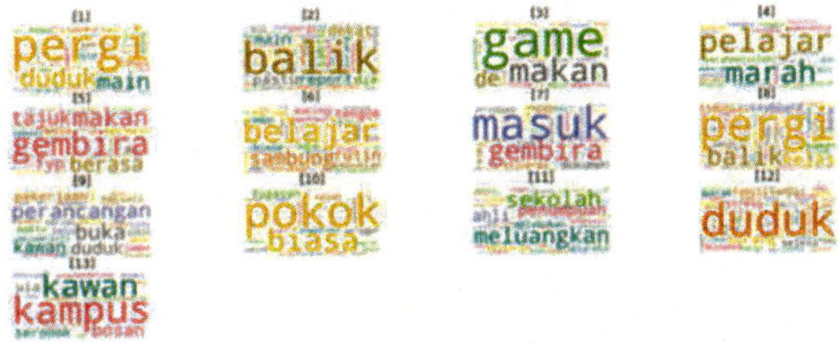

Fig. 4 Word Cloud of non-depressed male subjects

pressure, and tiredness. Moreover, at least one in both male and female depressed participants will mention "ubat" in their transcribed speech. Last observation that can be seen is that the male depressed participants never talk about the playing game and having fun, in their transcribed speech, unlike the non-depressed male participants. All these observations are related to the depression symptom such as medication description and negative feelings.

4.2 NLP Classification Analysis

TF-IDF feature was then input into classifiers model to identify subjects with depression and healthy. The performance of the classifiers was compared based on these parameters,

Table 1 Results of classification model

Classifier	Precision	Recall	F1-score	Accuracy (%)
Extra Tree	0.58	0.56	0.53	57
AdaBoost	0.67	0.60	0.57	62
Random Forest	0.71	0.65	0.64	67
Multinomial Naïve Bayes	0.96	0.95	0.95	95
Logistic Regression	0.89	0.85	0.85	86

i. Accuracy of estimations (Acc.): The rate of accurate classification.
ii. Precision (P): Estimation of true positive identified samples.
iii. Recall (R): Approximate the number of positive samples that was accurately detected.
iv. F1-score (F1): Harmonic average of P and R.

Referring to Table 1, there are five models of classifier that were implemented with NLP features. Each of them has precision, recall, F1-score and accuracy values as the result. The best classification model is the Multinomial Naïve Bayes classification model with an accuracy of 95% and 0.95 F1 score. The second-best model is the model with Logistic Regression as its classifier with the accuracy of 86% and 0.85 F1 score. Meanwhile, for the other three classification models, their accuracy is less than the targeted value which is 80%.

5 Conclusion

We have identified common words that are used by depressed subjects. Evaluating the performance of all five classification models, the model with Multinomial Naïve Bayes classifier and Logistic Regression are more suitable for this type of database, the transcribed speeches in Bahasa Malaysia. This also shows the possibility of using text to classify between the depressed and healthy for Bahasa Malaysia language. However, in the future, more data should be gathered to strengthen and conclude this finding. It should be noted that there is also a possibility that if other features such as Word2Vec instead of TF-IDF were to be implemented, the performance of the model can be enhanced.

Acknowledgements This work is supported by the Fundamental Research Grant Scheme (FRGS19-051-0659).

References

1. Nadeem, M.: Identifying depression on Twitter, pp. 1–9 (2016). Available: http://arxiv.org/abs/1607.07384
2. MonkeyLearn: text classification (2020). https://monkeylearn.com/text-classification/
3. Tadesse, M.M., Lin, H., Xu, B., Yang, L.: Detection of depression-related posts in reddit social media forum. IEEE Access **7**, 44883–44893 (2019). https://doi.org/10.1109/ACCESS.2019.2909180
4. Al Asad, N., Mahmud Pranto, M.A., Afreen, S., Islam, M.M.: Depression detection by analyzing social media posts of user. In: IEEE International Conference on Signal Processing, Information, Communication and Systems, SPICSCON 2019, pp. 13–17 (2019). https://doi.org/10.1109/SPICSCON48833.2019.9065101
5. Burdisso, S.G., Errecalde, M., Montes-y-Gómez, M.: A text classification framework for simple and effective early depression detection over social media streams. Expert Syst. Appl. **133**, 182–197 (2019). https://doi.org/10.1016/j.eswa.2019.05.023
6. Oyong, I., Utami, E., Luthfi, E.T.: Natural language processing and lexical approach for depression symptoms screening of Indonesian twitter user. In: 2018 10th International Conference on Information Technology and Electrical Engineering: Smart Technology for Better Society, ICITEE 2018, pp. 359–364 (2018). https://doi.org/10.1109/ICITEED.2018.8534929
7. Nadzirah, Interviewee, Depression among Malaysian. 30 Dec 2020
8. Zhou, L., et al.: Identifying patients with depression using free-text clinical documents. Stud. Health Technol. Inform. **216**(Aug), 629–633 (2015). https://doi.org/10.3233/978-1-61499-564-7-629
9. Vaci, N., et al.: Natural language processing for structuring clinical text data on depression using UK-CRIS. Evid. Based. Ment. Health **23**(1), 21–26 (2020). https://doi.org/10.1136/ebmental-2019-300134
10. Stasak, B., Epps, J., Goecke, R.: Automatic depression classification based on affective read sentences: opportunities for text-dependent analysis. Speech Commun. **115**(September), 1–14 (2019). https://doi.org/10.1016/j.specom.2019.10.003
11. Wolohan, J.T., Hiraga, M., Mukherjee, A., Sayyed, Z.A.: Detecting linguistic traces of depression in topic-restricted text: attending to self-stigmatized depression with NLP. Workshop, pp. 11–21, 2018. Available: https://doi.org/10.18653/v1/P17
12. Ameisen, E.: How to solve 90% of NLP problems: a step-by-step guide (2019). https://www.kdnuggets.com/2019/01/solve-90-nlp-problems-step-by-step-guide.html
13. Zhao, A.: Github: adashofdata. Github Web site (2020). https://github.com/adashofdata
14. Shaikh, J.: Machine learning, NLP: Text Classification using scikit-learn, python and NLTK. towards data science Web site (2017). https://towardsdatascience.com/machine-learning-nlp-text-classification-using-scikit-learn-python-and-nltk-c52b92a7c73a
15. Elboukkouri, H.: Text classification: the first step toward NLP mastery. Medium Web site (2018). https://medium.com/data-from-the-trenches/text-classification-the-first-step-toward-nlp-mastery-f5f95d525d73
16. Pietro, M.D.: Text Classification with NLP: Tf-Idf vs Word2Vec vs BERT (2020). https://towardsdatascience.com/text-classification-with-nlp-tf-idf-vs-word2vec-72vs-bert-41ff868d1794

A Preliminary Study of IVOCT-Based Atherosclerosis Plaque Classification Technique

Sanjiv Rajkumar, Muhammad Safwan Soaib, Yih Miin Liew, Kok Han Chee, Ho Kin Tang, Kanendra Naidu, Nooranida Arifin, and Chow Khuen Chan

Abstract Atherosclerosis is a type of cardiovascular disease (CVD) that affects the coronary artery by build-up of plaque, which can potentially cause stroke or ischemic damage to the surrounding tissue. Intravascular Optical Coherence Tomography (IVOCT), an imaging modality, is able to capture detailed images of arteries affected by atherosclerosis that contain identifiable characteristics. These characteristics can assist clinicians to differentiate certain plaque types such as, fibrous, calcific and lipid, and provide diagnosis appropriately. However, clinicians face challenges in manual visual plaque identification from IVOCT images such as fatigue and IVOCT artifacts. Hence, the aim of this study is to produce an automated IVOCT-based plaque segmentation method to assist clinicians in their diagnosis. This preliminary study investigated only two plaque types, which are fibrous and calcified plaque as they are much more prominent to be labelled manually. The image dataset was pre-processed with Gabor filters before training the Random Forest (RF) and XGBoost models. The results demonstrated that the XGBoost model performed slightly better than the Random Forest model with 82.0% and 80.9% accuracy respectively. This shows that machine learning techniques can be applied conveniently to assist, automate and reduce the time for clinician's visual assessment in the overall diagnosis workflow.

S. Rajkumar · M. S. Soaib · Y. M. Liew · N. Arifin · C. K. Chan (✉)
Department of Biomedical Engineering, Faculty of Engineering, Universiti Malaya, Kuala Lumpur, Malaysia
e-mail: ckchan@um.edu.my

K. H. Chee
Department of Medicine, Faculty of Medicine, Universiti Malaya, Kuala Lumpur, Malaysia

H. K. Tang
Shenzhen JL Computational Science and Applied Research Institute, Guangdong, People's Republic of China

K. Naidu
School of Electrical Engineering, College of Engineering, Universiti Teknologi Mara, Selangor, Malaysia

J. Usman et al. (eds.), *6th Kuala Lumpur International Conference on Biomedical Engineering 2021*, IFMBE Proceedings 86,
https://doi.org/10.1007/978-3-030-90724-2_18

Keywords Atherosclerosis · Intravascular optical coherence tomography · Plaque classification · Image segmentation · Machine learning

1 Introduction

According to the World Health Organization (WHO), cardiovascular disease (CVD) are among the main cause of deaths globally in 2016. Ischemic heart disease is also a prevailing cause of Malaysian deaths in 2018 [1]. Atherosclerosis is a type of cardiovascular disease that affects the coronary artery in which the artery is narrowed down with plaque build-up [2]. Among various imaging methods introduced to assist clinicians in diagnosing atherosclerosis is Intravascular Optical Coherence Tomography (IVOCT), which can be considered as a highly detailed light-based counterpart to Intravascular Ultrasound (IVUS). IVOCT provides high resolution imaging of the coronary artery of about 10–20 μm, which is approximately 10 times higher than IVUS [3].

Objective grading criteria has been established based on certain visual and morphological characteristics from IVOCT images to primarily identify three main types of atherosclerosis plaque in the coronary artery, which are fibrous, calcified and lipid. Although classification criteria can be established to identify plaque, IVOCT image interpreters and pathologists may not reach immediately reach a consensus [4]. Additionally, speckle noise and image artifacts present in IVOCT images may complicate visual assessment of plaque [5]. Therefore, expert assessment of IVOCT images can often be time-consuming and burdensome for clinicians.

IVOCT-based classification methods have been previously implemented before to tackle the challenge of plaque classification. Plaque characterization utilizing optical coefficients, such as attenuation and backscattering coefficients, have been successfully carried out [6, 7]. Machine learning techniques such as, Support Vector Machines (SVM) and Random Forest (RF), has also been used for plaque classification with decent accuracy [8–10]. Although there are published methods, there is still much to explore in terms of implementation and further improving large-scale consistent plaque assessment of IVOCT pullbacks. This objectives of this study are threefold; (1) to analyze output of image enhancement methods that highlight atherosclerotic plaque characteristics from IVOCT images, (2) measure effectiveness of segmentation methods for atherosclerosis plaque from IVOCT images and (3) determine viability of machine learning implementation towards automated atherosclerotic plaque segmentation. This preliminary study serves to highlight the capabilities of machine learning techniques as viable plaque segmentation methods in terms of accuracy.

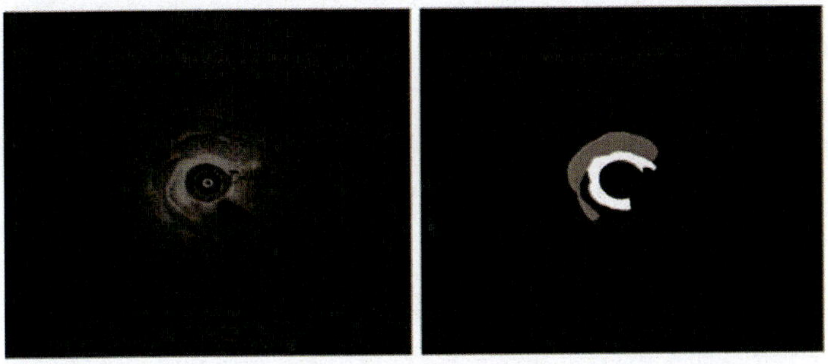

Fig. 1 **a** Original image, **b** labeled image/Ground truth produced with MATLAB labelling tool in which the white and grey regions represent fibrous and calcified plaque respectively

2 Methodology

2.1 Dataset

Three IVOCT pullbacks, each containing approximately 370 frames, were obtained from Universiti Malaya Medical Centre (UMMC). The pullbacks contain images of coronary arteries with fibrous and fibrocalcific plaque. All the IVOCT pullbacks have been provided with the approval of an ethics committee and personal patient information was not included. For this preliminary study, 30 frames were prepared for training while 20 frames were only selected for testing.

Manual segmentation was carried out to label the fibrous and calcified plaque appropriately according to the guidance of UMMC cardiologists using the image labelling tools provided in MATLAB 2020b. MATLAB's Video Labelling Tool provides the ability to label pixel areas accordingly to the type of plaque corresponding in the image. Figure 1 below illustrates a sample of the labelling result and its original image.

2.2 Pre-processing

Pre-processing was carried out to facilitate image processing through the machine learning models. Gabor filters are used for feature extraction and its usage in the 2D image domain is described by a sinusoidal plane wave contained within a 2D Gaussian envelope [11, 12]. These filters have shown effectiveness at edge and texture discrimination similar to Canny, Roberts, Sobel, Scharr and Prewitt filters [11, 12]. Parameters such as frequencies and orientations are defined in Gabor filters as well [11].

2.3 Training and Validation

The features extracted using the Gabor filters were fed into the classifier model for training and testing. Grayscale conversion was performed and the images reshaped into one dimension prior to training. The labelled ground truth images were not processed using Gabor filters as performed with the original images for training.

2.3.1 Performance Metrics

Confusion matrix was used to evaluate the classifications. Class 1 and Class 2 are labelled as fibrous and fibrocalcific respectively. The confusion matrix can be described in terms of true positive (TP), true negative (TN), false positive (FP) and false negative (FN) pixels. The confusion matrix format can be observed in Table 1.

Training and validation dataset size were defined by allocating 30% for training and the remaining 70% for validation. The number of estimators, maximum depth and random state was iteratively adjusted to find optimal performance for the XGBoost classifier. Average accuracy can be defined using the formula below:

$$Accuracy = \frac{TP + TN}{TP + TN + FP + FN} \tag{1}$$

Accuracy metrics are meant to indicate classification performance across all classes and the ratio of correct prediction over total number of predictions. Higher average accuracy can indicate classification result [13].

The average accuracy however does not reflect the model's individual classification class scores accurately. Each segmented class accuracy can also examined by calculating their precision, recall and F1-score. Formula for precision class can be defined below:

$$Precision = \frac{TP}{TP + FP} \tag{2}$$

Precision is used to calculate pixels that were correctly classified (TP) over total number of positive pixels correctly (TP) or incorrectly classified (FP). Another metric that can is used is recall, which calculates the number of positive pixels correctly classified (TP) over total number of positive samples correctly classified or negative

Table 1 Confusion matrix table format

Ground truth	Predicted		
		Class 1	Class 2
	Class 1	True +ve	False −ve
	Class 2	False +ve	True −ve

Positive (+ve) and negative (−ve) classified pixels are indicated samples incorrectly classified. The closer the recall score is to one indicates better classification effect [13]. The formula that defines recall is as follows:

$$Recall = \frac{TP}{TP + FN} \tag{3}$$

An additional metric used in this study to validate accuracy is Intersection over Union (IoU) which calculates the predicted segmented area over the labelled ground truth image. The IoU formula can be defined as follow:

$$IoU = \frac{Area\ of\ Overlap}{Area\ of\ Union} \tag{4}$$

2.3.2 Random Forest and XGBoost Classifiers

The Random Forest (RF) model is based on an ensemble of decision trees, whereby each split in every decision tree is based on a feature. The generalization error minimizes as the number of trees in an RF model increases and this characteristic enables the RF model to perform well over a dataset [14]. On the other hand, bootstrap aggregating or bagging is a training technique used to improve the classification capabilities of the RF model whereby random sampling is performed on the dataset with replacement and done in parallel [14]. Boosting, however, is a training technique where models are trained sequentially. The error weights are optimized accordingly to the loss function from model to model trained each time [15]. In comparison, XGBoost utilizes boosting while Random Forests typically utilize bagging for training. XGBoost also features regularization and exact greedy algorithm to acquire optimal classification results [15].

3 Results

The segmentation results can be illustrated in Figs. 2 and 3 in comparsion with the ground truth label (Tables 2, 3, and 4).

The above results indicate that XGBoost classifier achieved slightly higher average accuracy and the precision compared to Random Forest with 82.0% and 80.9% overall respectively. Additionally, the same number of decision trees and random state were used for both classifiers.

One method to cross check the average accuracy was by comparing it against Intersection over Union (IoU) score across both classifiers. Fibrous and calcified plaque segmentation performance in terms of IoU score and average accuracy obtained were similar. Therefore, the above classification report is consistent between these two metrics for comparison purposes.

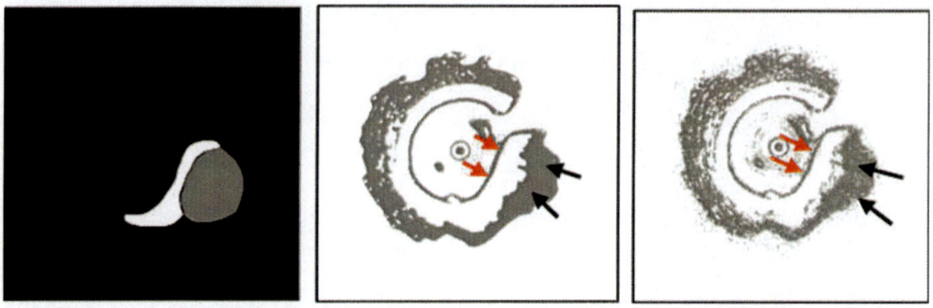

Fig. 2 Ground truth image (left), XGBoost segmentation result (middle), Random Forest segmentation result (right) of frame/slice number 14 shown. Grey and white colour areas represent calcified and fibrous respectively in the ground truth image. Red arrows and black arrows indicate fibrous and calcified plaques segmented areas respectively for the segmentation results

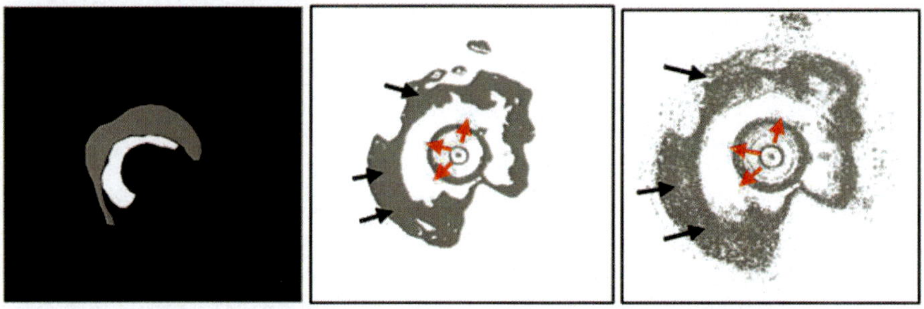

Fig. 3 Ground truth image (left), XGBoost segmentation result (middle), Random Forest segmentation result (right) of frame/slice number 269 shown. Grey and white colour areas represent calcified and fibrous respectively in the ground truth image. Red arrows and black arrows indicate fibrous and calcified plaques segmented areas respectively for the segmentation results

Table 2 Intersection over Union for each plaque across both classifiers

Class	Intersection over Union (%)	
	Random Forest	XGBoost
Fibrous	61.5	63.5
Calcified	72.7	73.7

Table 3 Model classification performance

Model	Class	No. of pixels	Precision	Recall	F1 score
XGBoost	Calcified	34,501	0.73	**0.83**	0.78
	Fibrous	21,787	**0.89**	0.81	**0.85**
Random Forest	Calcified	34,501	0.72	0.81	0.76
	Fibrous	21,787	0.87	0.81	0.84

The significance of the bold is to reveal the respective classification performance is the highest for a particular model. For instance, with XGBoost, fibrous plaque classification with the no of pixels of 21,787 reported the highest precision compared with other models and no of pixels

Table 4 Confusion matrix for both models result

Model		Predicted		
XGBoost	Ground truth		Fibrous	Calcified
		Fibrous	51,835	10,626
		Calcified	19,217	83,618
Random Forest		Fibrous	50,291	12,170
		Calcified	19,251	83,584

4 Discussion

Machine learning techniques, such as Random Forest and XGBoost, in this preliminary study show promising results as the average accuracy alongside other metrics such as precision, recall and F1 score indicate promising segmentation ability. It is seen that Random Forest and XGBoost models have similar performance and that XGBoost performs only slightly better compared to the Random Forest model.

The results shown are limited in dataset size and testing should be expanded over a larger dataset. Additionally, this preliminary study has utilized Gabor to pre-process the dataset for training and has not made a comparison between the performance of feeding the classifier models non pre-processed data or using different pre-process methods. Both mentioned aspects can be taken into account as this study continues.

5 Conclusion

In conclusion, machine learning techniques such as XGBoost show promising atherosclerostic plaque segmentation and classification capability on IVOCT images. It has been shown although the difference in between performance capabilities between Random Forest and XGBoost classifier models were minimal, XGBoost performed better in terms of average accuracy, precision, recall and F1-score overall. Further research should include testing the whole dataset as to determine the viability of machine learning techniques to be included into clinical settings. Additionally, deep learning methods, a subset of the machine learning field, can be implemented to further explore the viability of utilizing deep learning models, such as U-Net and State-of-The-Art (SOTA) CNNs, in classifying and segmenting plaque from IVOCT images.

Acknowledgements This research was funded by the Malaysia Ministry of Higher Education Fundamental Research Grant Scheme (FRGS/1/2018/SKK03/UM/02/1) and Faculty Research Grant GPF (GPF026A-2019).

References

1. Department of Statistics Malaysia Press Release: Statistics on Causes of Death, Malaysia, 2019. Dep. Stat. Malaysia (Oct 2019)
2. George, S.J., Johnson, J.: Atherosclerosis: Molecular and Cellular Mechanisms (2010)
3. Bezerra, H.G., Costa, M.A., Guagliumi, G., Rollins, A.M., Simon, D.I.: Intracoronary optical coherence tomography: a comprehensive review: clinical and research applications. JACC: Cardiovasc. Interven. (2009). https://doi.org/10.1016/j.jcin.2009.06.019
4. Patwari, P., et al.: Assessment of coronary plaque with optical coherence tomography and high-frequency ultrasound. Am. J. Cardiol. **85**(5), 641–644 (2000). https://doi.org/10.1016/S0002-9149(99)00825-5
5. Van Soest, G., et al.: Pitfalls in plaque characterization by OCT: image artifacts in native coronary arteries. JACC Cardiovasc. Imaging (2011). https://doi.org/10.1016/j.jcmg.2011.01.022
6. Xu, C., Schmitt, J.M., Carlier, S.G., Virmani, R.: Characterization of atherosclerosis plaques by measuring both backscattering and attenuation coefficients in optical coherence tomography. J. Biomed. Opt. (2008). https://doi.org/10.1117/1.2927464
7. van Soest, G., et al.: Atherosclerotic tissue characterization in vivo by optical coherence tomography attenuation imaging. J. Biomed. Opt. (2010). https://doi.org/10.1117/1.3280271
8. Lu, H., et al.: Application and evaluation of highly automated software for comprehensive stent analysis in intravascular optical coherence tomography. Sci. Rep. (2020). https://doi.org/10.1038/s41598-020-59212-y
9. Ughi, G.J., Adriaenssens, T., Sinnaeve, P., Desmet, W., D'hooge, J.: Automated tissue characterization of in vivo atherosclerotic plaques by intravascular optical coherence tomography images. Biomed. Opt. Express (2013). https://doi.org/10.1364/boe.4.001014
10. Athanasiou, L.S., et al.: Methodology for fully automated segmentation and plaque characterization in intracoronary optical coherence tomography images. J. Biomed. Opt. (2014). https://doi.org/10.1117/1.jbo.19.2.026009
11. Li, W., Mao, K.Z., Zhang, H., Chai, T.: Selection of Gabor filters for improved texture feature extraction. In: Proceedings—International Conference on Image Processing, ICIP, pp. 361–364 (2010). https://doi.org/10.1109/ICIP.2010.5653278
12. Fogel, I., Sagi, D.: Gabor filters as texture discriminator. Biol. Cybern. **61**(2), 103–113 (1989). https://doi.org/10.1007/BF00204594
13. Huang, C., et al.: A deep segmentation network of multi-scale feature fusion based on attention mechanism for IVOCT lumen contour. IEEE/ACM Trans. Comput. Biol. Bioinforma. **18**(1), 62–69 (2021). https://doi.org/10.1109/TCBB.2020.2973971
14. Breiman, L.: Random forests. Mach. Learn. (2001). https://doi.org/10.1023/A:1010933404324
15. Chen, T., Guestrin, C.: XGBoost: a scalable tree boosting system. In: Proceedings of the ACM SIGKDD International Conference on Knowledge Discovery and Data Mining, Aug 2016, vol. 13–17-August-2016, pp. 785–794 (2016). https://doi.org/10.1145/2939672.2939785

Biomechanics, Rehabilitation, and Education

The Effects of Prosthetic Knee Joints During Walking on Different Types of Surfaces: A Preliminary Study

Nur Amira Adlan, Nooranida Arifin, Noor Azuan Abu Osman, Hasif Rafidee Hasbollah, Saari Mohamad Yatim, Yusniza Mohd Yusof, and Chan Chow Khuen

Abstract Individuals with transfemoral amputation continue to face mobility challenges despite the advancements in prosthetics technology. Generally, a mechanical prosthetic knee joint is prescribed to replace the important role of the anatomic knee joint in providing an effective walking process. However, research on assessing the biomechanical advantages or disadvantages of various mechanical knee joint designs is yet to be conducted. The objective of this study was to analyze the dual-task gait assessment of transfemoral amputees between two groups of prosthetic knees (polycentric, TFA_P; and fluid-controlled, TFA_{FC}) on different types of surfaces (even and uneven), by comparing them to the age-matched able-bodied group. All participants walked at their self-selected pace along a 5-m walkway. Primary outcomes consisted of temporal-spatial, kinetics, kinematics of the lower limb and descriptive analysis was performed in this study. The findings demonstrated that people with TFA walked slower with longer stride and step times, shorter stride and step lengths, with reduced vertical GRF and range of motion compared to the able-bodied participants in all conditions. The effects were much greater in the TFA_P group than the TFA_{FC} group in most conditions. In comparison between types of surfaces, the performance in dual-task gait assessment on the even surface is better than the uneven surface for all participants. The stance phase duration of the prosthetic leg was shorter than

N. A. Adlan · N. Arifin (✉) · N. A. A. Osman · C. C. Khuen
Department of Biomedical Engineering, Universiti Malaya, Kuala Lumpur, Malaysia
e-mail: anidaum@um.edu.my

N. Arifin · N. A. A. Osman
Center for Applied Biomechanics, Faculty of Engineering, Universiti Malaya, Kuala Lumpur, Malaysia

H. R. Hasbollah
Faculty of Hospitality, Tourism and Wellness, University of Malaysia Kelantan, Pengkalan Chepa, Malaysia

S. M. Yatim
Department of Rehabilitation, Serdang Hospital, Serdang, Malaysia

Y. M. Yusof
Department of Rehabilitation, Cheras Rehabilitation Hospital, Kuala Lumpur, Malaysia

J. Usman et al. (eds.), *6th Kuala Lumpur International Conference on Biomedical Engineering 2021*, IFMBE Proceedings 86,
https://doi.org/10.1007/978-3-030-90724-2_19

the able-bodied. Results indicated that the quality of gait deteriorates in challenging walking conditions for both able-bodied and people with TFA, but fluid-controlled prosthetic knee users have better performance compared to polycentric prosthetic knee users.

Keywords Transfemoral · Dual-task · Gait analysis

1 Introduction

People with transfemoral amputation (TFA) experience mobility restrictions due to the loss of a lower limb. The severe consequence of the missing limb completely alters the physical anatomy of the leg. Even though the development of the modern prosthetic device has been performed to imitate and replace the missing physical limb due to amputation, it still could not afford to restore the peripheral or sensory feedback of the users.

The lack of information affecting the walking ability of people with TFA in terms of biomechanical aspects such as kinetics and kinematics [1]. The assessment of walking ability in prosthetics users usually involves walking speed, symmetry in gait, and energy expenditure [2–6].

People with lower limb amputation often prevent themselves from doing activities due to the fear of falling and it stated that at least one fall per year was reported [7]. Stability and control of movement during standing are also reduced due to the loss of the knee joint [8]. Adaptations of the prosthetic device and beneficial treatment based on individuals with TFA need to be improved to obtain satisfactory walking stability.

An individual with TFA needs to have a functional prosthetic knee. Previous research has shown a connection between technical advancements in prosthetic knee design and better gait dynamics [9, 10]. The development of prosthetic knee joints is crucial in helping people with TFA to accommodate their daily life necessities while achieving normative gait. Over time, prosthetic knees have progressed significantly, including the variable-damping, computer-controlled knees [10]. Nevertheless, passive prosthetic knee devices are still a huge market and especially suited for people in developing countries when it comes to financial value [11, 12].

The main purpose of rehabilitation after amputation is to ensure the amputee to be able to ambulate successfully with the use of a prosthesis. Walking is a challenging task for amputees, and it is one of the demanding activities of daily living. When people with TFA learned to ambulate with the prosthetic device during the rehabilitation process, they will eventually need to adapt to the more challenging environmental factor, such as uneven surfaces.

Walking on an uneven surface involves unpredictable circumstances such as inclines, declines, while concurrently performing cognitive or motor interference tasks. Biomechanical assessment based on walking on an uneven surface is still insufficient contrary to the assessment of walking on an even surface and other conditions such as over obstacles, stairs, ramps, etc. The research of walking assessment on even surface, however, extensive gait research on an uneven surface is needed to test lower limb amputees' ability to navigate more difficult terrains that mimic outdoor walking [13].

This study investigated the effects of prosthetic knee joints during dual-task walking on even and uneven surfaces in people with TFA wearing a non-microprocessor-controlled prosthetic knee compared to age-matched controls. The uneven surface was designed to simulate the regular outdoor walking condition in daily life that would distort subjects' peripheral sensory feedback. Dual-task gait assessment involves in this study will determine the effects of a cognitive process during walking in terms of temporal-spatial, kinetic, and kinematics parameters.

The lack of information affecting the walking ability of people with TFA in terms of biomechanical aspects such as kinetics and kinematics [1]. The assessment of walking ability in prosthetics users usually involves walking speed, symmetry in gait, and energy expenditure [2–6].

People with lower limb amputation often prevent themselves from doing activities due to the fear of falling and it stated that at least one fall per year was reported [7]. Stability and control of movement during standing are also reduced due to the loss of the knee joint [8]. Adaptations of the prosthetic device and beneficial treatment based on individuals with TFA need to be improved to obtain satisfactory walking stability.

An individual with TFA needs to have a functional prosthetic knee. Previous research has shown a connection between technical advancements in prosthetic knee design and better gait dynamics [9, 10]. The development of prosthetic knee joints is crucial in helping people with TFA to accommodate their daily life necessities while achieving normative gait. Over time, prosthetic knees have progressed significantly, including the variable-damping, computer-controlled knees [10]. Nevertheless, passive prosthetic knee devices are still a huge market and especially suited for people in developing countries when it comes to financial value [11, 12].

The main purpose of rehabilitation after amputation is to ensure the amputee to be able to ambulate successfully with the use of a prosthesis. Walking is a challenging task for amputees, and it is one of the demanding activities of daily living. When people with TFA learned to ambulate with the prosthetic device during the rehabilitation process, they will eventually need to adapt to the more challenging environmental factor, such as uneven surfaces.

Walking on an uneven surface involves unpredictable circumstances such as inclines, declines, while concurrently performing cognitive or motor interference tasks. Biomechanical assessment based on walking on an uneven surface is still insufficient contrary to the assessment of walking on an even surface and other conditions such as over obstacles, stairs, ramps, etc. The research of walking assessment on even surface, however, extensive gait research on an uneven surface is needed to test lower limb amputees' ability to navigate more difficult terrains that mimic outdoor walking [13].

This study investigated the effects of prosthetic knee joints during dual-task walking on even and uneven surfaces in people with TFA wearing a non-microprocessor-controlled prosthetic knee compared to age-matched controls. The uneven surface was designed to simulate the regular outdoor walking condition in daily life that would distort subjects' peripheral sensory feedback. Dual-task gait assessment involves in this study will determine the effects of a cognitive process during walking in terms of temporal-spatial, kinetic, and kinematics parameters.

2 Methods

2.1 *Participants*

Seven individuals, all males, who had undergone a transfemoral amputation were recruited in the study. The eligible criteria for people with TFA were one-sided amputation, 18 years of age or older, able to walk without any aid assistance, and average hearing ability. Fifteen able-bodied participants (8 males, 7 females) were selected as controls. Participant details are presented in Table 1. Transfemoral participants had been amputated for an average of 4.86 years (range: 2–8) due to trauma. All transfemoral participants were selected based on their passive mechanical prosthesis and were categorized into two groups: polycentric (TFA_P) and fluid-controlled which consisted of pneumatic and hydraulic (TFA_{FC}). Among the seven subjects, four wore polycentric knee joints whereas the other three wore fluid-controlled knee

Table 1 Participant demographics/characteristics

Subject	Sex	Age (y)	Mass (kg)	Height (cm)	Time since amputation (y)	Aetiology	Prosthetic knee
Transfemoral							
T1	M	24	96	169	2	Trauma	Polycentric
T2	M	21	58	163	2	Trauma	Polycentric
T3	M	44	68	168	2	Trauma	Polycentric
T4	M	27	105	176	5	Trauma	Pneumatic
T5	M	25	54.5	165	8	Trauma	Hydraulic
T6	M	35	76	178	5	Trauma	Polycentric
T7	M	29	77	174.5	8	Trauma	Pneumatic
Mean		29.29	76.36	170.29	4.86		
SD		7.85	18.67	5.88	2.61		
Able-bodied							
Mean		29.33	79.73	163.80			
SD		5.31	20.80	9.21			

joints, respectively. The study was approved by the Medical Research and Ethics Committee (MREC) [Reference Number: KKM/NIHSEC/P19-2206(11)].

2.2 Procedure

All participants attended one session of a lab visit. The participants were given forms that contain study details, and consent before conducting the research. Demographic information of participants was collected beforehand to characterize participants. The participants were verbally informed about experiment protocols and were given forms such as participant information sheet and consent form were distributed before the data was collected. All participants were required to wear shoes and transfemoral amputees wore their prostheses during gait analysis.

Motion data were collected using a 5-camera motion capture system (Vicon Nexus, Oxford, UK) with two Kistler force plates. The sampling rate used for force measurement and marker trajectories were 1000 Hz and 100 Hz, respectively. Total 16 reflective markers were attached to the torso over the iliac crest, and to the hips, thighs, knees, shanks, ankles, and feet of both lower limbs as well as to the prosthesis for amputees using self-adhesive, non-allergenic tape. Participants performed straight-line walking along five meters walkway (even and uneven surfaces) in the laboratory at their self-selected walking speed by wearing their own prosthetic feet and shoes. The force plates are located at the center of the walkway.

The gait assessment consisted of two main conditions: single task (walking alone), and dual-task (walking while performing a cognitive task) for both even and uneven surfaces. The uneven surface was performed over a 65 kg/m^3 density of foam surface as a base, layered by 50 mm thickness of grass and gravels in random order. The length and width of the designed surface were 5 m $\times$ 2 m, respectively. Adequate rest between walking trials was allowed if necessary. Three successful trials were recorded and processed for each assessment.

The Auditory Stroop Test (AST) was selected as the cognitive assessment in this study [14]. The stimuli were programmed using a custom PsychoPy program (Version 3.1.5, Jonathan Peirce, UK) and were administered using a Bluetooth headset (to produce the AST; Sony CH500). The auditory stimuli contained the words "high and "low" pronounced in either a high or low pitch. Participants were instructed to verbally name the pitch as quickly and accurately as possible after each stimulus was produced. The assessment was performed during single-task (while participants were seated) and dual-task (while participants were walking) conditions. Three successful trials were collected and extracted for further analysis. Descriptive analysis was performed for biomechanical assessment.

3 Results

3.1 Temporal-Spatial

Participants with TFA had lower walking speed and cadence, longer stride and step times, shorter stride length, and step length for temporal-spatial measurement compared to the able-bodied group under both even and uneven walking conditions. The results shows also that subjects with fluid-controlled knee joints obtained overall higher values compared to the subjects with polycentric knee joints (Table 2).

3.2 Joint Kinematics of the Lower Limb

The illustration of joint kinematic parameters of the hip, knee, and ankle in the sagittal plane are represented in Fig. 1 and summarized in Table 2. Individuals with TFA had a shorter stance phase and longer swing phase compared to able-bodied subjects. The amputee group with fluid-controlled knee joints had an almost similar range of hip extension at HA1, while the amputee group with polycentric knee joints had a lower hip extension at that phase.

The hip extension for the able-bodied group did not show much difference between even and uneven surfaces, however, the difference between the amputee group can be observed when walking on both surfaces. People with TFA had lower maximum early-stance knee flexion [KA1] compared to the able-bodied group. The maximum swing ankle plantarflexion [AA3] in people with TFA also very minimal and the value is closer to neutral.

3.3 Joint Kinetics of the Lower Limb

In comparison to the able-bodied group, the joint moments and powers in people with TFA were reduced. The prosthetic leg of the TFA group had reduced hip moments, at HM1 and HM2, reduced knee moment range at KM3, plantarflexion moment, at AM2, compared to the controls in all conditions (Fig. 1; Table 2). The prosthetic leg when walked on the even surface had reduced knee power range and reduced hip power generation, at HP1 and HP3, and reduced hip power generation at HP1 and HP2 compared to the able-bodied.

However, the able-bodied group and amputee group with polycentric prosthetic knee joints had greater power generation during the early-stance phase [HP1] when walking on the uneven surface. The amputee group with fluid-controlled knee joints had power absorption during walking on the even surface, contradict to power generation of the able-bodied group during the early-stance phase [KP1], and the amputee group had less power absorption during the early-swing phase [KP3] and late-swing

Table 2 Means of temporal-spatial, kinematic, and kinetics parameters for all participants during walking on even and uneven surfaces

	Even surface			Uneven surface		
Parameter	AB	TFA_P	TFA_{FC}	AB	TFA_P	TFA_{FC}
Temporal-spatial						
Walking speed (m/s)	1.01	0.68	0.81	0.87	0.59	0.63
Cadence (steps/min)	99.34	86.96	92.08	84.52	78.68	81.71
Stride time (s)	1.13	1.38	1.306	1.232	1.54	1.48
Stride length (m)	1.16	0.93	1.053	1.14	0.88	0.95
Step time (s)	0.58	0.77	0.744	0.62	0.89	0.89
Step length (m)	0.58	0.45	0.544	0.58	0.45	0.52
Kinematic						
HA1 (°)	9.10	4.65	8.26	10.13	4.98	3.51
KA1(°)	29.58	38.78	21.28	30.67	29.37	62.24
KA2 (°)	62.24	48.41	38.79	75.06	47.51	42.75
AA1 (°)	5.19	18.67	3.42	2.69	12.04	1.59
AA2 (°)	11.78	19.94	8.15	10.47	23.23	8.74
AA3 (°)	10.85	0.34	0.48	8.68	5.25	0.16
Kinetic						
HM1 (Nmm)	875.88	229.13	274.65	940.25	444.16	444.80
HM2 (Nmm)	1194.35	643.38	604.89	283.41	343.45	352.88
HP1 (W)	0.89	0.31	0.36	1.67	2.68	0.41
HP2 (W)	0.60	0.27	0.33	0.94	0.37	0.16
HP3 (W)	1.10	0.22	0.19	0.95	0.37	0.16
KM1 (Nmm)	46.30	142.82	28.18	8.76	148.34	30.43
KM2 (Nmm)	149.18	40.64	125.79	5.89	186.39	149.18
KM3 (Nmm)	455.82	51.38	89.29	364.22	66.56	143.94
KP1 (W)	0.12	0.05	0.39	0.20	0.14	0.05
KP2 (W)	0.04	0.03	0.06	0.02	0.02	0.07
KP3 (W)	2.00	0.23	0.36	1.30	0.24	0.24
KP4 (W)	1.18	0.20	0.33	1.18	0.22	0.21
AM1 (Nmm)	27.76	181.04	81.25	25.57	13.40	43.74
AM2 (Nmm)	1107.91	365.48	731.71	900.47	424.56	564.24
AP1 (W)	0.43	0.07	0.33	0.18	0.05	0.11
AP2 (W)	1.27	0.21	0.40	0.49	0.14	0.11

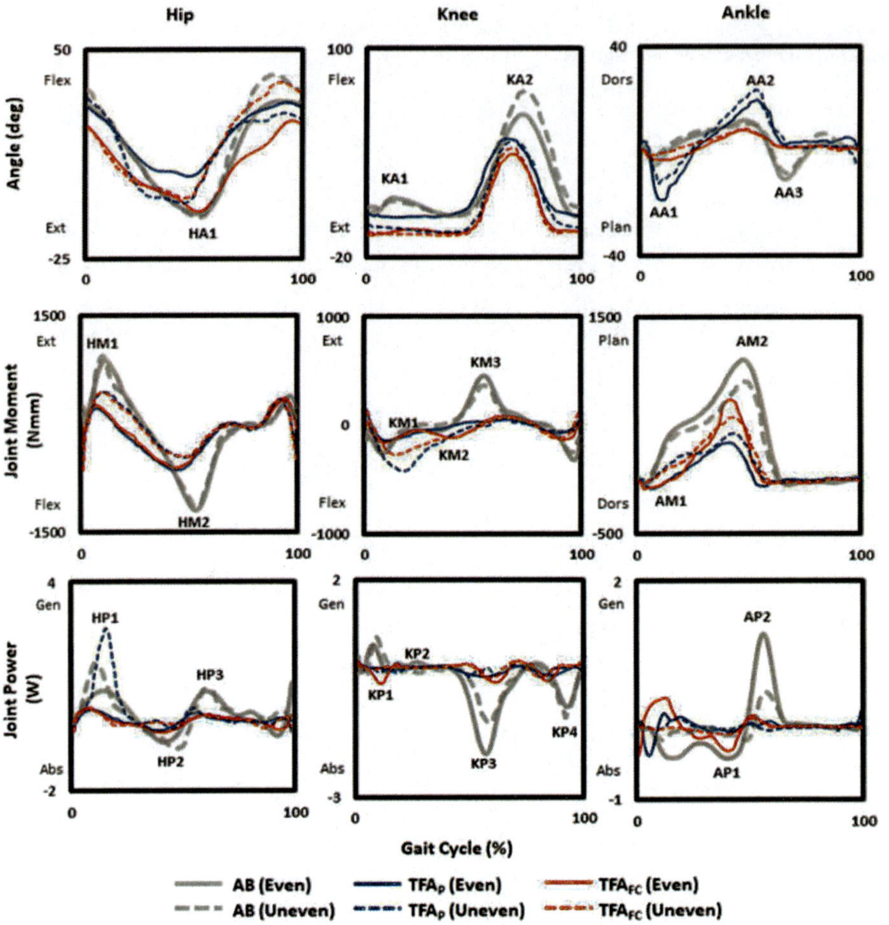

Fig. 1 The comparison of the kinematics and kinetics of the prosthetic leg TFA_{FC} (red and dash), TFA_P (blue and dash), and the able-bodied leg (grey and dash). A plot of the mean of the able-bodied limb in the angle, moment, and power for hip, knee, ankle joints as a percentage of a gait cycle, where 0% is initial contact and 100% is subsequent initial contact

phase [KP4]. The dominant leg of the able-bodied group had less power generation, at AP2, when walked on the uneven surface, and the amputee group had much lesser ankle power generation, at AP2 than the able-bodied group, coinciding with toe-off.

For the kinematic parameters: HA1, maximum hip extension; KA1, maximum early stance knee flexion; KA2, maximum swing knee flexion; AA1, maximum early stance ankle plantarflexion; AA2, maximum stance ankle dorsiflexion; AA3, maximum swing ankle plantar flexion.

For the kinetic parameters: HM1, maximum stance hip extension moment; HM2, maximum hip flexion moment; HP1, maximum early-stance hip concentric power;

HP2, maximum late-stance hip eccentric power; HP3, maximum swing hip concentric power; KM1, maximum stance knee extension moment; KM2, maximum stance knee flexion moment; KM3, maximum swing knee flexion moment; KP1, maximum early-stance knee eccentric power; KP2, maximum stance knee concentric power; KP3, maximum early-swing knee eccentric power; KP4, maximum late-swing knee eccentric power; AM1, maximum ankle dorsiflexion moment; AM2, maximum ankle plantarflexion moment; AP1, maximum ankle eccentric power; AP2, maximum ankle concentric power [15, 16].

3.4 Ground Reaction Forces

Time-histories for vertical GRF in the stance phase are presented in Fig. 2 and their peaks are summarized in Table 3. The vertical GRF patterns of the dominant leg of the able-bodied and transfemoral group at their preferrable speeds show the typical M-shape (two-peak pattern) found in human walking. TFA_P and the able-bodied groups had a higher active peak [FZ_{Max2}] than the impact peak [FZ_{Max1}] when walking on the even surface, opposite to the TFA_{FC} group which had a larger FZ_{Max2} than FZ_{Max1}.

All groups have larger FZ_{Max1} than FZ_{Max2} when walking on uneven surfaces. The prosthetic leg had a significantly decreased vertical GRF at FZ_{Max1} during weight acceptance. People with TFA had decreased vertical GRF at Fz_{Max1} and Fz_{Max2}, compared to the controls during the stance phase. The spike at heel contact can be observed for the TFA group when walking on the even surface. The vertical GRF

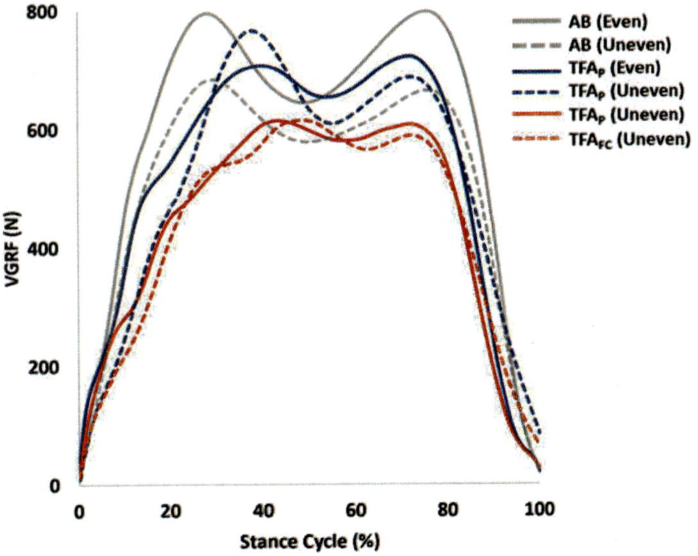

Fig. 2 Average vertical ground reaction force when walking on even and uneven surfaces

Table 3 Means of vertical ground reaction forces for all participants during walking on even and uneven surfaces

	Even surface			Uneven surface		
Parameter	AB	TFA_P	TFA_{FC}	AB	TFA_P	TFA_{FC}
vGRF						
Fz_{Max1} (N)	794.53	706.20	613.50	682.90	765.91	614.30
Fz_{Min} (N)	643.53	652.86	543.17	577.37	608.40	526.07
Fz_{Max2} (N)	797.55	721.74	606.97	663.67	686.84	588.21

of the able-bodied increased steeper compared to the amputees with fluid-controlled knee joints in both conditions. The difference of vertical force maxima [Fz_{Max}] can be observed when all subjects walked on the different types of surfaces.

4 Discussion

The goal of the present study was to assess the gait pattern of amputees with different types of prosthetic knee joints, by comparing them to the able-bodied participants in terms of temporal-spatial, kinetics, and kinematics. The effects of a cognitive and mechanical disturbance such as walking on an uneven surface were investigated apart from walking on an even surface.

People with TFA were hypothesized to be affected by the cognitive and mechanical perturbation compared to the able-bodied group with more irregularity and less stability [1]. The effects were observed to be greater in the amputee group with the polycentric knee joints.

In comparison between the transfemoral amputees and able-bodied individuals' gait, the cadence was found to be decreased resulting from the increased cycle time as the duration of the stance phase seemed to be shorter while the swing phase was longer on the amputated side. It indicated that individuals with TFA have less stability compared to normal healthy people and therefore spend longer time in the swing phase during the gait cycle.

The previous study reported that the duration of the stance phase of the prosthetic leg in people with TFA was shorter than the sound leg, which is suggesting that the sound leg bears most of the load during walking [17–20]. The stance phase for people with TFA in this study seemed to be shorter during walking on the uneven surface. In comparison between different types of prosthetic knee joints, the amputee group with polycentric knee joints had a shorter stance cycle than the amputee group with fluid-controlled knee joints.

The measurement of walking speed in gait assessment is proven to be reliable and people with lower extremity amputation were reported to have lower speed when performing dual-task conditions. Participants with TFA walked slower with shorter step lengths and longer step times, which is related to the walking speed of subjects [21].

Forces play a large role in influencing the motions. In the case of walking, it is both the supporting force which would be the vertical ground reaction force as well as the frictional force which enables us to walk the way we do. Supporting the body weight, in static and dynamic conditions, is one of the main functions of the lower limb. Symmetrical weight shifting over the limbs during stance and gait is a relevant clinical problem for people with a lower limb amputation. Through limb loss, the center of gravity is shifted laterally to the side of the non-amputated limb, a shift that is not fully compensated for by the mass of the prosthesis. Thus, the decrease in vertical loading on the amputated side is not only related to the difference between the weight of the prosthesis and the weight of the anatomical segment.

For kinematic findings in this study, the knee range during loading response or maximum early-stance knee flexion [KA1] among amputees with passive prosthetic knee joints was reported to be limited in the previous literature. The knee flexion at the swing phase was closer to normal. Similar results were shown for the hip movement, however, there was a sudden increment of flexion in the swing phase, as the component comes to its expansion halt and the energy of the swinging prosthetic leg was exchanged to the femur. The heel-rise phase of individuals with TFA during the stance phase also appeared to be earlier than in the able-bodied group, due to the ability to dorsiflex using their prosthetic ankle were reduced.

The ankle range of motion during the gait cycle in people with TFA was very restricted, with no plantarflexion around toe-off [AA3]. The moment shows that the prosthesis attempted to retain a neutral position, resisting plantarflexion during the loading response phase, resisting dorsiflexion during the mid-stance phase and terminal stance phase, when the ankle absorbed a little power in becoming maximally dorsiflexed. Part of this was returned in power generation as the moment reduced and the ankle returned towards the neutral position. However, the power generation involved was very small, when compared with the able-bodied group.

The loss of active plantar flexion at the end of the stance phase showed that the muscle power cannot be used to provide an active ‘push off’ and the effective length of the prosthetic leg is shorter than the able-bodied so that it had to be lifted clear of the ground sooner. The ankle angle was also nearly normal, although the movement into plantarflexion at the end of the stance phase was the relatively low magnitude and occurred a little late. This is because of passive movement which resulting from the removal of loading from the elastic foot mechanism, rather than the active plantarflexion seen in able-bodied subjects.

This preliminary study was limited to a small sample size of the homogeneous amputee group. The significant effect between groups could not be determined. The increase in sample size may show the greater effect of dual-task gait assessment on the performance of amputees with different types of prosthetic knees.

Hence, the preliminary results from this study may act as supplementary evidence for gait rehabilitation of the transfemoral amputees by analyzing the performance of prosthetic leg based on dual-task walking assessment. Applying these measures to larger patient populations may enhance fundamental gait analysis and could provide a useful diagnostic tool to reveal differences in the gait patterns between patients and controls and their responses.

5 Conclusion

Results of this quantitative gait analysis study evaluate the way prosthetic users walk compared to healthy individuals. It is well known that bodyweight transfer over the prosthesis when standing and walking is an important goal in the rehabilitation of people with a lower limb amputation. Based on the preliminary results in this study, it can be concluded that kinetic measures of walking are useful because they convey information that cannot be discerned visually by an observer, and they may directly relate to what the prosthetic user perceives while they walk.

Changes in terrain modify the gait characteristics of able-bodied and transfemoral amputee subjects. In both subject groups, self-selected walking speed and cadence decreased. The amputee's locomotion disability becomes a significant factor when exposed to a particularly difficult environment, such as uneven ground where the transfemoral amputees walked slightly slower with a reduced range of motion. This study reports a preliminary result on the effects of transfemoral amputees with different types of prosthetic knees while performing dual-task walking on the different types of surfaces. Further research should be prioritized on the effects between dual-task activities and different types of surfaces with a larger sample size of people with TFA.

Acknowledgements This project is supported by the Ministry of Education Malaysia through the Fundamental Research Grant Scheme (FRGS/1/2017/SKK06/UM/02/1).

References

1. Lamoth, C.J., Ainsworth, E., Polomski, W., Houdijk, H.: Variability and stability analysis of walking of transfemoral amputees. Med. Eng. Phys. **32**(9), 1009–1014 (2010)
2. Jaegers, S.M., Vos, L.D., Rispens, P., Hof, A.L.: The relationship between comfortable and most metabolically efficient walking speed in persons with unilateral above-knee amputation. Arch. Phys. Med. Rehab. **74**(5), 521–525 (1993)
3. Silverman, A.K., et al.: Compensatory mechanisms in below-knee amputee gait in response to increasing steady-state walking speeds. **28**(4), 602–609 (2008)
4. Chow, D.H., Holmes, A.D., Lee, C.K., Sin, S.W.: The effect of prosthesis alignment on the symmetry of gait in subjects with unilateral transtibial amputation. **30**(2), 114–128 (2006)
5. Houdijk, H., Pollmann, E., Groenewold, M., Wiggerts, H., Polomski, W.: The energy cost for the step-to-step transition in amputee walking. Gait and Posture **30**(1), 35–40 (2009)
6. Chin, T., et al.: % VO2max as an indicator of prosthetic rehabilitation outcome after dysvascular amputation. **26**(1), 44–49 (2002)
7. Miller, W.C., Speechley, M., Deathe, B.: The prevalence and risk factors of falling and fear of falling among lower extremity amputees. Arch. Phys. Med. Rehab. **82**(8), 1031–1037 (2001)

8. Ku, P.X., Osman, N.A.A., Abas, W.A.B.W.: Balance control in lower extremity amputees during quiet standing: a systematic review. Gait and Posture **39**(2), 672–682 (2014)
9. Chin, T. et al.: Effect of an intelligent prosthesis (IP) on the walking ability of young transfemoral amputees: comparison of IP users with able-bodied people. **82**(6), 447–451 (2003)
10. Johansson, J.L., Sherrill, D.M., Riley, P.O., Bonato, P., Herr, H.A.: A clinical comparison of variable-damping and mechanically passive prosthetic knee devices. Am. J. Phys. Med. Rehab. **84**(8), 563–575 (2005)
11. Arelekatti, V.M., Winter, A.G.: Design of a fully passive prosthetic knee mechanism for transfemoral amputees in India. In: 2015 IEEE International Conference on Rehabilitation Robotics (ICORR), pp. 350–356. IEEE (2015)
12. Narang, Y.S.: Identification of design requirements for a high-performance, low-cost, passive prosthetic knee through user analysis and dynamic simulation. Massachusetts Institute of Technology (2013)
13. Muessig, J.A., et al.: Variability in trunk and pelvic movement of transfemoral amputees using a C-leg system compared to healthy controls. **68**, 102539 (2019)
14. Morgan, S.J., Hafner, B.J., Kelly, V.E.: The effects of a concurrent task on walking in persons with transfemoral amputation compared to persons without limb loss. Prosthet. Orthot. Int. **40**(4), 490–496 (2016)
15. Kobayashi, T., Hisano, G., Namiki, Y., Hashizume, S., Hobara, H.: Walking characteristics of runners with a transfemoral or knee-disarticulation prosthesis. Clin. Biomech. **80**, 105132 (2020)
16. Okita, Y., et al.: Kinetic differences between level walking and ramp descent in individuals with unilateral transfemoral amputation using a prosthetic knee without a stance control mechanism. **63**, 80–85 (2018)
17. Hof, A.L., van Bockel, R.M., Schoppen, T., Postema, K.: Control of lateral balance in walking: experimental findings in normal subjects and above-knee amputees. Gait Posture **25**(2), 250–258 (2007)
18. Creylman, V., Knippels, I., Janssen, P., Biesbrouck, E., Lechler, K., Peeraer, L.: Assessment of transfemoral amputees using a passive microprocessor-controlled knee versus an active powered microprocessor-controlled knee for level walking. **15**(3), 53–63 (2016)
19. Nolan, L., Lees, A.: The functional demands on the intact limb during walking for active trans-femoral and trans-tibial amputees. **24**(2), 117–125 (2000)
20. Nolan, L., et al.: Adjustments in gait symmetry with walking speed in trans-femoral and trans-tibial amputees. **17**(2), 142–151 (2003)
21. Sturk, J.A., et al.: Maintaining stable transfemoral amputee gait on level, sloped and simulated uneven conditions in a virtual environment. **14**(3), 226–235 (2019)

Ground Reaction Force of Trilateral Amputee During Walking With and Without Upper Limb Prosthesis: Case Report

Nur Afiqah Hashim, Nasrul Anuar Abd Razak, and Noor Azuan Abu Osman

Abstract Background: Human walking has been extensively studied but less research has been done on the gait of trilateral amputee. Trilateral amputee is a person with three missing limbs. This study investigates the effect of upper limb prostheses on vertical ground reaction force of a trilateral amputee during level walking. A subject with bilateral transradial and unilateral transtibial amputation participated in this study. The subject wore prostheses both for upper and lower limb. Kristler force platform was used to collect data while the subject walked with and without upper limb prosthesis. The determined mean values of normalized components of trajectory of vertical ground reaction force were compared with able-bodied data. Three vertical GRF measures (F1, the first peak force; F2, minimum force; and F3, the second peak force) were extracted and analyzed. Ground reaction force, loading rate and unloading rate generated by the trilateral amputee is greater than able-bodied person. When donning upper limb prosthesis, the value of F1 and F3 increased by 11.93% and 9.90% respectively, but the value of F2 reduced by 8.75%. The gait of trilateral amputee wearing upper limb prosthesis were characterized by high impact peak, low force value during mid stance and steeper loading rate and unloading rate. The use of upper limb prostheses affects the vertical ground reaction force of trilateral amputee subject in this study during walking.

Keywords Adaptive gait · Amputee gait · Ground reaction force · Multiple amputation · Prosthetic hand · Trilateral amputee

1 Introduction

The prevalence of limb loss in the United States was estimated to be 1.6 million in 2005 and is anticipated to more than double by the year 2050, at which point it will affect nearly 1 in every 120 individuals [1]. The most common causes of amputation include vascular disease, trauma, cancer, and congenital deformities [2] and it is

N. A. Hashim (✉) · N. A. A. Razak · N. A. A. Osman
Department of Biomedical Engineering, Faculty of Engineering, Universiti Malaya, Kuala Lumpur, Malaysia

J. Usman et al. (eds.), *6th Kuala Lumpur International Conference on Biomedical Engineering 2021*, IFMBE Proceedings 86,
https://doi.org/10.1007/978-3-030-90724-2_20

estimated that approximately 7.3% of individuals with trauma-associated amputation have multiple limb loss [3]. Although there are large number of pathologies in which the effectiveness of gait analysis was assessed, high quality literature evidences exist only for cerebral palsy, acquired lesions of the central nervous system such as stroke, traumatic brain injury and lower limb amputations [4]. Multiple limb amputation is one of the interesting topics that received less attention. There have been few reports about a multiple amputee because such cases are very uncommon [5–10] and very few of them discussing about gait analysis. The effect of upper-limb loss on lower-limb gait biomechanics is not fully understood [11]. Monitoring human gait is essential to quantify gait issues [12] associated with fall-prone individuals as well as other gait-related movement disorders [13].

In this article, the gait analysis of 33 years old trilateral amputee donning upper and lower limb prosthesis was discussed. Trilateral amputee is a person with multiple limb amputations who had three limbs amputated. This paper aims to examine the effect of upper limb prostheses on vertical ground reaction force of a trilateral amputee during walking. In order to access the influence of upper limb prostheses on trilateral amputee during walking, this study compares the data of vertical ground reaction force (GRF) of a trilateral amputee who walks with and without prosthesis with able-bodied gait data from the previous study by Winiarski et al. [14].

2 Methods

The experiment was carried out at Human Performance & Motion Analysis Lab, Faculty Engineering University of Malaya. The research protocol of this study was approved by the Medical Research Ethics Committee and the Ministry of Health Malaysia, with an Approval ID: NMRR-16-2106-32880. The Medical Research Ethics Committee decided that the data collection for this study would involve physical evaluation. The subject was required to sign a written consent form prior to the tests. The study was conducted under the supervision of Certified Prosthetist and Orthotist Category 1.

2.1 Participants

A 32 years old trilateral amputee, who has a bilateral transradial and a unilateral transtibial (left) amputation was selected to participate in the study (Fig. 1). The subject was amputated from electrical injury in 2010 and started to use prosthetic hands and leg two months after amputation until now, 2021. The amputation of both upper limbs was made at approximately 40% of level of short below elbow amputation. The subject had changed his prosthetic hands and leg twice after his first prosthesis. For upper limb prothesis the subject use MyoHand VariPlus Speed from Ottobock, made of aluminium and plastic, weighted 632 g, with 2 internal socket

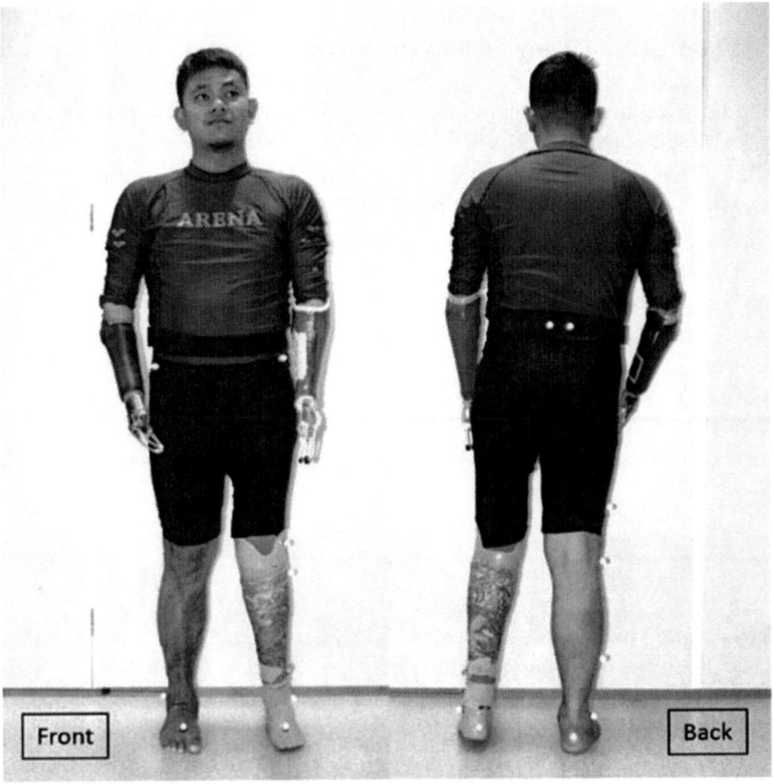

Fig. 1 Trilateral amputee subject with two upper limb prostheses

electrodes, 1 myo battery on the laminated forearm, and a terminal device without a myo-glove. Meanwhile for lower limb prosthesis, subject used patella tendon bearing socket with locking liner and Solid Ankle Cushioned Heel type of feet. Recently, the subject stopped using one of his prosthetic hands for about five months due to the problem with the sensors. The subject has the ability to walk 10 m without an assistive device or undue fatigue, and no other reported conditions or medication use that would affect walking or balance.

2.2 Data Collection

The goal of this study is to compare the vertical ground reaction force of a trilateral amputee during walking with and without upper limb prosthesis. The participants performed six successful walking trials (barefoot walking) and the mean data were used for analysis. The subject was asked to walk leisurely, according to their comfortable speed of walking at two conditions of wearing and not wearing upper limb prosthesis. The subject was asked to practice walking for 3 m, and the walking speed was monitored using a timer in order to ensure the speed would be similar for every trial. The measurements of vertical GRF were obtained with two 6-degrees of freedom force plates, Kistler 9286A (Kistler, Switzerland) embedded in the middle of the pathway. Force plates were able to measure the GRF generated by a body moving across them, in order to quantify balance, gait and other parameters of biomechanics. The system was calibrated at every session to ensure its accuracy. The GRF were calculated using the Vicon clinical manager software (Oxford Metrics). The average data for all the trials were normalized with respect to the body weight (BW) of subject to objectively compare the results with the data from able-bodied subject from Winiarski et al. [14]. Relative difference was conducted to compare the GRF parameters of able-bodied subject found from previous study by Winiarski et al. [14]. The vertical component of the GRF [15] vector was parameterized by the following indicators:

- F_{HS}—magnitude of force at heel strike.
- F_1—maximal value of force between 0 and 40% of stance time.
- F_2—minimal value of force between 40 and 60% of stance time.
- F_3—maximal value of force between 60 and 100% of stance time.
- F_{TO}—magnitude of force during toe off.
- tF_1—the time occurrence of F_1.
- tF_2—the time occurrence of F_2.
- tF_3—the time occurrence of F_3.

3 Results

The analysis revealed a close correspondence between the measured parameters. The parameters F_1, F_2 and F_3 followed by loading rate (LR) and unloading rate (ULR) demonstrated some differences (Table 1). For the trilateral amputee, the GRF value at the end of initial double stance (F_{HS}) was greater (4.88%) than normal person. No differences were noted between F_{HS} of person wearing and not wearing upper limb prostheses.

Similar relations were found in the GRF value at the beginning of terminal double stance (F_{TO}). The force during toe off by trilateral amputee subject was slightly greater than the normal person both when wearing (3.66%) and not wearing prosthesis (2.44%). Compared to able-bodied data, trilateral amputee produced 4.27% more F_1 when walking with upper limb prosthesis but 6.84% less without upper limb prosthesis. The first maximal value of GRF (F_1) increased considerably (11.93%) when the subject walked with upper limb prosthesis. The local minimum of GRF in the middle of single stance (F_2) of trilateral amputee was less than able-bodied person.

Table 1 Comparison of gait parameter between able-bodied individual and trilateral amputee

Indicators	Able-bodied	Trilateral		Relative difference (%)		
		√[a]	X[b]	Normal versus √[a]	Normal versus X[b]	√[a] versus X[b]
F_{HS} [BW]	0.82 (SD 0.05)	0.86 (SD 0.16)	0.86 (SD 0.25)	−4.88	−4.88	0.00
F_1 [BW]	1.17 (SD 0.09)	1.22 (SD 0.05)	1.09 (SD 0.11)	−4.27	6.84	−11.93
Δt_{F1} [s]	0.15 (SD 0.05)	0.19 (SD 0.08)	0.18 (SD 0.03)	−26.67	−20.00	5.26
LR [BW/s]	8.0 (SD 0.1)	23.72 (SD 0.05)	10.31 (SD 0.04)	−196.50	−28.88	56.53
F_2 [BW]	0.81 (SD 0.05)	0.73 (SD 0.01)	0.80 (SD 0.03)	9.88	1.23	8.75
F_3 [BW]	1.11 (SD 0.03)	1.11 (SD 0.05)	1.01 (SD 0.10)	0.00	9.01	−9.90
T_{sw}—t_{F3} [s]	0.16 (SD 0.01)	0.16 (SD 0.04)	0.15 (SD 0.05)	0.00	6.25	6.25
ULR [BW/s]	7.0 (SD 0.1)	13.64 (SD 0.07)	10.13 (SD 0.05)	−94.86	−44.71	25.73
F_{TO} [BW]	0.82 (SD 0.08)	0.85 (SD 0.11)	0.84 (SD 0.09)	−3.66	−2.44	1.18

[a] √: trilateral amputee walks with upper limb prosthesis
[b] X: trilateral amputee walks without upper limb prosthesis

The value of F_2 reduced (8.75%) when the subject walked with upper limb prostheses. Second maximal value of GRF (F_3) were similar for both able-bodied and trilateral amputee with upper limb prostheses but decreased considerably (9.90%) when trilateral amputee subject walked without upper limb prostheses. The LR demonstrated clear difference between normal and trilateral amputee subject. Steeper LR was noted for the trilateral amputee. Without upper limb prostheses, trilateral amputee subject's LR increased about 28.88% but 196% with upper limb prostheses when compared to able-bodied LR. Upper limb prosthesis affected subject's gait as its LR doubled (56.53%) when subject walked with upper limb prosthesis. Similar relations were found for ULR force. ULR for trilateral amputee was greater than able-bodied data but it increased only 25.73% when the subject walked with upper limb prostheses.

4 Discussion

The The three-dimensional kinematic gait analysis was conducted on trilateral amputee subject when the subject walked with and without upper limb prostheses.

This study measure how different this study from the parameter of able-bodied subject found from previous study by Winiarski et al. [14]. The vertical GRF data collected from able-bodied were selected to be compared with the data from this experiment.

Two obvious peaks were observed in vertical GRF called the Impact peak (F_1) and Active peak (F_3) which separated by valley (F_2). The impact peak corresponded to the time just after the heel touched the force plate and at the same time the centre of gravity travelled down towards the ground caused increased force from the ground in vertical direction meanwhile active peak corresponded to the toe pushing off the ground. The value of vertical GRF reduced between the 1st and 2nd peaks. This dip (F_2) occurred as the centre of gravity was moving away from the ground. Impact peak occurred in phase I (0–40% St), the dip in phase II (40–60% St) and active peak in phase III (60–100 St).

In Wang et al. [16] study proved that increased mass of carriage lead to increased peak GRF and reaction LR during walking while assessing the influences of load carriage and muscular fatigue on GRF and ground reaction LR during walking. The result from this study is corresponded to the findings of the research. When the subject wore upper limb prosthesis, it was clear that the mass of the carriage increased. Although the additional weight is less than 1 kg, this could be the reason of the increments of F_1 and F_3 value during walking.

Mathematically, based on impulse $I = \int F\,dt$ formula, impulse was calculated by multiplying the impact force by the time over which the impact force acted. Subject reported that he was less stable while walking with upper limb prostheses and walked 3.58% faster as seen in Fig. 2. The kinematic and kinetic characteristics were proven to be influenced by the gait speed [17]. It has been stated that the margins of stability

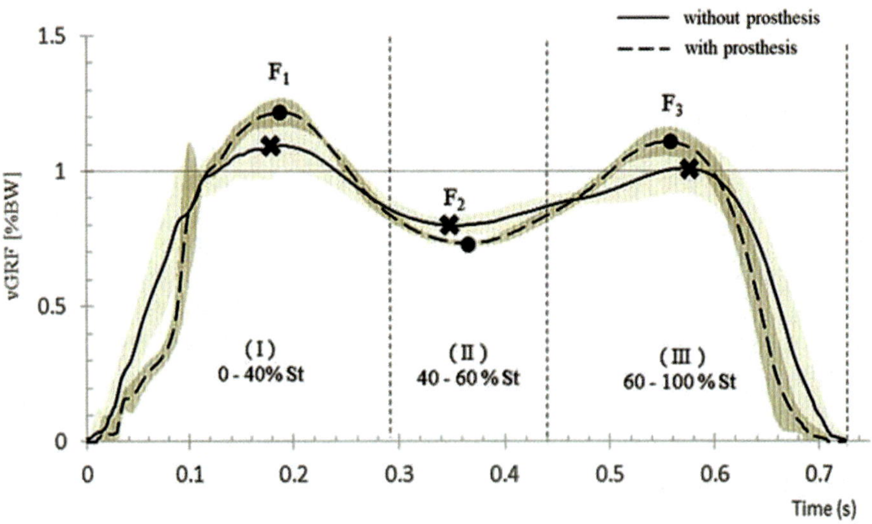

Fig. 2 The vertical ground reaction force (vGRF) of trilateral amputee walking with and without both upper limb prostheses

can be increased by increasing walking speed or decreasing stride length [18, 19]. As the subject increased the speed to increase margin of stability, the stance time reduced. Reduced stance time leads to less time to produce an impulse to the ground, so the peak forces (F_1 and F_2) became greater.

The LR of the GRF in human gait was the degree of the slope of the GRF curve determined by the change of force (ΔF) divided by the time interval at which the change of force occurred. LR occurred at the time interval $\Delta tF1$ while ULR occurred measured at the time interval ΔtF_3. As expected, the LR and ULR of trilateral subject proved to be greater than the able-bodied subject also because of shorter support time at ΔtF_1 and ΔtF_3. This can be reduced by shock absorbing material to compensate for the absence of impact-absorbing mechanisms in an amputee's lower limb [20].

Investigators have further observed that increased gait variability was associated with significantly higher energy expenditure during walking [21]. Walking required metabolic energy, primarily to generate muscle force and work for body weight support, propulsion and leg swing [22]. It was reported that increase in vertical GRF and LR result in increased muscle activities [23]. These changes were accompanied by increase in energy cost as an attempt to enhance gait stability and/or the selection of alternative balance control strategies. From the results, it can be said that the usage of upper limb prosthesis requires extra energy during walking.

The limitation of this study was that the subject reported that he was more comfortable walking with his shoes compared to barefoot walking. In order to follow common approach in the literature to have participant walking barefooted, however this may not accurately represent their natural movement patterns in everyday life. The conclusions drawn from this case study may not be transferable to other settings as it deals only with one person. In addition, different prostheses weight will influence the gait of a trilateral amputee differently. Although it is not convenient to find the similar sample of a trilateral amputee, further study should incorporate greater number of participants. With that, an adequately powered statistical analysis of the main effect can be performed.

5 Conclusion

This result obtained in this paper discovered that the gait of a trilateral amputee was influenced by upper limb prosthetic usage. The gait of trilateral amputee wearing upper limb prosthesis were characterized by high impact peak, low force value during mid stance and steeper LR and ULR. The data collected from this experiment showed that the trilateral amputee utilized more energy when walking with upper limb prostheses. The authors believed that this gap can be minimized with reduction of upper limb prosthesis mass.

References

1. Ziegler-Graham, K., MacKenzie, E.J., Ephraim, P.L., Travison, T.G., Brookmeyer, R.: Estimating the prevalence of limb loss in the United States: 2005 to 2050. Arch. Phys. Med. Rehabil. **89**(3), 422–429 (2008)
2. Pasquina, P.F., Miller, M., Carvalho, A., Corcoran, M., Vandersea, J., Johnson, E., et al.: Special considerations for multiple limb amputation. Curr. Phys. Med. Rehabil. Rep. **2**(4), 273–289 (2014)
3. Barmparas, G., Inaba, K., Teixeira, P.G., Dubose, J.J., Criscuoli, M., Talving, P., et al.: Epidemiology of post-traumatic limb amputation: a National Trauma Databank analysis. Am. Surg. **76**(11), 1214–1222 (2010)
4. Baker, R., Esquenazi, A., Benedetti, M.G., Desloovere, K.: Gait analysis: clinical facts. Eur. J. Phys. Rehab. Med. **52**(4), 560–574 (2016). PubMed PMID: 27618499. Epub 2016/09/13. eng
5. Davidson, J., Jones, L., Cornet, J., Cittarelli, T.: Management of the multiple limb amputee. Disabil. Rehabil. **24**(13), 688–699 (2002)
6. Kitowski, V.J., Leavitt, L.A.: Rehabilitation of a quadruple amputee. South. Med. J. **61**(9), 912 (1968)
7. Park, J.M., Kim, Y.J., Kim, I.S., Lee, Y.T., Kim, S.H., Kim, Y.H., et al.: Rehabilitation for ambulation of triple amputee: a case report. J. Korean Acad. Rehab. Med. **31**(1), 123–126 (2007)
8. Shaw, M., Kaplow, M., Mitchell, N., Stillwell, D.: Traumatic triple amputation: psycho-social problems in rehabilitation. Arch. Phys. Med. Rehabil. **58**(10), 460–462 (1977)
9. Shin, J.C., Park, C.I., Kim, Y.C., Jang, S.H., Bang, I.K., Shin, J.S.: Rehabilitation of a triple amputee including a hip disarticulation. Prosth. Orth. Int. **22**(3), 251–253 (1998)
10. Wilken, J.M., Marin, R.: Gait analysis and training of people with limb loss. Care o the Combat Amputee. 535–552 (2009)
11. Armstrong, K., Brinkmann, J.T., Stine, R., Gard, S.A., Major, M.J.: Do upper limb loss and prosthesis use affect lower limb gait dynamics? J. Prosth. Orth. JPO (2019)
12. Alam, M.N., Garg, A., Munia, T.T.K., Fazel-Rezai, R., Tavakolian, K.: Vertical ground reaction force marker for Parkinson's disease. PloS one **12**(5), e0175951 (2017)
13. Liu, J., Lockhart, T., Kim, S.: Prediction of the spatio-temporal gait parameters using inertial sensor. 1840002 (2018)
14. Winiarski, S., Rutkowska-Kucharska, A.: Estimated ground reaction force in normal and pathological gait. Acta Bioeng. Biomech. **11**(1), 53–60 (2009). PubMed PMID: 19739592. Epub 2009/09/11. eng
15. Webster, J., Murphy, D.: Atlas of Orthoses and Assistive Devices E-Book. Elsevier Health Sciences (2017)
16. Wang, H., Frame, J., Ozimek, E., Leib, D., Dugan, E.L.: Influence of fatigue and load carriage on mechanical loading during walking. Military Med. **177**(2), 152–156 (2012). PubMed PMID: 22360059. Epub 2012/03/01. eng
17. Benedetti, M.G., Catani, F., Leardini, A., Pignotti, E., Giannini, S.: Data management in gait analysis for clinical applications. Clin. Biomech. **13**(3), 204–215 (1998)
18. Kwon, M.-S., Kwon, Y.-R., Park, Y.-S., Kim, J.-W.: Comparison of gait patterns in elderly fallers and non-fallers. Technol. Health Care **26**(S1), 427–436 (2018)
19. Hak, L., Houdijk, H., Beek, P.J., van Dieen, J.H.: Steps to take to enhance gait stability: the effect of stride frequency, stride length, and walking speed on local dynamic stability and margins of stability. PloS one **8**(12), e82842 (2013). PubMed PMID: 24349379. Pubmed Central PMCID: PMC3862734. Epub 2013/12/19. eng
20. Berge, J.S., Czerniecki, J.M., Klute, G.K.: Efficacy of shock-absorbing versus rigid pylons for impact reduction in transtibial amputees based on laboratory, field, and outcome metrics. J. Rehabil. Res. Dev. **42**(6), 795 (2005)
21. Sebastiao, E., Bollaert, R.E., Hubbard, E.A., Motl, R.W.: Gait variability and energy cost of overground walking in persons with multiple sclerosis: a cross-sectional study. Am. J. Phys. Med. Rehabil. **97**(9), 646–650 (2018). PubMed PMID: 29595583. Epub 2018/03/30. eng

22. Grabowski, A, Farley, C.T., Kram, R.: Independent metabolic costs of supporting body weight and accelerating body mass during walking. J. Appl. Physiol. (Bethesda, Md: 1985). **98**(2), 579–583 (2005). PubMed PMID: 15649878. Epub 2005/01/15. eng.
23. Dufek, J.S., Bates, B.T.: The evaluation and prediction of impact forces during landings. Med. Sci. Sports Exer. **22**(3), 370–377 (1990). PubMed PMID: 2381305. Epub 1990/06/01. eng

A Low-Cost Human Gait Analysis System

Siow Cheng Chan, Yu T'ng Chan, and Yu Zheng Chong

Abstract To analyze the gait movement in detail, assistance of software-based motion analysis systems is required as some parameters such as forces and moments of the joints are not directly measurable. However, most of the software systems require certain level of technical expertise to operate and expensive tools such as motion capture systems to collect the input parameters. The goal of this project is to develop a simple and cost-effective gait analysis system to compute the ankle joint moments of lower extremities in the sagittal plane with available tools and software. The proposed gait analysis system involves three devices which are a digital camera, an instrumented treadmill embedded force plates (H/P Cosmos™ Instrumented Treadmill), a personal computer equipped with Gaitway software and SkillSpector software. The digital camera and SkillSpector software were served as motion capture system to acquire the trajectories of the markers and perform knee and ankle kinematic analysis to obtain linear and angular kinematic parameters. The ankle joint moment was calculated based on the coordinates of the markers and the vertical ground reaction force (VGRF) data measured from the treadmill. Two healthy subjects (one male and one female) were recruited and the outputs of the system were then validated against existing data. In overall, the system produces kinematic and kinetic results comparable to those experimental results.

Keywords Gait · Kinematic · Kinetic

S. C. Chan (✉) · Y. T. Chan · Y. Z. Chong
Department of Mechatronics and Biomedical Engineering, Universiti Tunku Abdul Rahman, Sg. Long, Malaysia
e-mail: chansc@utar.edu.my

Y. T. Chan
e-mail: yutng08@1utar.my

J. Usman et al. (eds.), *6th Kuala Lumpur International Conference on Biomedical Engineering 2021*, IFMBE Proceedings 86,
https://doi.org/10.1007/978-3-030-90724-2_21

1 Introduction

Human gait is a pattern of locomotion associated with their posture, and gait analysis refers to research related to human walking. It is a way to disclose how human walk by evaluating factors that controls the performance of the lower extremities.

Gait studies have two main tracks: clinical gait analysis and biometric goal of human gait analysis. Clinical gait analysis depends on data acquisition in controlled environment [1] while biometric goal of human gait analysis performs data acquisition in different areas and scenario [2]. Clinical gait analysis includes five elements: videotape examination, temporal-spatial analysis, kinematic analysis, kinetic analysis and electromyography [3]. Temporal-spatial analysis identifies the parameters such as step length, stride length, cadence, walking speed etc. Kinematic analysis describes the motion of the joints in the lower limb without any reference to forces and kinetic analysis determines the power and moment exerted by the joints while walking [4].

In recent years, numerous gait models have been developed to study the behavior of human locomotion in different application such as biomechanics research, ergonomics, sport biomechanics, medical device design and orthopedics [5–8]. The major reason behind this development is due to the possibility of quantitative prediction, hypothesis testing and estimation of dynamic parameters such as forces and moments of the joints that are not directly measurable [9].

Software-based motion analysis plays an important role in assess motion or movement in a quicker and more reliable way. To achieve this, motion data needs to be processed, and maps the tracked information to motion description [10]. Over the years, numerous software systems such as AnyBody, Kinovea, MSMS, OpenSim, SIMM, SkillSpector and Visual3D that offer the capability to perform modelling and analysis gradually emerge in the market.

Unfortunately, most of the systems are either not freely available [11, 12] or do not provide complete source code to public which causes the researches difficult to improve their capabilities [13] as well as require 3D motion data as input. 3D motion capture systems are expensive, space consuming and require technical expertise to operate. The system proposed in this research aims to produce quantitative kinematics and kinetic data of human gait using simple and affordable tools. The proposed system can assist in future research in better understanding of the experimental subject's gait pathology and the activity occurred at the joint during gait.

2 Methodology

2.1 Subjects Recruitment

Two young (between age of 20 and 25) and healthy subjects were recruited in the experiment. One female subject (height of 163 cm and mass of 49.0 kg) and one

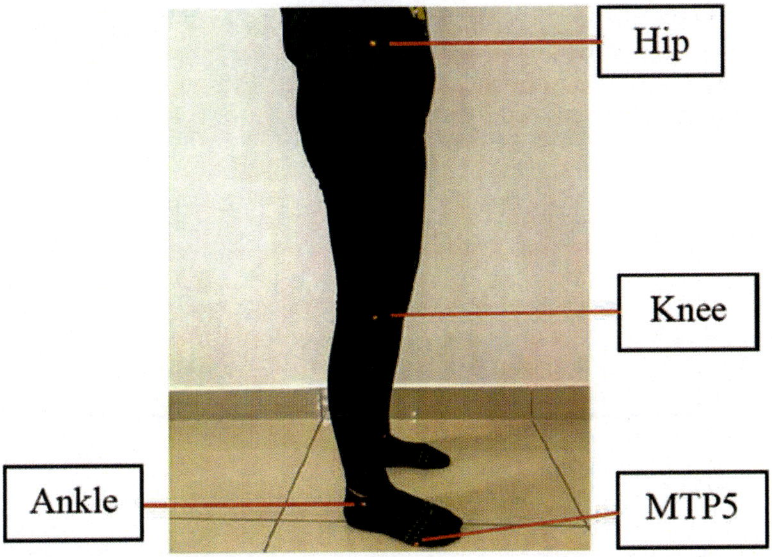

Fig. 1 Marker placement

male subject (height of 170 cm and mass of 58.3 kg). Both do not suffer from any cardiovascular disease and any postural deformity.

2.2 *Experiment Protocol*

Before the experiment, four markers were placed on the MTP5, ankle joint, knee joint and hip joint respectively as shown in Fig. 1. Then, the subject was instructed to walk at his own preferable speed (2.5 km/h for female subject 3.2 km/h for male subject) on the treadmill for 30 s. The paths of the markers were then recorded through a digital camera located at 1.0 m away from the treadmill providing a sagittal view of the subject. At the same time, the VGRF data were acquired using the Gaitway software.

2.3 *Kinematic Analysis*

SkillSpector software was used as a motion capture system to acquire the trajectories of the markers and perform kinematic analysis to obtain linear and angular kinematic parameters such as joint angle, velocity and acceleration. Before performing the kinematic analysis, the human model and object calibration need to be defined. The number of marker points attached at the joints as well as the movement need to be digitized. Due to the presence of noise caused by skin movement artefacts and improper digitization of markers [14], the kinematic data are filtered at cut-off frequency of 6 Hz. The linear and angular data produced in the kinematic analysis were then export as text file for further analysis.

2.4 Kinetic Analysis

Newton–Euler equations and the sagittal plane link-segment model combined with free body diagram (FBD) of the right leg proposed by Kirtley [15] was adopted in this work to calculate proximal joint moment. The FBD consists of three segments (foot, shank and thigh) linked together by the joints where the markers were located at the MTP5, ankle, knee and hip.

$$R_{xp} = m_z a_x - R_{xd} \tag{1}$$

$$R_{yp} = m_z a_y + m_z g - R_{yd} \tag{2}$$

$$\begin{aligned} M_{zp} = {} & I_z \alpha_z - M_{zd} - R_{xp}\left(Y_p - Y_{CoM}\right) + R_{yp}\left(X_{CoM} - X_p\right) \\ & - R_{xd}(Y_{CoM} - Y_d) - R_{yd}(X_d - X_{CoM}) \end{aligned} \tag{3}$$

where m_z = segment mass (kg); R = reaction force (N); x = x-direction; y = y-direction; p = proximal; d = distal; a = acceleration of CoM $\left(\frac{\text{m}}{\text{s}^2}\right)$; $g = 9.81\,\text{m/s}^2$; M_z = joint moment (Nm); I_z = segment mass moment of inertia (kg m^2); α_z = segment angular acceleration $\left(\frac{\text{rad}}{\text{s}^2}\right)$; CoM = Centre of Mass; CoP = Centre of Pressure; X = x-coordinate; Y = y-coordinate. Before substitute these parameters into the inverse dynamics method, some of the anthropometric parameters such as segment mass, length, distance of segment CoM to proximal or distal joint were estimated [16].

3 Results and Discussion

The graphs of ankle joint angle against gait cycle plotted from analysis are shown in Fig. 2. Initially the ankle experience plantarflexion and slowly convert into dorsiflexion until midstance to move body forward. Maximum dorsiflexion is achieved at the middle of push off period. Although the magnitude of angles might be different due to age of the subjects, gender of the subjects and gait speed [17], it is more important to focus on changes of variables, rather than the absolute values.

The changes of knee joint angle against gait cycle plotted from analysis is shown in Fig. 3. The curve pattern describes the knee joint angle during where initially

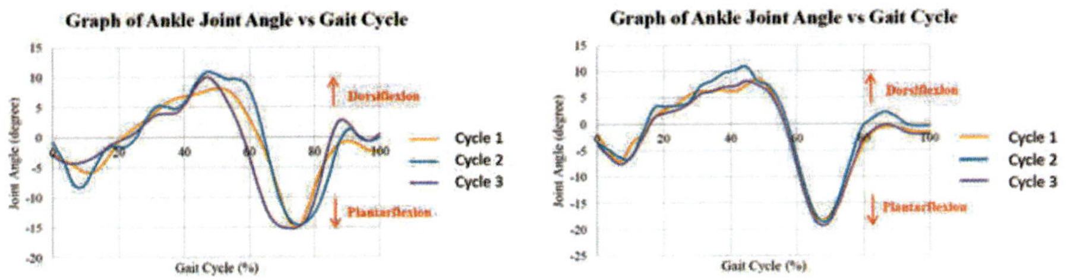

Fig. 2 The graph of ankle joint angle against percentage of gait plotted from analysis for female (left) and male (right) subjects

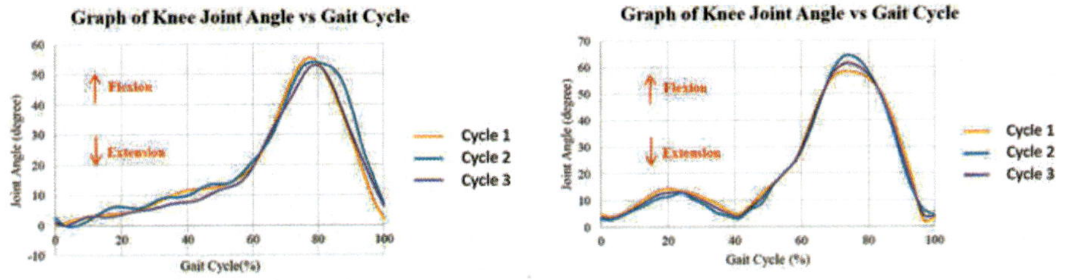

Fig. 3 The graph of knee joint angle against percentage of gait plotted from analysis for female (left) and male (right) subjects

the knee joint experience flexion and maximum extension during at the heel rise. Maximum flexion is achieved during swing phase and maximum knee extension at second heel strike. Both female and male subjects showed maximum knee flexion during swing phase and maximum knee extension at the second contact of foot with ground.

Figure 4 shows the graphs of ankle joint moment against gait cycle plotted from analysis. From the curve patterns, it was observed that after initial contact, there is a small ankle dorsiflexion moment due to eccentric contraction of ankle dorsiflexors to pull the foot towards the shank to avoid foot from slapping onto the ground. A negative value was used to represent this anticlockwise rotation dorsiflexion moment. Then followed by ankle plantarflexion moment as the shank move towards the foot.

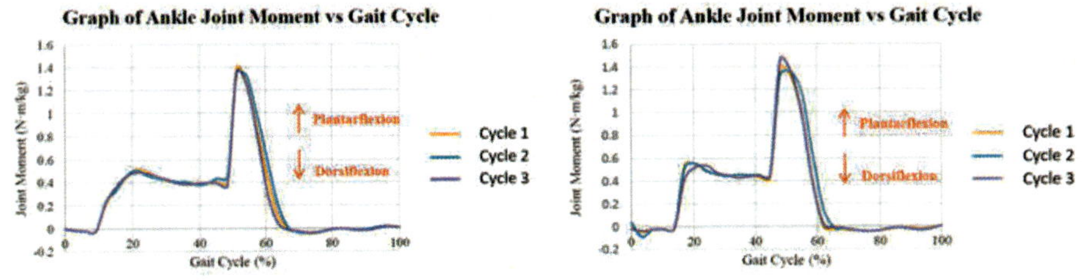

Fig. 4 The graph of ankle joint moment against percentage of gait plotted from analysis for female (left) and male (right) subjects

During toe-off, large ankle plantarflexion moment was observed. The large ankle plantarflexion moment was due to concentric contraction of the ankle plantarflexors to push the body upwards.

4 Conclusion

In a nutshell, the system proposed in this paper comprise a digital camera, a split-belt instrumented treadmill (H/P Cosmos™ Instrumented Treadmill) and a personal computer equipped with Gaitway software and SkillSpector Software. Inverse dynamic model was incorporated to perform the kinetic analysis. This project provides an alternative method for human gait modelling and analysis using low cost resources. Nevertheless, the proposed model can reproduce the outputs that are comparable to the existing results.

References

1. Katiyar, R., Pathak, D., Kumar, V.: Clinical gait data analysis based on spatio-temporal features. Int. J. Comp. Sci. Inf. Secur. **7**(2) (2010)
2. Nandy, A., Bhowmick, S., Chakraborty, P., Nandi, G.C.: Gait biometrics: an approach to speed invariant human gait analysis for person identification. In: Proceedings of the Second International Conference on Soft Computing for Problem Solving (SocProS 2012), pp. 729–737. Springer, New Delhi (2014)
3. Fandaklı, S.A., Okumuş, H.İ., Öztürk, M.: A study of human walking biomechanics for ankle-foot prosthesis design. In: International Conference on Control Engineering and Information Technology (CEIT), pp. 1–5. IEEE (2018)
4. Pfister, A., West, A.M., Bronner, S., Noah, J.A.: Comparative abilities of Microsoft Kinect and Vicon 3D motion capture for gait analysis. J. Med. Eng. Technol. **38**(5), 274–280 (2014)
5. Thomas, G.W., Johns, B.D., Marsh, J.L., Anderson, D.D.: A review of the role of simulation in developing and accessing orthopaedic surgical skills. IOWA Orthop. J. **34**, 181 (2014)
6. Debaere, S., Delecluse, C., Aerenhouts, D., Hagman, F., Jonkers, I.: Control of propulsion and body lift during the first two stances of sprint running: a simulation study. J. Sports Sci. **33**(19), 2016–2024 (2015)
7. Abad, J.D.: Ergonomics and simulation-based approach in improving facility layout. J. Ind. Eng. Int. 1–9 (2018)
8. Brown, N.P., Bertocci, G.E., Levine, G.J., Levine, J.M., Howland, D.R.: Development of a canine rigid body musculoskeletal computer model to evaluate gait. Front. Bioeng. Biotechnol. **8**, 150 (2020)
9. Siegler, S., Seliktar, R., Hyman, W.: Simulation of human gait with the aid of a simple mechanical model. J. Biomech. **15**(6), 415–425 (1982)
10. Nunes, J.F., Moreira, P.M., Tavares, J.M.R.: Human motion analysis and simulation tools: a survey. In: Handbook of Research on Computational Simulation and Modeling in Engineering. IGI Global (2016)
11. Bajelan, S., Azghani, M.R.: Musculoskeletal modeling and simulation of three various sit-to-stand strategies: an evaluation of the biomechanical effects of the chair-rise strategy modification. Technol. Health Care **22**(4), 627–644 (2014)

12. Noehren, B., Schmitz, A., Hempel, R., Westlake, C., Black, W.: Assessment of strength, flexibility, and running mechanics in men with iliotibial band syndrome. J. Orthop. Sports Phys. Ther. **44**(3), 217–222 (2014)
13. Delp, S.L., Anderson, F.C., Arnold, A.S., Loan, P., Habib, A., John, C.T., Guendelman, E., Thelen, D.G.: OpenSim: open-source software to create and analyze dynamic simulations of movement. IEEE Trans. Biomed. Eng. **54**(11), 1940–1950 (2007)
14. Winter, D.A., Quanbury, A.O., Hobson, D.A., Sidwall, H.G., Reimer, G., Trenholm, B.G., Steinke, T., Shlosser, H.: Kinematics of normal locomotion—a statistical study based on TV data. J. Biomech. **7**(6), 479–486 (1974)
15. Kirtley, C.: Clinical gait analysis: theory and practice. Elsevier Health Sciences (2006)
16. Dempster, W.T., Gabel, W.C., Felts, W.J.: The anthropometry of the manual workspace for the seated subject. Am. J. Phys. Anthropol. **17**(4), 289–317 (1959)
17. Oberg, T., Karsznia, A., Oberg, K.: Joint angle parameters in gait: reference data for normal subjects, 10–79 years of age. J. Rehabil. Res. Dev. **31**(3), 199–213 (1994)

Qualitative Study of Prosthetic Liner Materials on Transtibial Amputees' Satisfaction in Term of Positional Pain and Discomfort

M. A. Mohamed Nizam, N. A. Abd Razak, N. A. Abu Osman, and R. A. Mohd Jaladin

Abstract Objectives: The objective of this study is to find out the relationship of the type of prosthetic liner materials and the usage of the prosthesis on the satisfaction of the transtibial prosthesis user in term of positional pain and discomfort. Patients and Methods: This study included 50 transtibial amputees that using transtibial prosthesis (29 males, 21 females; mean age 55.4 ± 14.7 years; range, 18–78 years). The respondents were required to answer a set of questionnaire regarding the types of liner used, the prosthesis usage, and the positional pain experienced. Results: Based on the result obtain, the most prone area that experienced pain and discomfort is the end of the residual limb for both liners. Which Pelite liner users shows a greater amount over silicone liner users by 18% and 6% respectively. Prosthetist can reduce the discomfort and pain experienced by the user by prescribing softer material as the prosthetic liner. This study gathered that silicone liner users rate their prosthesis higher than Pelite liner user, 18% silicone liner users rate 5 for their prosthesis and only 8% for Pelite liner user. Conclusion: The prosthetic liner materials is one of the factors affecting the satisfaction with prosthesis use which in this study shows that the user prefer silicone liner over Pelite liner.

Keywords Discomfort · Positional pain · Prosthetic liner · Transtibial prosthesis · User satisfaction

1 Introduction

Prosthesis is a device that acts as an artificial extension that replaces a missing limb; upper or lower body extremity [1]. Hence, the prosthesis should be comfortable to

M. A. M. Nizam · N. A. A. Razak (✉) · N. A. A. Osman
Department of Biomedical Engineering, Faculty of Engineering, Universiti Malaya, Kuala Lumpur, Malaysia
e-mail: Nasrul.anuar@udu.edu.my

R. A. M. Jaladin
Department of Educational Psychology and Counselling, Faculty of Education, Universiti Malaya, Kuala Lumpur, Malaysia

J. Usman et al. (eds.), *6th Kuala Lumpur International Conference on Biomedical Engineering 2021*, IFMBE Proceedings 86,
https://doi.org/10.1007/978-3-030-90724-2_22

wear, light weight, durable, offer easy maintenance and serve the function well [2]. A transtibial prosthetic limb characteristically consist of a liner, a socket, a pylon and a prosthetic foot as the main parts. The prime objective for any prosthesis is to provide function in a comfortable manner, but comfort is mainly subjective and difficult to standardise [3]. Comfort primarily involves the pressures between the socket and residual limb. The socket fit, type of prosthetic suspension, and alignment of the prosthesis can alter pressures on the residual limb [4]. But the most important factor that affect user's comfort is the type or material of the liner. Therefore, the liner design and materials are the most important in determining the satisfaction of the user while wearing the prosthesis.

Advanced technologies, environmental, social, and economic factors have led to considerable improvements in prostheses. There are various types of prosthetic liner currently used globally. The most common material used as prosthetic liner in Malaysia are Pelite foam and silicone. The differences between Pelite foam and silicone despite of their materials are; the practicality and the cost. In the production of the prosthesis, it is easier for the prosthetist to work with silicone rather than Pelite foam. In addition, the time consume for prosthesis with silicone liner is relatively short than Pelite foam. But in term of the cost, Pelite foam is way cheaper than silicone [5]. A prosthetist should be wise in prescribing type of liner to the patient.

Malaysia is located near the equator making the weather hot and humid. So it is important for the user to use a liner that can withstand the weather and not making them uncomfortable. Pelite foam relatively more suitable for transtibial prosthesis user than silicone liner. It is because silicone liner tends to make the residual limb sweaty [6].

The type of suspension also affect the user's comfort and satisfaction [7]. Mainly there are three different type of suspensions that commonly used; anatomical suspension, pin and lock suspension, and vacuum suspension. Different suspension caters for different individuals. As an example, for an active user, it is appropriate to prescribe pin and lock suspension other than anatomical or vacuum suspension. In addition, the socket fitting also important when user ambulating with the prosthesis [8].

Most of transtibial prosthesis users always experience pain sensation at the distal of the residual limb [9–11]. The main cause of this phenomenon is the present of bony prominences and nerve endings at the residual limb. Many initiatives have been taken to resolve this problem which include using softer material such as silicone or gel liner and by designing a distal off load prosthetic socket [11, 12].

The prosthesis is worn by the user everyday with the maximum of time in a day to carry activities of daily living [13]. The average period of wearing the prosthesis is 12 h a day [14]. Hence, the prosthesis should be comfortable and caters the needs of the user. The average lifespan of a transtibial prosthesis is 3 years [15]. So the user is required to change the prosthesis after that period of time or when some components of the prosthesis are no longer working normally. In addition, it is extremely dangerous for the user to use the defected prosthesis.

Based on the previous literature in this field, the most common method to overcome the pain is to prescribe a liner with softer materials to the users [16]. There are various types of soft materials that have been used as prosthetic liner, such as silicone, gel and polyurethane foam [17]. However other method such as pain management is also encourage for the user to ease the pain. The objective of this study is to find out the relationship between the type of prosthetic liner materials and the satisfaction of the transtibial prosthesis user in term of positional pain and discomfort.

2 Patients and Methods

2.1 Ethics Approval

This research is conducted with the approval of permission by National Medical Research Register Secretariat 37,912.

2.2 Subject Recruitment

This study included 50 transtibial amputees (29 males, 21 females; mean age 55.4 ± 14.7 years; range, 18–78 years). The respondents were randomly chosen from University Malaya Medical Centre. The study required the respondents to meet certain criteria to be considered as respondents for the study. The study was conducted under the supervision of the Certified Prosthetics and Orthotics (CPO) of the International Society of Prosthetics and Orthotics (ISPO) Category 2.

The 50 respondents were randomly selected from all ages and genders and regardless of left or right amputation side. The selection was selected only after the participants met the following criteria:

1. Transtibial amputee.
2. Were able to communicate efficiently.

2.3 Questionnaire

Data were collected using a set of questionnaires which were filled in by the respondents. The types of information included in the questionnaire was: demographic data (age and sex) (Refer Appendix A for the set of questionnaire).

The second parts of the questionnaire consist of the information about the respondents' usage. The first question is about how many prostheses the respondents had worn after the amputation. The second question asked how long in term of years had the respondents worn their current prosthesis. Next, followed by how long the respondents wear the prosthesis in a day. Other questions asked include the type of liner the respondents currently used and had used previously.

In addition, the respondents were also asked about the pain or discomfort experienced while using the prosthesis. After that the respondents need to choose which the area that experienced pain or discomfort at the residual limb as shown in Fig. 1 and Table 1. The areas are; (A) the patellar tendon bearing, (B) the end of the residual limb, (C) the fibula head, (D) the suprapatellar, and (E) the medial and lateral parts of the residual limb. The area selected were chosen after verbal interview with the transtibial prosthesis user.

Then the respondents were asked for any complaint and future recommendation about the prosthesis. Finally the respondents were required to rate the prosthesis from 1–5 scale, which 1 is very poor and 5 is very good.

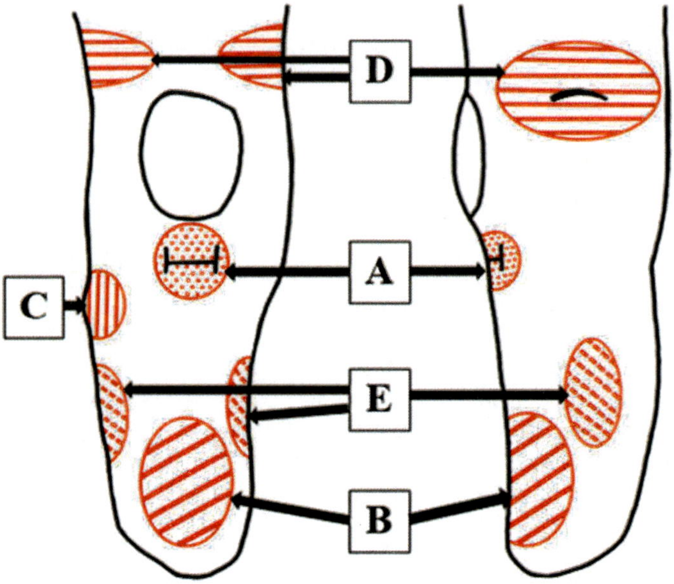

Fig. 1 The areas at the residual limb that prone to experience pain and discomfort (A: the patellar tendon bearing; B: the end of the residual limb; C: the fibula head; D: the suprapatellar; E: the medial and lateral parts of the residual limb

Table 1 Areas at the residual limb that experienced pain and discomfort

Area	Pelite	Silicone
The patellar tendon bearing (A)	1 (2%)	0 (0%)
The end of the residual limb (B)	9 (18%)	3 (6%)
Fibula head (C)	1 (2%)	1 (2%)
The suprapatellar (D)	0 (0%)	1 (2%)
The medial and lateral parts of the residual limb (E)	1 (2%)	0 (0%)

3 Results

The respondents chosen are transtibial prosthesis user with different demographics and characteristics. Majority of the respondents are first time user, 69% of Pelite liner user and 58% of silicone liner user portrays it. As shown in Table 2 data obtained, 2 of silicone liner user have used 5 transtibial prostheses within 20 years. While the others are second and third times users. But none of the respondents were forth times users.

Typically a transtibial prosthesis user usually wears the prosthesis number maximum 3 years prior changing into a new one. Based on the data obtained in Table 3, most of the respondents have used their prosthesis for one year. However, only one respondent have used the prosthesis for 3 years.

Based on Table 4, 60% of respondents used their prosthesis more than 8 h in a day to conduct their daily activities which both Pelite liner and silicone liner users

Table 2 Information about prosthesis usage comparing Pelite liner and silicone liner users in term of number of prosthesis used

Number of prosthesis used	Pelite	Silicone
1	18 (36%)	14 (24%)
2	6 (12%)	7 (14%)
3	2 (4%)	1 (2%)
4	0 (0%)	0 (0%)
5	0 (0%)	2 (4%)

Table 3 Information about prosthesis usage comparing Pelite liner and silicone liner users in term of period of using the prosthesis after amputation

Period of using the prosthesis after amputation (n = year)	Pelite	Silicone
<1n	9 (18%)	5 (10%)
1n	6 (12%)	10 (20%)
2n	2 (4%)	5 (10%)
3n	0 (0%)	1 (2%)
>3n	9 (18%)	3 (6%)

Table 4 Information about prosthesis usage comparing Pelite liner and silicone liner users in term of prosthesis wearing duration in a day

Prosthesis wearing duration in a day (n = hour)	Pelite	Silicone
<4n	1 (2%)	1 (2%)
4n to 6n	2 (4%)	2 (4%)
6n to 8n	8 (16%)	6 (12%)
>8n	15 (30%)	15 (30%)

Table 5 Pain and discomfort experienced by the respondents

Variables		Pelite	Silicone
Pain	Yes	5 (10%)	3 (6%)
	No	21 (41%)	21 (41%)
Discomfort	Yes	8 (16%)	5 (10%)
	No	18 (36%)	19 (38%)

Table 6 Rating of the prosthesis by the respondents

Rate	Pelite	Silicone
1	0 (0%)	0 (0%)
2	0 (0%)	0 (0%)
3	5 (10%)	3 (6%)
4	17 (34%)	12 (24%)
5	4 (8%)	9 (18%)

shows 30%. While only 2 respondents used their prosthesis less than 4 hours. This is more likely because they are first time prosthesis user.

In this study we gathered that the Pelite liner user experienced pain more statistically than silicone liner user. Based on the data obtained in Table 5, 10% Pelite liner user experienced pain while using the prosthesis while the rest 90% did not experienced it. On the other hand, only 6% silicone liner user experienced pain and 94% of the did not. The pain experienced by the user while using the prosthesis can be at various parts of the stump. In addition, we obtained that Pelite liner user experienced discomfort when using the prosthesis more than silicone liner user. 16% of Pelite liner user experienced discomfort and only 10% of silicone liner experienced discomfort while using the prosthesis.

Furthermore, the respondents were asked to rate from 1 to 5 how comfortable the prosthesis is. This study gathered that silicone liner users rate their prosthesis higher than Pelite liner user, 18% silicone liner users rate 5 for their prosthesis and only 8% for Pelite liner user as shown in Table 6.

4 Discussion

A prosthesis should be serve the function well but at the same time provide comfort to the user since it will be worn the majority of time in a day. Sometimes comfort could affect the function as well, when the user feel uncomfortable or pain, they will not wear the prosthesis. Prosthetic satisfaction is a multifactorial issue [7, 18]. These aspects mainly include prosthetic alignment, prosthetic components, prosthetist's skill, residual limb condition, level of activity, and socket fit [7].

Two type of liners that discussed in this study are Pelite liner and silicone liner. Pelite foam is a polyethylene closed cell foam that widely used as a prosthetic liner

[19]. Pelite is usually prescribed to a patient that have water retention due to vascular disease. The residual limb of the user will fluctuate in size throughout the day. By using Pelite liner, the user can add on stump socks when the residual limb shrinks. On the other hand, silicone liner is commonly prescribed to a patient with bony prominences at the residual limb because of the soft nature of silicone that lessen the shear pressure onto the skin [20].

Pelite liner can last longer than silicone liner [2]. Based on the data obtained, silicone liner user tends to change their liner more frequent in a short period of time. In this study, two of the respondents who use silicone liner had changed their prosthesis within average of 12 years. This means that one prosthesis was roughly used for 2.4 years. While the average of transtibial prosthesis is 3 years [15]. This shows that silicone liner is not sustainable as Pelite liner. Plus silicone liner cost more than Pelite liner [21].

The wearing duration of the prosthesis is matter to the transtibial prosthesis user. Most of the transtibial prosthesis user prefer to wear the prosthesis as maximise as they can since the prosthesis function is to replace the missing limb. Based on the study by Morlock et al., the average period of wearing the prosthesis is 12 h a day [14]. But discomfort and pain can affect the wearing duration. When the user experienced discomfort or pain they prefer not to wear the prosthesis which can affect their quality of life [22].

The condition has significant impacts on the prosthesis users. Based on Fig. 2a, more Pelite liner user experienced pain at the residual limb than silicone liner user.

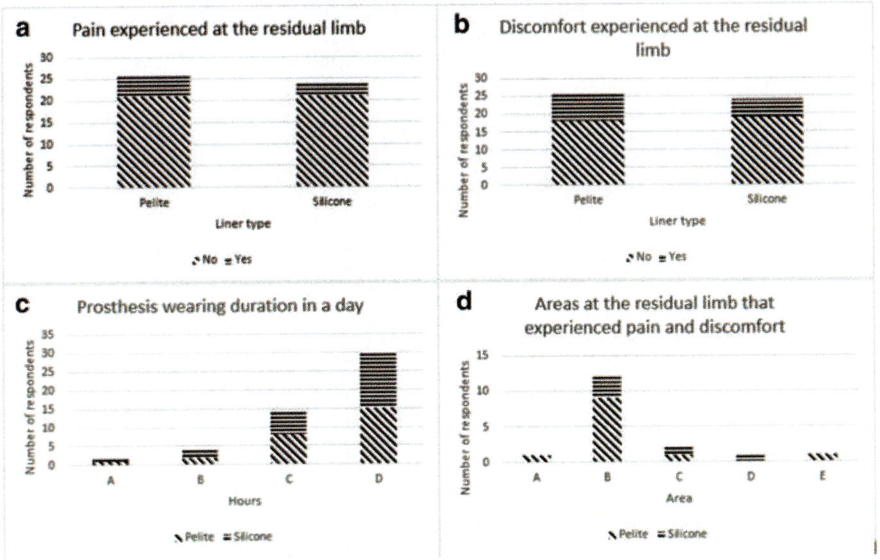

Fig. 2 **a** Pain experienced at the residual limb; **b** discomfort experienced at the residual limb; **c** prosthesis wearing duration in a day (A: Less than 4 h; B: 4 to 6 h; C: 6 to 8 h; D: More than 8 h); **d** area at the residual limb that experienced pain and discomfort (A: Patellar tendon bearing; B: End of the residual limb; C: Fibula head; D: Suprapatellar; E: Medial and lateral sides of the stump)

The presence of the pain at distal part of the residual limb may prevent them from achieving optimum prosthesis usage. The reason for this is that the pain disrupts the gait of the users which could lead to a number of complexities during walking, such as gait deviations [23, 24].

Moreover, in this study we found out that the majority of transtibial user experienced discomfort and pain at the end of the residual limb [4]. The data in Fig. 2a, b shows that Pelite liner users are more likely to experienced pain and discomfort rather than silicone liner user. The pain and discomfort experienced are more likely because the presence of tibia bone at the end of the residual limb [25, 26]. When the user donning and ambulating using the prosthesis, there will be pressure pushed at the end of the residual limb that can cause discomfort and pain. Prosthetist can reduce the discomfort and pain experienced by the user by prescribing softer material as the prosthetic liner [5].

The temperature of the residual increases when the user is wearing the prosthesis causing moisture buildup and sweating inside the liner [23]. In addition, Demir et al. also reported that more than half of the subjects experienced excessive perspiration at the residual limb when using the prosthesis [6]. The sweating and moistures buildup inside the liner can cause a major effect on user comfort and satisfaction. Based on previous literatures, Pelite liner user experienced less sweating compared to silicone liner user [4]. This condition is similar with one of silicone liner user in this study, she complained about the sweat build up in the liner and she had to doff the prosthesis regularly to remove the sweat.

There are various areas that a prosthesis user experienced pain and discomfort at the residual limb. Based on Fig. 1, the areas are the patellar tendon bearing, the end of the residual limb; which end of tibia bone located, the fibula head, the suprapatellar, the medial and lateral parts of the residual limb. It is not abnormal for a transtibial prosthesis user to experience pain and discomfort at those areas. This is because the residual limb is not designed to bear weight as the sole of the foot is. In addition, the end of the residual limb is more likely to experienced pain and discomfort because of the presence of end of tibia bone. In fact, one of the respondents had to change his Pelite liner to silicone liner because he had blister at the distal end of the residual limb. Based on Fig. 2 (D), most of the respondents from both Pelite liner and silicone liner users experienced pain and discomfort at the end of the residual limb. But the pain and discomfort experienced by the user can be overcome by prescribing a suitable prosthetic liner to the transtibial prosthesis user [27].

5 Conclusion

The prosthetic liner materials is one of the factors affecting the satisfaction with prosthesis use which in this study shows that the user prefer silicone liner over Pelite liner. In addition, the most prone area to experienced pain and discomfort is the end of the residual limb for both liners.

Funding Acknowledgement The author(s) disclosed receipt of the following financial support for the research, authorship, and/or publication of this article: This work was supported by University of Malaya (IIRG004B-19SAH).

Declaration of Interest The Author(s) declare(s) that there is no conflict of interest.

Appendix A

Transtibial (below knee) prosthesis user survey.
Personal information.

1. Name: ____
   ____
2. Age: ______________
3. Sex: ☐ Male ☐ Female

Prosthesis experience.

1. How many prostheses have you used?

   ☐ 1 ☐ 2 ☐ 3 ☐ More than 3 (state :______)
2. How long have you used your current prosthesis?

   ☐ Less than 1 year ☐ 1 year ☐ 2 years ☐ 3 years ☐ More than 3 years (state :_____)
3. How many hours in a day you use the prosthesis?

   ☐ Less than 4 hours ☐ 4 to 6 hours ☐ 6 to 8 hours ☐ More than 8 hours
4. What type of liner you currently use?

   ☐ Pelite ☐ Silicone ☐ Others (state :__________________________)
5. If you had used more than one prosthesis, state previous type of liner.

   ____
6. Is there any pain experienced while using current prosthesis?

   ☐ Yes ☐ No

7. Is there any discomfort experienced while using current prosthesis?

☐ Yes ☐ No

8. Please choose the areas that you feel pain or uncomfortable if any.

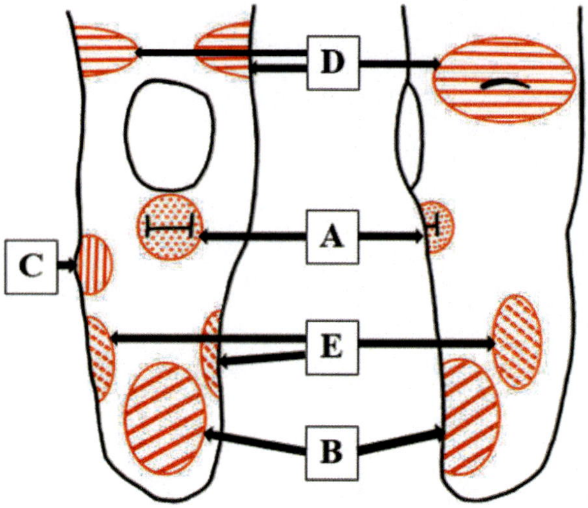

9. Any complaint for your current prosthesis?

____

____

____

10. Any future recommendation?

____

____

____

11. Rate your prosthesis. (1=very poor, 5=very good)

☐ 1 ☐ 2 ☐ 3 ☐ 4 ☐ 5

References

1. McGimpsey, G., Bradford, T.C.: Limb prosthetics services and devices. Bioengineering Institute Center for Neuroprosthetics Worcester Polytechnic Institution (2008)
2. Mohd Hawari, N., Jawaid, M., Md Tahir, P., Azmeer, R.A.: Case study: survey of patient satisfaction with prosthesis quality and design among below-knee prosthetic leg socket users. Disabil. Rehabil. Assist. Technol. **12**(8), 868–874 (2017)

3. Pirouzi, G., Abu Osman, N.A., Eshraghi, A., Ali, S., Gholizadeh, H., Wan Abas, W.A.: Review of the socket design and interface pressure measurement for transtibial prosthesis. Sci. World J. (2014)
4. Ali, S., Abu Osman, N.A., Arifin, N., Gholizadeh, H., Abd Razak, N.A., Wan Abas, W.A.: Comparative study between dermo, pelite, and seal-in x5 liners: effect on patient's satisfaction and perceived problems. Sci. World J. (2014)
5. Coleman, K.L., Boone, D.A., Laing, L.S., Mathews, D.E., Smith, D.G.: Quantification of prosthetic outcomes: elastomeric gel liner with locking pin suspension versus polyethylene foam liner with neoprene sleeve suspension. J. Rehabil. Res. Dev. **41**(4), 591–602 (2004)
6. Demir, Y., Atar, N.M., Güzelküjük, Ü., Aydemir, K., Yaşar, E.: The use of and satisfaction with prosthesis and quality of life in patients with combat related lower limb amputation, experience of a tertiary referral amputee clinic in Turkey. Age (Years). **1**(36), 7–10 (2019)
7. Ali, S., Osman, N.A., Naqshbandi, M.M., Eshraghi, A., Kamyab, M., Gholizadeh, H.: Qualitative study of prosthetic suspension systems on transtibial amputees' satisfaction and perceived problems with their prosthetic devices. Arch. Phys. Med. Rehabil. **93**(11), 1919–1923 (2012)
8. Klute, G.K., Berge, J.S., Biggs, W., Pongnumkul, S., Popovic, Z., Curless, B.: Vacuum-assisted socket suspension compared with pin suspension for lower extremity amputees: effect on fit, activity, and limb volume. Arch. Phys. Med. Rehabil. **92**(10), 1570–1575 (2011)
9. Lee, W.C., Zhang, M., Mak, A.F.: Regional differences in pain threshold and tolerance of the transtibial residual limb: including the effects of age and interface material. Arch. Phys. Med. Rehabil. **86**(4), 641–649 (2005)
10. Lee, W.C., Zhang, M., Jia, X., Cheung, J.T.: Finite element modeling of the contact interface between trans-tibial residual limb and prosthetic socket. Med. Eng. Phys. **26**(8), 655–662 (2004)
11. Portnoy, S., Yizhar, Z., Shabshin, N., Itzchak, Y., Kristal, A., Dotan-Marom, Y., Siev-Ner, I., Gefen, A.: Internal mechanical conditions in the soft tissues of a residual limb of a trans-tibial amputee. J. Biomech. **41**(9), 1897–1909 (2008)
12. Rankin, K., Steer, J., Paton, J., Mavrogordato, M., Marter, A., Worsley, P., Browne, M., Dickinson, A.: Developing an analogue residual limb for comparative DVC analysis of transtibial prosthetic socket designs. Materials **13**(18), 3955 (2020)
13. Cordella, F., Ciancio, A.L., Sacchetti, R., Davalli, A., Cutti, A.G., Guglielmelli, E., Zollo, L.: Literature review on needs of upper limb prosthesis users. Front. Neurosci. **10**, 209 (2016)
14. Morlock, M., Schneider, E., Bluhm, A., Vollmer, M., Bergmann, G., Müller, V., Honl, M.: Duration and frequency of everyday activities in total hip patients. J. Biomech **34**(7), 873–881 (2001)
15. Verhoeff, T.T., Poetsma, P.A., Gasser, L., Tung, H.: Evaluation of use and durability of polypropylene trans-tibial prostheses. Prosth. Orth. Int. **23**(3), 249–255 (1999)
16. Boutwell, E., Stine, R., Tucker, K.: Effect of prosthetic gel liner thickness on gait biomechanics and pressure distribution within the transtibial socket. J. Rehabil. Res. Dev. **49**(2), 227 (2012)
17. Al-Fakih, E.A., Abu Osman, N.A., Mahmad Adikan, F.R.: Techniques for interface stress measurements within prosthetic sockets of transtibial amputees: a review of the past 50 years of research. Sensors **16**(7), 1119 (2016)
18. Gholizadeh, H., Osman, N.A., Eshraghi, A., Ali, S., Razak, N.A.: Transtibial prosthesis suspension systems: systematic review of literature. Clin. Biomech. **29**(1), 87–97 (2014)
19. Sanders, J.E., Daly, C.H.: How does vacuum forming affect Pelite mechanical properties?. Prosth. Orth. Int. **18**(1), 43–48 (1994)
20. Bertels, T., Kettwig, T.: Breathable liner for transradial prostheses. In: Proceedings of the Myoelectric Symposium 2011 (2011)
21. Edwards, M.L.: Below knee prosthetic socket designs and suspension systems. Phys. Med. Rehabil. Clin. **11**(3), 585–594 (2000)
22. Meulenbelt, H.E., Dijkstra, P.U., Jonkman, M.F., Geertzen, J.H.: Skin problems in lower limb amputees: a systematic review. Disabil. Rehabil. **28**(10), 603–608 (2006)
23. Caldwell, R., Fatone, S.: Technique for perforating a prosthetic liner to expel sweat. JPO: J. Prosth. Orth. **29**(3), 145–147 (2017)

24. Zhang, L.Q., Dobson, S., Shiavi, R., Peterson, S., Limbird, T.: Changes in knee kinematics caused by ACL deficiency during fast walking. Gait and Posture **7**(2) (1998)
25. Dou, P., Jia, X., Suo, S., Wang, R., Zhang, M.: Pressure distribution at the stump/socket interface in transtibial amputees during walking on stairs, slope and non-flat road. Clin. Biomech. **21**(10), 1067–1073 (2006)
26. Lin, C.C., Chang, C.H., Wu, C.L., Chung, K.C., Liao, I.C.: Effects of liner stiffness for transtibial prosthesis: a finite element contact model. Med. Eng. Phy. **26**(1), 1–9 (2004)
27. McGrath, M., McCarthy, J., Gallego, A., Kercher, A., Zahedi, S., Moser, D.: The influence of perforated prosthetic liners on residual limb wound healing: a case report. Can. Prosth. Orth. J. **2**(1) (2019)

Restoration of Gait Spatio-temporals After Anterior Cruciate Ligament Reconstruction

Maryam Hadizadeh, Hamidreza Mohafez, Khin Wee Lai, and Saidon Bin Amri

Abstract The purpose of this study was to evaluate symmetrical alternations in gait spatio-temporal parameters among athletes after ACL reconstruction. Motion analysis was used to analyze the gait of 22 athletes with ACL reconstruction at three different times of rehabilitation program and 15 healthy subjects. Asymmetry indexes of cadence, step length, weight acceptance time, and stance time (STT) were assessed. One way and repeated measure multivariate analyses of variance were applied to analyze the data. There was a significance difference ($P = 0.007$) in combination of measured variables of patients comparing to control group. Stance time asymmetry index was the only parameter that demonstrated a significant reduction from initial to final test ($P = 0.004$). By performing the rehabilitation program, asymmetry restoration of the gait spatio-temporal parameters towards the range of control group was achieved three months after ACL reconstruction. The results also suggested to consider the inter-correlation of parameters for gait improvement evaluation.

Keywords Step length · Stance time · Cadence · Weight acceptance time · Symmetry · ACL reconstruction

1 Introduction

Anterior cruciate ligament (ACL) provide an important role in the knee joint biomechanics as it restricts the sliding of anterior tibial over the femur and prevent knee joint hyperextension [1]. One of the common knee injuries in sport activities is ACL

M. Hadizadeh (✉)
Centre for Sport and Exercise Sciences, Universiti Malaya, Jalan Universiti, 50603 Kuala Lumpur, Malaysia

H. Mohafez · K. W. Lai
Department of Biomedical Engineering, Faculty of Engineering, Universiti Malaya, Jalan Universiti, 50603 Kuala Lumpur, Malaysia

S. B. Amri
Department of Sport Studies, Faculty of Educational Studies, Universiti Putra Malaysia, 43400 Serdang, Selangor, Malaysia

J. Usman et al. (eds.), *6th Kuala Lumpur International Conference on Biomedical Engineering 2021*, IFMBE Proceedings 86,
https://doi.org/10.1007/978-3-030-90724-2_23

tear [2] that cause instability of the knee thereby surgical reconstruction is required to help subjects for returning to active sport life [3, 4]. Following an ACL reconstruction, usually subjects experience gait abnormalities, knee kinematic and kinetic alteration which lead to lack of stability during gait [5, 6]. Commonly, rehabilitation program after ACL surgery is to reduce the risk of re-injury, increase the chance of return to sport successfully [7–9] and knee stability [10]. Typically, by using clinical tests it is assumed that on completion of three- months rehabilitation program gait of subjects with ACL reconstruction should become normal [11]; However, such measures do not quantify the biomechanical changes of lower extremity during walking and may lead to uncertain evaluation regarding the appropriate time for releasing athletes to progressive activities of rehabilitation, post reconstruction.

Gait analysis has recently become more prevalent as a reliable technique to quantify baseline gait measurements and symmetry in athletes with ACL reconstruction before advancing to progressive activities. Among multiple parameters have been used to describe the gait, the spatio-temporals are indicative of appropriate human gait specifications. Although in the past studies changes of gait spatio-temporals has been reported in different time intervals post ACL reconstruction [5, 6, 11–14], but comprehensive evaluation of gait changes in athletes shortly after ACL reconstruction has not been investigated yet. Gait asymmetry may have serious indications for re-injury; hence, quantifying asymmetry of gait parameters may predict the risk of second injury and helps clinical experts in following up recovery after surgery. Moreover, no study was found to consider the inter-relationship exists between gait variables which may increase the power of the analysis. The purpose of this study was quantitative assessment of changes in asymmetry index of gait spatio-temporals in athletes with ACL reconstruction during rehabilitation program, using motion analysis system and considering the correlation among variables.

2 Details Experimental

2.1 Participants and Rehabilitation

Twenty-two athletes (13 males, 9 female) with ACL reconstruction (hamstring graft) were recruited for the study (mean age: 23.6(±5.4) years, mean height: 168.8(±8.8) cm, mean body weight: 66(±13.7) kg, and average time since injury to surgery: 65(±15) days. They were included if never had history of knee and other ligamentous injuries and were free from neurological injury. They were excluded if they had fractures and posterior cruciate ligament injury; however, presence of some cartilage damage and meniscal injury was acceptable. Fifteen healthy athletes (9 males, 6 female) were also recruited as the control group (mean age: 21.5(±1) years, mean height: 166.3(±7.1) cm, and mean body weight: 61.71(±11.3 kg)). All subjects provided informed consent form to sign before participation. The patients completed a similar rehabilitation program for the first three-months post reconstruction and none of them went through any more surgery after the reconstruction process. The aim of exercises was to obtain painless range of motion (ROM), full weight bearing, and the knee joint stability; increase the muscle strength and endurance; perform activities of daily living; and walk at least 20 min without pain. The study was approved by the Ethics Committee of University Putra Malaysia (Reference number: FPP(EX14)P036).

2.2 Data Collection Procedure

Both control and patient groups participated in the same testing protocol once and three times respectively. Gait analysis of patients was performed at the end of the 1st, 2nd, and 3rd months post ACL reconstruction using 8-camera three-dimensional (3-D) motion analysis system (CORTEX 2.5) at 60 Hz. Twenty-four markers were attached on the subjects' bony landmarks [15] (Fig. 1). After capturing a static

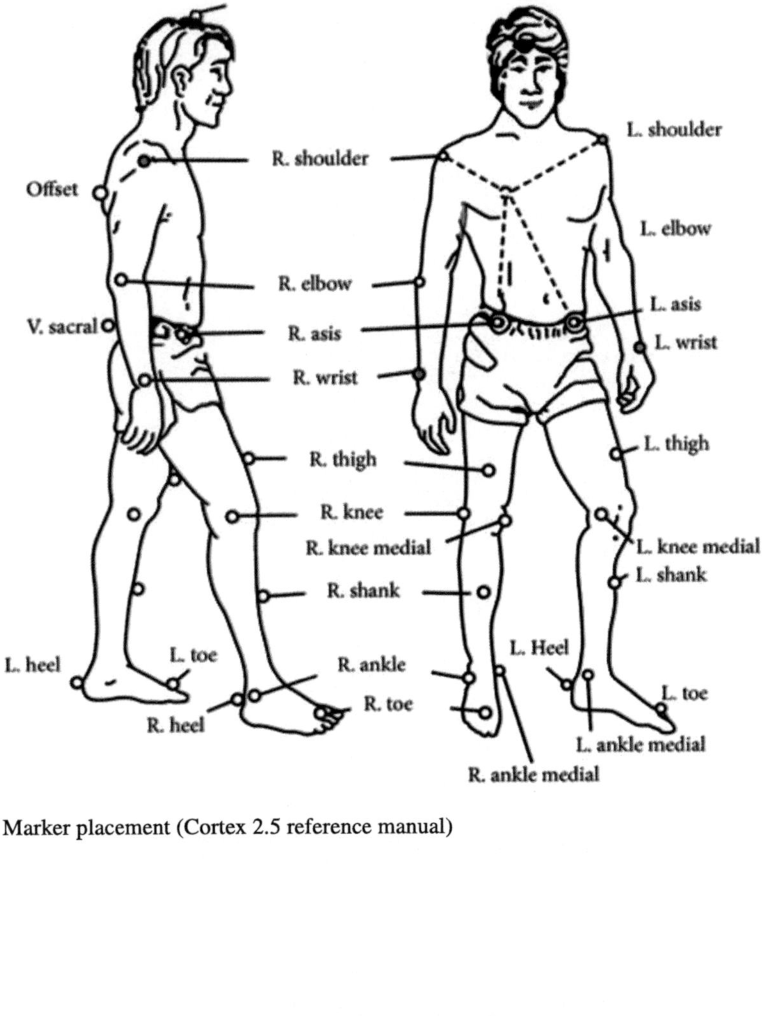

Fig. 1 Marker placement (Cortex 2.5 reference manual)

trial, subjects walked barefoot along x-axis walkway which two force plates were embedded in its center, until they reached to a constant walking speed. In each test, fifteen walking trials were captured bilaterally. Cortex software was used to digitized reflective markers from right heel contact prior to the force plate until left heel contact after the force plate. To process the 3-D trajectory outputs as Excel profile an Orthotrak software (6.6) was used. Timing for all measurements was normalized as percentage of a gait cycle (100%). The spatio-temporal parameters, including stance time (STT), step length (STL), weight acceptance time (WAT%GC), and cadence were derived from foot contact events. Step length was measured as the distance from initial contact of one foot to the initial contact of the opposite foot and stance time was measured as the period of time from heel contact to toe off of the same foot. WAT during the stance phase was measured from initial contact to peak knee flexion. The number of steps taken in a minutes was evaluated as cadence. The parameters were calculated from all successful walking trials for both limbs of subjects. For each subject, seven best trials were averaged for further analysis. Asymmetry index (AI) equation was used to measure the gait asymmetries [16].

2.3 Statistical Analysis

SPSS, version 24 was used to perform statistical analyses. One-way multivariate analysis of variance (MANOVA) was used to determine the differences of the studied parameters between control and patients group. A repeated measure MANOVA was used to assess the changes of variables within three tests. Post hoc comparisons were used to find out the differences between the tests.

3 Results and Discussion

Table 1 presents mean and standard deviation of the studied variables for the control group and the three tests of patients. A significant mean difference was found between control group and patients' test 1 on combination of AIs of gait parameters. Among all studied variable, stance time AI was the only that demonstrated remarkable difference

Table 1 Mean and standard deviation of gait spatio-temporals

Measurements	Test 1	Test 2	Test 3	Control
AI of STL	5.04 ± 3.8	4.4 ± 2.5	3.1 ± 2.6	2.9 ± 1.4
AI of cadence	1.8 ± 0.6	1.6 ± 1.2	1.6 ± 0.96	1.37 ± 0.6
AI of STT	2.8 ± 1.6	1.97 ± 0.9	1.5 ± 0.9	1.65 ± 1.2
AI of WAT	10.7 ± 5.3	9.8 ± 4.4	8.75 ± 6.2	8.33 ± 4.1

AI Asymmetry index, *STL* Step length, *STT* Stance time, *WAT* Weight acceptance time among groups at significant level of 0.0125 ($P = 0.01$) (Table 2). No significant difference was found in AIs of STL, cadence, and WAT among groups confirmed compensatory motion pattern of the unaffected limb in order to adjust to the affected limb. It can be also concluded that the combination of AIs of gait variables was significantly affected due to ACL surgery, but not individual ones. The results of test 1 were not in line with the study that reported significant differences in AIs of STL and WAT between control group and ACL patients two weeks after surgery [14]. Time from injury to surgery and surgery to data collection, and patients' characteristics might be highlighted as the factors for differences in findings. The reason that we did not find asymmetry in some of spatio-temporals might be because of the enough body preparation of subjects who were athletes and limited time (<3 months) from injury to surgery which may cause to provide better recovery following reconstruction.

Results of multivariate analysis demonstrated significant effects of time on AIs of the measured variables ($P < 0.05$). From the univariate analysis only stance time AI showed significant improvement across three tests at 0.0125 alpha level, with 30.63% at test 2 and 46.48% at test 3. Post hoc comparison of this variable demonstrated significant difference between tests 1 and 3 ($P = 0.017$) (Table 3). Asymmetries of cadence, WAT, and STL reduced by 10.87%, 38.3%, and 17.84% from initial to final test respectively; however, since both limbs showed increment the value of both limbs increased simultaneously lead to negligible alterations in the value of AI.

Table 2 Results of one-way MANOVA for test 1 and control

Results	Variables	F	Sig	η_p^2
Multivariate		4.4	0.007*	0.41
Univariate	AI of STL (%)	5.96	0.021	0.17
	AI of cadence (%)	4.7	0.04	0.14
	AI of STT (%)	5.3	0.011**	0.26
	AI of WAT (%)	1.9	0.184	0.06

*$P < 0.05$
**$P < 0.0125$

Table 3 Results of repeated measure MANOVA

Results	F	Sig	Post hoc	η_p^2
Multivariate	3.6	0.04*		0.78
Univariate				
AI of STL (%)	4.0	0.029		0.2
AI of cadence (%)	0.4	0.69		0.02
AI of STT (%)	6.6	0.004**	Tests 1 and 3 ($P = 0.017$)	0.31
AI of WAT (%)	0.5	0.59		0.03

*$P < 0.05$
**$P < 0.0125$

Table 4 Results of one-way MANOVA for test 3 and control

Results	Variables	F	Sig	η_p^2
Multivariate		0.23	0.92	0.04
Univariate	AI of STL (%)	0.11	0.75	0.004
	AI of cadence (%)	0.86	0.36	0.03
	AI of STT (%)	0.33	0.57	0.01
	AI of WAT (%)	0.05	0.83	0.002

(Sig. value >0.05)

Simultaneous improvement in the affected and unaffected limbs may suggest bilateral adaption as a result of unilateral injury. The findings were in harmony with the outcomes of the previous study revealed a decrement in AI of spatio-temporal parameters 12 weeks after reconstruction [14]. However, the large variation in surgical and rehabilitation procedures, patients' characteristics and their adaptation with rehabilitation, and methodological differences such as measurement techniques limit the comparison of the results. Such differences have become more highlighted when the inter-relationship between variables has been taken into account. After 12 weeks, no significant difference was found among patients and control group on combination of AI of gait variables ($P > 0.05$) (Table 4).

Findings of the study revealed that gait spatio-temporal of athletes can be restored in three months following ACL reconstruction using gait motion analysis system. Access to quantitative gait measures affected by ACL reconstruction and evaluating their changes through three-months rehabilitation, may highlight gait deficits of athletes and provide a proactive rehabilitation program which enables rehabilitators to modify the early return protocol based on the improvement in gait spatio-temporal parameters. While this research provided valuable results regarding the changes of gait spatio-temporal parameters among athletes with ACL reconstruction, the type of sport that they were involved prior to the injury was not same for all. Future studies with considering the type of sport is needed to support the current results.

4 Conclusion

The study outcomes revealed that ACL reconstruction leads to alteration in symmetry of studied gait parameters of athletes. However, by applying the rehabilitation program, they could improve the parameters toward the normal values and restore normal gait spatio-temporal characteristics three months following reconstruction. Considering the characteristics of the study subjects who were athletes, it can be summarized that the best results regarding the gait spatio-temporals is assured within the first three months of rehabilitation, before to start aggressive strengthening.

References

1. Marieswaran, M., Jain, I., Garg, B., Sharma, V., Kalyanasundaram, D.: A review on biomechanics of anterior cruciate ligament and materials for reconstruction. Appl. Bionics Biomech. **2018**, 1–14 (2018)
2. Montalvo, A.M., Schneider, D.K., Webster, K.E., Yut, L., Galloway, M.T., Heidt, R.S., Jr., Kaeding, C.C., Kremcheck, T.E., Magnussen, R.A., Parikh, S.N., Stanfield, D.T., Wall, E.J., Myer, G.D.: Anterior cruciate ligament injury risk in sport: a systematic review and meta-analysis of injury incidence by sex and sport classification. J. Athl. Train. **54**(5), 472–482 (2019)
3. Alswat, M.M., Khojah, O., Alswat, A.M., Alghamdi, A., Almadani, M.S., Alshibely, A., Dabroom, A.A., Algarni, H.M., Alshehri, M.S.: Returning to sport after anterior cruciate ligament reconstruction in physically active individuals. Cureus **12**(9), e10466 (2020)
4. Paschos, N.K., Howell, S.M.: Anterior cruciate ligament reconstruction: principles of treatment. EFORT Open Rev. **1**(11), 398–408 (2017)
5. Arhos, E.K., Capin, J.J., Buchanan, T.S., Snyder-Mackler, L.: Quadriceps strength symmetry does not modify gait mechanics after anterior cruciate ligament reconstruction, rehabilitation, and return-to-sport training. Am. J. Sports Med. **49**(2), 417–425 (2021)
6. Hart, H.F., Culvenor, A.G., Collins, N.J., Ackland, D.C., Cowan, S.M., Machotka, Z., Crossley, K.M.: Knee kinematics and joint moments during gait following anterior cruciate ligament reconstruction: a systematic review and meta-analysis. Br. J. Sports Med. **50**(10), 597–612 (2016)
7. Beynnon, B.D., Uh, B.S., Johnson, R.J., Abate, J.A., Nichols, C.E., Fleming, B.C., Poole, A.R., Roos, H.: Rehabilitation after anterior cruciate ligament reconstruction a prospective, randomized, double-blind comparison of programs administered over 2 different time intervals. Am. J. Sports Med. **33**(3), 347–359 (2005)
8. Joreitz, R., Lynch, A., Popchak, A., Irrgang, J.: Criterion-based rehabilitation program with return to sport testing following ACL reconstruction: a case series. Int. J. Sports Phys. Ther. **15**(6), 1151–1173 (2020)
9. Webster, K.E., Feller, J.A.: A research update on the state of play for return to sport after anterior cruciate ligament reconstruction. J. Orthop. Traumatol. **20**, 10 (2019)
10. Trąbka, R., Maicki, T., Kamiński, P., Pawełczyk, A., Zieliński, P., Wilk-Frańczuk, M.: Outcomes following arthroscopic single and double bundle anterior cruciate ligament (ACL) reconstruction supported by the comprehensive early rehabilitation program (CERP). Medical science monitor: Int. Med. J. Exp. Clin. Res. **26**, e921003 (2020)
11. Minning, S.J., Myer, G.D., Mangine, R.E., Eifert-Mangine, M., Colosimo, A.J.: Serial assessments to determine normalization of gait following anterior cruciate ligament reconstruction. Scand. J. Med. Sci. Sports **19**(4), 569–575 (2009)
12. Gao, B., Zheng, N.N.: Alterations in three-dimensional joint kinematics of anterior cruciate ligament-deficient and-reconstructed knees during walking. Clin. Biomech. **25**(3), 222–229 (2010)
13. Leporace, G., Metsavaht, L., Zeitoune, G., Marinho, T., Oliveira, T., Pereira, G.R., Oliveira, L.P., Batista, L.A.: Use of spatiotemporal gait parameters to determine return to sports after ACL reconstruction. Acta Ortop. Bras. **24**(2), 73–76 (2016)
14. Winiarski, S., Czamara, A.: Evaluation of gait kinematics and symmetry during the first two stages of physiotherapy after anterior cruciate ligament reconstruction. Acta Bioeng. Biomech. **14**(2), 91–100 (2012)
15. Hadizadeh, M., Amri, S., Roohi, S.A., Mohafez, H.: Assessment of gait symmetry improvements in national athletes after anterior cruciate ligament reconstruction during rehabilitation. Int. J. Sports Med. **37**(12), 997–1002 (2016)

16. Kadaba, M.P., Ramakrishnan, H.K., Wootten, M.E.: Measurement of lower extremity kinematics during level walking. J. Orthop. Res. **8**(3), 383–392 (1990)
17. Robinson, R.O., Herzog, W., Nigg, B.M.: Use of force platform variables to quantify the effects of chiropractic manipulation on gait symmetry. J. Manipulative Physiol. Ther. **10**(4), 172–176 (1987)

Surface Electromyography: A New Indicator of Fatigue Level

Fauzani Jamaluddin, Fatimah Ibrahim, and Siti Anom Ahmad

Abstract Prolonged high intensity physical activity induces fatigue at the central and peripheral system, and inadequate recovery process lead to the emergence of maladaptation symptoms. Usually in tracking fatigue level, lactate test, heart rate and self-evaluation questionnaire are utilized. Surface EMG is known as one of the electrophysiological techniques, which physiological information of human body can be extracted from sEMG signals. This paper proposes a new indicator known as surface electromyography (EMG) to track fatigue level with the existence of maladaptation symptoms muscle soreness, unexplained lethargy and performance reduction. An experiment has been conducted on twenty participants to investigate the behavior of surface EMG during five days of intensive training that was based on Bruce Protocol treadmill test. The intension was to induce maladaptation signs on biceps femoris (BF), rectus femoris (RF), vastus lateralis (VL) and vastus medialis (VM). Results demonstrate that ΔFmed of BF, RF, VL and VM tend to decrease under normal fatigue condition, and increase under fatigue with maladaptation signs ($P < 0.05$) for RF and VL. Thus, this study successfully demonstrated that inception of maladaptation signs can be observed based on surface EMG.

Keywords Surface electromyography · Fatigue level · Maladaptation

F. Jamaluddin (✉) · F. Ibrahim
Center for Innovation in Medical Engineering, Faculty of Engineering, Universiti Malaya, 50603 Kuala Lumpur, Malaysia
e-mail: nfauzani@um.edu.my

F. Ibrahim
Department of Biomedical Engineering, Faculty of Engineering, Universiti Malaya, 50603 Kuala Lumpur, Malaysia

S. A. Ahmad
Institute of Gerontology, Universiti Putra Malaysia, 43400 Serdang, Selangor, Malaysia

J. Usman et al. (eds.), *6th Kuala Lumpur International Conference on Biomedical Engineering 2021*, IFMBE Proceedings 86,
https://doi.org/10.1007/978-3-030-90724-2_24

1 Introduction

In general, physical activities involve central and peripheral mechanism chain processes. It starts with the brain (central) giving commands for movements, to the formation of actin-myosin (peripheral) in producing a movement [1]. The peripheral system refers to the motor units, which consists of motor neurons and muscle fibers. Prolonged physical activity or force induces fatigue at the central and peripheral system. First, fatigue at the central system occurs when neurochemical in the brain are altered and stress hormones [2] are secreted. When this happens, central gives command to modify peripheral information in the contracting muscles. The modification causes muscle to lose the recruitment of high threshold motor units, decreases the force output and reduces the discharge of motor neurons [3]. This reflex phenomenon occurs as a protective mechanism to prevent organ failure if the physical activity continues at the same intensity [4].

Second, fatigue at the peripheral system takes place. It refers to the alteration or failure of neuromuscular transmission and muscle action potential propagation [3]. During muscle contraction, a biological process within muscle fiber emerges, which is known as peripheral regulation. Fatigue at the peripheral system arises from the muscle itself when there is an impairment of the peripheral mechanism due to high-intensity exercise.

Prolonged fatigue occurs due to inadequate rest and recovery. When hormone level during physical activity is unable to return to its normal condition, this hormonal change leads to maladaptation on musculoskeletal, psychological, physiological, immunologic and endocrine elements [3]. The situation may get worse and destroy an individual's life if the maladaptation signs keep accumulated, prolonged, persistent and are not treated. In sports, this is known as chronic fatigue or overtraining syndrome.

Diagnosing chronic fatigue syndrome is a complex procedure; in fact, there is no specific tools to identify it [5, 6]. Most of the methods utilized to identify fatigue level include blood test, biopsies, heart rate, and self-evaluation questionnaire. Among those, blood test and biopsies are considered as reliable indicators. Nevertheless, most subjects find them invasive, uncomfortable and painful. Moreover, these methods require numbing medicine and cannot be applied frequently. The non-invasive available method used currently is questionnaires. It is used to monitor training stress and response. However, it demands high cooperation between subject and health professional. In addition, some of the terms are impossible to quantify like the amount of stress and emotion. Hence, identifying fatigue level is getting more complex since individual fatigue responses are substantially variable [6, 7]

Other than blood test and questionnaire, surface electromyography (EMG) can also be used to measure fatigue level. Surface EMG, which was discovered in 1912, records electrical energy of muscles from human skin. This recording is able to indicate fatigue. The electrical energy changes due to ionic diffusion within muscle and mechanical responses during muscle force to contract [8]. As a result, surface EMG behavior indicates the stage of fatigue as experienced by the subject. There are advantages of using surface EMG in fatigue detection. These include its features of being non-invasive, inexpensive, simple and easy procedure, not requiring lab environment or applicability, enabling real-time fatigue monitoring and enabling specific muscle fatigue monitoring and its correlation with biochemical and physiological changes in muscles during [9].

Unfortunately, limitation discovered from previous findings does not encourage surface EMG to be the main choice in fatigue identification. However, new findings demonstrate that strong characteristic of surface EMG is able to identify fatigue with maladaptation signs. Therefore, the aim of this paper is to investigate surface EMG behavior under mild maladaptation symptoms. Nonetheless, the mechanism of fatigue and its relation to surface EMG signals are discussed in the earlier sections of the paper.

2 Methodology

A sample of twenty participants (Age $\pm$ standard deviation (SD): 24.2 $\pm$ 3.74 years old, body mass index $\pm$ SD: 22.7 $\pm$ 2 kgm^2) had participated in the study. Physical Activeness questionnaire (Par-Q and You) was employed as a screening tool. It was utilized to detect cardiovascular, pulmonary disease and orthopedic problems. Only participants who answered 'NO' to all questions in Par-Q and You were allowed to participate in the study. The participants who had diabetes, high blood pressure, heart disease, any of the chronic diseases, joint or bone problem and were on any medication to control blood pressure and blood sugar were excluded from the study. It is important to note that the experiment protocol was approved by the institution's ethical committee.

2.1 Experiment

The experiment was conducted based on Bruce Protocol treadmill test. The protocol chosen as it may provide high intensity of training and induce maladaptation signs faster. The total duration of the protocol was 21 min. In the protocol, inclination and speed of the treadmill were increased for every three minutes, and it was start from 10° with speed 2.7 km/h. The participants were required to improve their performance on a daily basis. As individual fatigue response is highly variable; no specific distance and time duration are fixed.

Physiological measurements collected from the participants to determine the intensity of the running activities and maladaptation condition. The intensity of training will indicate running effort performed by the participants. It was determined based on percentage of maximal heart rate (HRmax) during running. Running at >80% of HRmax is consider as hard and very exhausting, and may cause muscular fatigue. The maladaptation symptoms of the participants observed in the study was muscle soreness, endurance time, and unexplained lethargy. These symptoms were determined by using short interview and training log. Due to ethical reasons and potential risk endured by the participant, only five-day experiment was allowed by the Ethical Committee.

Throughout the experiment, four muscles were observed via custom made surface EMG acquisition system. These muscles were biceps femoris (BF), rectus femoris (RF), vastus medialis (VM) and vastus lateralis (VL). These muscles were selected based on the criteria that they were the most activated muscles during running and suffered the highest rate of injury in sports [10, 11]. In the experiment, electrodes placement was according to SENIAM recommendation. Data were collected from the aforementioned muscles during the pre and post exercises. Participants were asked to stand and flex left knee to activate BF muscles, and sit on chair and extend left knee to activate RF, VL and VM muscles.

2.2 *Signals Analysis*

Surface EMG then analyzed the input using stationary wavelet transform to eliminate 20 Hz corner frequency and baseline noises. Information, such as mean absolute value (MAV) and median frequency (Fmed), was extracted from the collected data. Fatigue was traced due to the changes of features between post and pre-exercise:

$$\Delta\text{Feature} = \text{Feature(post exercise)} - \text{Feature(pre - exercise)}$$

Then, features were normalized before statistical analysis. Afterwards, the extracted features were differentiated to two groups: Maladapted (features during the existence of maladaptation symptoms) and Adapted (features during the non-existence of maladaptation symptoms). All the extracted parameters were tested using paired t-test to investigate the significant difference between ‘Maladapted’ and ‘Adapted’ signals. Daily trends of ΔFmed and ΔMAV were also plotted for ‘Adapted’ and ‘Maladapted’ signals to investigate the behavior.

3 Results and Discussion

Table 1 indicates the mean of ΔFmed and ΔMAV between adapted and maladapted groups based on the combination of individual muscles of BF, RF, VL and VM, and daily average value of the four muscles. While Table 2 shows the results of statistical analysis namely paired T-test of the muscles.

Results in Table 1 demonstrate that ΔFmed under maladaptation condition tended to shift towards positive value compared to the adapted condition. As shown in Table 2, this characteristic was only significant at $p < 0.05$ for features with the combination

Table 1 Mean of ΔFeatures between adapted and maladapted condition

Muscle(s)	Feature	Adapted (mean)	Maladapted (mean)
Combination of individual muscles	ΔFmed	−0.11	0.90
	ΔMAV	−0.19	0.24
BF	ΔFmed	−0.10	0.44
	ΔMAV	0.01	−0.32
RF	ΔFmed	−0.11	0.83
	ΔMAV	0.2	0.81
VL	ΔFmed	−0.08	1.03
	ΔMAV	−0.32	0.13
VM	ΔFmed	−0.04	0.46
	ΔMAV	−0.06	−0.01
Daily average value	ΔFmed	−0.19	1.89
	ΔMAV	0.15	0.74

Table 2 *p*-values based on paired T-test

Muscle(s)	Feature	*p*-value
Combination of individual muscles	ΔFmed	$*p < 0.00001$
	ΔMAV	$*p$ is 0.000987
BF	ΔFmed	$p = 0.05491$
	ΔMAV	$p = 0.248165$
RF	ΔFmed	$*p = 0.00027$
	ΔMAV	$*p = 0.029631$
VL	ΔFmed	$*p = 0.000119$
	ΔMAV	$*p = 0.049458$
VM	ΔFmed	$p = 0.071109$
	ΔMAV	$p = 0.801501$
Daily average value	ΔFmed	$*p < 0.00001$
	ΔMAV	$*p$ is 0.005276

*Significant at $p < 0.05$

of individual muscles, RF, VL and daily average value of muscles. On the other hand, the results on BF and VM muscles were not significant although both demonstrate similar trends. The different features between adapted and maladapted conditions on ΔMAV also indicate that it was significant for features combination of individual muscles, RF, VL and daily average value of muscles, but it was insignificant for BF and VM muscles. Table 1 illustrates that ΔMAV had more positive value during maladaptation compares to ΔMAV under adapted condition.

Different statistical results presented by the respective muscles demonstrate that every muscle had different capabilities and projects different responses [12]. Insignificant outcomes of previous studies on maladaptation sign in Hedayatpour et al. [13] and Bajaj et al. [14] may due to the fact that they studied the wrong muscles. Meanwhile, different experimental design performed by Hedayatpour et al. [13] and Bajaj et al. [14] also might have contributed to similar findings.

Although stages of fatigue proposed by Dimitrova and Dimitrov [21] did not include frequency shifting towards positive value as part of fatigue stages, results demonstrate that center of frequency have increased. However, the increasing center of frequency was similar to the findings by Petrofsky [15] and Osborne [16]. The increasing center of frequency was proposed to have caused by temperature increment, accumulation of lactic acid and glycogen reduction in the muscle [15, 16]. In Tenan [17], it was mentioned that there was a weak relation to correlate potassium concentration to surface EMG, but there were possibilities [17]. Results in Tenan [17] demonstrate that the recovering duration period taken for potassium and frequency to return at resting value was quite similar.

ΔFmed and ΔMAV for Adapted and Maladapted daily trends had merged as shown in Fig. 1. The trend indicates that median frequency had shifted on lower value earlier, and tended to shift to positive value during the emergence of soreness, unexplained lethargy and performance decrement. The negative changes showed an agreement with previous studies on the center of spectral during fatigue, while positive changes caused by biochemical changes in response to maladaptation condition.

It was a slightly different trend showed by the amplitude behavior. The trend showed that the participants had ran on treadmills under maximal voluntary contraction from the first day of the experiment. It was demonstrated by the negative of ΔMAV as shown in 'Adapted' trend. ΔMAV showed negative changes on the first day of maladaptation, and followed by the positive changes. The positive changes at this stage showed that muscles were unable to contract at maximum voluntary

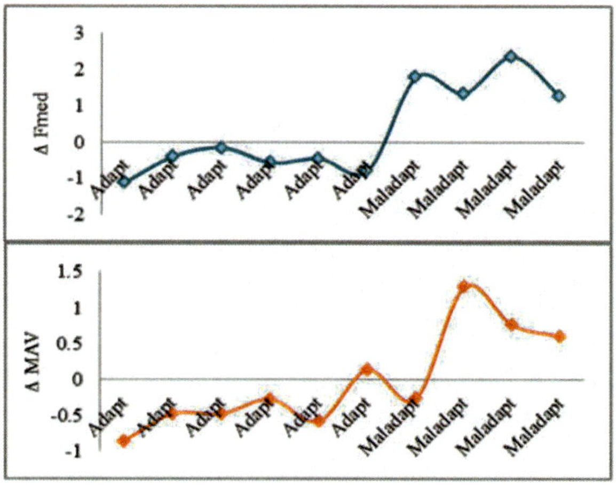

Fig. 1 Daily trend of ΔFmed and ΔMAV

contraction. The positive changes also might have caused by the elevation of lactate concentration as suggested by Loss et al. [18] or due the glycogen reduction as proposed by Tenan [18, 19]. These behaviors may also refer to protective adaptation to response for harmful stimuli [20].

At the moment, stages of fatigue proposed by Dimitrova and Dimitrov [21] is as follows:

Stage 1: Spectral shifted to lower, Amplitude increase.
Stage 2: Spectral shifted to lower, Amplitude increase.
Stage 3: Spectral shifted to lower, Amplitude unchanged.
Stage 4: Spectral shifted to lower, Amplitude decrease.

Trend in Fig. 1 also demonstrated that, new fatigue index can be added to update stages of fatigue profile suggested by Dimitrova and Dimitrov [21]. Therefore, this paper proposes two more stages to indicate fatigue level based on surface EMG behavior, with the assumption that maladaptation signs observed in the study are the highest level of fatigue at the moment.

Stage 5: Spectral shifted to upper, Amplitude decrease (indicate really heavy exercise and sign of early mild maladaptation may have developed).
Stage 6: Spectral shifted to upper, Amplitude increase (more maladaptation signs may have developed).

4 Conclusions

Results presented in the paper indicate that surface EMG can be used to indicate fatigue level. The combination of individual features and average features of investigated muscles demonstrate significant results compared to individual muscle. This study also shows that the experimental design based on Bruce Protocol is suitable to observe surface EMG behavior for maladaptation investigation. The study also indicates that both frequency and amplitude information are significant in determining fatigue level. Every change of the center of frequency and amplitude of surface EMG may demonstrate fatigue experience by the subject.

References

1. Boyas, S., Guével, A.: Neuromuscular fatigue in healthy muscle: underlying factors and adaptation mechanisms. Ann. Phys. Rehabil. Med. **54**(2), 88–108 (2011).https://doi.org/10.1016/j.rehab.2011.01.001
2. Kreher, J.B., Schwartz, J.B.: Overtraining syndrome: a practical guide. Sports Health **4**(2), 128–138 (2012). https://doi.org/10.1177/1941738111434406
3. Sesboüé, B., Guincestre, J.-Y.: Muscular fatigue. Annales de Readaptation et de Medecine Physique: Revue Scientifique de La Societe Francaise de Reeducation Fonctionnelle de Readaptation et de Medecine Physique **49**(6), 257–264, 348–354 (2006). https://doi.org/10.1016/j.annrmp.2006.04.020

4. González-Izal, M., Malanda, A., Gorostiaga, E., Izquierdo, M.: Review electromyographic models to assess muscle fatigue. J. Electromyography Kinesiol.: Official J. Int. Soc. Electrophysiol. Kinesiol. **22**(4), 501–512 (2012). https://doi.org/10.1016/j.jelekin.2012.02.019
5. Pearce, P.Z.: A practical approach to the overtraining syndrome. Curr. Sports Med. Rep. **1**(3), 179–183 (2002). Retrieved from http://www.ncbi.nlm.nih.gov/pubmed/12831711
6. Purvis, D., Gonsalves, S., Deuster, P.A.: Physiological and psychological fatigue in extreme conditions: overtraining and elite athletes. J. Injury, Func. Rehabil. **2**(5), 442–450 (2010).https://doi.org/10.1016/j.pmrj.2010.03.025
7. Jamaluddin, F.N., Ahmad, S.A., Bahari, S., Noor, M., Zuha, W., Hassan, W.: Future direction of the electromyography based method to evaluate muscle fatigue. In: 2014 4th International Conference on Engineering Technology and Technopreneurship (ICE2T), pp. 314–319 (2014)
8. Massó, N., Rey, F., Romero, D., Gual, G., Costa, L., Germán, A.: Surface electromyography applications in the sport. **45**(165), 121–130 (2010)
9. Cifrek, M., Medved, V., Tonković, S., Ostojić, S.: Surface EMG based muscle fatigue evaluation in biomechanics. Clin. Biomech. **24**(4), 327–340 (2009). https://doi.org/10.1016/j.clinbiomech.2009.01.010
10. Armfield, D.R., Kim, D.H.-M., Towers, J.D., Bradley, J.P., Robertson, D.D.: Sports-related muscle injury in the lower extremity. Clin. Sports Med. **25**(4), 803–842 (2006). https://doi.org/10.1016/j.csm.2006.06.011
11. Sloniger, M.A., Cureton, K.J., Prior, B.M., Evans, E.M., Carrier, D.R., Anders, C., … Batterham, M.: Lower extremity muscle activation during horizontal and uphill running. J. Appl. Physiol. **83**, 2073–2079 (1997)
12. Kamaruddin, N.A., Khalid, P.I., Shaameri, A.Z.: The use of surface electromyography in muscle fatigue assessments—a review. Jurnal Teknologi **6**(74), 1–5 (2015)
13. Hedayatpour, N., Falla, D., Farina, D.: Effect of delayed-onset muscle soreness on muscle recovery after a fatiguing isometric contraction. Scand. J. Med. Sci. Sports **20**(1), 1–9 (2008). https://doi.org/10.1111/j.1600-0838.2008.00866.x
14. Bajaj, P., Madeleine, P., Sjøgaard, G., Arendt-nielsen, L.: Assessment of postexercise muscle soreness by electromyography and mechanomyography. J. Pain **3**(2), 126–136 (2002). https://doi.org/10.1054/jpai.2002.122945
15. Petrofsky, J.S.: Frequency and amplitude analysis of the EMG during exercise on the bicycle ergometer. Eur. J. Appl. Physiol. **15**(41), 1–15 (1979)
16. Osborne, M.A., Schneider, D.A.: Muscle glycogen reduction in man: relationship between surface EMG activity and oxygen uptake kinetics during heavy exercise. Physiol. Soc. **91**(1), 179–189 (2006).https://doi.org/10.1113/expphysiol.2005.031450
17. Tenan, M.S.: The relationship between blood potassium, blood lactate, and electromyography signals related to fatigue in a progressive cycling exercise test, ATC A thesis submitted to the faculty of the University of North Carolina at Chapel Hill (2009)
18. Loss, J.F., Melo, D.O., Torre, M.L., Pasini, M., Arau, L., De Oliveira, L.N., Pinto, L.: Comparing the lactate and EMG thresholds of recreational cyclists during incremental pedaling exercise. Can. J. Physiol. Pharmacol. **86**(2008), 272–278 (2008). https://doi.org/10.1139/Y08-020
19. Tenan, M.S., Blackburn, J.T., Robert, G.: Exercise-induced glycogen reduction increases muscle activity. Int. J. Exerc. Sci. **9**(3), 336–346 (2016)
20. Nie, H., Arendt-nielsen, L., Kawczynski, A., Madeleine, P.: Gender effects on trapezius surface EMG during delayed onset muscle soreness due to eccentric shoulder exercise. J. Electromyogr. Kinesiol. **17**, 401–409 (2007). https://doi.org/10.1016/j.jelekin.2006.04.006
21. Dimitrova, N.A., Dimitrov, G.V.: Interpretation of EMG changes with fatigue: facts, pitfalls and fallacies. J. Electromyogr. Kinesiol. **13**(1), 13–36 (2003)

Relationship Between Handedness and Cognition Performance of University Undergraduates

Yin Qing Tan, Si Yun Tee, and Hong Kiat Ooi

Abstract Human were born to be left-or right-handers. Left-handedness is rare and only consists of around 10% of population. Some lefties facing problems in daily life and may need to declare their left-handedness as one of the disabilities, however, there are also some lefties show excel in music and mathematics. One of the common theories about left-handers is their brain are structure differently than common right-handers, and thus resulted in different cognition ability. This study aimed to investigate the relationship between handedness and cognition performance among 108 young adults in a local university using MATRICS Consensus Cognitive Battery. Results are considered to support the hypothesis that handedness may have significant impact on two cognition tests, Symbol Coding and Maze test, with *p*-value 0.04 and 0.005, respectively. There was no significant difference has been found on Trail Making Test, Working Memory and Social Cognition test. This study suggested that right-handed participants able to complete the timed cognition tests faster than left-handers which indicates their better ability in speed of processing and problem-solving skills.

Keywords Handedness · Cognition · MCCB

1 Introduction

There are myths that passed on from the older generations which saying that the left-handed is unique and smarter than the right-hander. There are many famous left-handers that excel in various field, such as philosopher Aristotle, French emperor Napoleon Bonaparte, physicist Albert Einstein, artist Leonardo da Vinci, scientist

Y. Q. Tan (✉) · S. Y. Tee · H. K. Ooi
Department of Mechatronics and Biomedical Engineering, Universiti Tunku Abdul Rahman, Sungai Long, Selangor, Malaysia
e-mail: tanyq@utar.edu.my

Y. Q. Tan
Center for Healthcare Science and Technology, Universiti Tunku Abdul Rahman, Sungai Long, Selangor, Malaysia

J. Usman et al. (eds.), *6th Kuala Lumpur International Conference on Biomedical Engineering 2021*, IFMBE Proceedings 86,
https://doi.org/10.1007/978-3-030-90724-2_25

Nicola Tesla, former US president Barack Obama, Microsoft founder Bill Gates, and many more.

Smart is not only referring to intelligence, but also can be related to the cognition. Cognition is defined as the mental performance that involve in memory, understanding, acquiring knowledges and problem-solving. As our hand motions are control by left and right hemisphere of motor cortex, it may be interesting to find out is there any differences among left- and right-hander in their cognition performance? It is also a need for more studies to correct (or may be to confirm) the myths of lefties with convincible statistical data.

1.1 Handedness

According to the study, there are about 10% of individual are left hand preference for most of their daily activities, and 1% have no hand preference which can used both hands to perform certain task, the rest of about 89% of individuals are right hand preference [1]. In general, individuals can be classified into 3 groups of handedness: the left handers, right handers and mixed handers [2].

1.2 Cognition

The definition of the word "cognition" that defined by Oxford Languages is *the mental action or process of acquiring knowledge and understanding through thought, experience, and the senses.* To make it simple, cognition refer to the ability to think, learn, comprehend and remember. Therefore, cognition or cognitive process is extremely important in routine life. There are a few major domains of cognition which included judgement, memory, attention, intelligence, social cognition and executive functions [3].

There are various cognitive performance tests available, some of the tests can easily assess online, and some were launch as cognition test kits. The MATRICS Consensus Cognitive Battery (MCCB) was developed in 2004 by the National Institute of Mental Health (NIMH) and has been recommended by the United States Food and Drug Administration (FDA) to assess cognitive impairment as the primary outcome measure in the registry trials of Schizophrenia [4]. Yet, MCCB is also been widely use not only to improve cognition performance of various mental health patients but also to assess the cognition performance of healthy subjects.

1.3 Handedness Versus Cognition

There are a lot of studies had been carried out to investigate the relationship between handedness and health. Left-handedness has been connected with innovative [5], homosexualism [6], diseases e.g., hearing disability [7], cerebral palsy [8], Schizophrenia [9] and other mental health issues [10–12].

As early from 1960s, various studies had been carried out to investigate the differences between left- and right-handers' intelligence and cognition performance. However, there are various outcome been found from these studies. Some studies had confirmed that right-hander beat left-handers in the cognition test [13–16], in opposite, some studies support the theory that left-handers can perform better [17–20] and also studies proof there is no significant differences due to handedness [21–23].

Still there is no firm conclusion on the relationship between handedness and cognition performance. One of the reasons may due to the cognition tests use by previous studies are not standardize. Since the MCCB had served as a standardized battery of cognitive tests to use in clinical trials for schizophrenia and healthy controls, we present a study to examine the cognition performance of healthy young undergraduates in Malaysia using MCCB Cognitive Tests. Our goal is to investigate the influence of handedness on test performance.

2 Methodology

Study was conducted in a local university; ethical approval had been obtained from University Scientific and Ethical Review Committee (U/SERC/02/2019).

2.1 Subject Recruitment

Targeted population were undergraduate students, thus able to avoid the biasing due to age and education level. There was total 108 undergraduates participated the study, demographic data as show in Table 1. All participants were self-declared in good health without any mental health illness. Exclusion criteria include those who had suffered serious accident, trauma, hospitalized, surgery or had loss of consciousness in the past six months, alcohol and / or substance abuse. Written consent was obtained from participants prior the conduct of test.

Table 1 Demographics of participants

	Left-hander (LH) (N = 47)	Right-hander (RH) (N = 61)
Age (year old)	21.00 ± 1.68	21.61 ± 1.54
Education level (years)	17.36 ± 2.01	17.61 ± 1.72

2.2 Cognition Test

Five cognition tests from MCCB were adapted to the study, as shown in Table 2.

In Trail Making Test, participant is requested to connect the numbers from 1 to 25 using pen as fast as possible, without lifted the pen from paper throughout the process, raw data collected from this test is total time (in seconds) to complete the task.

There are 9 pairs of Symbol-Number Keys been given under Symbol Coding test, participant is required to fill in the number base on the given keys, complete as much as they can in 90 s, 1 mark is given for each correct answer.

There are 7 paper-and-pen maze tests, increasing in difficulties been provided. Participant been requested to keep they pen on the paper throughout the test, if they find the wrong way in the maze, they must trace back to find the correct way, and total time needed to complete each maze is recorded. Scoring is based on the time recorded, for example, if participants able to complete the Maze Set G in less than 99 s, 5 marks will be rewarded, 4 marks for 100–129 s, 3 marks for 130–168 s, 2 marks for 169–201 s, 1 mark for 202–240 s, if participants complete in more than 240 s, no mark been given.

In Working Memory test, a block with 10 cubes place in irregular pattern put in between coordinator and participants, participants need to tap the cubes in same.

sequence as coordinator, start from 2 cubes in a row, gradually increase until 9 cubes in a row, then restart the test by tapping the cube in reverse sequence as the coordinator, 1 mark will be rewarded for each correct answer given by the participants.

A paper-and-pencil multiple-choice test is provided for Social Cognition test, participants choose the answer base on their own judgement after reading the text, then coordinator will key in the answer into the MCCB scoring program, to convert the data to numbering score.

2.3 Data Analysis

Raw score collected will then key into the MCCB Scoring Program to convert to standard t-score for further data analysis, which range between 0 and100.

Statistical test was performed with SPSS. Comparison between LH and RH group is carried out with independent sample t-test, to determine significant different between LH and RH cognition performances, significant level was set at $p < 0.05$.

Table 2 Cognition tests

Test	Task	Example
Trail making test	Link the number according to the sequence as soon as possible	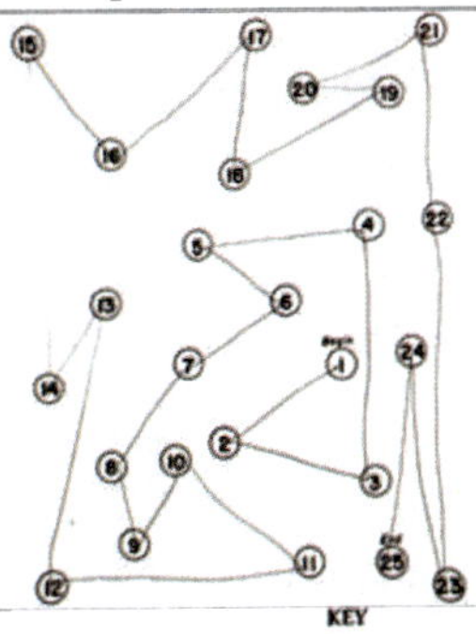
Symbol coding	Pair the symbol with their corresponding number as many as possible in 90 s	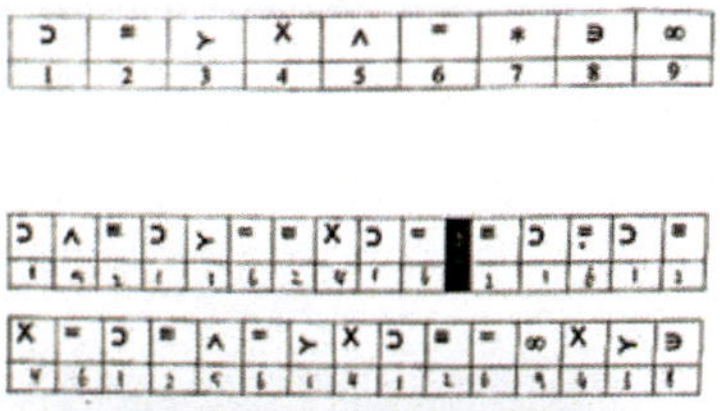
Working memory	The coordinator taps the cubes of a series of numbers, participants need to repeat to tap the cubes correctly, and then in reverse order	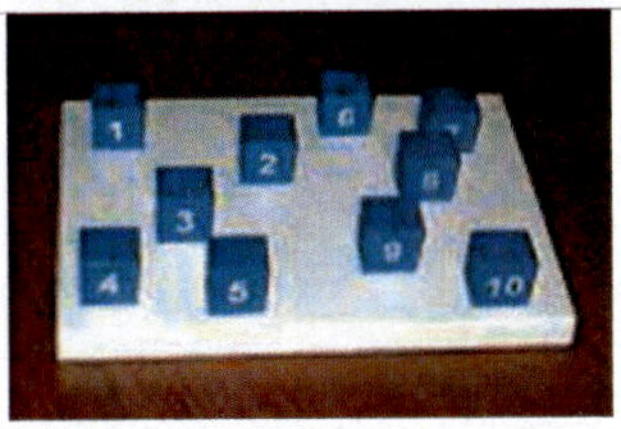
Maze	There were 7 mazes in this test, from easiest to hardest. Participants need to complete the maze in the given time as soon as possible	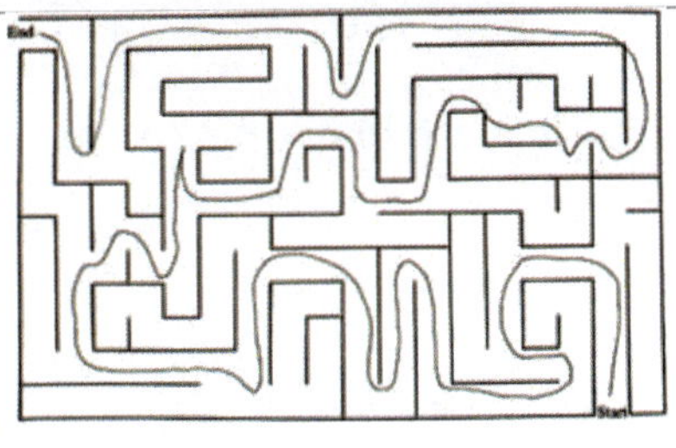
Social cognition	Participants choose the action after read the passage	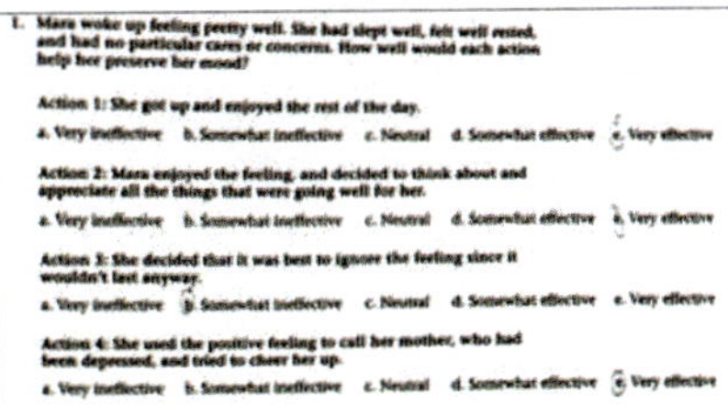1. Mara woke up feeling pretty well. She had slept well, felt well rested, and had no particular cares or concerns. How well would each action help her preserve her mood? Action 1: She got up and enjoyed the rest of the day. a. Very ineffective b. Somewhat ineffective c. Neutral d. Somewhat effective e. Very effective Action 2: Mara enjoyed the feeling, and decided to think about and appreciate all the things that were going well for her. a. Very ineffective b. Somewhat ineffective c. Neutral d. Somewhat effective e. Very effective Action 3: She decided that it was best to ignore the feeling since it wouldn't last anyway. a. Very ineffective b. Somewhat ineffective c. Neutral d. Somewhat effective e. Very effective Action 4: She used the positive feeling to call her mother, who had been depressed, and tried to cheer her up. a. Very ineffective b. Somewhat ineffective c. Neutral d. Somewhat effective e. Very effective

3 Results and Discussions

The results of this study shows that left-handers can perform better than right-handers in Trail Making Test and Social Cognition, but right-handers beat lefties in another 3 cognition tests, which are Symbol Coding, Working Memory and Maze. Among these 5 cognition performances, only Symbol Coding and Maze shows significant differences between the handedness group (Table 3).

Three of the cognition test Trail Making Test, Symbol Coding and Maze were timed, participants were requested to complete the task as fast as they can, this will indirectly give pressure to the participants. According to the instruction given in MCCB, participants were requested to keep the pencil on the paper while completing the tasks Trail Making Test and Maze, therefore the participants may block the view with their own hand. In trail making test, the next sequence number will appear at the right side for 11 times, while appear at the left side for 9 times, in other words, the right-handers will face more vision blocking during the test compared with left-handers, to accommodate the problem the participants will need to raise their hand from the paper or shift their hand position to have more complete view, and thus may delay the time to complete the test. The result from this study shows left-handers score slightly better than right-handers in Trail Making Test, and this result may due to the vision blocking and not to present the cognition ability. The same observation also been reported by Beratis et al. [20] and Bracken et al. [24].

Maze is a cognition test where participants need to plan and foresight the pathway in 2D maze. This test able to train the spatial ability, organization and problem-solving skill. Study had confirmed that left-handers have a more developed right hemisphere cerebrum than right-handers [25], and thus had advantages in spatial reasoning [26] such as Mathematics problem solving ability [27, 28]. However, some recent studies had overturned this theory, suggested that there is no relationship in between handedness and spatial ability [23, 29, 30]. However, the result current study shows significant different between handedness group, where right-handed beat the

Table 3 MCCB cognitive test score

	Group	N	Mean ± S.D	*p*-value
Trail making test	LH	47	45.26 ± 5.72	0.29
	RH	61	43.83 ± 5.92	
Symbol coding	LH	47	48.54 ± 5.90	0.04*
	RH	61	51.19 ± 5.54	
Working memory	LH	47	72.16 ± 7.37	0.209
	RH	61	74.37 ± 7.25	
Maze	LH	47	47.13 ± 5.95	0.005*
	RH	61	51.27 ± 6.48	
Social cognition	LH	47	50.36 ± 7.41	0.231
	RH	61	48.05 ± 8.52	

*significant difference $p < 0.05$

left-handers in speed. This may due to the vision blocking problem like Trail Making Test as explained above. Even though the both left- and right-handers will face the same blocking issue during the test, but most of the maze were started at the right side and participants need to trace the way out towards left side, thus no surprise to reflect in the result where left-handers will complete the task with longer time requested compared with right-handers. Study from Jones et al. [31] states that handedness is not a predictor or indicator of creative thinking and problem-solving ability.

Right-handers had shown significant better performance than left-handers in Symbol Coding, combined with the result of Maze, which also timed test, we may suggest that right-handers are generally perform better in the timed cognition tests than left-handers. The results indicate their better ability in speed of processing and problem-solving skills.

Result of Working Memory shows that there are no significant differences between the handedness group, but right-handers are generally performed slightly better than left handers, which is tally with the previous findings [32, 33].

Social cognition refers to how an individual deal with others members, the processes involve are encoding, storage, retrieval and processing. From our finding, there is only slightly different in Social Cognition score and not able to give any conclusive evidence. However, this result is persuasive as all human are unique, right-handers are not all identical in their pattern with others right-handers and left-handers are probably more variable in nature to adapt to the environment, as suggested by study [34]. Therefore, handedness should not able to predict an individual's reaction, but the social cognition ability is more depends on culture, education and environment.

3.1 Limitations

There are number of limitations in the current study. The participants were recruited from same university, even though this is to limit the effect of age and education level, but also limited the demographics which not representative of the population. The relatively small sample size also might be reflected in the not significant different presented in result. The study does not check the effect of gender on cognition level, which according to studies, gender may correlate with certain cognition abilities.

3.2 Future Works

Since cognition performance test could not represent significant indicators for handedness, the study may be expanded to genetic profiling to investigate the impact of handedness and genetic variance. As known, genetics is one of the major factors contribute to human handedness, thus it may be an interesting topic to study the correlation between handedness, genetic variance and cognition performance, for both males and females.

4 Conclusion

In conclusion, the finding of this study indicate there is a significant effect of handedness on certain cognition test, namely Symbol Coding and Maze, which engage processing time and problem-solving skills. These cognition functions may contribute in a person's daily life to manage well with daily goal, organizing lifestyle and decision making. Current study result may help in better understanding about the relationship among handedness and cognition ability or behavioral pattern.

Acknowledgements This study was fully funded by the Universiti Tunku Abdul Rahman Research Fund Project No. IPSR/RMC/UTARRF/2018-C1/T02 and Malaysia Toray Science Foundation (MTSF) Science and Technology Research Fund Project No. 4417/T06.

References

1. De Kovel, C.G., Carrión-Castillo, A., Francks, C.: A large-scale population study of early life factors influencing left-handedness. Sci. Rep. **9**(1), 1–11 (2019)
2. Zheng, M., McBride, C., Ho, C.S.H., Chan, J.K.C., Choy, K.W., Paracchini, S.: Prevalence and heritability of handedness in a Hong Kong Chinese twin and singleton sample. BMC Psychol. **8**, 1–12 (2020)
3. Kar, S.K., Jain, M.: Current understandings about cognition and the neurobiological correlates in schizophrenia. J. Neurosci. Rural Pract. **7**(3), 412 (2016)
4. Liang, S., Yu, W., Ma, X., Luo, S., Zhang, J., Sun, X., ... Zhang, Y.: Psychometric properties of the MATRICS consensus cognitive battery (MCCB) in Chinese patients with major depressive disorder. J. Affect. Disorders **265**, 132–138 (2020)
5. Badzakova-Trajkov, G., Häberling, I.S., Corballis, M.C.: Magical ideation, creativity, handedness, and cerebral asymmetries: a combined behavioural and fMRI study. Neuropsychologia **49**(10), 2896–2903 (2011)
6. Lalumiere, M.L., Blanchard, R., Zucker, K.J.: Sexual orientation and handedness in men and women: a meta-analysis. Psychol. Bull. **126**(4), 575 (2000)
7. Papadatou-Pastou, M., Sáfár, A.: Handedness prevalence in the deaf: meta-analyses. Neurosci. Biobehav. Rev. **60**, 98–114 (2016)
8. Vlachos, F., Andreou, E., Delliou, A., Agapitou, P.: Dyslexia and hand preference in secondary school students. Psychol. Neurosc. **6**(1), 67–72 (2013)
9. Sommer, I., Aleman, A., Ramsey, N., Bouma, A., Kahn, R.: Handedness, language lateralisation and anatomical asymmetry in schizophrenia: meta-analysis. Br. J. Psychiatry **178**(4), 344–351 (2001)
10. Cheng, B., Liang, C., Li, P., Liu, L., Cheng, S., Ma, M., ... Zhang, F.: Evaluating the genetic correlations between left-handedness and mental disorder using linkage disequilibrium score regression and transcriptome-wide association study. Biochem. Genet. **58**(2), 348–358 (2020)
11. Wiberg, A., Ng, M., Al Omran, Y., Alfaro-Almagro, F., McCarthy, P., Marchini, J., ... Furniss, D.: Handedness, language areas and neuropsychiatric diseases: insights from brain imaging and genetics. Brain **142**(10), 2938–2947 (2019)

12. Schmitz, J., Packheiser, J., Birnkraut, T., Hinz, N.A., Friedrich, P., Güntürkün, O., Ocklenburg, S.: The neurophysiological correlates of handedness: Insights from the lateralized readiness potential. Behav. Brain Res. **364**, 114–122 (2019)
13. Briggs, G.G., Nebes, R.D.: The effects of handedness, family history and sex on the performance of a dichotic listening task. Neuropsychologia **14**(1), 129–133 (1976)
14. Calnan, M., Richardson, K.: Developmental correlates of handedness in a national sample of 11-year-olds. Ann. Hum. Biol. **3**(4), 329–342 (1976)
15. Johnston, D.W., Nicholls, M., Shah, M., Shields, M.A.: Handedness, health and cognitive development: evidence from children in the NLSY (2010)
16. Hatta, T.: Associations between handedness and executive function in upper-middle-aged people. Laterality: Asymm. Body, Brain Cogn. **23**(3), 274–289 (2018)
17. Heim, A.W., Watts, K.P.: Handedness and cognitive bias. Q. J. Exp. Psychol. **28**(3), 355–360 (1976)
18. Johnson, O., Harley, C.W.: Handedness and sex differences in cognitive tests of brain laterality. Cortex (1980)
19. Levander, M., Schalling, D., Levander, S.E.: Birth stress, handedness and cognitive performance. Cortex **25**(4), 673–681 (1989)
20. Beratis, I.N., Rabavilas, A.D., Kyprianou, M., Papadimitriou, G.N., Papageorgiou, C.: Investigation of the link between higher order cognitive functions and handedness. J. Clin. Exp. Neuropsychol. **35**(4), 393–403 (2013)
21. Hardyck, C., Petrinovich, L.F., Goldman, R.D.: Left-handedness and cognitive deficit. Cortex **12**(3), 266–279 (1976)
22. Inglis, J., Lawson, J.S.: Handedness, sex and intelligence. Cortex **20**(3), 447–451 (1984)
23. Sala, G., Signorelli, M., Barsuola, G., Bolognese, M., Gobet, F.: The relationship between handedness and mathematics is non-linear and is moderated by gender, age, and type of task. Front. Psychol. **8**, 948 (2017)
24. Bracken, M.R., Mazur-Mosiewicz, A., Glazek, K.: Trail making test: comparison of paper-and-pencil and electronic versions. Appl. Neuropsychol.: Adult (2018)
25. Gutwinski, S., Löscher, A., Mahler, L., Kalbitzer, J., Heinz, A., Bermpohl, F.: Understanding left-handedness. Deutsches Ärzteblatt Int. **108**(50), 849 (2011)
26. Ganley, C.M., Vasilyeva, M.: Sex differences in the relation between math performance, spatial skills, and attitudes. J. Appl. Dev. Psychol. **32**(4), 235–242 (2011)
27. Casey, M.B., Pezaris, E., Nuttall, R.L.: Spatial ability as a predictor of math achievement: the importance of sex and handedness patterns. Neuropsychologia **30**(1), 35–45 (1992)
28. Levander, M., Levander, S.: Cognitive performance among left-handers differing in strength of handedness and familial sinistrality. Intelligence **14**(1), 97–108 (1990)
29. Leone Ganado, K.: Examining the role of handedness in visual-spatial abilities. Bachelor's thesis, University of Malta (2020)
30. Papadatou-Pastou, M.: Handedness and cognitive ability: using meta-analysis to make sense of the data. Prog. Brain Res. **238**, 179–206 (2018)
31. Jones, T., Caulfield, L., Wilkinson, D., Weller, L.: The relationship between nonclinical schizotypy and handedness on divergent and convergent creative problem-solving tasks. Creat. Res. J. **23**(3), 222–228 (2011)
32. Sahu, A., Christman, S.D., Propper, R.E.: The contributions of handedness and working memory to episodic memory. Mem. Cognit. **44**(8), 1149–1156 (2016)
33. Powell, J.L.: An investigation of the association between handedness, cognition, brain structure and function. Doctoral dissertation, University of Liverpool (2011)
34. McManus, I.C., Buckens, G., Harris, N., Flint, A., Ng, H.L.A., Vovou, F.: Faking handedness: individual differences in ability to fake handedness, social cognitions of the handedness of others, and a forensic application using Bayes' theorem. Lateral.: Asymm. Body, Brain Cogn. **23**(1), 67–100 (2018)

Parents Involvement in Young STEM Learners and Talent Development: A Pilot Study

Nur Azah Hamzaid, Juliana Usman, Jegalakshimi Jewaratnam, Chan Chow Khuen, Suzieleez Syrene Abdul Rahim, and Mohd Faiz Azmi

Abstract The need to promote genuine interest for learning is especially required for STEM based understanding, knowledge and skills in very young learners. Parents involvement in STEM learning has been established as a critical factor that would move the students' interest and adoption into STEM field and STEM related careers later in the future. This is critical even in the early childhood years where curiosity and interest are at its peak. Play based learning at home and in informal settings are one of the most effective way to experience STEM and this has been reflected in the literature especially where parents are involved. While the efficacy and usefulness of play-based learning is clear among children, the acceptance and thorough adoption among parents still requires clear method and direction. This research aims to explore and identify key factors of effective STEM learning for young children. Parents' background and STEM career could influence their children's interest and ability in STEM, while utility values by parents are key in nurturing children's interest as children are independently evoked and may be influenced by their perceived utility-values by the parents.

Keywords Parents · STEM · Children · Talent

N. A. Hamzaid (✉) · J. Usman · C. C. Khuen · M. F. Azmi
Department of Biomedical Engineering, Faculty of Engineering, Universiti Malaya, 50603 Kuala Lumpur, Malaysia
e-mail: azah.hamzaid@um.edu.my

J. Jewaratnam
Department of Chemical Engineering, Faculty of Engineering, Universiti Malaya, 50603 Kuala Lumpur, Malaysia

S. S. A. Rahim
Department of Mathematics and Science Education, Faculty of Education, Universiti Malaya, 50603 Kuala Lumpur, Malaysia

M. F. Azmi
Faculty of Economics and Administration, Universiti Malaya, 50603 Kuala Lumpur, Malaysia

J. Usman et al. (eds.), *6th Kuala Lumpur International Conference on Biomedical Engineering 2021*, IFMBE Proceedings 86,
https://doi.org/10.1007/978-3-030-90724-2_26

1 Introduction

1.1 The Move Away from Examination-Based Assessments

The need for non-examination-based assessment was highlighted to promote genuine interest for learning. This is especially true and required even more for science, technology, engineering and mathematics (STEM)-based understanding, knowledge and skills in very young learners. The adoption of play-based learning with 3H principle (Heads on, Hands on, Hearts on) in young children has been established as one of the most effective approach in instilling the passion and curiosity [1] to build solid foundation to master future STEM disciplines.

While the efficacy and usefulness of play-based learning is clear among children, the acceptance and thorough adoption among parents are still weak and lacks clear method and direction. Parents, while with good intentions may impose route learning exercises for their children, could be open to more authentic learning approach and scaffolding roles [2].

This research explored and identified key factors of effective STEM learning for young children, and model the most significant approach. Mixed-method investigation was conducted with children in primary schools and their parents. Parents interview and case studies were crucial observations to extract real interaction and responses with the children.

2 Methodology

2.1 Participants

Thirty (30) respondents were recruited for this study. The participants were recruited by invitation through emails and through the WhatsApp platform. The inclusion criteria for participation in the study were: 1. Must be a parent, 2. Have at least one child, and 3. Since the questionnaires are in English language, participants must have a basic understanding in English Language. The respondent's participation in this study is entirely voluntary. The study was approved by the Universiti Malaya Research Ethics Committee (UMREC) UM.TNC2/UMREC_1157.

2.2 Study Instrument and Procedures

A series of questionnaires were used during the study. The questionnaires were adapted and adopted from A Validation of the Family Involvement Questionnaire-High School Version [3], Family-Friendly Science: Increasing Family Engagement in STEM Education [4], 'Ikigai' in older Japanese people [5] and Sense of Life Worth Living (Ikigai), Mortality in Japan: Ohsaki Study [6] and Ikigai Worksheets [7].

There are two parts of questionnaires. Part I of the questionnaires are related to Science, Technology, Engineering and Mathematics (STEM) while Part II of the questionnaires are related to *Ikigai* which is the "Sense of Life Worth Living". A total of 50 questions were used with 25 questions in both parts, respectively. The questionnaires were distributed to the participants online via Google Form. Once completed, the participants were given the "Bermain dengan STEM" e-book [8] as a token of appreciation. The average and standard deviation (SD) was obtained and analysed for each question.

3 Results

After data preprocessing, 25 responses were used for data analysis. Figure 1 shows the demographic of the participants. The participants were parents of young children.

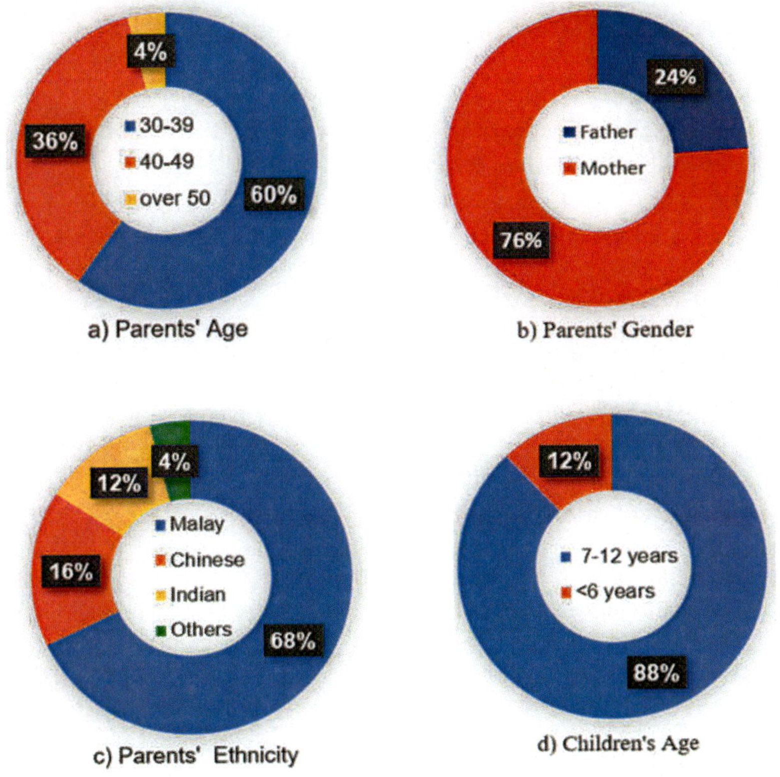

Fig. 1 Participants' demography

The majority of the parents' age is 30–39 years old. As for gender, 76% of mothers and 24% of fathers participated in this survey. The majority of parents were of Malay ethnicity. 88% of the participants' children are aged between 7 and 12 years old. 12% of the children are 6 years and below. From the 25 children, 72% and 24% goes to government and private schools, respectively. 4% is not schooling yet.

Tables 1 and 2 show the average and standard deviation for each question in the Part 1 and 2 of the questionnaires, respectively. The overall average for Table 2 is higher than Table 1. Parents definitely have high desires for their children's

Table 1 Parents present involvement in STEM

Questions	Ave	SD
Part I: STEM (Science, Technology, Engineering and Mathematics)	3.2	0.4
(1) I attend meeting/parents-teacher meeting to discuss about my child's learning behavior	3.4	0.8
(2) I make contact with school (teacher or principal) to get information regarding my child	3.3	0.8
(3) I converse with my child's teacher	3.4	0.6
(4) I monitor my child's TV and Internet usage	3.5	0.6
(5) I review my child's school work OR I ensure my child's school work are reviewed	3.6	0.6
(6) I send my child to school	3.5	0.7
(7) I keep a regular schedule (studying, morning, bedtime) for my child	3.3	0.6
(8) I praise my child for doing/completing his/her schoolwork	3.8	0.4
(9) I share my experience of studying back in my time	3.1	0.9
(10) I take my child to other learning centers to learn specific things	2.8	0.9
(11) I contact the school when my child tells me something about school that concerns me	3.2	0.6
(12) I participate and volunteer in my child's classroom	2.6	0.8
(13) I praise my child for his/her accomplishments	3.7	0.5
(14) I read and do STEM-related activity with my child	2.8	0.9
(15) I participate in my child's school activities	3.0	0.8
(16) I ask about my child's day / difficulties at school	3.6	0.6
(17) I discuss with other parents about my child's school events	2.6	1.0
(18) I ask my child to do home chores	3.3	0.6
(19) I do singing, drawing and storytelling with my child to enhance her/his creativity	3.1	0.8
(20) I help my child with work and problem solving related to Science, Technology, Engineering, Mathematics skills	3.3	0.8
(21) I do STEM activities with my child and we enjoy it	2.8	0.8
(22) I attend my child's school STEM event(s)	2.7	0.9
(23) I believe that by joining school events in STEM, I can contribute to my child's STEM education	3.3	0.6
(24) I prepare more home resources to engage STEM learning with my child	2.9	0.7
(25) I have the desire to see my child pursue a STEM-related field	3.4	0.6

Table 2 Parents desire for their children's future

Questions	Ave	SD
Part II: Ikigai or "Sense of Life Worth Living"	3.7	0.2
(1) I want my child to grow up with a healthy lifestyle	4.0	0.0
(2) I want my child to grow up with a sense that 'life is worth living'	4.0	0.2
(3) Creativity is related to a person's well being	3.7	0.5
(4) I want my children to grow up feeling that their lives are valuable	4.0	0.2
(5) I want my child to be concerned with his/her future	3.8	0.4
(6) I want my child to have a desire or goal for the future	3.8	0.4
(7) I want my child to willingly do spontaneous activities	3.8	0.4
(8) I want my child to behave/take actions which they are forced to take	3.6	0.6
(9) I want my child to reflect their inner self and express it honestly/faithfully	3.8	0.4
(10) I want my child to be able to establish a unique mental world in which he/she can feel at ease	3.8	0.4
(11) I want my child to grow up and experience the pleasure of living through EITHER work, family or communication with neighbors	3.8	0.4
(12) I want my child to be able to go through the process of cultivating his/her inner potential that makes his/her life significant	4.0	0.2
(13) I believe we should consider how our lifestyle effects our functional, societal and psychological well-being	3.9	0.3
(14) I believe that the sense of "life worth living" is associated with mortality risks	3.5	0.8
(15) I believe that health, socioeconomic status or health-related lifestyle are not associated with the negative psychological factors and mortality risk	3.0	1.0
(16) I believe that sense of "life worth living" reflects an individual's motivation for living or "purpose in life" or "reason for living."	3.8	0.4
(17) I want my child to have a sense of "joy and a sense of well-being from being alive"	3.8	0.6
(18) I want my child to have a sense of "realizing the value of being alive"	4.0	0.2
(19) I believe that the lack of 'ikigai' or the sense of "life worth living" was associated with poorer psychosocial status and poorer physical health status	3.4	0.7
(20) I believe my child should be able to grow up doing what he/she loves	3.9	0.3
(21) I believe that my child should be able to grow up doing what he/she is good at	3.9	0.3
(22) I believe that my child should be able to grow up doing what the world needs	3.2	0.9
(23) I believe that my child should be able to grow up doing what he/she can be paid for	3.4	0.6
(24) I believe that my child is able to achieve all of the above in item 20, 21, 22, 23	3.6	0.5
(25) I believe that my child should have a strong personal value	3.8	0.4

future and wellbeing. However, their actual involvement in STEM activities with children and school is rather low. As shown in Table 1, parents scored highest for praising their children's achievement. Parents are also committed to review their children's homework and monitor their media usage. Parents pay attention to their children's account on their daily school activities. The parents seem to be lacking in communication with other parents about school events, as the score is the lowest. Subsequently, the scores for attendance to STEM events in school and classroom were also low.

4 Discussion

From the results obtained through this study, parents who intend for their children to have a good future will focus on several of these considerations. Parents might go to the extent of registering and sending their children to the best school possible. Parents seem to prefer a school with good academic achievement and reputation. Other considerations by parents were distance from home to school, finances (low expenses and availability of financial aids and scholarships), and school philosophy or mission. Our findings show that there are slight differences though between parents of private school going children and government school-goer children (Fig. 2). Responses of parents' STEM involvement were more varied compared to their Ikigai responses, which indicate that both groups have undoubtedly greater desire for their children's future and wellbeing compared to their actual involvement in their child's learning.

From our study, parents could play a role in contributing to the learning curve of their children. Nonetheless, there are challenges that might appear from the parents' viewpoint. One of the obstacles for parents in contributing significantly to their children's learning-related activities is to find the time to attend school events or support their children. This is significantly shown in families with low economic

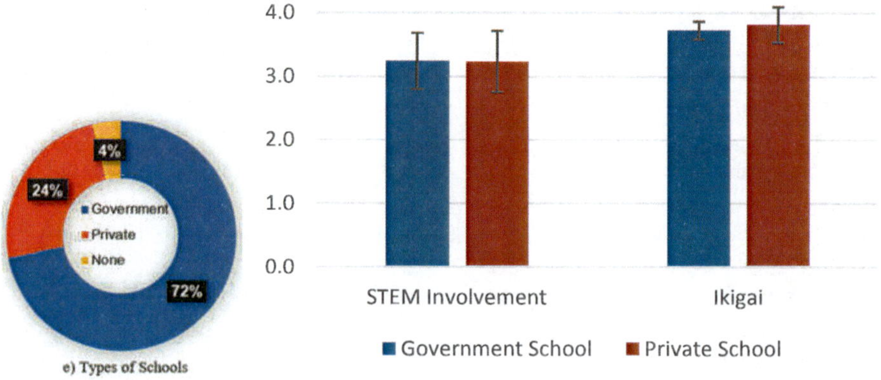

Fig. 2 Types of schools and parents responses respectively

resources, which causes the parents to work hard to make ends meet. Moreover, teachers might face difficulties when the children are expected to perform in academic while receiving less to no effort from their parents.

Another challenge is the socioeconomic statuses of the family. It could not be denied that some of the parents are illiterate, or perhaps using their mother tongues in educating or communicating with their children. Hence, this makes the parents feel uneasy and not comfortable when attending events and meetings in school. Hence, parents would feel unwelcomed or unaccepted in schools, which will further make the parents put in less effort in educating their children. Due to this, children might feel that their parents are not interested in their well-being, contribution, and achievement in schools.

Parents who contribute sufficiently to their children's learning-related activities will positively influence the children's future. Parents can ask how the children fair in school and attend school meetings as well as annual school events. Additionally, the best indicator of a student's accomplishment is the extent to which families are involved in their education. Children will be more motivated and cultivate affection in learning if there is support from their parents.

The learning environment in classes will change accordingly when there is involvement from parents. Additionally, working together with parents can assist in determining the needs and objectives that parents may consider contributing towards.

Hence, involvement from parents would contribute to the advantages for everyone, including the school, the teachers, the parents, and students.

5 Conclusion

In conclusion, parents are concerned of their children's wellbeing. They have high hopes for their children to live a happy and fulfilling life. However, parents' actual involvement toward ensuring promising future, needs more effort. The convenience sampling conducted in this study clearly shows some intervention is needed to increase parents involvement in STEM activities with their children, both at home and in school. The paper is concluded with some Ikigai quotes for readers consumption.

Ikigai refers to situations whereby the following quotes apply [9]:

> **Existential crisis**, is typical of modern societies in which people **do what they are told to do**, or what others do, rather than what they want to do. They often try to fill the gap between what is expected of them and what they want for themselves with economic power or physical pleasure, or by numbing their senses.
>
> Those who give up the things they love doing and do well will lose their purpose in life. That's why it's so important to keep doing things of value, making progress, bringing beauty or utility to others, helping out, and shaping the world around you, even after your 'official' professional activity has ended.
>
> The happiest people are not the ones who achieve the most. They are the ones who spend more time than others in a state of flow.

In order to achieve this optimal experience, we have to focus on increasing the time we spend on activities that bring us to this state of flow, rather than allowing ourselves to get caught up in activities that offer immediate pleasure.

Acknowledgements This work was funded by University Malaya under grant number IIRG033A-2019 "The Science of Play: Role of Parents Scaffoldings in Young Stem Learners".

References

1. Lee, Y.L., Hamzaid, N.A.: Promoting hands-on, heads-on, hearts-on (3Hs) biomedical engineering education among first graders through Let's go to Mummie's Lab. In: Fadzil, H.M., Sathasivam, R.V., Ithnin, R., Mohktar, M.S. (eds.) Best Practices in STEM Mentor Mentee, pp. 62–74. UM STEM Centre, Kuala Lumpur (2019)
2. Lee, Y.L., Hamzaid, N.A.: Parents' perspectives on elementary engineering education using hands-on, heads-on, and hearts-on (3HS) approach. Malay. Online J. Educ. Sci. (MOJES) **7**(4), 15–29 (2019)
3. Grover, K.A., Houlihan, D.D., Campana, K.: A Validation of the family involvement questionnaire-high school version. Int. J. Psychol. Stud. **8**(2), 28 (2016). https://doi.org/10.5539/ijps.v8n2p28
4. Bixler, A.: Family-friendly science: increasing family engagement in STEM education (2016)
5. Nakanishi, N.: 'Ikigai' in older Japanese people. Age Ageing **28**(3), 323–324 (1999)
6. Sone, T., Nakaya, N., Ohmori, K., Shimazu, T., Higashiguchi, M., Kakizaki, M., … Tsuji, I.: Sense of life worth living (Ikigai) and mortality in Japan: Ohsaki study. Psychosom. Med. **70**(6), 709–715 (2008)
7. Kemp, N.: Ikigai Worksheets (2020). Retrieved 30 Oct 2020, from https://ikigaitribe.com/
8. Hamzaid, N.A., Abdul Rahim, S.S., Chan, C.K., Usman, J., Jewaratnam, J., Azmi, M.F., Chinatamby, P.: Bermain dengan STEM. Panduan Untuk Ibu Bapa, pp. 1–96. UM STEM Centre, Kuala Lumpur (2020)
9. García, H., Miralles, F.: Ikigai: The Japanese secret to a long and happy life. Penguin (2017)

Practice Analysis: The Service Delivery and Domains of Prosthetic and Orthotic Practitioners in Malaysia

Hasif Rafidee Hasbollah and Nooranida Arifin

Abstract Malaysia has a database for physiotherapist and occupational therapist, however, the statistic for manpower in Prosthetic and Orthotic (P&O) practitioners are yet to be reported. The aim of this research is to establish the database of P&O practitioners in Malaysia according to the Standards of Prosthetics and Orthotics of service delivery and domains using Practice Analysis (PA). PA is a strategy or technique used to explore and expand the content and description of the profession P&O practitioners. A total of fifty-one (51) respondents were selected in this research by using purposive sampling via hospitals and private practices companies in Malaysia. This number of respondents are divided into two which were twenty-one (21) Certified Prosthetists Orthotists (CPOs) and thirty (30) technicians. The data is collected using a questionnaire adapted from American Board for Certification in Orthotics, Prosthetics and Orthotic. The findings of the questionnaire are analyzed and interpreted via descriptive statistics such as percentages and frequency. Prosthetic Fabrication (PF) has recorded the highest total frequency of CPOs and Technicians with 48 practitioners. The result of this study showed that the top three domains are patient assessment (Domain 1), implementation of the treatment plan (Domain 3), promotion of competency and enhancement of professional (Domain 4) were the most domains performed by the practitioners. These elementary findings of this study are useful for higher education and training providers in planning for a proper clinical and technical programme for future and existing practitioners as well as serve as a support evidence for the policy maker in ensuring the high quality of P&O service provision. This study has concluded that, P&O Practitioners have practiced the PA according to the Standards of Prosthetics and Orthotics of nine primary service delivery based on the four main domains.

H. R. Hasbollah (✉)
Wellness Department, Faculty of Hospitality, Tourism and Wellness, Universiti Malaysia Kelantan, Kota Bharu, Malaysia
e-mail: rafidee@umk.edu.my

N. Arifin
Biomedical Engineering Department, Faculty of Engineering, Universiti Malaya, Kuala Lumpur, Malaysia
e-mail: anidaum@um.edu.my

J. Usman et al. (eds.), *6th Kuala Lumpur International Conference on Biomedical Engineering 2021*, IFMBE Proceedings 86,
https://doi.org/10.1007/978-3-030-90724-2_27

Keywords Practice analysis · Service delivery · Domains · Prosthetic · Orthotic · Malaysia

1 Introduction

Since 1937, Prosthetic and Orthotic (P&O) in Malaysia has started when the orthopaedic appliance workshop in the National Leprosy Control Center in Sungai Buloh was established by British. The first P&O centre was built at University Hospital (currently known as University of Malaya Medical Centre) in 1967. After 1969, the General Hospital Kuala Lumpur has administered the National Limb Fitting Centre [1].

P&O is the combination between policy (financing), products (parts and material), practitioners, prepares the suitable prostheses, orthoses and others related treatment that is aimed to achieve the good quality services in manufacturing and fitting P&O devices [2, 3].

In general, P&O practitioners were divided into clinicians and non-clinicals. For the clinicians, the practitioner is required to have a deep understanding of medical and technical subjects, where in non-clinicals, the practitioner is required to able to use and handle tools, machines, and material for plastic, metal and plaster for manufacturing the devices [4]. Only prosthetists, orthotists and assistants were involved in clinicians, where technicians and support staff are in non-clinicians [3].

Each year, the demands of P&O practitioners increased especially in low-income and developing countries. Over than six (6) million amputees need P&O devices in Africa, Asia and Latin America. However, it is estimated about 180,000 practitioners are needed in P&O services. Conversely, it is only 40,000 trained Certified Prosthetist Orthotist (ISPO Category I) and technologist (ISPO Category II) are available [5].

Therefore, the availability of competent and well-trained clinicians and non-clinicians are vital to achieve a high-quality P&O practitioner as stated in the Standards of Prosthetics and Orthotics, the services must conduct by competent and adequately trained personnel in the related areas [3].

Each of the country provides the P&O services, but it may differ in terms of quantity and quality of services and devices. Unfortunately, certain practitioners of P&O were not practicing patient safety as their priority due to the insufficient number of practitioners [6, 7].

Malaysia has a database for physiotherapist and occupational therapist, however, the statistic for manpower in P&O practitioner is yet to be reported. Thus, the aim of this research is to establish the database of P&O practitioners in Malaysia according to the Standards of Prosthetics and Orthotics of service delivery and domains using Practice Analysis (PA).

American Board for Certification in Orthotics, Prosthetics and Orthotic stated that Practice Analysis (PA) is a strategy or technique used to explore and expand the content and description of the profession. In the other word, practice analysis

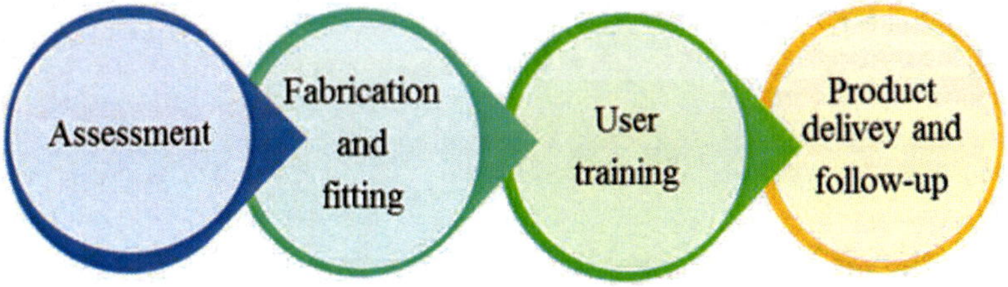

Fig. 1 Steps in service delivery of P&O practitioner

comprises a group of job analysis, role analysis, role delineation study and the process analysis [8].

According to UN there are the four (4) steps in service delivery of P&O practitioner in ensuring the consistency, successful and competent at all level of care [9] (Fig. 1).

For the first step, P&O practitioner should assess the patient (user) holistically with taking into account the user lifestyle, living environment condition and physical condition of the user. Then, the P&O practitioner must stress on the fabrication and fitting process. The caregiver must abide every instruction meticulously from the manufacturer and supplier regarding the instructions on the use of components and materials to ensure the device is beneficial towards the user and thereby reducing the danger. Next step is providing sufficient training towards the user in order to increase the benefits of using the device. The final step is, P&O practitioner must check all the features of the device in the best quality and well-function before delivering prostheses and orthoses service. Evaluation of the result of medical care and in follow-up sessions will allow real benefits of prostheses and orthoses service, thus the achieved the objective of treatment is achieved. The aim of this research is to establish the database of P&O practitioners in Malaysia according to the Standards of Prosthetics and Orthotics of service delivery and domains using Practice Analysis (PA).

2 Methodology

This study adopted quantitative method in order to collect data the practice analysis of P&O practitioners in Malaysia. The function of quantitative method is to find the answer to every question based on the facts, general knowledge and their intention [10].

A total of fifty-one (51) respondents were selected in this research by using purposive sampling via hospitals and private practices companies in Malaysia. This number of respondents are divided into two which were twenty-one (21) Certified Prosthetists Orthotists (CPOs) and thirty (30) technicians. Purposive sampling is a non-random technique that does not need any theories and a set number of participants to find people who are willing to provide the information based on their knowledge and experience [11].

The data is collected using a questionnaire. The collection of data conducted based on the set time and it is cost effective when using a questionnaire.

The findings of the questionnaire are easily identified and quantified [12]. The questionnaire was adapted from American Board for Certification in Orthotics, Prosthetics and Orthotics which is stress on the Practice Analysis of certified practitioners in the disciplines of orthotics and prosthetics. It is then analysed and interpreted via descriptive statistics such as percentage and frequency in order to report the general outcomes of the study.

3 Results and Discussion

Based on the Table 1, the result indicated the frequency of P&O practitioners according to the primary service delivery performed according to the function of the position. While, Fig. 2 showed the comparison of primary service performed for CPO and technician.

Prosthetic Fabrication (PF) has recorded the highest total frequency of CPOs and Technicians with 48 practitioners. It is clear that, most of the Prosthetic and Orthotic (P&O) service centre in Malaysia were focused on the Primary Work in PF. From this number, 28 of them are Technicians and the rest of this task is done and monitored by CPOs. After the Primary Work in PF, Orthotic Fabrication (OF) is a common field of work in the P&O. The findings showed that number of CPOs are fewer (19) than Technicians (27) who were engaged in OF. There were three types of Primary Work that indicated the same total number of practitioners namely as Clinical Prosthetic Patient Care (CPPC), Clinical Orthotic Patient Care—Custom

Table 1 Frequency of primary service performed by the practitioners

Primary service	Frequency of CPO	Frequency of technician	Total (n)
Clinical prosthetic patient care (CPPC)	20	11	31
Clinical orthotic patient care (Custom fabricated) (COPCCF)	19	12	31
Clinical orthotic patient care (Pre-fabricated) (COPCPF)	17	10	27
Prosthetic fabrication (PF)	20	28	48
Orthotic fabrication (OF)	19	27	46
Education (EDU)	12	19	31
Research (RES)	3	5	8
Administration (ADM)	10	6	16
Other (OTHER)	9	4	13

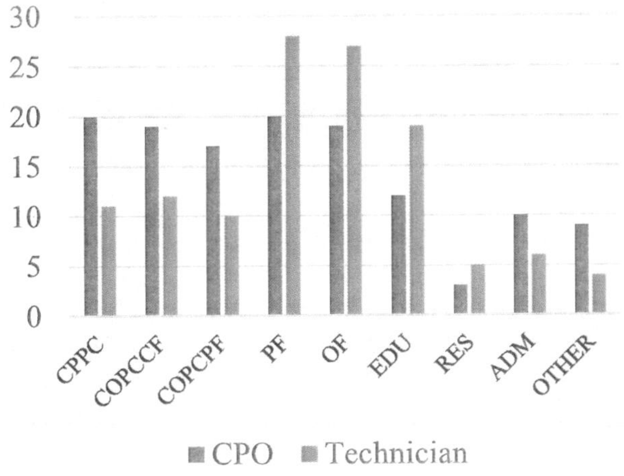

Fig. 2 Comparison of primary service performed for CPO and technician

Fabricated (COPCCF), and Education (EDU). The total amount for each Primary Work were 31 practitioners per work field. As for CPPC, this field is dominated by CPOs with 20 practitioners and 11 practitioners for the Technicians. Meanwhile, COPCCF was set to less than one practitioner for CPO which were 19 practitioners and 12 Technicians. In contrast to the Primary Work in Education indicated that the Technicians showed a higher number (19) while the CPOs were less (12).

The Primary Work of Clinical Orthotic Patient Care—Pre-Fabricated (COPCPF) recorded a total of 17 practitioners for CPOs and 10 practitioners for Technicians. CPOs recorded a significant number in this Primary Work because of its specialisation job. In P&O industry, there were an area specifically for Administration (ADM), whereby it was dominated by the CPOs. The number of Technicians showed a small number because in Malaysia, there were P&O centres that only consists of Technicians.

Table 2 presented the results of the average percentages of service delivery based on different domains. As can be seen, CPOs indicated that they spend the most time performing tasks associated with Patient Assessment for both disciplines with the respective percentages of 27.95% and 27.24%. Compared to the Technicians, most of the time, they are spending on Implementation of the Treatment Plan which indicates 37.0% and 38.33% respectively for both disciplines.

Table 2 Average percentages of service delivery based on the domains

Domain	Percentage prosthetic		Percentage orthotic	
	CPO	Technician	CPO	Technician
One (1): Patient assessment	27.95	15.60	27.24	15.67
Two (2): Formulation of the treatment plan	18.95	13.37	18.52	12.87
Three (3): Implementation of the treatment plan	18.95	37.00	21.14	38.33
Four (4): Follow-up to the treatment plan	14.43	8.87	13.76	7.80

Referring to **Domain 1—Patient Assessment**, both CPOs and Technician most commonly performed task such as reviewed patient's prescription as referral in both P&O discipline. The practitioners were also using established record-keeping requirements to documented the patient assessment. Usually, the practitioners collected the data based on patient background such as demographic characteristics, family dynamics, previous use of orthopedic devices and medical history.

Based on the findings of **Patient Assessment** in **Domain 1**, the practitioners will **Formulate Treatment (Domain 2)** to identify which design, materials and components are needed based on their physical condition and daily activity.

Domain 3 is about **Implementation of the Treatment Plan** towards patient or orthopedic user. Both practitioners informed user, relatives and caregivers regarding to the measurement taken, future obstacle and time taken in fabricated the devices. It is important to provide optimum strength; durability and it function by selecting an appropriate material for the devices.

After **Implementation of the Treatment Plan**, it is vital for the practitioners to **Follow-up to the Treatment Plan (Domain 4)**. User's feedback is valuable in determining their satisfaction and recommendation for the future treatment.

These elementary findings of this study are useful for higher education and training providers in planning for a proper clinical and technical programme for future and existing practitioners. Additionally, this finding serves as a support evidence for the policy maker in ensuring the high quality of P&O service provision [13, 14].

4 Conclusion

This study has concluded that, P&O Practitioners have practiced the PA according to the Standards of Prosthetics and Orthotics of nine (9) primary service delivery based on the four (4) main domains. The frequency of Primary Service and average percentages of services delivery by the CPOs and Technicians were presented in establishing the database for this research.

References

1. Arifin, N., Hasbollah, H.R., Hanafi, M.H., Ibrahim, A.H., Wan Abdul Rahman, W.A, Che Aziz, R.: Provision of prosthetic services following lower limb amputation in Malaysia. Malay. J. Med. Sci. **24**(5), 106–111 (2017)
2. LSN.: Prosthetics and orthotics programme guide (2006). Retrieved from Landmine Survivors Network: http://landminesurvivors.org/documents/indicator_bosnia.pdf. Last accessed 14 Feb 2020
3. WHO: Standards for Prosthetics and Orthotics Part 1: Standards. World Health Organization, France (2017)
4. ISPO: Prosthetics and Orthotics Programme Guide: Implementing P&O Services in Low-Income Settings. International Society for Prosthetics and Orthotics, Geneva (2006)

5. WHO.: Guideline for Training Personnel in Developing Countries for Prosthetics and Orthotics Services (2005)
6. Hughes, R.G.: Patient Safety and Quality: An Evidence-Based Handbook for Nurses. Agency for Healthcare Research and Quality, Rockville (MD) (2008)
7. Magnusson, L.: Prosthetic and Orthotic Services in Developing Countries. School of Health Sciences, Jonkoping University, Sweden (2014)
8. ABC.: Practice Analysis of Certified Practitioners in the Discipline of Orthotics and Prosthetics. American Board for Certification in Orthotics, Prosthetics & Orthotics, Virginia (2015)
9. WHO: Standards for Prosthetics and Orthotics Part 2: Implementation Manual. World Health Organization, France (2017)
10. Leedy, P.D.: Practical Research: Planning and design. Prentice-Hall, New Jersey (1993)
11. Bernard, H.R.: Research Methods in Anthropology: Qualitative and Quantitative Approaches. 3rd Alta Mira Press, Walnut Creek, CA (2002)
12. Stefan, D.: 9 Advantages and disadvantages of questionnaires. In: Survey Anyplace (2016). https://surveyanyplace.com/questionnaire-pros-and-cons, Last accessed 14 Feb 2020
13. Choong, M., Chau, T., Chy, D., Ross, A.: Clinical management of quadriplegia in low and middle-income countries: a patient's road to physiotherapy, prostheses and rehabilitation. BMJ case reports (2018)
14. Shahabi, S., Pardhan, S., Ahmadi Teymourlouy, A., Skempes, D., Shahali, S., Mojgani, P., Jalali, M., Lankarani, K.B.: Prioritizing solutions to incorporate Prosthetics and Orthotics services into Iranian health benefits package: Using an analytic hierarchy process. PLoS One. **16**(6), e0253001 (2021)

A Conceptual Design and Control of a Novel Powered Ankle–Foot Prosthesis (RoMicP™) for Heavy Amputees

Jingjing Liu, Noor Azuan Abu Osman, Mouaz Al Kouzbary, Hamza Al Kouzbary, Nasrul Anuar Abd Razak, Hanie Nadia Shasmin, and Nooranida Arifin

Abstract A novel powered ankle–foot prosthesis (RoMicP™) is designed for heavy amputees. A novel elastic actuator, namely, a unidirectional parallel elastic actuator with series elastic element (SE+UPEA), is implemented by the employment of a harmonic reducer and a two-level cable-drive system and the application of planar torsional springs. The results of mechanical design declare that the designed structure can achieve outstanding performance on both the height of installation position and the motion range of the ankle joint. The mass of all mechanical components can meet the requirements of design. A double-loop impedance control system is developed with two constant parameters and two time-varying parameters. With optimal parameters of parallel and series springs and tuned parameters of the control system, RoMicP™ is verified by simulation under different loads. The simulation results show that the performance is remarkable in tracking the ankle position reference with small errors during walking on level ground, where the torque load on the ankle is equivalent to that of an amputee whose weight is 100 kg.

Keywords Powered ankle–foot prosthesis · Mechanical design · Control system

1 Introduction

Being one of the most straightforward ways to recover functional mobility, wearing an ankle–foot prosthesis is accepted by increasing below-knee amputees. Obviously, compared to passive or semi-active prostheses, powered ankle–foot prosthesis, which can provide net power during the operation, has more potential to help users to return to the level of non-amputees in walking or some other activities.

J. Liu · N. A. Abu Osman (✉) · M. Al Kouzbary · H. Al Kouzbary · N. A. A. Razak · H. N. Shasmin · N. Arifin
Centre for Applied Biomechanics, Department of Biomedical Engineering, Faculty of Engineering, Universiti Malaya, 50603 Kuala Lumpur, Malaysia
e-mail: azuan@um.edu.my

J. Usman et al. (eds.), *6th Kuala Lumpur International Conference on Biomedical Engineering 2021*, IFMBE Proceedings 86,
https://doi.org/10.1007/978-3-030-90724-2_28

In the past two decades, the development of powered ankle–foot prosthesis is incredibly accelerated thanks to related technologies. According to our statistic data, there are 94 powered ankle–foot prostheses designed and developed from 2000 to 2019. More than 40% of these designs employ motorized elastic actuators [1]. However, different combination of elastic elements in motorized actuators needs to be explored to achieve a better performance of powered ankle–foot prosthesis.

In addition, the other problem that should be noticed is that most powered prostheses are designed for amputees with regular weights. Some examples are compared as follows. Users whose weight is less than 75 kg are targeted by a majority of designs, such as [2, 3]. A minority of prostheses are designed for users with a weight from 75 to 85 kg, such as [4, 5]. In this case, it is difficult for heavier amputees to select an appropriate powered ankle–foot prosthesis.

Solving the abovementioned problems, this work will introduce a novel powered ankle–foot prosthesis (RoMicP™) for heavy amputees with an available control system named double-loop impedance control. To ease understanding, the design of the mechanical structure and control system will be shown in the next section, and then the third part will report the simulation verification.

2 Conceptual Design and Control Scheme

2.1 Design of Mechanical Structure

According to our previous comparison of seven kinds of elastic actuators [6], the unidirectional parallel elastic actuator with series elastic element (SE+UPEA) is the best in optimizing the output requirement of motor mechanical power during the gait cycle of walking on level ground. Based on the concept of SE+UPEA, the virtual model of RoMicP™ and some details are shown in Fig. 1.

Figure 1a shows the overall appearance of RoMicP™. The form of double steps is adopted to reduce the vertical distance from the top of the standard pyramid adapter to the heel, which is only 149.8 mm. In addition, the motion range of RoMicP™ is large enough, up to 54° for both dorsiflexion and plantarflexion. In Fig. 1b, the cover parts and the adapter are hidden to show the transmission clearly. The transmission mechanism consists of a harmonic reducer and a two-level cable-drive system. The output pulley of the second level cable-drive system connects to the housing that works as the rack in the prosthesis with unidirectional parallel spring (UPE) and to the ankle axis with series spring (SE). Both springs are designed in the style of planar torsional spring, in which the primary curve of flexible part is based on the Archimedes helix, and Fig. 1c, d show the differences between the free end and fixed end.

The permanent magnet synchronous motor (PMSM) is Maxon, EC i-52 with a 48 V nominal voltage. The brake that can provide 0.6 Nm is selected from MIKI PULLEY Co., Ltd. The 6 mm cable is woven with ultra-high molecular weight

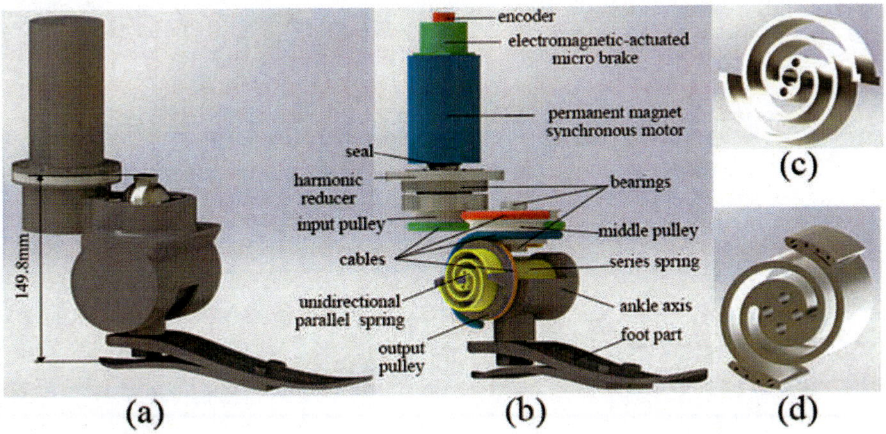

Fig. 1 Model of mechanical design of RoMicP™

polyethylene, which is a kind of material with extremely high strength. The foot part employs ÖSSUR, Flex-Symes™ without an adapter, and the adapter accords to Ottobock's product. The housing, pulleys, the coupler between the motor output shaft and the wave generator of harmonic reducer, and the ankle axis are proposed to be manufactured via the 3-dimensional print technology with a kind of high-strength material, that is, polyether ether ketone (PEEK). The total weight of the mechanical parts of RoMicP™ is 2.32 kg without battery and electrical components.

2.2 *Design of Control System*

Most current control system of powered ankle–foot prostheses are based on a finite-state machine, which works with impedance controller [7–9], admittance controller [10], or artificial neural networks [11].

In this design, a novel control system named double-loop impedance control is based on the dynamic model of SE+UPEA on the platform of Simulink (MathWorks). Excluding the complete model of PMSM in the library of Simulink, all other parts are regarded as the mechanical system and constructed in the way of differential equations.

The novel control system includes two levels. The inner level is a torque/current control for the motor, shown in Fig. 2a. The implementation of the current controller is based on two proportional–integral (PI) controllers and the space vector pulse width modulation (SVPWM) [12]. Because of the almost perfect linear relationship between electromagnetic torque and current of PMSM, the torque reference is easy to convert into the reference of q-phase stator current by dividing the torque constant from Maxon official datasheet [13].

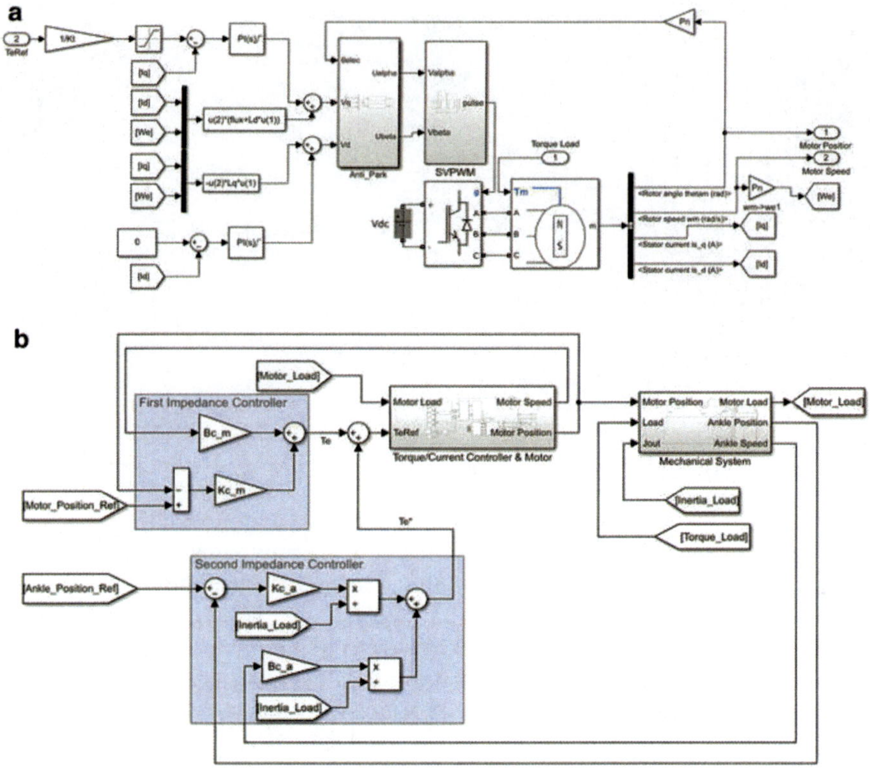

Fig. 2 Simulink model of double-loop impedance control system

The outer level of the control system is the main part of the design, shown in Fig. 2b. The traditional impedance control can be described as follows.

$$\tau = K\left(\theta_{ref} - \theta\right) + B\dot{\theta} \tag{1}$$

where K and B are the parameters to be adjusted, which mean the stiffness and damping characteristics that controlled system performs, τ is the torque command signal output by the controller, θ_{ref} is the reference of angular displacement, θ and $\dot{\theta}$ are the angular displacement and velocity feedback of controlled system, respectively.

The first impedance controller of the double-loop impedance control system is utilized to adjust the behaviour of motor output, and its parameters are termed as K_{c_m} and B_{c_m}, respectively. The angular displacement reference of the motor is obtained from a reverse solution of the dynamic model of SE+UPEA. The first controller outputs the main part of the electromagnetic torque command signal.

The second impedance controller is engaged to complete the final control of the prosthesis output after the primary control of the first one, and K_{c_a} and B_{c_a} are the parameters correspondingly. The feedback of ankle joint motion and the normal ankle position during the gait are the input parameters, and the controller will output an amendment to the output of the first controller. It is very significant to note that the parameters in the second controller are designed in a time-varying format instead of constant as usual, and the method to construct these two time-varying parameters is to make a constant divided by the dynamic inertia of the load end.

3 Simulation Verification

3.1 Simulation Conditions

Gait data from sound subjects during walking works as a significant target and conditions for simulation. The data of ankle position during walking from [14] is utilized as the reference of angular displacement output by ankle axis, shown in Fig. 3a; The dynamic inertia on ankle joint is merged from [15–17] as the inertia of the load end, shown in Fig. 3b; Including these two sets of data, the ankle torque from [14] and the dynamic stiffness and damping from [15–17] are also utilized in the calculation of the torque load on the mechanical system, and the result is from [6], shown in Fig. 3c.

Including the abovementioned biomechanical data, parameters of SE and UPE, and parameters of control system can be determined. With the specific torque load on the mechanical system, an optimal stiffness of SE can be obtained to minimize the absolute maximum of the angular velocity of the motor. Then, the target of minimizing the absolute maximum of the torque load on the motor is applied to optimize the stiffness of UPE and its equilibrium position. The optimisation process is completed by applying Response Optimizer in Simulink with a specified requirement on a signal property. For the convenience of spring design, the stiffness of both springs is required in multiples of 10 Nm/rad.

The tuning of the designed double-loop impedance control system is also based on the application of Response Optimizer, and the output signals of angular displacement

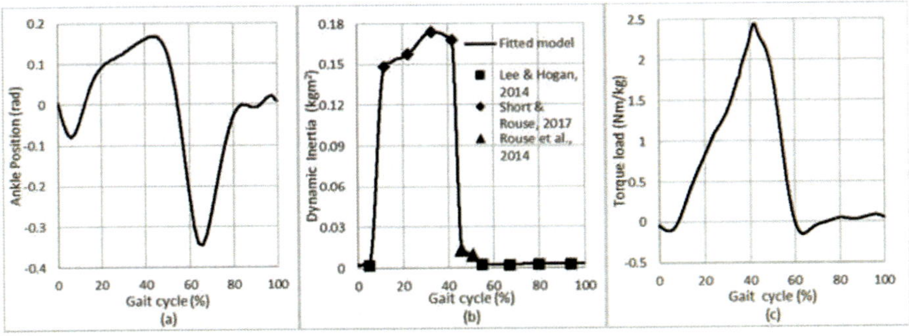

Fig. 3 Biomechanical data for simulation

are optimized in the function of Signal Tracking to minimize the Sum of the Squared Errors (SSE) compared to the corresponding reference.

The simulation period is decided as 1.13 s for one gait cycle and the fundamental sample time is 1×10^{-5} s. When the SSE is less than 11.3, which means the average error on each sample time is less than 1%, the optimal results are accepted.

3.2 *Results*

With the simulation in Simulink, it is verified that RoMicP™ can provide enough power for walking on the level ground at the speed of 1.5 m/s to subjects whose weight is up to 100 kg, with the absolute value of the q-phase current reference is limited to be less than 25 A. Under this situation, the optimized parameters of two springs and the tuned parameters of the double-loop impedance control system are listed in Table 1.

Based on the optimal parameters, all the outputs of the ankle position of RoMicP™ under all different loads tracks the reference from [14] with small errors in one walking gait cycle. Because results under different loads have tiny differences, only the output under the load of 100 kg, as an example, is shown in Fig. 4.

The principal fluctuation happens in the initial 6% of the gait cycle, where the errors are less than 0.012 rad, and the error ratios at each sample time are high (from −66.9 to 17.5%). The other fluctuation is much slighter in the period of 20–45% gait cycle. The maximum error and error ratio are less than 0.0035 rad and 3.6%, respectively. After the load peak appears at 45% of the gait cycle approximately, there is almost no error between the simulation result and the reference from the sound ankle.

Table 1 Parameters of springs and control system under different loads

Load	75 kg	80 kg	85 kg	90 kg	95 kg	100 kg
θ_0 (rad)	−0.778	−0.774	−0.774	−0.774	−0.774	−0.774
K_S (Nm/rad)	260	280	300	310	330	350
K_P (Nm/rad)	90	100	100	110	120	120
K_{c_m}	2187.906	1964.344	2520.375	963.813	631.625	12,651.125
B_{c_m}	−0.878	−0.821	−1.124	−1.181	−0.905	−16.615
K_{c_a}	0.314	0.123	0.629	0.559	7.614	0.885
B_{c_a}	−0.144	−0.129	−0.157	−0.296	−0.187	−3.128

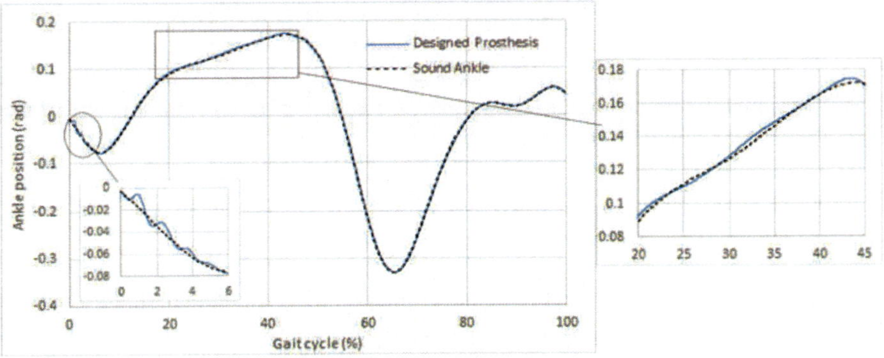

Fig. 4 Simulation output of RoMicP™ under the load of 100 kg

4 Discussion

On the aspect of the mechanical design of RoMicP™, the features of the installation height and motion range are outstanding compared to previous prostheses. The former benefits from the design of the double-step form. The latter is achieved by employing rotary transmissions in the design, instead of translational ones, such as lead screw applied in [2, 3], so the motion range is expanded to a large extent. Both the harmonic reducer and the cable-drive mechanism are the lightest compared to other kinds of transmission with the same reduction ratio and the same mechanical strength. In this case, although the mass of mechanical components without battery and electric components is still as much as 2.32 kg, for users whose weight is 100 kg, the mass is less than 2.5% of the user's weight, which is available. The planar torsional springs, which can be manufactured via laser cutting easily, guarantees the implementation of the novel elastic actuator, SE+UPEA. Because of the preload of UPE, the motor needs to hold its position with the consumption of electric energy. Therefore, an electromagnetic-actuated micro brake is installed to reduce the total amount of current during the standby time.

On the aspect of the control system, the double-loop impedance control system is a significant development of the traditional impedance control algorithm. When the traditional one is applied to operate a powered ankle–foot prosthesis, it usually needs to divide the whole gait cycle into five different stages, and in each stage, two parameters need to be tuned [18]. However, without needing the detection of gait stage, there are only four parameters in the double-loop impedance control system, which is also convenient to complete the fuzzification of the novel control system, such as the process to a genetic algorithm-based control system [19]. In addition, the transformation of two outer-loop parameters from constants into the time-varying format also improves the performance of the control system in dealing with the problem that the inertia from the human body during walking changes periodically.

On the aspect of parameters optimization, it can be found that the optimal stiffness of series spring increases significantly with the augment of the torque load on the ankle, however, the counterpart of UPE is not obvious. For the four tuned parameters of control system, the results reported in this work are only a possibility, neither the best ones nor the unique ones. Because of the randomness of initial values, there is no obvious pattern among parameters. However, it is worth noting that the absolute values of two outer-loop parameters under different loads are small, and it demonstrates that the final performance of compliance of the system is outstanding, which contributes to protecting the users and the prosthesis itself in an unknown environment.

Finally, it infers that the appearance of the apparent fluctuation at the beginning of the gait cycle is caused by the instability of the PMSM launched from a state of rest, therefore, it will be improved in consecutive gaits. However, because of the imperfection of the data from [14], that is, the values of ankle position at 0% and 100% gait cycle are not consistent, it is impossible to simulate more periods to complete further verification without a more accurate set of data.

5 Conclusion

A novel powered ankle–foot prosthesis (RoMicP™) for heavy amputees is designed, employing a novel elastic actuator—SE+UPEA. The transmission includes a harmonic reducer and a two-level cable-drive mechanism. A double-loop impedance control system is designed and tuned to complete the operation of the designed prosthesis. The simulation verifies the performance of the SE+UPEA with the control system can track the reference data very well under loads up to 100 kg, although there are still few errors.

In future work, more accurate biomechanical data of walking in various terrain will be collected as the reference for further bench-top and clinical experiments to verify the design of mechanical structure and control system.

References

1. Liu, J., Abu Osman, N.A., Al Kouzbary, M., Al Kouzbary, H., Abd Razak, N.A., Shasmin, H.N., Arifin, N.: Classification and comparison of mechanical design of powered ankle–foot prostheses for transtibial amputees developed in the 21st century: a systematic review. J. Med. Dev. **15**(1), 010801 (2021)
2. Eilenberg, M.F., Geyer, H., Herr, H.: Control of a powered ankle–foot prosthesis based on a neuromuscular model. IEEE Trans. Neural Syst. Rehabil. Eng. **18**(2), 164–173 (2010)
3. Agboola-Dobson, A., Wei, G., Ren, L.: Biologically inspired design and development of a variable stiffness powered ankle-foot prosthesis. J. Mech. Robot. **11**(4), 041012 (2019)
4. Bartlett, H.L., Lawson, B.E., Goldfarb, M.: Design, control, and preliminary assessment of a multifunctional semipowered ankle prosthesis. IEEE/ASME Trans. Mechatron. **24**(4), 1532–1540 (2019)
5. Jimenez-Fabian, R., Flynn, L., Geeroms, J., Vitiello, N., Vanderborght, B., Lefeber, D.: Sliding-bar MACCEPA for a powered ankle prosthesis. J. Mech. Robot. **7**(4), 041011 (2015)

6. Liu, J., Abu Osman, N.A., Al Kouzbary, M., Al Kouzbary, H., Abd Razak, N.A., Shasmin, H.N., Arifin, N.: Optimization and comparison of typical elastic actuators in powered ankle-foot prosthesis. Int. J. Control, Autom. Syst. (Accepted)
7. Zhu, J., Wang, Q., Wang, L.: On the design of a powered transtibial prosthesis with stiffness adaptable ankle and toe joints. IEEE Trans. Industr. Electron. **61**(9), 4797–4807 (2014)
8. Yuan, K., Wang, Q., Zhu, J., Wang, L.: A hierarchical control scheme for smooth transitions between level ground and ramps with a robotic transtibial prosthesis. IFAC Proc. **47**(3), 3527–3532 (2014)
9. Gao, F., Liu, Y., Liao, W.H.: Implementation and testing of ankle-foot prosthesis with a new compensated controller. IEEE/ASME Trans. Mechatron. **24**(4), 1775–1784 (2019)
10. Ficanha, E.M., Rastgaar, M., Kaufman, K.R.: Control of a 2-DOF powered ankle-foot mechanism. In: 2015 IEEE International Conference on Robotics and Automation (ICRA), pp. 6439–6444 (2015)
11. Mai, A., Commuri, S.: Intelligent control of a prosthetic ankle joint using gait recognition. Control. Eng. Pract. **49**, 1–13 (2016)
12. Yuan, L., Hu, B., Wei, K. and Chen, S.: Control principle of modern permanent magnet synchronous motor and simulation in MATLAB. Beihang University Press, Beijing, China (2016)
13. EC-i 52 Datasheet. https://www.maxongroup.com/medias/sys_master/root/8882560892958/EN-21-281.pdf
14. Winter, D.A.: Biomechanics and Motor Control of Human Gait: Normal, Elderly and Pathological. University of Waterloo Press, Waterloo, Canada (1991)
15. Rouse, E.J., Hargrove, L.J., Perreault, E.J., Kuiken, T.A.: Estimation of human ankle impedance during the stance phase of walking. IEEE Trans. Neural Syst. Rehabil. Eng. **22**(4), 870–878 (2014)
16. Shorter, A.L., Rouse, E.J.: Mechanical impedance of the ankle during the terminal stance phase of walking. IEEE Trans. Neural Syst. Rehabil. Eng. **26**(1), 135–143 (2017)
17. Lee, H., Hogan, N.: Time-varying ankle mechanical impedance during human locomotion. IEEE Trans. Neural Syst. Rehabil. Eng. **23**(5), 755–764 (2014)
18. Al Kouzbary, M., Abu Osman, N.A., Abdul Wahab, A.K.: Sensorless control system for assistive robotic ankle-foot. Int. J. Adv. Rob. Syst. **15**(3), 1729881418775854 (2018)
19. Al Kouzbary, M., Abu Osman, N.A., Al Kouzbary, H., Shasmin, H.N., Arifin, N.: Towards universal control system for powered ankle-foot prosthesis: a simulation study. Int. J. Fuzzy Syst. **22**(4), 1299–1313 (2020)

The Treatment Impact of Partial Body Weight Supported Treadmill (PBWST) on Cerebral Palsy Kid Using Physio-Treadmill (*PhyMill*): A Case Study

Rabiatul Aisyah Ariffin, Mohd Azrul Hisham Mohd Adib, Nurul Shahida Mohd Shalahim, Narimah Daud, and Nur Hazreen Mohd Husni

Abstract Cerebral Palsy (CP) prevalence has remained stable in the global population over the last few years. This case study aims to examine the impact of the Partial Body Weight Supported Treadmill (PBWST) on gait control in kids with cerebral palsy. Kids with CP completed a gait training protocol two-session between two weeks' intervals. Outcome measures included a Berg balancing scale, Dynamic gait index, Katz index of independence in activities of daily living, and several steps. The individual results indicated there were improvements in balance, dynamic gait, and step count. After the second session, the number of steps improved. The step length of the second session is better. There were more active movements during the second session. Additional research is needed to determine the treatment parameters and the long-term effects of PBWST on gait performance in CP children.

Keywords Cerebral palsy · Treadmill training · Rehabilitation · Gait · *PhyMill*

R. A. Ariffin (✉) · M. A. H. M. Adib (✉)
Medical Engineering and Health Intervention Team (MedEHiT), Department of Mechanical Engineering, College of Engineering, Universiti Malaysia Pahang, Lebuhraya Tun Abdul Razak, 26300 Kuantan, Pahang, Malaysia
e-mail: azrul@ump.edu.my

N. S. M. Shalahim
Department of Industrial Engineering, College of Engineering, Universiti Malaysia Pahang, Lebuhraya Tun Abdul Razak, 26300 Kuantan, Pahang, Malaysia

N. Daud
Kuantan Physical Therapy, Physiotherapy Center, Lot B1.10, Ground Floor, Block B, Bangunan Al-Tabari, IM 7/3, Bandar Indera Mahkota 7, 25582 Kuantan, Pahang, Malaysia

N. H. M. Husni
Family Health Unit, Pahang State Health Department, Jalan IM 4, Bandar Indera Mahkota, 25582 Kuantan, Pahang, Malaysia

J. Usman et al. (eds.), *6th Kuala Lumpur International Conference on Biomedical Engineering 2021*, IFMBE Proceedings 86,
https://doi.org/10.1007/978-3-030-90724-2_29

1 Introduction

Cerebral palsy (CP) is referred to as a group of neurological disorders that begin in infancy or early childhood and impair body movement and muscle coordination permanently [1–6]. CP is commonly classified into four types: spastic, dyskinetic, ataxic, and mixed. The most difficult challenge for children with cerebral palsy is a lack of coordination, interaction, manipulation, balance, and understanding. Since there is no known cure, the goal of treatment is to help patients to be as much as possible to be the only way to help with their personal development. Evidence shows that appropriate rehabilitation can benefit them in improving motor impairment and improving quality of life. In the rehabilitation of children with CP, repetitive exercise is an important factor.

Partial body weight supported treadmill (PBWST) has expanded its wing for rehabilitation purposes. As a rehabilitation assistance tool, there is an increasing interest in the treadmill. PBWST is thought to promise better experience to motor skills for CP children. PBWST allows the kids to use guidance from the therapist as well as the surface to vary differently and feel the effects of this variability [7]. For example, a child will take smaller steps and expect a real fall, but in a controlled environment. In the adaptation stage of locomotion, the child can choose to increase the step length and take advantage of more effective torque generation to contribute to overall performance. Therapists can increase demand for and use certain muscles by changing speed and inclination. Physiotherapy-Treadmill (*PhyMill*) is one of the areas in PBWST which assists to improve gait performance [8–10]. PBWST has been reported to be a benefit to task-oriented exercise, allowing patients to perform a high number of repetitions with an almost null risk of falling while improving balance, gait, and symmetry in people who have suffered a stroke, spinal cord injury, or traumatic brain injury.

Previous studies have shown that PBWST improves gait function in people with stroke or the backbone, but there is no application and effectiveness of PBWST in children with CP. These case studies were intended to investigate the effect of PBWST in children with CP on gait function.

2 Materials and Methods

This was an unregulated open-label pretest–posttest experimental. It started with a series of assessments, then a PBWST procedure, and finally another series of assessments at the end of the treatment. The participant received written consent.

Table 1 Personal characteristics

Characteristics	Participant
Gender	Male
Age	6
Height (cm)	100
Weight (kg)	14
BMI (kg/m^2)	14

Note BMI: body mass index

2.1 Participant

Participant across the study was diagnosed with CP. An individual with ambulatory movement disorders from a local physical therapy center was invited to participate. The individual characteristics of the participants are summarised in Table 1.

2.2 Intervention Procedures

The study was performed at the rehabilitation center 'Kuantan Physical Therapy—Physiotherapy Centre' at Kuantan, Pahang. During the first visit, the *PhyMill* product was adjusted to the participant's characteristics, and participants practiced a selection of the experimental conditions to determine whether they could be included in the study.

Firstly, all participants underwent four types of assessment. After the assessment was complete, the PBWST protocol was performed by participants. At this stage, the interaction between a child and *PhyMill* will be supervised by a Physiotherapist (PT) and/or clinician. They will observe the type of interaction shown by the children. Each training session lasts for 30 min per session. The session will be repeated once every 2 weeks interval. After the PBWST training protocol has been completed, the children will undergo an exit assessment. Again, the children need to complete the Berg balancing scale (BBS), Dynamic Gait Index (DGI), Katz index of independence in activities of daily living (Katz ADL), and step count conducted by physiotherapy and/or clinician as shown in Fig. 1. The final assessment results will be used to compare pre-test and post-test interaction between product and CP children. Figure 2 shows the *PhyMill* product which can lift to 30 kg [11]. The participant was connected to the harness equipment, which was fixed to the *PhyMill* product through a series of

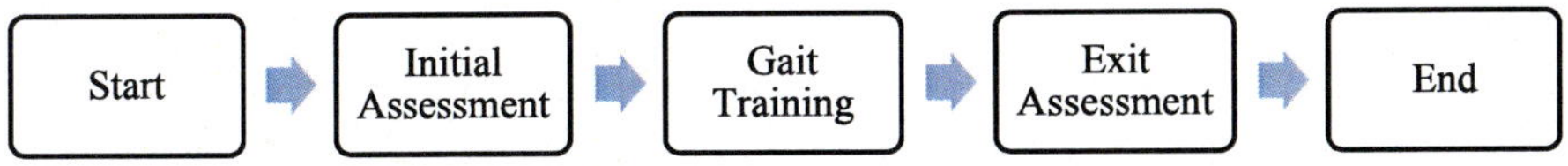

Fig. 1 Experimental flowchart

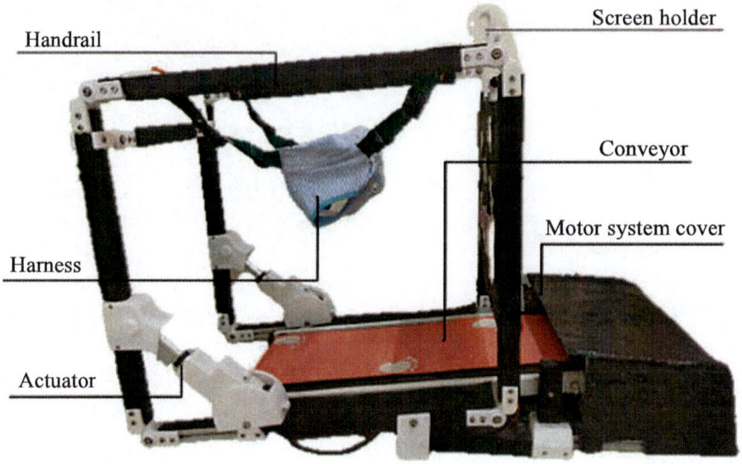

Fig. 2 *PhyMill* product

straps and fittings. The harness was firmly positioned around the participant's lower trunk, which enabled the hip to bend and stretch as shown in Fig. 3.

The treadmill walking training sessions lasted about 30 min. For the first training session, the treadmill was set at a low pace so that the child will demonstrate proper skill during the adaptation phase to sustain an upright lower limb posture, ankle push-off, and toe clearance. The treadmill speed was progressively increased in each session to increase the number of steps practiced by the child. The gradual speed changes, on the other hand, were determined by the child's capacity to control their movement patterns.

2.3 Outcome Measures

In terms of balance and gait, functional capability and quality of life were assessed. The balance was evaluated with the Berg balancing scale (BBS) which offers clinicians a standardized tool for measuring balance among individuals ranging between 0 and 56 [12]. The greater the BBS score, the better the postural stability. A score of 56 points to a balance of functions. Muir et al. [13] suggested that a score of less than 45 shows that people are at a higher risk of falling. The same criterion has been used here. The Dynamic Gait Index (DGI) evaluated participants' capability to respond to demands on the walk, with values from 0 (high risk of fall) to 24 (low risk of fall) [14]. Scores equivalent to or smaller than 19 are linked to a higher risk of falling. The Katz index of independence in activities of daily living (Katz ADL) has been used to evaluate the quality of life, an instrument that measures the capacity

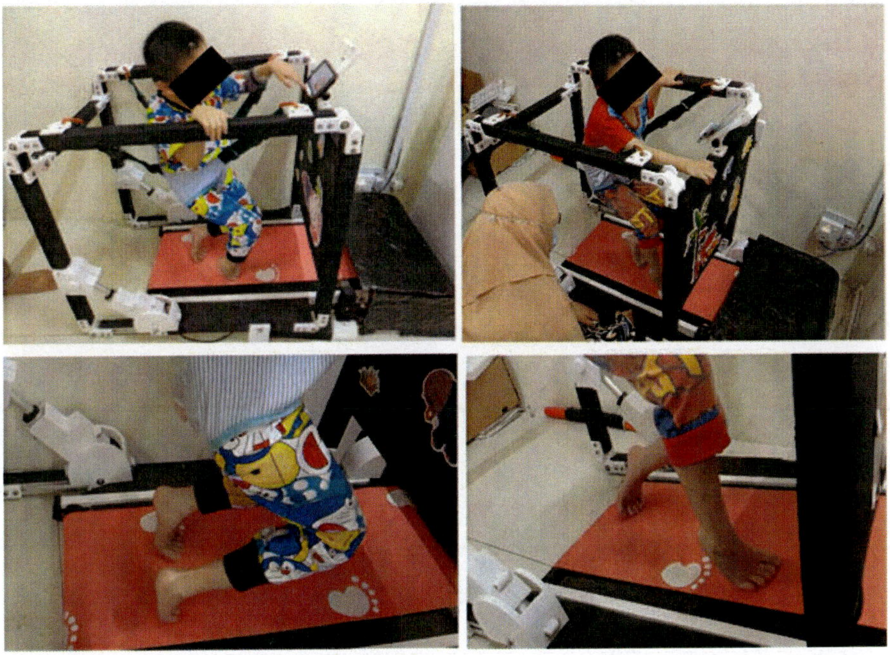

Fig. 3 Participant during the gait training using *PhyMill*

of a person to carry out daily life activities independently from 6 (independent) to 0 (very dependent) [15]. The number of steps was counted by video recorded using a camera. After the study process is completed, the captured video will be analyzed.

3 Results

Table 2 displays the findings for the various outcome variables.

The chart in Fig. 4 illustrates the outcome measure for BBS in both sessions. The colored lines represent different sessions. Blue indicates the first session while red

Table 2 Measures of the outcome before and after the balance dynamic training stage

Session	BBS		% Change	DGI		% Change	Step count (step/min)	% Change
	Pre	Post		Pre	Post			
1	5	5	0	1	1	0	10	23
2	5	6	17	1	2	50	13	

Comments % Change step count (reported as change between sessions). *Abbreviations* BBS = Berg balance scale; DGI = Dynamic gait index

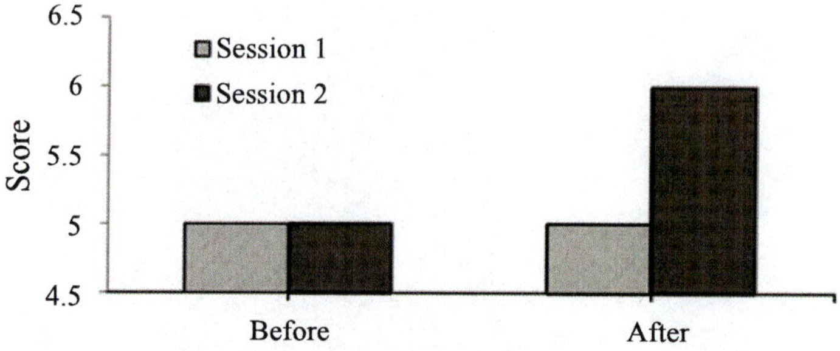

Fig. 4 The outcome measure for the berg balance scale

indicates the second session. The gradual increase in mentions of BBS score for the second session means reduced risk of fall. The first session stays at the same level with a score of 5. While the percentage of change during the second session is 17%.

The gait training also affected postural demands during the walk, as seen in the DGI results as shown in Fig. 5 compared to before the intervention. The percentage of changes during the second session is 50%. Even though, the score is still less than 19 which participants are predicted to fall.

The bar chart illustrates the number of steps during the walking treatment for initial and exit sessions. It can be seen that the number of steps counted on the first and second sessions are 10 and 13 steps, respectively. Overall, we can see a clear upward trend of steps counted (see Fig. 6). The percentage of changes is 23% which is a huge improvement. The number of steps increases influence by repetitive movement during participant on gait training using *PhyMill*. It helps to keep track

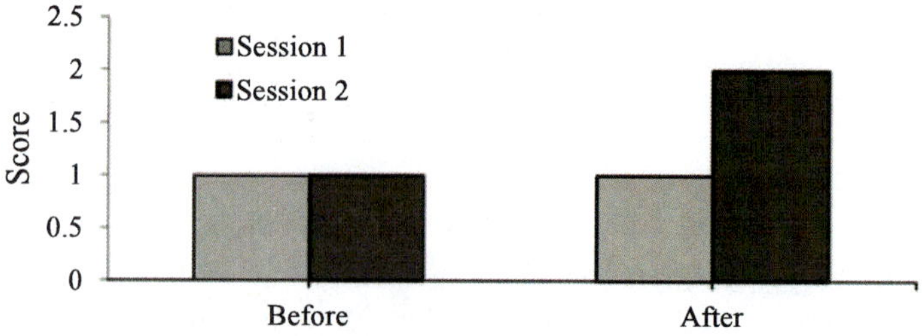

Fig. 5 The outcome measure for the dynamic gait index

Fig. 6 The outcome measures the number of steps

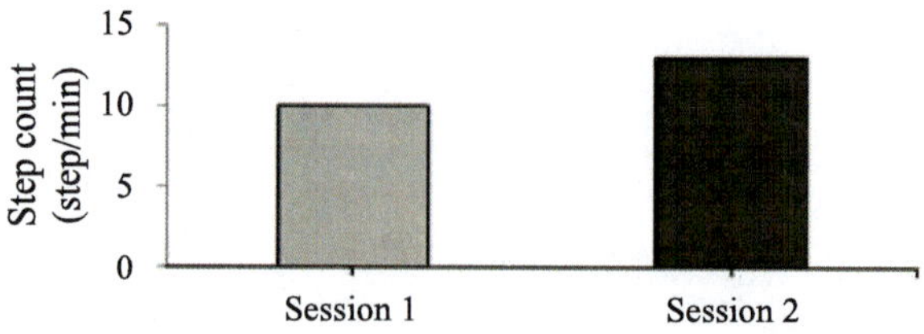

of strength. While Katz ADL results showed no improvements after the procedure, perhaps because it is still in the early stage of intervention.

4 Discussion

This study supports the growing clinical interest in using treadmills in CP rehabilitation by indicating that treadmill retraining of gait can improve functional mobility as well as gait and that these improvements may be aided by the utilization of partial body weight supported treadmill. From the results, the number of steps improved after the second session. The stride and step length are better in the second session. During the second session, there was more interactive movement. Participants are likely to be familiar with *PhyMill*.

There is evidence that *PhyMill* has a beneficial impact on children with cerebral palsy. The reviewed studies that used *PhyMill* to examine the possible use of *PhyMill* for children with CP are few and have not been thoroughly explored. Most previous studies employed a small sample size focused on a single exposure, or were theoretical [16]. The size of the sample was small because limited availability of respondents (with specific criteria) and time constraints to complete the study. To fully realize this opportunity, engineers and clinicians must actively participate in the transfer of expertise and progress from the technological arena to medical situations. Researchers must determine the number of subjects and evaluate the range of impairment in the sample of children with CP.

However, the majority of the studies mentioned here have the potential for clinical application. Since it can combine all criteria of conventional walking therapy in one customize therapeutic tool of physiotherapy treadmill. However, future research and wider trials are needed to optimize this therapeutic utility for children with CP.

5 Conclusion

Results indicate that the two sessions of physical therapy interventions have had good results in motor control and walking skills improvement. More study is needed with the use of higher-level architecture, increased numbers, and relevant results in particular populations to both validate the efficacy and explain training schedules. The beneficial effects of PBWST in children with CP were shown in these case studies. Further research is required into the parameters of treatment and the long-term effects of PBWST on the function of gait in CP children.

Acknowledgements A big thank you dedicated to MOHE under grant FRGS/1/2021/TK0/UMP/02/25. Also to University Malaysia Pahang (UMP) under grant RDU210332 and PGRS2003199 and Medical Engineering and Health Intervention Team

(MedEHiT) are gratefully acknowledged for providing us with a good environment and facilities to complete these research activities.

References

1. Stuberg, W.A.: Considerations related to weight-bearing programs in children with developmental disabilities. Phys. Ther. **72**(1), 35–40 (1992). https://doi.org/10.1093/ptj/72.1.35
2. Body-Weight-Supported Treadmill Training: Using Evidence to Guide Physical Therapy Intervention Definition. [Online]. Available: www.hocoma.ch/en/
3. Buchwald, J., Graciana, O., Hayes, K., Thomsen, C.: Pediatric Body-Weight Supported Treadmill Training
4. Ross, S.M., Macdonald, M., Bigouette, J.P.: Effects of strength training on mobility in adults with cerebral palsy: a systematic review. Disabil. Health J. **9**(3), 375–384 (2016). https://doi.org/10.1016/j.dhjo.2016.04.005
5. Ismail, I.: "Physiotherapy Management For Cerebral Palsy—PORTAL MyHEALTH. http://www.myhealth.gov.my/en/physiotherapy-management-cerebral-palsy/
6. Ameer, M.A., Fayez, E.S., Elkholy, H.H.: Improving spatiotemporal gait parameters in spastic diplegic children using treadmill gait training. J. Bodyw. Mov. Ther. **23**(4), 937–942 (2019). https://doi.org/10.1016/j.jbmt.2019.02.003
7. Lowe, L., McMillan, A.G., Yates, C.: Body weight support treadmill training for children with developmental delay who are ambulatory. Pediatr. Phys. Ther. **27**(4), 386–394 (2015). https://doi.org/10.1097/PEP.0000000000000172
8. Ariffin, R.A., Azrul, M., Mohd, H., Mohd, N.S.: Ergonomics Study on Visual Contribution of Postural Stability Using Physio-Treadmill (*PhyMill*) for Kid with Cerebral Palsy, pp. 1–12.
9. Ariffin, R.A., Adib, M.A.H.M., Shalahim, N.S.M., Daud, N., Hasni, N.H.M.: An ergonomic perspective of user need on physio-treadmill (PhyMill) criteria: knowledge and awareness of cerebral palsy among future parents. J. Phys. Conf. Ser. **1529**(5) (2020). https://doi.org/10.1088/1742-6596/1529/5/052071
10. Ariffin, R.A., Hisham Mohd Adib, M.A., Mohd Shalahim, N.S., Daud, N., Mohd Hasni, N.H.: Physio-treadmill (PhyMill): ergonomics evaluation of posture impact on kids with cerebral palsy using digital human modeling (DHM) simulation. In: 2020 IEEE-EMBS Conference on Biomedical Engineering and Sciences (IECBES), pp. 1–6, 2021. https://doi.org/10.1109/IECBES48179.2021.9398764
11. Azrul, M., Mohd, H., Arifin, R.A., Abdul, M.H.: Development of Physiotherapy-Treadmill (*PhyMill*) as Rehabilitation Technology Tools for Kid with Cerebral Palsy, pp. 1–10
12. Berg, K., Wood-Dauphine, S.L., Wiliams, J.L.: Berg Balance Tests and Rating Scale, pp. 2–5 (1992) [Online]. Available: http://www.chiropractic.on.ca/wp-content/uploads/fp-berg-balance-scale.pdf
13. Muir, S.W., Berg, K., Chesworth, B., Speechley, M.: Use of the berg balance scale for predicting multiple falls in community-dwelling elderly people: a prospective study. Phys. Ther. **88**(4), 449–459 (2008). https://doi.org/10.2522/ptj.20070251
14. Dynamic Gait Index
15. Wallace, M.: Katz index of independence in activities of daily living (ADL). Accessed 29 April, 2021. [Online]. Available: www.ConsultGeriRN.org
16. Malik, N.A., Hanapiah, F.A., Rahman, R.A.A., Yussof, H.: Emergence of socially assistive robotics in rehabilitation for children with cerebral palsy: a review. Int. J. Adv. Robot. Syst. **13**(3) (2016). https://doi.org/10.5772/64163

Design and Testing of an Interim Transtibial Prosthetic Leg for Amputees Living in Rural Areas: A Case Study

Nur Azah Hamzaid, Mohamad Hasmizan Halim, and Chung Tze Yang

Abstract An interim prosthesis is proposed to be used by amputees living in rural environment in situations where the amputee is in between prescribed prosthesis by an endorsed organization. The design and development of using the Polyvinyl Chloride (PVC) pipe as socket, bamboo to replace the common aluminum pylon and hand-crafted foot prostheses for people living in the rural area was performed and its performance were tested. Corn starch flour were used inside the socket to provide pressure distribution and cushioning effect in place of silicon gel. Tensile test on bamboo specimens revealed that the bamboo with tape could hold higher flexural load than bamboo without tape, and approximately 6 kN higher in the compression test. An amputee from a rural village performed gait testing with the interim prosthesis. The gait test revealed that despite the high strength of the bamboo pylon and the wooden foot, the breaking point of the prosthesis during gait was at the adapted which connected the socket and the pylon. Better load bearing adapter materials should be considered for the interim prosthesis, and further investigation is required in the actual rural setting to determine whether the prosthesis is appropriate for a rural patient to use.

Keywords Amputee · Prosthesis · Rural · Lower limb · Gait

N. A. Hamzaid (✉) · M. H. Halim
Biomechatronics and Neuroprosthetics Laboratory, Department of Biomedical Engineering, Faculty of Engineering, Universiti Malaya, 50603 Kuala Lumpur, Malaysia
e-mail: azah.hamzaid@um.edu.my

C. T. Yang
Department of Rehabilitation Medicine, Faculty of Medicine, Universiti Malaya, 50603 Kuala Lumpur, Malaysia

M. H. Halim
Return to Work Unit, Malaysia Social Security Organisation (SOCSO), 50538 Kuala Lumpur, Malaysia

J. Usman et al. (eds.), *6th Kuala Lumpur International Conference on Biomedical Engineering 2021*, IFMBE Proceedings 86,
https://doi.org/10.1007/978-3-030-90724-2_30

1 Introduction

1.1 An Interim Prosthesis: A Potential Solution for Amputees Living in Rural Areas

Rural area are the area where the community live outside the urban area in which access to affordable prosthesis care, services and maintenance are limited. In an effort to clearly define it, researchers in South Africa [1] came to the assumption that there is no definite definition of 'rural'. A person who underwent amputation are always confronted with low confidence level. This is due to the loss of their ability to walk as normal people. For some of them, their mental health might be affected as they might set their mind as themselves being 'useless' after their leg was amputated. One of the most important factor of prosthesis use is their confidence in balance, which has been reported to be a better predictor of an individual's engagement in physical, daily, and social activities than actual measures of physical performance among lower limb amputees [2]. These effects can be greater among amputees living in rural areas as they are faced with rough terrain and uneven surfaces even more than amputees living in urban or semi-urban areas on a daily basis. They may also have difficulties in maintaining their prosthesis as they do not have enough access to general utility. Therefore, it is important to provide reasonable options for them to gain back their confidence in using a prosthesis device, with the ability for them to care and mend for it themselves when required.

For a whole basic prosthesis, the cost is estimated to be in the thousands [3, 4]. That high price is why some patients in the rural cannot afford them, particularly if they do not have access to relevant social security coverage. The price of a prostheses is very expensive because the materials and components was imported from foreign country. In addition, the limited transportation ability to move about from rural to urban areas may add to reasons of why rural amputees may not be using a prosthetic leg. This study identified this issue and proposed an interim prosthesis made from affordable and materials that could be sources from rural areas to be used. Amputees living in rural areas could use and self-care for this temporary prosthesis in between access to a certified provision prosthetic leg. In specific, this study designed a combination of a complete device build from assembling components of a prosthetic leg which are socket, liner, adapter, shank and also the foot. Those components are crucial to a below knee prosthesis device to make them able to walk again and undergo their routine life.

2 Methodology

2.1 Designing and Manufacturing of the Prosthesis

The main considerations for the development of the new interim prostheses are (i) comfort, (ii) cost, (iii) weight, (iv) safety, and (v) other limitations. Few design sketches were made and one was chosen to be drawn in Fusion360 [5] part by part. Suitable materials that are easily available in rural areas were identified to manufacture the interim prosthesis (Fig. 1). Bamboo material was chosen for the Pylon. The bamboo was left at room temperature for about 3 months until its green colour turned to brownish yellow, indicating it has fully dried up. We ensured that the bamboo had no cracks at all. The diameter of bamboo was chosen nearly about the diameter of aluminium pylon tube.

For the socket, PVC water pipe was selected. This was based on its ability to withstand high temperature of up to 90 °C. For the foot, wooden craft was identified as the best option. A few rectangular wooden blocks was cut from a tree trunk. Strong wood was selected as it cannot easily rust at room temperature. A white PVC was used as tube adapter and screwed onto the wood in the socket and passed through the grey PVC. A few modifications were made to the foot design considering its ability to hold high force.

For the bamboo, cloth tape was used to wrap around it in order to increase the strength of bamboo when force is applied onto it. It also serves to bind the structure of fibre in the bamboo for it to not easily break. Steel bar was added to reinforce the pylon thus preventing it from breaking easily. For the socket liner, the use of pelite was replaced by corn flour mixture which behaves as a force distributor inside the socket [6].

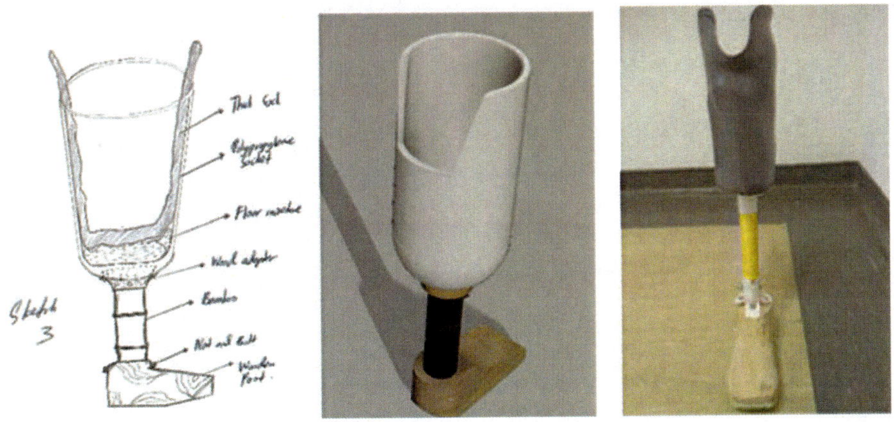

Fig. 1 Design sketch of the interim prosthesis (left), 3D drawing (middle) and completed prototype (right)

2.2 Material Strength Test

Three types of pylon materials; i.e. raw bamboo, taped bamboo and common aluminium pylon tube, were tested for their compressive strength. The Instron was set to operate at 1 mm/min for the rate of compressive extension with 700 N compression load. Flexural test were conducted to determine the strength of pylon from the side. The rate of extension applied during the test was 30 mm/min with 700 N flexural load. The specimens' material dimensions such as thickness, length and diameter were keyed into the Bluehill software prior to the analysis which also calculated and recorded the output data throughout the test directly.

2.3 Participants

The first study participant was an amputee from a village in Jitra, Kedah, Malaysia (male, 69 years old, 173 cm height, 63 kg weight). He was 3 years left leg post amputation due to diabetes mellitus. He has been using a below knee prosthesis for about 2 years, however, has stopped using it to walk 7 months prior to the study. His level of ambulation was limited to K2, with walking frame. His skin of his sound leg was dry, while his residual limb was slightly flabby with pain at the stump end (Fig. 2).

The second participant was also a below knee amputee with 2 year post amputation (male, 60 years old, 176 cm height, 63 kg weight) who lives in a palm oil plantation area in Tanjung Karang, Selangor, Malaysia. The cause of his amputation is diabetes mellitus and he used a prosthesis leg for about 4 months provided by Selangor Zakat Board. For the experimental trial session, only the second amputee was able to participate and thus the new interim prostheses prototype was custom made only for him.

2.4 Pre-testing Evaluation

Upon completing the development of the interim transtibial prosthesis (Fig. 1), the device was tested on amputee subject. Before testing, the researchers had some discussion with the amputee while assessing his history and also condition on the current prosthesis that he was currently wearing. With the current health condition of the patient, he could walk with his current prosthesis but not for a long time. His endurance and stamina during wearing the proper prosthesis is roughly for 30 min. The researchers explained to the amputee about the final interim prosthesis he was going to use in the trial was made from some materials which are steel, bamboo, pipe and wood. The amputee provided his written consent to participate.

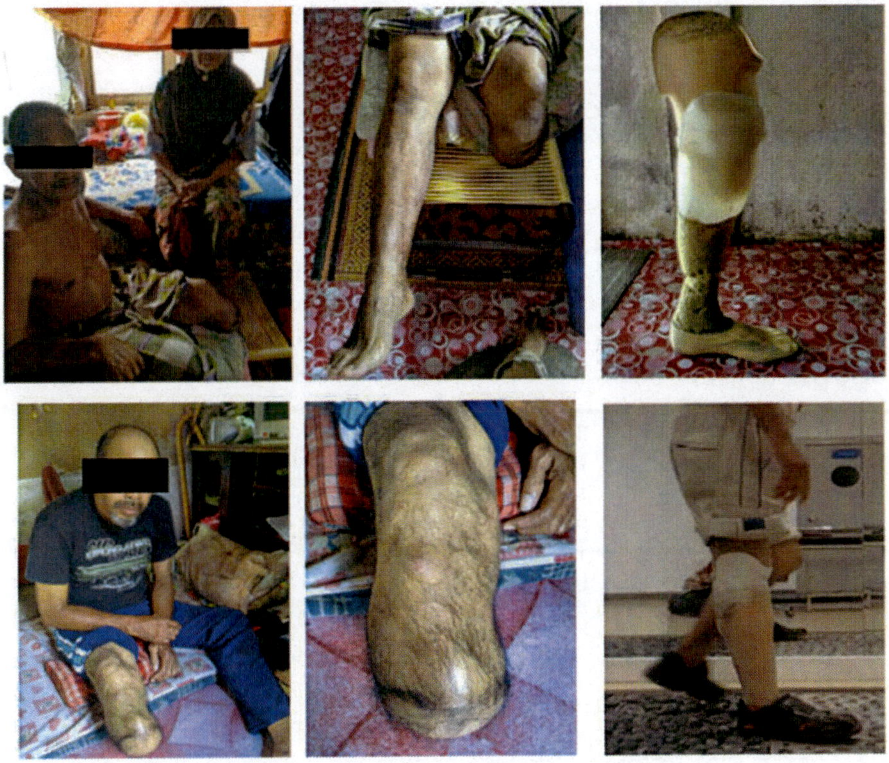

Fig. 2 First amputee participant (top) and second amputee participant (bottom)

During this discussion, the main discussion revolves around the part where the socket and the bamboo was attached i.e. the adapter. The adapter was white color surface which was made from Polyvinylchloride (PVC) pipe that is commonly used in the water piping system. The concern was because, during the production of the adapter, it needed go through heating process to take shape. If the heat is too much for this adapter, it would be fragile and may break when patient put weight onto the device.

2.5 *Gait Trial*

Gait performance tests conducted were the timed up and go test and 3 min-walk test using his current prosthesis. The amputee was requested to perform all tests with his own prosthesis as well as the interim prosthesis made for him. The subject also performed a short gait test with parallel bars using the interim prosthesis.

Table 1 Characteristics of potential pylon material

	Bamboo	Taped bamboo	Aluminum
Compressive load (N)	14,919.32	21,312.96	42,701.83
Compressive stress (N/m^2)	23.06	29.44	60.24
Compressive Young's Modulus (MPa)	217.45	410.02	21,025.55
Maximum flexure load (N)	2909.54	4561.56	7196.97
Maximum flexure stress (MPa)	29.85	41.48	88.25
Flexion Young's Modulus (GPa)	1.35	1.65	4.87

Table 2 Characteristics of potential socket material

	Polypropylene (PP)	Polyvinyl Chloride (PVC)
Tensile stress at break (MPa)	18.64	16.76
Elongation at break (%)	~224	~200
Tensile stress at break (MPa)	18.64	16.76

3 Results

3.1 *Material Strength Test Outcome*

Tables 1 and 2 shows the characteristics of pylon and socket tested materials. Taped bamboo was chosen as the final pylon material and PVC was selected as the final socket material based on its acceptable strength and ease of access.

3.2 *Amputee's Walking Performance with Existing Prosthesis*

For the set up in this test, a 3-m length was measured and was marked for the patient. A chair was provided. The time taken for the patient to complete this test will determine the fall risk that may happen. The time was separated into two type which high risk where the time taken to complete were 13.5 s above and the other risk was *none/low/moderate* where it was considered within 13.5 s and below. However, in this test, the amputee took 14.5 s to complete the test which means, he was at high risk of falling using this current prosthesis.

For the 3-min' walk test, the amputee was requested to walk around for 3 min. The covered distance was measured roughly after the test. A normal healthy person will walk around 1000 m per 10 min which means 300 m for 3 min. This patient wore a prosthesis device where he only can walk about roughly 91 m during the

3 min and he became very exhausted at the end of the 3 min-walk test. The amputee could not afford to undergo 6 min-walk test. This was assumed to be due to his unfit condition, his old age with less energy thus he gets tired easily. However, this patient has no problem in keeping his balance and performed well in completing the test. The K-level for this patient was improved from K2 to K3 when using his current prosthesis.

3.3 *Outcome of Gait Trial with the Interim Prosthesis*

When walking with the interim prostheses, he needed to wear at least 5 layers of socks for the test because of the shrinkage of his stump size to fit in the socket.

The walking path for the patient to walk was set up by the technician using two parallel bars. The length of the path was about 2 m with 30-degree inclined and decline slope at the start and end of the walking path respectively. The use of corn flour powder solution as liner to fill in the gap between the socket and the stump was unable to overcome the large difference in size of the socket and the stump.

At the start of the gait, the normal leg side make the first step where the heel strike phase occurs followed by loading response until the terminal stance where the single support happened when walking up the parallel bar path. Until the midstance phase of the amputated side, the device start to bend posteriorly and laterally making some angle between the socket and the 'bamboo shank'. The adapter started to break at the moment and the amputated side leg was further pushed laterally when the gait continued.

The trial revealed that the white PVC pipe which we used as the adapter, i.e. the connecting element, was fragile and could not hold the weight of the patient including the gravitational force that was applied on the handmade prosthesis. The lateral connector of the adapter broke after 2 s in midstance phase.

4 Discussion

The idea for using the white PVC as an adapter was challenged where it could not hold the force that was exerted on it. This caused the collapse during the gait. It needed reinforced support such as steel that was assembled at the posterior of the 'bamboo pylon'. Figure 3 shows the shape of PVC that was connected to the socket. The corner part of the 'adapter' was broken and could not hold the pylon that was place in the wood hole at the bottom of the socket. The attachment between the socket and pylon at breaking point during gait and the adapter after it was broken are presented in Fig. 3.

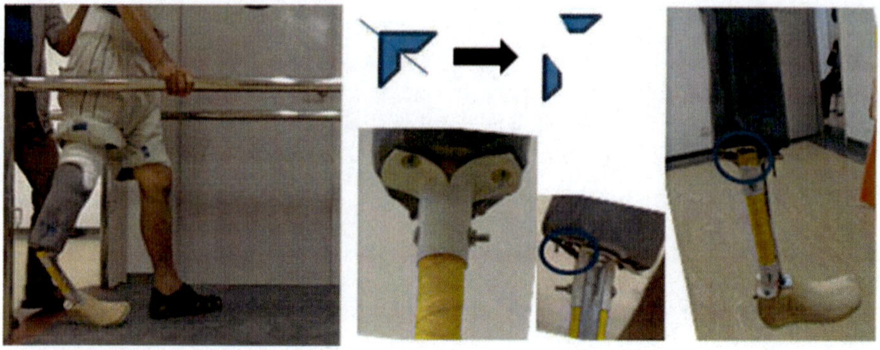

Fig. 3 Gait trial with the interim prosthesis failure point during toe-off (left). Breaking point at the connector (right)

5 Conclusion

The preliminary design of the newly developed interim prosthesis was successfully completed and trialed by a below knee amputee. However, it required further investigation to determine its full gait efficacy and long term suitability with amputees living in rural areas. In essence, a reliable interim prosthesis that is easy to care for and affordable are important for amputees living in the rural area.

Acknowledgements This work was funded by Case Writing Grant Scheme (CWGS) from the Ministry of Higher Education under grant number GA022-2016 "Prosthetic Intervention For Rural Amputees: Replacing A Limb, Regaining A Life". The authors would like to record their gratitude to The Administrator of Limbs For Life Prostheses Centre, Angeline Tan and her staffs; as well as Lazcorp Sdn. Bhd. for their assistance in providing information for analysis in this study.

References

1. Eagar, D., Versteeg-Mojanaga, M., Cooke, R.: RHAP (2014). Retrieved from rhap.org.za: http://rhap.org.za/wp-content/uploads/2014/08/RHAP_Defining_Rural_Version_1-060614-30th-June-2014.pdf
2. Miller, W.C., Speechley, M., Deathe, A.B.: Balance confidence among people. Phys. Therapy, 856–865 (2002)
3. Param.: Price of transtibial prosthesis (2016). (Halim, M.H., Interviewer)
4. Bakar, M.B.: Cost of a basic transtibial prostheses (2016). (Halim, M.H., Interviewer)
5. Yusof, N.H.B.M.: Structural design of a microcontroller based transfemoral prosthesis (2013)
6. Halim, M.H.: Design, development and experimental trials of transtibial prosthetic leg for amputees living in rural areas (2017)

Immediate Effect of Flexing the Toes During Performing Salat on Hemodynamic Status

Fatimah Ibrahim, Mas Sahidayana Mokhtar, Nur Fara Ateeka Jaafar, and Nurul Fauzani Jamaluddin

Abstract *Salat* is a routine for Muslims and involves some physical movement. The process of *Salat* promotes many physical and psychological benefits. One of the movements is the foot in flexion position during prostration and sitting. According to reflexology, flexing the foot and toes in foot massages techniques may increase blood flows and lead to the immediate hemodynamic effect. Thus, this paper investigates the immediate effect of flexing toes during performing prostration and sitting position in *Salat* on hemodynamic status. Fifty-two subjects have been recruited in this study and divided into two groups; control ($n = 33$) and uncontrolled ($n = 19$). Both groups were taught to perform *Salat* movement, but the proper movement and postures during prostrating were only emphasized in the control group, while it was not emphasized in the uncontrolled group. The subjects were required to perform two cycles of *Salat* movement. Systolic and diastolic blood pressure, heart rate, and electrocardiograph signals were recorded before and after the *Salat* movement. Our finding indicates that the toes flexion movement shown a significant effect on the hemodynamic status by lowering blood pressure both systolic and diastolic. Thus, it can be suggested as a supplementary to mimic the effect of reflexology massage.

Keywords Salat · Foot flexion · Bending toes · Blood pressure · Heart rate

---

F. Ibrahim (✉) · M. S. Mokhtar · N. F. A. Jaafar
Department of Biomedical Engineering, Faculty of Engineering, Universiti Malaya, 50603 Kuala Lumpur, Malaysia
e-mail: fatimah@um.edu.my

F. Ibrahim · M. S. Mokhtar · N. F. A. Jaafar · N. F. Jamaluddin
Faculty of Engineering, Center for Innovation in Medical Engineering, Universiti Malaya, 50603 Kuala Lumpur, Malaysia

F. Ibrahim
Center for Printable Electronics, Universiti Malaya, 50603 Kuala Lumpur, Malaysia

J. Usman et al. (eds.), *6th Kuala Lumpur International Conference on Biomedical Engineering 2021*, IFMBE Proceedings 86,
https://doi.org/10.1007/978-3-030-90724-2_31

1 Introduction

Reflexology is an alternative medical therapy by applying some pressure to any particular points on our body such as feet and hands. Each of the pressure points can be linked with different parts of the body organ specifically. Foot reflexology itself is believed to bring relaxation and healing to the corresponding area of the body by improves blood and energy circulation. Department of Thai Traditional and Alternative Medicine under the Ministry of Public Health, Thailand recommends this alternative medical therapy for lowering blood pressure and promotes health. However, there is a fee for each treatment session and the efficiency of foot reflexology in improving blood circulation is highly dependent on the skills possessed by the masseur [9]. Therefore, an alternative activity that could mimic the effect of reflexology upon the hemodynamic system would be an advantage to the practitioner.

Salat is a daily routine for every Muslim and involves some physical movement. The process of *Salat* promotes many physical and psychological benefits. A complete sequence in one cycle of *Salat* includes standing, bowing, prostrating, and sitting. *Salat* can be categorized as slow moderate exercise [12], and the practice of the right posture in completing the sequence of *Salat* may be beneficial to the body [4, 7, 8]. In the prostration and the sitting position, while performing the *Salat*, it is recommended that the toes are to be bent. Ones can activate the metatarsophalangeal articulations; which is stimulating the joints between the metatarsal bones of the foot and the proximal bones during flexing the foot by bending the toes. A certain physiological reaction is hypothesized when the foot is stimulated [6].

A physiological reaction such as hemodynamic effects status is measured through blood pressure (BP) and heart rate (HR). BP determines the value of blood force that is exerted on the artery walls as it travels through the body. The average normal pressure is about 120/80 mmHg. A person who has reading diastolic and systolic reading of 140/90 mm Hg or greater and this reading sustained and consistent over a long period is classified as having high BP. They will face the risk of long-term health problems and serious complications including heart attack, heart failure, aneurysms, stroke, kidney failure, and impaired vision [3]. Resting HR is an independent forecaster of cardiovascular disease. Studies indicate that a fairly high HR has direct unfavorable effects on the development of cardiovascular diseases, consequently lowering HR is an important mechanism [5].

A study by Doufesh et al. discovered that the HR value measured during the standing position is higher than the HR value measured during the prostration position of *Salat*. Moreover, the study also stated that the systolic and diastolic BP values decreased significantly after the performance of *Salat* [4]. However, the study does not discuss in detail the effect of foot flexion before and after the *Salat* performance. Hence, this study aims to investigate the immediate effect of foot flexion during sitting and prostrating (two of the positions in *Salat*) on BP and HR of healthy individuals, with an incentive of promoting this movement as an alternative or supplementary exercise to a reflexology massage.

2 Materials and Methods

2.1 Subjects

About 52 healthy volunteers (24 males and 28 females) were recruited in the study. This research complied with ethical standards as laid down in the 1964 Declaration of Helsinki. Consent forms were taken from each participant before the experiment procedure is conducted.

2.2 Groups

Controlled group

Subjects assigned into this group were taught to perform the *Salat* encompassing all the correct postures and movements, which are; standing straight, bowing at a 90° angle, flexing their foot by bending both toes (right and left feet) during prostrating (Fig. 1), and bending right toes during sitting (Fig. 2).

Uncontrolled group

Subjects assigned to this group were taught to perform the *Salat* that encompasses all the correct posture except flexing of the foot during the prostrating and sitting position.

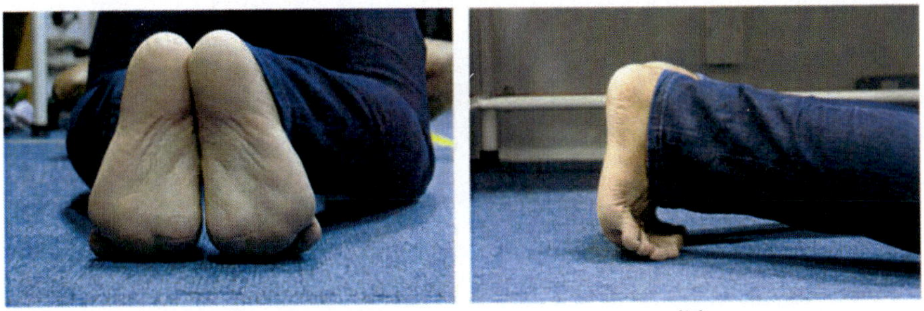

(a) (b)

Fig. 1 Foot flexion by bending both toes during prostrating position; **a** view from behind, and **b** view from the side

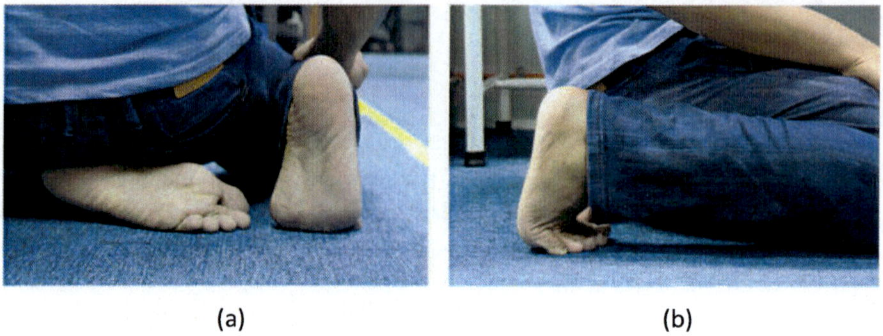

Fig. 2 Bending of the toes during sitting position; **a** view from behind, and **b** view from the side

2.3 *Salat* Movement

Salat consists of the posture and movement of standing, bowing, prostration, and sitting as standing again to complete as one cycle. This posture and movement are repeated for two cycles.

2.4 Measurement

Consents forms were obtained from the subjects or the subject's guardian before conducting the measurements. The subjects were asked to avoid doing any heavy or strenuous exercise a day before the test being conducted. Each subject in both the controlled and uncontrolled group was required to perform the procedure as described in Fig. 3. The anthropometric measurements such as height and weight, body circumference, and skinfold thickness were measured by using the Healthcare

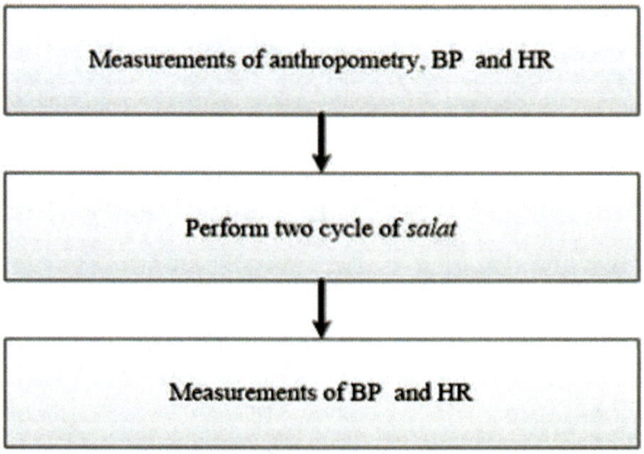

Fig. 3 Flow procedure during conducting experiment

height and weight scale, measuring tape, and skinfold caliper respectively. Systolic and diastolic BP and HR were measured using the OMRON, SEM 1, Green Tact Solution BP monitor. The signal of the heart is recorded by using the electrocardiograph device, CARDIOVIT AT-102 brand of Schiller. Subjects were asked to perform two cycles of the *Salat*; one cycle of *Salat* includes standing, bowing, prostrating, and sitting before and after prostrating [4].

2.5 Statistical Analysis

SPSS 20.0 (IBM SPSS Statistics) statistical software package was used for statistical analysis. Continuous data were expressed as mean ± standard deviation. Changes in hemodynamic parameters between groups before and after performed the *Salat* movement were tested using the non-parametric Sign Test and Wilcoxon Signed Rank Test. The significant *p*-value was set at below 0.05.

3 Results and Discussion

The controlled group consists of 33 subjects including 15 males and 18 females. The mean ± standard deviation (SD) of the weight for the male and females were 69.0 ± 11.2 kg and 56.5 ± 11.4 kg respectively. While the height for males and females were 166.8 ± 4.7 cm and 153.8 ± 6.5 cm respectively. There are 19 subjects in the uncontrolled group which consists of 9 males and 10 females. The mean ± SD weight of the male and female were 60.8 ± 10.7 kg and 52.2 ± 6.3 kg respectively. While the height of the male and female were 168.4 ± 6.1 cm and 155.6 ± 5.6 cm respectively. The anthropometry data for the subjects in the controlled and uncontrolled groups are summarized in Table 1.

Table 2 shows the result for the subjects before and after performing 2 cycles of *Salat*. The results from Table 2 also illustrate that BP components (systolic and diastolic levels) show an obvious decrement after performing the *Salat*. The differences were more significant among the female subjects, where 14 out of 18 and 12 out of 18 subjects demonstrated a reduction in their systolic and diastolic reading respectively. On the other hand, BP data in the uncontrolled group did not show any significant immediate changes. Even though there are no significant differences in the HR value before and after performing the two cycles of *Salat*, 22 out of the 33 subjects in the controlled group were shown to experience a lowering in their HR levels (Table 2).

Figure 4 shows the reflexology 'maps' of the feet. Comparing the 'maps' [1], and Fig. 1, by bending the right and left toe during the prostration position, the heart, the thalamus (a structure situated between the cerebral cortex and the midbrain), the lung, the brain, the throat, the nose, the glands, the eye, the ear, and the shoulder are

Table 1 Summary of subject's anthropometry data

Parameters	Controlled group		Uncontrolled group	
	Male (n = 15)	Female (n = 18)	Male (n = 9)	Female (n = 10)
	Mean (SD)			
Age (years)	32.7 (14.3)	29.2 (11.4)	17.3 (2.6)	22.7 (0.8)
Height (cm)	166.8 (4.7)	153.8 (6.5)	168.4 (6.1)	155.6 (5.6)
Weight (kg)	69.0 (11.2)	56.5 (11.4)	60.8 (10.7)	52.2 (6.3)
Body mass index (BMI) (kg/m^2)	24.7 (3.7)	23.9 (4.6)	21.4 (3.6)	21.7 (3.2)
Circumference (cm)				
Chest	89.9 (7.2)	86.0 (9.9)	82.6 (5.8)	82.6 (6.4)
Arm	30.0 (7.8)	26.6 (3.7)	26.0 (3.1)	25.7 (1.7)
Waist	85.0 (10.7)	75.7 (8.7)	74.1 (8.6)	70.8 (6.8)
Hip	98.4 (7.3)	97.0 (8.5)	93.2 (7.2)	91.0 (14.9)
Thigh	51.7 (6.8)	48.8 (6.4)	47.8 (4.5)	49.0 (14.9)

Table 2 Comparisons on subject's measurement data before and after performing two cycles of *Salat*

Parameters		Differences[a]		Controlled group		Uncontrolled group	
		Overall (n = 33)	Male (n = 15)	Female (n = 18)	Overall (n = 19)	Male (n = 9)	Female (n = 10)
Systolic	Negative	21*	9	14#	12	5	7
	Positive	8	4	4	5	4	1
	Ties	4	2	2	2	0	2
Diastolic	Negative	22*	10	12^	9	4	5
	Positive	8	5	3	9	4	5
	Ties	3	0	3	1	1	0
HR	Negative	21	11	10	11	5	6
	Positive	11	4	7	8	4	4
	Ties	1	0	1	0	0	0

[a] Differences are calculated by parameter's value after minus parameter's value before subject's performing two cycles of Salat movement

* The differences differ significantly tested using both Sign Test and Wilcoxon Signed Ranks Test at $p < 0.05$

The differences differ significantly tested using Wilcoxon Signed Ranks Test at $p < 0.05$

^ The differences differ significantly tested using Sign Test at $p < 0.05$

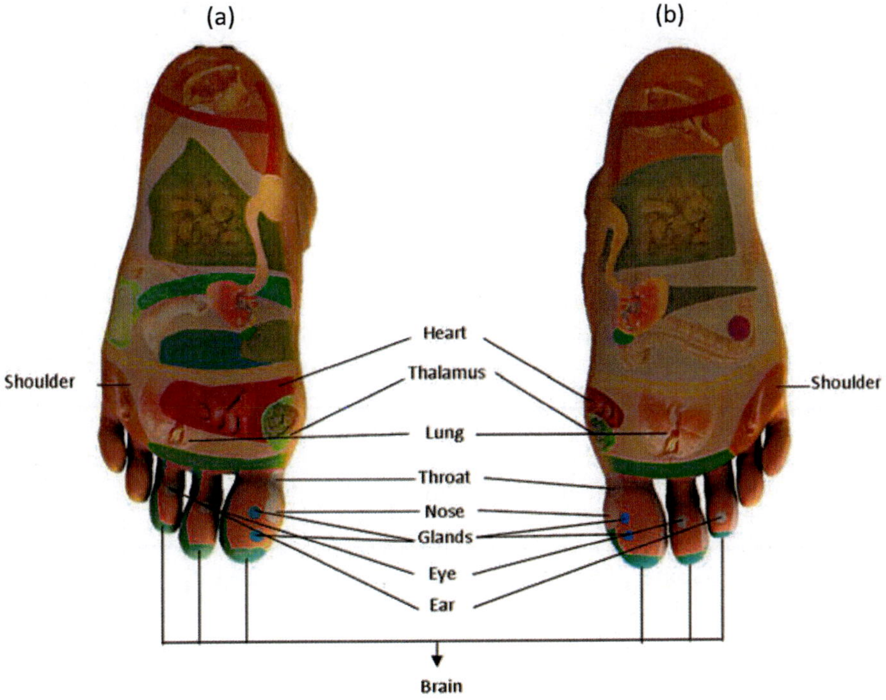

Fig. 4 Reflexology 'maps' of the feet; **a** right leg and **b** left leg

postulated to be stimulated. Also, the heart is further stimulated by bending the right toes during the sitting position of *Salat* as shown in Fig. 2.

The substantial decrease in the systolic and the diastolic value among subjects in the controlled group is probably since their heart was stimulated while performing the *Salat*. The process of pumping blood through the whole body using the contracting (systolic) and relaxing (diastolic) movements can be more efficient when the heart is motivated [13]. Studies have exhibited that BP can be lowered by blocking the renin–angiotensin–aldosterone enzyme that is produced by the glands [10]. When the controlled subjects flexed their foot during the prostration and the sitting positions, the glands enzyme productions might have been blocked temporarily and thus the immediate lowering in BP levels can be observed. In addition, foot flexion by bending the toes during *Salat* is also mimicking a gentle dorsiflexion stretch, one of the movements recommended in foot flexor strengthening exercises. This treatment has been used by Chiro-practitioner to treat a condition known as hallux rigidus [2].

According to the reflexology 'map', performing *Salat* in the most correct manners inclusive of flexed feet will also activate or stimulate parts of the brain. Hypothetically, the effect could be similar to scalp acupuncture. Where, according to a study by Park et al., the contralateral somatosensory association cortex, the postcentral gyrus, and the parietal lobe (parts of the brain) were activated after an acupuncture needling technique was performed [11].

Future work will include the study of the long-term effect of *Salat* on not only the hemodynamic system but also the effects on breathing, hormonal changes, and the brain. Larger cohorts of subjects are needed to confirm our findings.

4 Conclusions

Salat not only is necessary for the fulfillment of one's spiritual quest but also can be considered a natural exercise without any costs. By performing *Salat* in the most correct posture and movement manner such as flexing the toes during prostrating and sitting, the performer could achieve the benefits of performing reflexology. This study has shown that comprehensive foot flexion in *Salat* posture can give an immediately reduction of the systolic and diastolic measurement value.

Acknowledgements This research was supported and funded by the Prime Minister's Department, Malaysia, through a special grant Project No. 66-02-03-0061/H-00000-37039 and University of Malaya, Malaysia.

References

1. Botting, D.: Review of literature on the effectiveness of reflexology. Complement. Ther. Nurs. Midwifery **3**(5), 123–130 (1997). https://doi.org/10.1016/S1353-6117(97)80012-1
2. Brantingham, J.W., Chang, M.N., Gendreau, D.F., Price, J.L.: The effect of chiropractic adjusting, exercises and modalities on a 32-year-old professional male golfer with hallux rigidus. Clin. Chiropr. **10**(2), 91–96 (2007). https://doi.org/10.1016/j.clch.2007.03.001
3. Chobanian, A.V., Bakris, G.L., Black, H.R., Cushman, W.C., Green, L.A., Izzo, J.L., Jones, D.W., Materson, B.J., Oparil, S., Wright, J.T., Roccella, E.J.: Seventh report of the joint national committee on prevention, detection, evaluation, and treatment of high blood pressure. Hypertension **42**(6), 1206–1252 (2003)
4. Doufesh, H., Ibrahim, F., Ismail, N.A., Ahmad, W.A.W.: Assessment of heart rates and blood pressure in different Salat positions. J. Phys. Ther. Sci. **25**(2), 211–214 (2013)
5. Fox, K., Borer, J.S., Camm, A.J., Danchin, N., Ferrari, R., Lopez Sendon, J.L., Steg, P.G., Tardif, J.C., Tavazzi, L., Tendera, M., Tendera, M.: Resting heart rate in cardiovascular disease. J. Am. Coll. Cardiol. **50**(9), 823–830 (2007). https://doi.org/10.1016/j.jacc.2007.04.079
6. Grimby, L.: Normal plantar response: integration of flexor and extensor reflex components. J. Neurol. Neurosurg. Psychiatry **26**(1), 39 (1963)
7. Ibrahim, F., Ahmad, S.A., Woo, P.J., Abas, W.A.B.W.: Biomechanical response of the upper body during prostration in Salat and the child's pose: a preliminary study. J. Phys. Ther. Sci. **24**(10), 1021–1024 (2012)
8. Ibrahim, F., Sian, T.C., Shanggar, K., Razack, A.H.: Muslim prayer movements as an alternative therapy in the treatment of erectile dysfunction: a preliminary study. J. Phys. Ther. Sci. **25**(9), 1087–1091 (2013). https://doi.org/10.1589/jpts.25.1087

9. Jones, J., Thomson, P., Lauder, W., Howie, K., Leslie, S.J.: Reflexology has an acute (immediate) haemodynamic effect in healthy volunteers: a double-blind randomised controlled trial. Complement. Ther. Clin. Pract. (2012)
10. Mackay, J.A.: Blocking the renin-angiotensin-aldosterone system or lowering the blood pressure: does EUROPA help? J. Renin-Angiotensin-Aldosterone Syst. **4**(4), 205–206 (2003). https://doi.org/10.3317/jraas.2003.033
11. Park, S.-U., Shin, A.-S., Jahng, G.-H., Moon, S.-K., Park, J.-M.: Effects of scalp acupuncture versus upper and lower limb acupuncture on signal activation of blood oxygen level dependent (BOLD) fMRI of the brain and somatosensory cortex. J. Alternative Complement. Med. **15**(11), 1193–1200 (2009)
12. Reza, M.F., Urakami, Y., Mano, Y.: Evaluation of a new physical exercise taken from Salat (prayer) as a short-duration and frequent physical activity in the rehabilitation of geriatric and disabled patients. Ann. Saudi Med. **22**(3/4), 177–180 (2002)
13. Verrier, R.L., Thompson, P.L., Lown, B.: Ventricular vulnerability during sympathetic stimulation: role of heart rate and blood pressure. Cardiovasc. Res. **8**(5), 602–610 (1974)

Automatic Physio-Walker (*PhyWalk*) as a Rehabilitation Therapy for Children with Lower Disability

Mohd Azrul Hisham Mohd Adib, Mohd Hanafi Abdul Rahim, Rabiatul Aisyah Ariffin, Idris Mat Sahat, Mohd Hafiz Hasan, Nurul Anati Basirah Sulaiman, Siti Nurfarhana Mohamad Wahid, Mohd Firdaus Mak Nayan, Mohammad Fitri Abdullah, Suraya Najiha Mohd Ishak, Nurul Shahida Mohd Shalahim, and Narimah Daud

Abstract Nowadays, the number of cases of cerebral palsy (CP) is shown an increase. Commonly, CP is caused by abnormal development of the brain or damage to the developing brain that affects a child's ability to control his or her muscles. It is the most common cause of childhood disability and as individuals with CP grow, the children with greater physical involvement often have few options for functional mobility. Therefore, in this study, the physio-walker (*PhyWalk*) is well developed to provide rehabilitation therapy for CP kids. *PhyWalk* is used to maintain the balance of the trunk and pelvis for children. It's also can be used for forwarding and backward movement, speed control. *PhyWalk* is automatic control and comes with a multi-function device. The preliminary walking distance test on kid has been done once every two weeks. The results show a significant improvement in the number of steps from the first training to four sessions of training. It also provides opportunities to stand and bear weight in a safe, supported position using a combination of formal and informal user-centered design methods. However, the modest speed adjustments were dependent on the capacity of the child to control their gait balance. *PhyWalk*

M. A. H. M. Adib (✉) · M. H. A. Rahim · R. A. Ariffin · M. H. Hasan · N. A. B. Sulaiman · S. N. M. Wahid · M. F. M. Nayan · M. F. Abdullah · S. N. M. Ishak
Medical Engineering & Health Intervention Team (MedEHiT), Department of Mechanical Engineering, College of Engineering, Universiti Malaysia Pahang, 26300 Lebuhraya Tun Abdul Razak, Kuantan, Pahang, Malaysia
e-mail: azrul@ump.edu.my

I. M. Sahat · N. S. M. Shalahim
Human Engineering Group (HEG), Faculty of Mechanical & Automotive Engineering Technology, Universiti Malaysia Pahang, 26600 Pekan, Pahang, Malaysia

N. Daud
Department of Industrial Engineering, College of Engineering, Universiti Malaysia Pahang, 26300 Lebuhraya Tun Abdul Razak, Kuantan, Pahang, Malaysia

Kuantan Physical Therapy, Physiotherapy Center, Lot B1.10, Ground Floor, Block B, Banggunan Al-Tabari, IM 7/3, 25582 Bandar Indera Mahkota 7, Kuantan, Pahang, Malaysia

J. Usman et al. (eds.), *6th Kuala Lumpur International Conference on Biomedical Engineering 2021*, IFMBE Proceedings 86,
https://doi.org/10.1007/978-3-030-90724-2_32

was developed for children with special needs and offers greater balance support and weight support than a conventional walker.

Keywords Cerebral palsy · Walker training · Rehabilitation · Gait · *PhyWalk*

1 Introduction

Neurocognitive rehabilitation has become an integral component of pediatric rehabilitation. Within neurocognitive rehabilitation, the child may perform systematically presented and functionally-oriented therapeutic activities that are based upon an assessment and understanding of the child's brain-behavior deficits. From a clinical perspective, neurocognitive rehabilitation typically connotes methodical intervention intended to aid the child impacted by cognitive or behavioral deficits. In general, the goal is to enable children to increase their ability to perform activities of daily living.

Children with disabilities from the day they were born are not common in our daily life. However, denying treatment to disabled children is not how things work in this modern life. Care needs to be taken to disabled children as they are vulnerable to child abuse [1] until they achieve the age of normal adults. The advances of emerging technologies could help these children in improving themselves from neurocognitive impairments, which include attention, ability to memorize, reasoning, and making decisions. These technologies may aid the children to prepare themselves for future undertakings especially before they become adults and while their parents still can take care of them. These technologies are proven by many researchers. The disabled children in this context are those who need special care towards lower limbs as there are many types of disabilities training and exercises available throughout the topic. To allow for longer training sessions with more repetitions while maintaining a consistent movement pattern and reducing the burden of the therapists, new robotic rehabilitation technologies have emerged during the last 15 years and have increasingly been implemented in the clinical setting.

Initially, the lower limbs exoskeleton was proposed in 1956 by [2] and continued in 2014 [3]. Further developments were expanded by General Electric late in [4]. They began the research intending to amplify human strength and for military purposes [5]. Nevertheless, the application of the lower limb exoskeleton reaches for medical applications such as 12 kg Orthosis [6] and ReWalk [7]. These devices are wearable robotics and can help a patient that suffered from a stroke or spinal cord injury to regain lower limb abilities such as CUHK-EXO [8] as well as ExRoLEG [9]. A rehabilitation gait device is a wheeled device that assists a person who is unable to walk independently to learn or relearn to walk safely as part of gait training. Gait devices are intended for children to improve their walking ability.

This study focuses on the development of the *PhyWalk* and investigates the preliminary walking distance test on a kid patient using *PhyWalk*. *PhyWalk* was developed to help cerebral palsy kids improve their lower extremity become stronger by training using this product [10, 11].

2 Methods

2.1 Design and Development

This *PhyWalk* is a combination of a mechanical system and an electronic system. To develop this *PhyWalk* consists of two main parts which are the mechanical parts and the electronic parts. The mechanical parts are categorized into two which are design and fabrication. The main structure of the device is made from Aluminium extrusion profile 3030 which is strong, lightweight and has no sharp edges. As for the joints, they are made of 3D printed poly-acetic acid (PLA) with a minimum 3D printing infill of 50%. There are two actuators installed between the middle structure and the top structure. Two motorized front wheels and two back wheels are attached to the main structure for motion control. A harness bracket was installed at the top structure so the harness that will carry the patient can be attached to the harness bracket. Two holders and LCD parts are installed at the top structure as well. The main control box is installed at the bottom middle front section of the device.

2.2 Control System

For the electronic parts, Arduino Uno R3 is acting as the main controller. The 12 V motorized front wheel is used to control the moving direction of the device, such as moving forward, backward, and turning right or left. The 12 V actuators accompanied by two relays are used to control the height of the harness that will be attached to the patient as shown in Fig. 1.

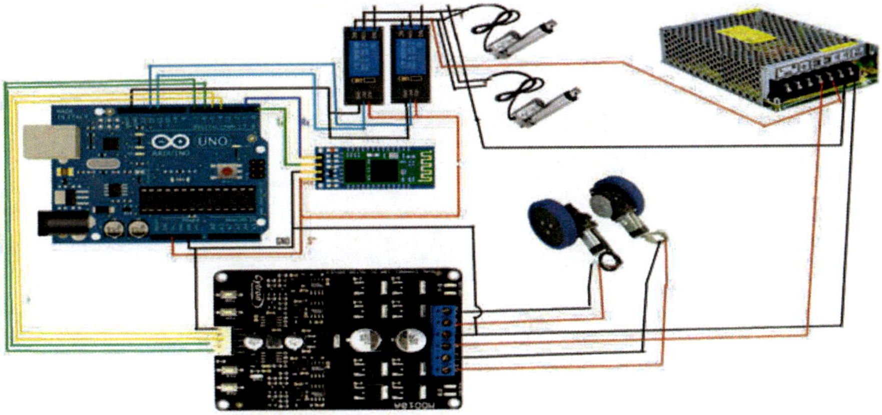

Fig. 1 Schematic diagram for the control system of *PhyWalk* product

Table 1 Bill of material (BOM)

Part name	Value (unit)
Aluminum profile	30 mm × 30 mm
Bracket 3D printing	500 g
Motor	24 V
Set sprocket	H25
Screen (Tab)	1.24 in
Arduino board	12–24 V
Power supply	24 V
Wire	1 set
Bold and nut	20 set
Actuator	1 hp
Children harness set	1 set
Flat board	1000 × 2000 mm
Button/switch	3 set

The adjustment of the harness is required as each patient has a different height. The top structure of the device is attached to bearings at the frontal section, thus it can move up and down freely according to the needs of the patient. A power supply of 12 V was attached to the main controller so it can supply enough power to the whole electronic system. The power supply can be changed to a battery system so that no wire is attached. A Bluetooth device is attached to the controller so that it can communicate with an android device. This is to make sure that the device can be controlled via smartphone. Detailed bill of material (BOM) details of the *PhyWalk* shows in Table 1.

Figure 2 shows details of the final prototype of the *PhyWalk*. The *PhyWalk* can lift less than a 30 kg load without a problem. The LCD panel is to help the patient

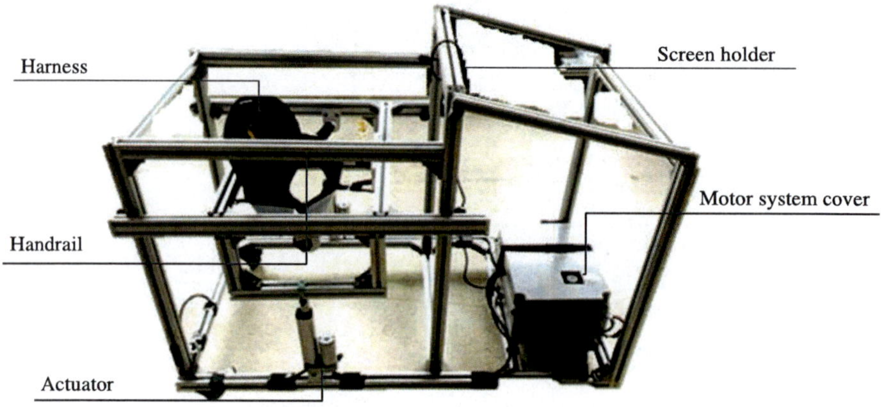

Fig. 2 The structure of *PhyWalk* product

focus on the gait training. The device speed can be controlled according to the needs of the patient training.

3 Results

The prototype of the *PhyWalk* for cerebral palsy kids is well developed [12]. This *PhyWalk* is intended for children aged from 6 to 9 years with cerebral palsy that could not walk on their own to improve their walking ability. Figure 3 shows the component involves in the development of the *PhyWalk*. This *PhyWalk* is attached with a motorized front wheel, so it can move easily according to the physiotherapist treatment which will be the operator of the *PhyWalk*. This could assist a patient who is unable to walk independently, to learn or relearn to walk safely as part of gait training [13].

Figure 4 shows the *PhyWalk* is tested on the normal kid as a preliminary study and the detailed information of the kid shows in Table 2.

The training sessions consisted of approximately 30 min of walking training using *PhyWalk*. The session is repeated once every 2 weeks. The *PhyWalk* was set to a low speed for the first training session so that the kid could show sufficient ability to maintain an upright lower limb stance, ankle push-off, and toe clearance during the adaptation process. A camera was used to count the number of steps. The recorded video will be examined once the research procedure is completed. The *PhyWalk* speed was progressively increased in each session to increase the number

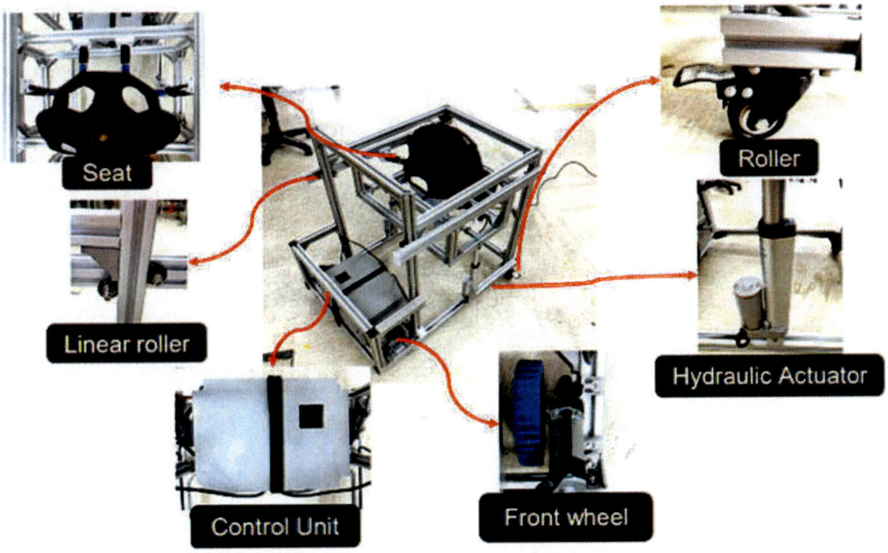

Fig. 3 The components involved in the *PhyWalk* product

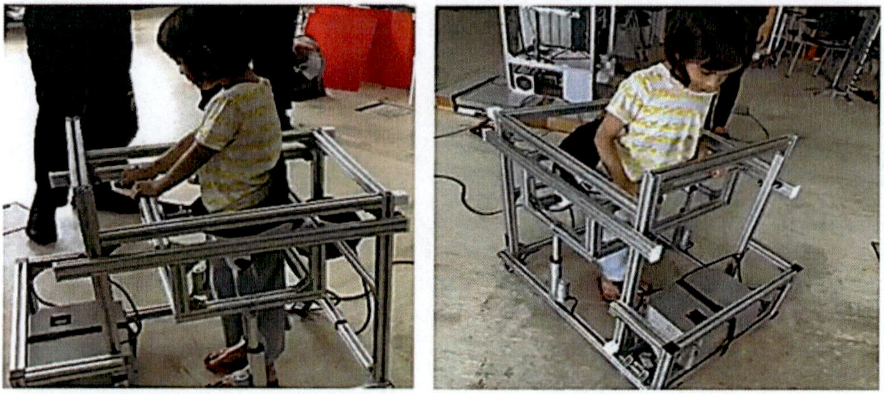

Fig. 4 Preliminary walking distance test on kid using *PhyWalk* product

Table 2 Demographics information

Patient	Details
Gender	Female
Age (years old)	7
Height (cm)	105
Weight (kg)	12
BMI (kg/m^2)	10.9

of steps. The gradual speed changes, on the other hand, were based on the kid's ability to regulate their gait pattern. As a result in Fig. 5, we obtained the kid shows a significant improvement in the number of steps from the first training to four sessions of training. The kid may take fewer steps to walk a given distance to increase step length, in which case fewer steps may indicate improvement. It may also increase their walking distance because it is easier for them. Where case more steps may indicate improvements.

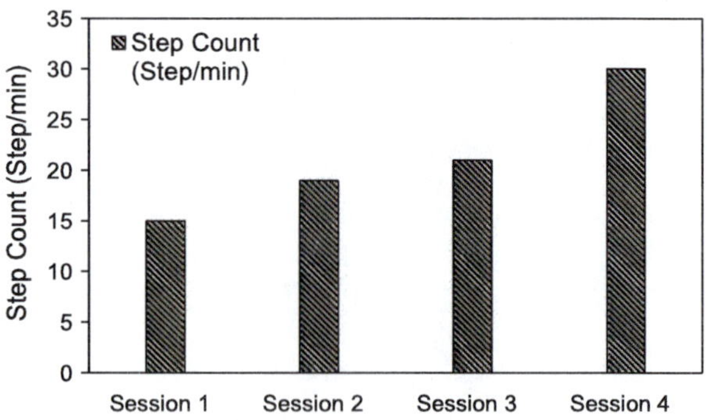

Fig. 5 The outcome measure for the number of steps using *PhyWalk* after 4 sessions

4 Discussion

The *PhyWalk* was generally found stability and safety. The development of *PhyWalk* was carried out to help cerebral palsy kids with their mobility issues, including problems with balance and posture. The *PhyWalk* chassis is rather large; thus, many centers have decided that the equipment is not suitable at home. Furthermore, the *PhyWalk* generally required therapists to assist the user over the seat and supervision during treatment. The height of the seat has to be modified before placement. Besides, there were certain limitations in the *PhyWalk* investigation. We have few limitations to test more kids. This might have led to inadequate reporting in our study and shows that our results cannot be applied to the community. Despite its limitations, our study provided important results to helps the population of cerebral palsy kids. These included physiotherapist treatment to improve their walking ability.

5 Conclusion

The *PhyWalk* is well designed and successfully developed as follows. The concept of designing the *PhyWalk* was obtained and practically produced. A support walker is specifically designed for children with special needs and provides more assistance for balance and weight-bearing, than does a traditional roller walker, or a walker with platform attachments. It also provides opportunities to stand and bear weight in a safe, supported position using a combination of informal and formal user-centered design methods. Additionally, the limitation of the rehabilitation device is understood as well. The *PhyWalk* is well secured and safe to use for children. Also, it gives the benefit to a person monitoring the child due to our automatic *PhyWalk* that can be controlled by the mobile application.

Acknowledgements A big thank you dedicated to University Malaysia Pahang (UMP) under grant RDU210332 and PGRS2003199 and Medical Engineering & Health Intervention Team (MedEHiT) are gratefully acknowledged for providing us with a good environment and facilities to complete these research activities.

References

1. Alwin, Y.D., Horridge, K.: Safeguarding disabled children and young people. Pediatr. Child Health **26**(11), 488–492 (2016)
2. Herr, H.: Exoskeletons and orthoses: classification, design challenges, and future directions. J. Neuroeng. Rehabil. **6**, 21–24 (2009)
3. Fontana, M., Vertechy, R., Marcheschi, S., Salsedo, F., Bergamasco, M.: The body extender: a full-body exoskeleton for the transport and handling of heavy loads. IEEE Robot. Autom. Mag. **21**, 34–44 (2014)

4. Fick, B.R., Makinson, J.B.: Final Report on Hardiman I Prototype for Machine Augmentation of Human Strength and Endurance (1971)
5. Kazerooni, H.: Hybrid control of the Berkeley lower extremity exoskeleton (BLEEX). Int. J. Robot. Res. **25**, 561–573 (2006)
6. Farris, M., Ryan, J., Hugo, A., Quintero, L., Michael, G.: Preliminary evaluation of a powered lower-limb orthosis to aid walking in paraplegic individuals. IEEE Trans. Neural Syst. Rehabil. Eng. **19**(6), 652–659 (2011)
7. Mukul, I., Alberto, E., Jorge, E.B.: Differentiating ability in users of the ReWalk TM powered exoskeleton: an analysis of walking kinematics. In: IEEE 13th International Conference on Rehabilitation Robotics (ICORR)
8. Chen, B., Zhong, C.H., Zhao, X., Ma, H., Guan, X., Li, X., Liao, W.H.: A wearable exoskeleton suit for motion assistance to paralyzed patients. J. Orthop. Transl. **11**, 7–18 (2017)
9. Adib, M.A.H.M., Han, S.Y., Ramani, P.R., You, L.J., Yan, L.M., Sahat, I.M., Hasni, N.H.M.: Restoration of kids leg function using exoskeleton robotic leg (ExRoLEG) device. In: Proceedings of the 10th National Technical Seminar on Underwater System Technology 2018 (2019), pp. 335–342
10. Ariffin, R.A., Adib, M.A.H.M., Shalahim, N.S.M., Daud, N., Hasni, N.H.M.: An ergonomic perspective of user need on physio-treadmill (PhyMill) criteria: knowledge and awareness of cerebral palsy among future parents. J. Phys. Conf. Ser. **1529**(5) (2020). https://doi.org/10.1088/1742-6596/1529/5/052071
11. Ariffin, R.A., Azrul, M., Mohd, H., Mohd, N.S.: Ergonomics Study on Visual Contribution of Postural Stability Using Physio-Treadmill (PhyMill) for Kid with Cerebral Palsy, pp. 1–12
12. M. Azrul, H. Mohd, R.A. Arifin, M.H. Abdul, Development of Physiotherapy-Treadmill (PhyMill) as Rehabilitation Technology Tools for Kid with Cerebral Palsy, pp. 1–10
13. Ariffin, R.A.: Physio-treadmill (PhyMill): Ergonomics Evaluation of Posture Impact on Kids with Cerebral Palsy Using Digital Human Modeling (DHM) Simulation

A Preliminary Study of Ankle Muscular Strategy During Single Leg Stance

Nureen Shahirah Ahmad Zaghlul, Siew Li Goh, Rizal Razman, Salmah Karman, and Chow Khuen Chan

Abstract Ankle contributes a significant role during dynamic movements in the double leg and single leg (SL) balance activities. The subject specific balance performance can be evaluated using SL stance as it has a small base of support, which is able to detect possible impairment during the balance abilities. Hence, the aim of this study was to comprehend the electromyographic (EMG) activity of muscles around the ankle, among healthy adults. This preliminary study was aimed at addressing muscle quantification during SL stance. Eight participants with sports background were recruited. Participants stood on their dominant leg on the Lafayette stability platform in two conditions: with eyes open (EO) and eyes close (EC). Three successful trials for 20 s were recorded respectively. The EMG data from three ankle stabilizer muscles namely Peroneus Longus (PL), Tibialis Anterior (TA) and Gastrocnemius Lateralis (GL) were compared during the SL stance. The results revealed greater balance performance in SL stance during EO compared to EC. PL was seen to be the most active among the three muscles in all conditions. Moreover, PL also demonstrated the highest frequency of total contractions followed by GL and TA during the 20 s task in EO and EC conditions. From this study, we can infer that PL imparts a role of evertor in balance control.

Keywords Single leg · Ankle muscle · Lafayette stability platform · Electromyography · Balance control

N. S. A. Zaghlul · S. Karman · C. K. Chan (✉)
Department of Biomedical Engineering, Faculty of Engineering, Universiti Malaya, 50603 Kuala Lumpur, Malaysia
e-mail: ckchan@um.edu.my

S. L. Goh (✉)
Sports Medicine Unit, Faculty of Medicine, Universiti Malaya, 50603 Kuala Lumpur, Malaysia
e-mail: gsiewli@um.edu.my

R. Razman
Centre for Sport & Exercise Sciences, Universiti Malaya, 50603 Kuala Lumpur, Malaysia

J. Usman et al. (eds.), *6th Kuala Lumpur International Conference on Biomedical Engineering 2021*, IFMBE Proceedings 86,
https://doi.org/10.1007/978-3-030-90724-2_33

1 Introduction

Human standing posture is controlled by muscle activations in propelling the body forward and backward [1]. The ability to sustain the body in equilibrium by maintaining the center of mass within the limits of the base of support is defined as a balance control [2]. Interestingly, interaction between somatosensory system and motor nerves contributes to postural balance, which includes vision and proprioception [2, 3]. In the lower limb muscles, muscles surrounding the ankle joint play an important part in controlling the balance over unstable conditions. Weak ligament of the ankle may lead to several sprains prior the initial injury in lateral ankle sprain (LAS) cases [4]. Previous study [5] reported that the ankle joint mechanisms contribute to the human posture.

Surface electromyography (surface EMG: sEMG) is a common research tool used to observe muscle physiology during human movements. sEMG is the most popular tool in understanding the neuromuscular system behaviours [6]. The intensity of muscle recruitment and its characteristics can also be attained from sEMG. A previous study demonstrated the magnitude of muscle activity depending on the stability of the used device. Approximately twice of the muscle activity would be required to control standing posture on an unstable platform compared to the stable platform [7]. Additionally, maximally stimulating muscle activity levels (such as standing on a balance platform) is expected to accelerate the rehabilitation process to pre-injury functional levels [8].

One of the most common assessments that potentially reveals impaired balance control is the single leg (SL) stance. Due to its narrow base of support, SL stance would better suit for detecting balance impairments compared to bilateral stance [8]. Lafayette stability platform is one of the balancing devices that utilizes the unstable base. However, there were lack of investigation of muscle activities reported using this platform. Additionally, the information on the muscle recruitment order and the relationship of the muscles with the tasks performed using Lafayette stability platform were scarce. Authors believe a better understanding of how the muscles control the posture and their direct connections represent important process in balancing mechanics. Therefore, this study aims to (1) compare the balance performance during eyes open (EO) and eyes close (EC) conditions on the Lafayette platform and (2) analyze the electromyographic activities of ankle stabilizer's muscles (Peroneus Longus: PL; Tibialis Anterior: TA; Gastrocnemius Lateralis; GL). It is hypothesized that the duration the participants maintain the SL stance on unstable platform were shorter in EC condition than in EO condition. We hypothesized that greater EMG magnitude will be obtained during EC rather than in EO conditions. This preliminary study serves to facilitate the understanding on how muscles control balance and would then enable physiotherapists and clinicians strategize better rehabilitation regime.

2 Methodology

2.1 Participants

Eight healthy university students (5 males, 3 females; age 22.8 ± 1.32 years; height 1.64 ± 0.11 m; weight 60.55 ± 17.85 kg) were recruited. The main inclusion criteria of the study were physically active and ages between 18 and 30 years old. Participants were excluded if they had lower extremity injury in the past three months, including fracture or surgery. No pain and musculoskeletal disorders that might affect the performance of the balance task were reported. Participants gave written consent prior to testing. The ethics of the study was approved by Medical Ethics Research Committee (MREC) of University of Malaya Medical Centre (GPF007C-2019).

2.2 Instrumentation

Lafayette Stability Platform Model 16030 (Lafayette, Indiana) was used to test the balance performance of the participants. The platform provided tilt angle, which represented the participant's error score, reflecting deviation (mediolateral) from the target horizontal platform position (0°). The stability platform consisted of a 65 × 107 cm wooden base, allowing a maximum deviation of 15° from the horizontal to either side of the platform. The participants are considered 'in balance' when the platform sway within ± 3° from the horizontal plane. A safety rail was mounted to the stability platform to allow the participants to hold onto if they lost the balance. Using the Psymlab software (Lafayette, Indiana), time in balance (TIB) was recorded, denoted by the duration the participants managed to stay within the range of deviation on the platform.

2.3 Protocol

The participants stood on their dominant leg barefooted on the stability platform (Fig. 1). The contralateral leg was slightly flexed with the foot minimally lifted approximately 10 cm above the platform. The dominant leg was determined from the preferences of the participants to kick a ball [9]. The arms were placed by the side during the SL stance task. The participants were required to balance in two conditions, in EO and EC. Three successful trials in each condition were recorded. The total duration for the SL stance was 20 s in each trial. During EO, the participants were instructed to focus on a mark placed on the wall about 2.5 m away. The participants were prohibited to speak, no distracting noise or conversation were allowed. The trials will be discarded and reconducted if the participants fall off the platform, touch the rail or the contralateral leg touched the platform.

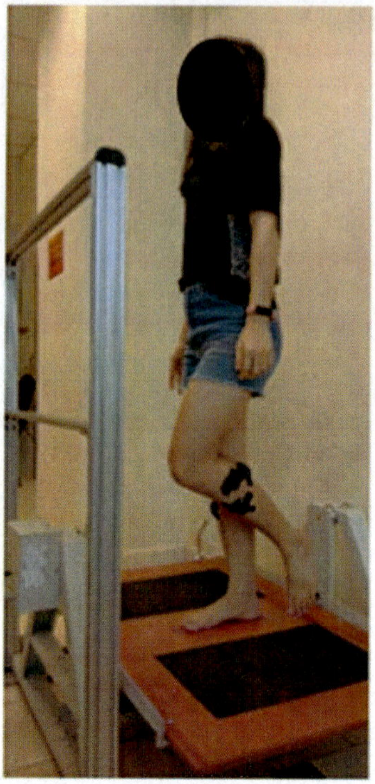

Fig. 1 Participant performed SL stance on Lafayette stability platform during EO condition

2.4 *Electromyography (EMG)*

Muscle activities of three muscles; Peroneus Longus (PL), Tibialis Anterior (TA), and Gastrocnemius Lateralis (GL) were recorded using sEMG (Delsys, USA). The skin was cleaned with isopropyl alcohol to reduce resistance prior attaching the electrodes [10]. The electrodes were further secured with adhesive tape to prevent slippage during testing and to minimize movement artifacts. EMG signals were recorded at a sampling rate of 2000 Hz. All EMG data were digitized, stored and analyzed using EMG Works Acquisition and Analysis software. Participants performed maximum voluntary contraction (MVC) prior to testing, in accordance with the Surface Electromyography for Non-Invasive Assessment of Muscles (SENIAM) guidelines. Data were normalized using the peak MVC values of tasks, namely dorsiflexion, plantarflexion and eversion for 5 s [11]. Normalized muscle activities were expressed in percentage of MVC (%MVC).

2.5 Data Analyses

The analysis was performed using Excel (Microsoft Corporation, USA). Data is presented as means and standard deviations. Using the means of EMG data in the Excel file, the frequency of peaks amplitudes above 70% of MVC were tabulated to determine the total contractions of the muscles. In addition, the highest peak of each muscle was observed in the first 5 s using computed graphs to determine the muscle reaction. The onset of muscle activity was further determined among the muscles. The difference in onset times between two muscles had to exceed 10 ms (measurement error) to represent a real time difference. If the difference did not exceed 10 ms, these muscles were considered to have similar onset time [12].

3 Results

The balance performance of participants during SL stance on Lafayette platform were recorded using TIB measurements. The TIB values for each participant during EO and EC conditions are tabulated in Table 1. It can be observed that, during EO condition, participants' balance performance on the Lafayette platform were consistent (19.88 s) in all eight participants. This indicated Lafayette platform was deviated within ± 3° for the entire 20 s period. However, during EC condition, the TIB values were varied. Four participants were able to maintain the platform within the angle provided with the longest duration of 19.88 s, followed by the other three participants with 19.60 s, 17.81 s, and 17.61 s respectively. Additionally, one participant had the shortest TIB value during EC condition, which was 3.48 s. The average TIB values for the eight participants were 19.88 ± 0.00 s in EO condition and 17.25 ± 5.65 s in EC condition respectively.

The muscles activities during SL stance on Lafayette stability platform were observed using the EMG signals recorded. The mean EMG amplitudes of the muscles in EO and EC conditions are illustrated in Figs. 2 and 3.

Table 1 Time in balance (TIB) of the participants in both EO and EC conditions

Subjects	Time in balance, s (EO)	Time in balance, s (EC)
1	19.88	19.88
2	19.88	19.88
3	19.88	17.81
4	19.88	19.88
5	19.88	19.60
6	19.88	19.88
7	19.88	17.61
8	19.88	3.48

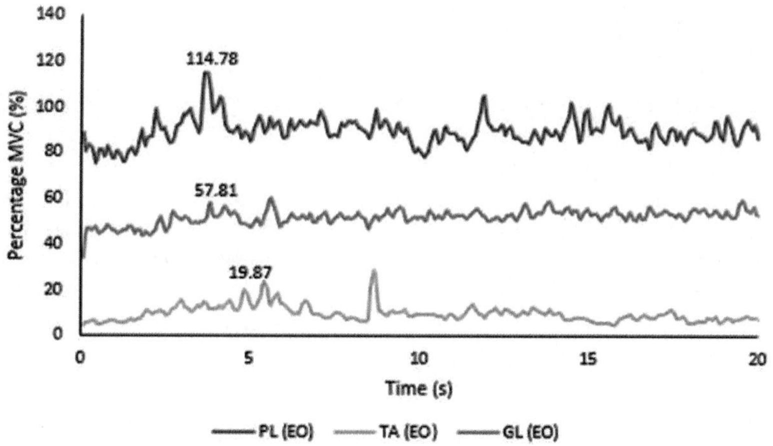

Fig. 2 The sEMG amplitudes of muscles during eyes open (EO) condition

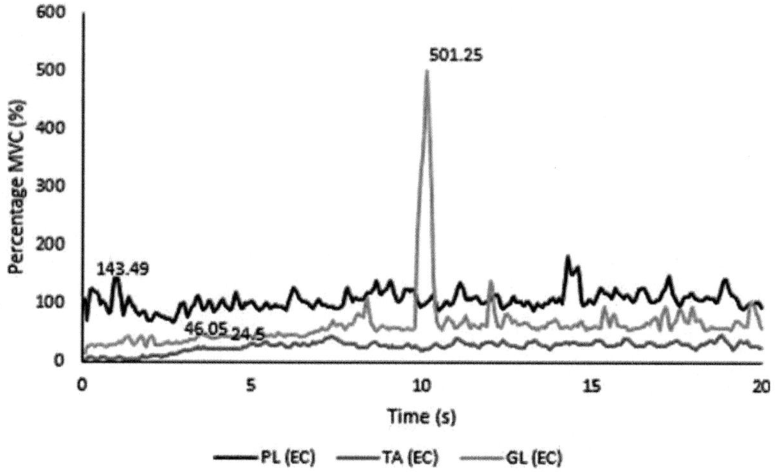

Fig. 3 The sEMG amplitudes of the muscles during eyes close (EC) condition

During EO, it can be seen that the three ankle muscles produced different percentages of MVC during the SL stance. PL demonstrated the highest percentage of EMG amplitudes (114.78%) at the earliest period (3.75 s), followed by GL (57.81%) at 3.88 s and lastly by TA (19.87%) at 4.88 s. The muscle recruitment order reflected from the finding was PL reacted initially during SL stance on Lafayette platform in EO condition, followed by GL and lastly by TA. The time difference between the muscles contractions was above 10 ms causing the finding to be acceptable.

In addition, the calculated total average peaks of each muscle during the 20 s showed the highest frequency demonstrated by PL with 320 peaks. Surprisingly,

GL and TA failed to reach EMG amplitudes of 70% of MVC value throughout the 20 s EO condition. However, EMG amplitudes for GL was higher than TA, with GL reaching above 50% of MVC value whereas EMG amplitudes for TA only reach nearly 30% of MVC.

During EC condition, there was a sudden increase of GL activities when approaching the 10 s point, before a protrude peak was recorded. Although the three muscles showed almost similar frequency of EMG signals in the first 10 s of EC condition, it should be highlighted that the %MVC values produced were greater compared in the EO condition for the two muscles, PL (EO: 114.78%; EC: 143.49%) and TA (EO: 19.87%; EC: 24.5%). However, GL revealed a decreased %MVC in the EC condition (46.05%) than in the EO condition (57.81%).

The total average peak calculated during the SL stance in EC condition showed 319 peaks in PL, 68 peaks in GL and still no peak value with the above 70% of MVC in TA.

4 Discussion

SL stance is able to distinguish between the ones that have normal balance from those that have balance impairment. The balance performance was clearly discriminated in both EO and EC conditions when on the unstable platform. In this study, it can be seen that the total duration in maintaining the balance during EC were relatively less compared to in EO condition. Among the healthy participants, the regular sEMG activity observed can be used to reflect the muscle behaviours whilst on the perturbation-based platform. Our finding showed that higher sEMG amplitudes from the SL stance during EC. This indicated that the muscle were more active when visual information was eliminated. Kwon et al. [3] enlightened that diminished of visual information lead to greater reliance on proprioception. As a result, increased muscle activities were generated to compensate the deficit. The greater recruitment of PL and GL during EC may result from the strategy to maintain the line of gravity in the sagittal plane slightly anterior to the axis of rotation of the ankle [1].

With regards to the muscle physiology, PL contributes to the balance of ankle. Although there were contradictions on actual PL function especially during ankle sprain, peroneal muscles will react first in the reaction towards perturbation [13]. From this study, PL contracted initially during the SL stance regardless of the conditions and the muscles. Furthermore, PL, the evertor muscle demonstrated the highest level of activation followed by GL and TA in both EO and EC. This finding was consistent with a previous study by Jung et al. [10] that demonstrated the highest muscle activation of PL and GL during SL stance. Additionally, a study proposed that plantar flexion moment should be contributed by PL and GL muscles in maintaining balance [10]. This is in line with our finding as PL was activated primarily followed by GL and TA. However, there were contradictory findings related to the LAS individuals. Significant results correlated with PL and TA showed lower sEMG amplitudes on both stable and unstable platforms [9]. In this case, researchers concluded there were impairment or alteration in these muscles after the sprain [8]. As the ankle plantar flexor, GL should contract frequently to maintain the balance, but this was not observed in this study as GL and PL contributed equally. Nonetheless, the findings for TA was against the prior studies as the dorsiflexor muscles should respond equally as the other muscles surrounding the ankle joint [7]. Lower sEMG was observed in TA during EO and EC.

SL stance on unstable platform was better in increasing the muscle activity around the ankle. The results revealed higher sEMG activity of the muscles during the SL stance on the Lafayette stability platform. This is in line with the previous study [3] that proposed dynamic tasks with narrower base of support that creates additional neuromuscular demand eliciting to the higher sEMG activity. The Lafayette stability platform was designated to deviate in mediolateral direction. Thus, investigation of LAS participants using this platform may benefit the improvement of balance control mechanism through SL stance training. It is also suggested to consider PL as the targeted muscle during the rehabilitation regime particularly for LAS individuals.

We note that the sample size in this preliminary study was small whereby the outcomes may not be able to be generalized to the general population. The authors suggest for future verifications of the findings using larger sample size and wider range of participants. Furthermore, it is proposed to compare the muscle activities in both dominant and non-dominant legs in future studies.

5 Conclusion

In conclusion, greater muscle activity were observed during the SL stance in EC condition in PL and GL muscles, which indicates higher neuromuscular demand with the absence of visual information. PL muscle demonstrated greater level of activation among the ankle stabilizers muscles when being assessed on unstable platform. Further, the muscle quantification outcomes can serve as a benchmark to the other research works that deal with the analyzation of muscle activities.

Acknowledgements We acknowledge support by the grants from university (GPF007C-2019 and GPF026A-2019) in the design of the study, recruitment of participants, collection, analysis, and interpretation of data, and in writing the manuscript.

References

1. Ogaya, S., Okita, Y., Fuchioka, S.: Muscle contributions to center of mass excursion in ankle and hip strategies during forward body tilting. J. Biomech. **49**(14), 3381–3386 (2016)
2. Bansbach, H.M., Lovalekar, M.T., Abt, J.P., Rafferty, D., Yount, D., Sell, T.C.: Military personnel with self-reported ankle injuries do not demonstrate deficits in dynamic postural stability or landing kinematics. Clin. Biomech. **47**, 27–32 (2017)

3. Kwon, J.W., Nam, S.M., Koo, D.K.: Electromyographic analysis of ankle muscles in chronic ankle instability during sudden inversion according to visual information provision. Sports Orthop. Traumatol. 1–6 (2021)
4. Kobayashi, T., Gamada, K.: Lateral ankle sprain and chronic ankle instability. Foot Ankle Spec. **7**(4), 298–326 (2014)
5. Cimadoro, G., Paizis, C., Alberti, G., Babault, N.: Effects of different unstable supports on EMG activity and balance. Neurosci. Lett. **548**, 228–232 (2013)
6. Vigotsky, A.D., Halperin, I., Lehman, G.J., Trajano, G.S., Vieira, T.M.: Interpreting signal amplitudes in surface electromyography studies in sport and rehabilitation sciences. Front. Physiol. **8**(985) (2018)
7. Hirono, T., Ikezoe, T., Taniguchi, M., Yamagata, M., Miyakoshi, K.: Relationship between ankle plantar flexor force steadiness and postural stability on stable and unstable platforms. Eur. J. Appl. Physiol. (2020)
8. Ridder, R.D., Willems, T., Vanrenterghem, J., Roosen, P.: Influence of balance surface on ankle stabilizing muscle activity in subjects with chronic ankle instability. J. Rehabil. Med. **47**, 632–638 (2015)
9. Mineta, S., Inami, T., Mariano, R., Hirose, N.: High lateral plantar pressure is related to an increased tibialis anterior / fibularis longus activity ratio in patients with recurrent lateral ankle sprain. Open Access J. Sports Med. **8**, 123–131 (2017)
10. Jung, Y., Yi, C., Baek, Y., Son, J., Lim, O.: Comparison of functional exercises on lower limb and trunk muscle activation in people with chronic ankle instability. Int. J. Ther. Rehabil. **24**(10), 435–442 (2017)
11. Merletti, R., Rainoldi, A., Farina, D.: Surface electromyography for noninvasive characterization of muscle. Exerc. Sport Sci. Rev. **29**(1), 20–25 (2001)
12. Van Deun, S., Stappaerts, K., Levin, O., Janssens, L., Staes, F.: Stability of measurement outcomes for voluntary task performance in participants with chronic ankle instability and healthy participants. J. Athl. Train. **46**(4), 366–375 (2011)
13. Slevin, Z.M., Arnold, G.P., Wang, W., Abboud, R.J., Wang, W.: Immediate effect of kinesiology tape on ankle stability. BMJ Open Sport Exerc. Med. 1–6 (2020)

The Prevalence of Lower Limb Musculoskeletal Pain Symptoms During Stop and Go Driving

Navien Arul Raj, Juliana Usman, Saad Jawaid Khan, and Siew-Li Goh

Abstract The prevalence of musculoskeletal pain among drivers during stop and go driving can be regarded as a common public health predicament. The action of frequent and prolonged driving in traffic congestion were distinguished as the prime contributors towards the musculoskeletal problem among drivers. This study emphasised on the importance to comprehend the relationship of the contributors towards the occurrence of musculoskeletal pain. Three hundred and twenty (N = 320) drivers responded in this cross-sectional survey study aimed to investigate the widespread of musculoskeletal pain symptoms specifically the knee pain symptom experienced by drivers during congested driving conditions. However, only one hundred and eighty (N = 180) drivers frequently drive during peak time and in congested driving conditions. The 180 drivers were segregated as targeted drivers and were tested for the relationship of two variables (frequency and prolonged driving in traffic) towards the prevalence of knee pain. The findings showed that the targeted drivers have experienced foot pain (64.4%) and knee pain (51.1%) more commonly while driving in the tested condition. A Pearson Chi Square statistical test was used to analyse the association of frequent and prolonged driving variables towards the prevalence of drivers experiencing knee pain had showed statistically non-significant relationship. Thus, other contributing risk parameters should be necessarily investigated for their influence towards the prevalence of knee pain among drivers to minimize and prevent the musculoskeletal pain symptoms.

N. A. Raj · J. Usman (✉)
Department of Biomedical Engineering, Faculty of Engineering, Universiti Malaya, Kuala Lumpur, Malaysia
e-mail: juliana_78@um.edu.my

S. J. Khan
Department of Biomedical Engineering, Faculty of Engineering, Science, Technology, and Management, Ziauddin University, Karachi, Pakistan

S.-L. Goh
Sports and Exercise Medicine Research and Education Group, Faculty of Medicine, Universiti Malaya, Kuala Lumpur, Malaysia

J. Usman
Centre for Applied Biomechanics, Universiti Malaya, Kuala Lumpur, Malaysia

J. Usman et al. (eds.), *6th Kuala Lumpur International Conference on Biomedical Engineering 2021*, IFMBE Proceedings 86,
https://doi.org/10.1007/978-3-030-90724-2_34

Keywords Knee pain · Prolonged driving · Repetitive movement

1 Introduction

Musculoskeletal disorder inflicting ache and pain have become a widespread condition especially among drivers. The severity of the traffic congestion was believed to have contributed for the drivers to experience musculoskeletal pain as stated in Golinko et al. [1]. Prolonged and repetitive driving conditions caused from traffic congestion can be categorized among the prime factors in contributing towards the prevalence of musculoskeletal pain for drivers.

Musculoskeletal conditions related to the lower extremity such as low back pain, knee pain, thigh pain and foot pain has been associated to the prolonged driving duration as observed in Abledu et al., which compels the drivers' lower extremity to repeat similar movement [2]. Repetitive frequent movement during driving causes muscle inflammation as stated in Punnett et al. especially during stop and go condition which subsequently result in muscle fatigue and knee pain symptoms [3].

Driving duration of about 6 h was noted with knee pain as observed in Chen et al., but Abledu et al. observed that the driving duration over 10 h for the drivers to have experienced knee pain in their study [2, 4]. Hence, the prevalence of knee pain varied with drivers' demographics and the presence of other impacting factors during the stop and go movement.

The objective of this study was to investigate and understand the prevalence of lower limb's musculoskeletal pain symptoms among drivers during stop and go movement due to the frequent and prolonged driving conditions.

2 Methodology

2.1 Survey Recruitment Procedure and Statistical Design

This study was designed to be a cross-sectional study that utilized a random sampling survey technique. Invitation to participate in the survey were sent out through multiple social platforms where a link connected to a Google Drive Document upon clicked was shared. The survey has adopted some useful ideas from Nordic Musculoskeletal Questionnaire along with other necessary rubrics of questions relevant to driving conditions. This survey comprised of 28 structured questions which were divided into 5 different sections.

The survey has two inclusion criteria for the drivers to fulfil if intended to take part in the study. The drivers have to be minimum of 18 years old or more and possessed a valid driving license. Those who fulfils the criteria will be subsequently served with the guidelines and information regarding the survey. If they agreed with the particulars outlined, they will proceed for consenting section within the survey itself. Otherwise, if they disagree, they can immediately withdraw themself from the survey without any further notice or reasons given.

The obtained responses from the drivers were statistically analysed with Statistical Package for Social Science (SPSS) version 25 software using descriptive statistics Pearson's Chi Square test. The statistical analysis finds the variables' association separately towards the prevalence of knee pain. The null hypothesis set was the variables have no association ($p > 0.05$) with the drivers' experience of knee pain. The alternative hypothesis was set otherwise ($p < 0.05$) to the null hypothesis.

2.2 *Informed Consent and Ethical Endorsement*

Prior before taking part in the survey study, an online consent form was filled by the respondents. The participation of the respondents were entirely voluntary. All of them read, verified and consented before getting into the subsequent sections within the survey.

This study has research ethics approval from the University of Malaya Research Ethics Committee (UM.TNC2/UMREC-208). All the particulars of the respondents were stored, protected and held in utmost confidentiality by the researcher and principal researcher.

3 Results

3.1 *Demographics*

A total of 320 drivers responded to the invitation for participation through multiple social media platforms. However, selective segregation was done to identify the targeted drivers by only choosing the drivers who ought to drive during peak time amidst the congested road conditions. The total targeted drivers chosen was 180 (56.3%) as depicted in Table 1 together with other demographics information.

Table 1 The demographics of the drivers responded to the survey (M: male and F: female)

	Total sample size, n = 320 (mean ± SD)	Targeted drivers, n = 180 (mean ± SD)
Genders	M:140; F:180	M:76; F:104
Weight (kg)	64.14 ± 14.30	64.23 ± 14.98
Height (m)	1.63 ± 0.09	1.63 ± 0.10
BMI (kg/m^2)	24.13 ± 5.20	24.15 ± 5.57

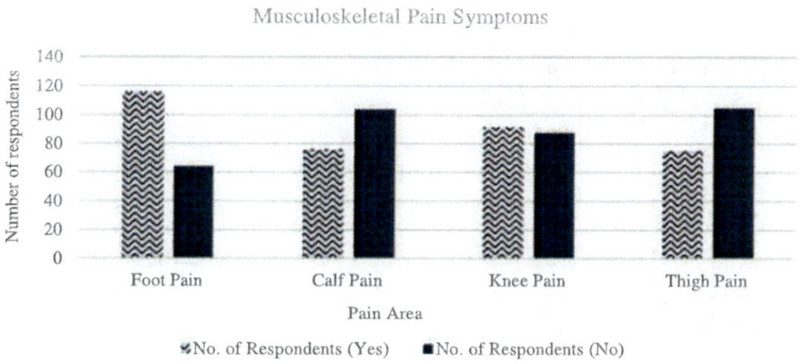

Fig. 1 The pain symptoms experienced by targeted drivers in traffic congestion

The average BMI for both the drivers' groups lied within normal range (18.5–24.9 kg/m^2) according to the guidelines suggested in Shafer et al. [5].

3.2 *Musculoskeletal Pain Symptoms*

The act of driving amidst congested road conditions often requires frequent prolonged stop and go movement that give rise to many pain symptoms. Referring to Fig. 1, the targeted drivers reported to have experienced musculoskeletal pain symptoms at different areas which included from thigh pain (41.7%) being the least experienced, followed with calf pain (42.2%), knee pain (51.1%) and foot pain (64.4%) being the most typical pain symptom experienced. Nevertheless, some studies reported the commonness of drivers who experienced knee pain and thigh pain were more compared to the other musculoskeletal pain symptoms [2, 4, 6].

3.3 *Analytics of Variables*

The frequency and period of targeted drivers stuck amidst congested road conditions were considered as the variables which may have contributed towards the prevalence of musculoskeletal pain. This study focussed on the prevalence of knee pain experienced among the targeted drivers. From 180 targeted drivers reported to be stuck amidst congested road conditions, 48.3% drivers as the majority reported to have stuck a few times per week meanwhile 25.0% drivers reported to have stuck every day.

As for the period of stuck, 56.7% drivers as the majority reported to have stuck for less than an hour whereas 39.4% drivers reported to have stuck for at least 1–2 h in traffic congestion. Hence, Pearson's Chi Square statistical test was carried out to test the relationship of both the variables separately with the experience of musculoskeletal pain among the targeted drivers. Despite the amount of targeted drivers' responses on the frequency, period and experience of knee pain amidst congested road conditions were moderately high, however the analysis revealed that the variables were statistically not significant ($p > 0.05$) towards the experience of knee pain among the targeted drivers.

4 Discussion

This self-administered survey study was carried out via Google Document in which the link to participate the survey was shared online through various social media tools. The aim of this study was to report the different musculoskeletal pain symptoms been experienced by targeted drivers, besides evaluating the relationship of frequent and prolonged driving amidst congested road conditions towards drivers' experience of knee pain. Hennessy et al. submitted that the prolonged and repetitive movement factors arise from traffic congestion could affect drivers' physiological health [7].

The targeted drivers were selected as they ought to drive during peak time amidst the congested road conditions that will force their lower extremity to undergo prolonged repetitive movement. Such prolonged repetitive movement can make the drivers susceptible of acquiring musculoskeletal pain. Previous studies have identified the repercussion of driving towards the development of musculoskeletal conditions such as of lower and upper extremity pain [2, 4, 8]. For this study, since we focussed on the knee pain, the symptoms can be in the form of ache or numbness when the patellar was engaged with prolonged repeated movement activity.

Despite 48.3% of the targeted drivers responded to have stuck a few times per week and 25.0% of them to have stuck every day, the statistical analysis revealed no significant relationship between frequency variable and drivers experiencing knee pain from traffic congestion. Nevertheless, Zhang et al. discussed the possibility of negative effects faced by drivers due to frequent fatigue driving amidst congested road conditions [9].

Similarly, 56.7% of the targeted drivers responded to have stuck for less than an hour and 39.4% of them to have stuck in between 1 and 2 h, the statistical analysis revealed no significant relationship between the period and drivers experiencing knee pain from the traffic congestion as well. However, Gyi and Porter uttered drivers tend to experience more musculoskeletal pain with more time taken for their journey [10].

In contrary to our expectation, both variables investigated showed no significant relationship with knee pain and this could be due to the consideration of only selecting targeted drivers for the analysis. However, this selection was regarded crucial as to specifically evaluate the repercussion of frequent prolonged stop go movement with respect to knee pain from congested driving condition. Different parameters that were not included such as loading forces, posture and fatigue might have contributed towards the knee pain symptoms among the targeted drivers.

5 Conclusion

This survey study portrayed the prevalence of musculoskeletal pain symptoms experienced by drivers who ought to engage in prolonged frequent stop and go movement. Consequently, the prolonged and period variables were statistically tested for knee pain prevalence among the targeted drivers. The outcome suggested the urgency to investigate other contributing driving risk variables to potentially minimize and prevent musculoskeletal pain among drivers.

Acknowledgements This study received financial support from the Malaysian Ministry of Higher Education's Fundamental Research Grant Scheme (FRGS No: FP130-2019A) and the Universiti Malaya's Faculty Research Grant (RF009A-2018).

Conflict of Interest The authors hereby believe and declare there is no any conflict of interest from this work.

References

1. Golinko, V., Cheberyachko, S., Deryugin, O., Tretyak, O., Dusmatova, O.: Assessment of the risks of occupational diseases of the passenger bus drivers. Saf. Health Work (2020). https://doi.org/10.1016/j.shaw.2020.07.005
2. Abledu, J.K., Offei, E.B., Abledu, G.K.: Occupational and personal determinants of musculoskeletal disorders among urban taxi drivers in Ghana. Int. Sch. Res. Not. (2014). https://doi.org/10.1155/2014/517259
3. Punnett, L., Wegman, D.H.: Work-related musculoskeletal disorders: the epidemiologic evidence and the debate. J. Electromyogr. Kinesiol. (2004). https://doi.org/10.1016/j.jelekin.2003.09.015
4. Chen, J.C., Dennerlein, J.T., Shih, T.S., Chen, C.J., Cheng, Y., Chang, W.P., Ryan, L.M., Christiani, D.C.: Knee pain and driving duration: a secondary analysis of the taxi drivers' health study. Am. J. Public Health (2004). https://doi.org/10.2105/AJPH.94.4.575
5. Shafer, K.J., Siders, W.A., Johnson, L.A.K., Lukaski, H.C.: Validity of segmental multiple-frequency bioelectrical impedance analysis to estimate body composition of adults across a range of body mass indexes. Nutrition (2009). https://doi.org/10.1016/j.nut.2008.07.004
6. Torén, A., Öberg, K., Lembke, B., Enlund, K., Rask-Andersen, A.: Tractor-driving hours and their relation to self-reported low-back and hip symptoms. Appl. Ergon. (2002). https://doi.org/10.1016/S0003-6870(01)00061-8
7. Hennessy, D.A., Wiesenthal, D.L.: Traffic congestion, driver stress, and driver aggression. Aggressive Behav. (1999). https://doi.org/10.1002/(SICI)1098-2337(1999)25:6%3c409::AID-AB2%3e3.0.CO;2-0
8. Kuijer, P.P.F.M., Van Der Beek, A.J., Van Dieën, J.H., Visser, B., Frings-Dresen, M.H.W.: Effect of job rotation on need for recovery, musculoskeletal complaints, and sick leave due to musculoskeletal complaints: a prospective study among refuse collectors. Am. J. Ind. Med. (2005). https://doi.org/10.1002/ajim.20159
9. Zhang, G., Yau, K.K.W., Zhang, X., Li, Y.: Traffic accidents involving fatigue driving and their extent of casualties. Accid. Anal. Prev. (2016). https://doi.org/10.1016/j.aap.2015.10.033
10. Gyi, D.E., Porter, J.M.: Musculoskeletal problems and driving in police officers. Occup. Med. (1998). https://doi.org/10.1093/occmed/48.3.153

The Effect of Physical Non-operative Modalities on Pain in Osteoarthritis of the Knee

Salma Mohamed Saad, Nor Hazwani Ibrahim, Anusha Nair, Norita Mohd Zain, and Juliana Usman

Abstract Knee osteoarthritis (OA) is the most common cause of a painful joint. To date, the main goals for knee OA therapies include relieving pain and maintaining the functional status. Transcutaneous electrical nerve stimulation (TENS) is proven to be effective for knee OA pain relief. It operates by transferring electrical pulses through the skin along the nerve fibers to help in relieving the pain in arthritis. However, some problems affect the conventional TENS performance such as electrode positioning, comfortability, and hygiene. An intervention called GNEEZAP was fabricated to solve these problems by having properties such as fixed electrodes points and the ability to be washed. Elastic knee sleeves help in relieving the knee OA symptoms by providing compression to increase blood flow and reduce pain and swelling. It is a cost-effective and easy solution. However, it is more effective when combined with other treatments. Previous researches indicated that improved proprioception and less pain can be achieved when electrical stimulation is combined with knee sleeves. Many physical functioning and performance tests, such as range-of-motion and strength, have been used as a proxy for objective pain measurement. This study aims to compare the efficacy of combined knee-sleeve and GNEEZAP TENS (intervention group) versus knee sleeve and traditional TENS (control group) in alleviating pain among knee OA patients using performance-based pre-post treatment tests on 18 patients divided into two groups. The research instruments include Stair Climbing Test, TUG Test, and 6MWT. At the end of this study, a comparison between both treatment combinations was done. The results indicated that both treatment combinations improve the knee OA patients' pain condition. However, the GNEEZAP TENS and knee sleeve combination was proven to have a larger effect than the traditional

S. M. Saad · N. H. Ibrahim · N. Mohd Zain · J. Usman (✉)
Department of Biomedical Engineering, Faculty of Engineering, Universiti Malaya, Kuala Lumpur, Malaysia
e-mail: juliana_78@um.edu.my

A. Nair
Nalika Ventures Sdn Bhd, Kuala Lumpur, Malaysia

J. Usman
Centre for Applied Biomechanics, Universiti Malaya, Kuala Lumpur, Malaysia

J. Usman et al. (eds.), *6th Kuala Lumpur International Conference on Biomedical Engineering 2021*, IFMBE Proceedings 86,
https://doi.org/10.1007/978-3-030-90724-2_35

TENS and knee sleeve combination since the difference in performance before and after treatment was much larger.

Keywords Knee osteoarthritis · TENS · GNEEZAP · Knee sleeve

1 Introduction

1.1 Knee Osteoarthritis

OA is the most common reason for physical disability in the elderly. Knee OA is a degenerative type of arthritis that occurs in the knee. It causes pain to the knee joint, in addition to functional disability and stiffness. Currently, there is no cure for this disease. Therefore, treatment strategies mainly focus on reducing pain in addition to preventing symptoms progression.

1.2 Knee Osteoarthritis Pain Management and Monitoring

Previous researches proved the effectiveness of TENS in improving knee OA patients' condition since it decreases the pain resulted from knee OA [2]. However, several factors affect TENS performance such as the accuracy of electrode positioning since the TENS effect decreases if an electrode is placed inaccurately. Moreover, there are hygiene problems associated with the conventional electrodes since they can be repeatedly used but can't be washed [6]. In addition to the fact that they are prone to fragmentation and uncomfortable due to their stickiness [9].

GNEEZAP (Patent number: 2018704119) is a therapeutic wearable device used as a replacement for conventional electrodes. It was fabricated to solve the conventional electrodes problems since it has fixed electrode points so it can be used easily without positioning confusions for the patients, it is reusable, and can be washed.

The knee sleeve can help in reducing the pain associated with knee OA and improving the patients' performance [13]. It is a cheap and easy solution compared to other knee OA treatments. Therefore, most people with knee problems prefer it. However, more pain relief will be achieved by combining it with other treatments. Some researches indicated that improved proprioception can be achieved when electrical stimulation is combined with knee sleeve [4].

Performance measures provide assessments of pain and function in people with knee OA [18]. The knee OA pain progression can be assessed by the performance-based tests (functional tests) since the patient's performance is improved when the pressure-pain threshold (PPT) increases [10].

1.3 Main Aim and Objectives

This research aims to assess the efficiency of physical non-operative modalities in knee OA pain management in order to derive the most effective intervention combination for reducing knee OA pain. The main objective of this study is to evaluate and compare the efficacy of combined knee-sleeve and GNEEZAP versus knee sleeve and traditional TENS in alleviating pain among knee OA patients using performance-based tests.

2 Methodology

2.1 Study Design

This is a pilot study; it was carried out in Clinic Genga since all the subjects were patients who came for treatment there. Before conducting the experiment, physical examinations (blood pressure, blood sugar level, and knee examination) were performed by a physician, and information about the patient's knee pain history was recorded, to ensure that the patients could be included in the study. Following this, the patients underwent a radiographic evaluation by doing an X-ray on their knee to identify the stages of knee OA.

Inclusion and Exclusion Criteria

The inclusion criteria involve Participants with knee OA fulfilling the ACR clinical criteria, with age between 50 and 75 and knee OA of stage 2 or 3 (according to KL grade), who haven't received TENS treatment before. The exclusion criteria include patients with a contraindication for TENS such as on pacemaker, open wound, or local skin lesion, and patients that had Previous knee surgery in the last six months, in addition to patients with severe medical or neurologic conditions.

Research Instruments

This experiment includes multiple treatment methods combined; the equipment used in this research are, a TENS machine, conventional electrodes (maintained with gel pads), GNEEZAP, and a pair of knee sleeves. The participants were randomly assigned to either intervention group—using TENS received by GNEEZAP, and knee sleeve, or control group—using TENS received by conventional electrodes, and knee sleeve. The TENS brand is Medichoice TENS-2000, with a frequency of 150 Hz and intensity that varies according to each patient preference. And the knee sleeve used is an open patella compressive knee sleeve; this type is chosen since it offers extra protection and stabilization to the knee.

2.2 Study Protocol

This experiment started by collecting information from subjects such as gender, age, weight, and height. Then the pre-treatment tests were conducted, which included the stairs climbing test, TUG test, and 6MWT. Patients were allowed to take a small rest between these tests.

The Osteoarthritis Research Society International (OARSI) is an organization that advocates the use of core outcome measures that assess the pain and function in people with OA. These three tests were used in this study because they are recommended by the OARSI to assess the knee OA patients' condition [5].

The first test was the Six Minute Walking Test; it was conducted by calculating the distance walked by the participants (at their own pace) in 6 min. Patients were permitted to slow down, stop, or even rest as necessary, but they were required to resume walking as soon as they were able to.

The Stairs Climbing Test required patients to climb up and down nine steps, where the time started from the point that the participant started ascending as fast as possible and stopped when the participant completed ascending and descending the nine steps for one time. The participants were allowed to use the handrail support.

The Timed Up and Go test required patients to be sitting on a chair in the beginning; when the time started, patients were required to stand up, walk as fast as possible till a mark on the ground which is 3 m away from the chair, then walk back to the chair and sit, the time stopped when the patient completely sat on the chair.

Next are the treatment sessions; the 18 patients were randomly divided into two groups where each group included nine patients. The first group of participants (Intervention) received treatment by TENS with the GNEEZAP device, and the second group of participants (control) received treatment by TENS with conventional electrodes. The treatment was carried out for one month, where two treatment sessions were conducted each week, and each treatment session lasted for 30 min (Fig. 1).

After all treatment sessions, the post-treatment tests were carried out; these tests had the same procedure as the pre-treatment tests, but all patients from both groups were required to wear a knee sleeve while conducting the tests. In the end, statistical analysis was done on the collected data using SPSS software, where a paired sample T-test was performed.

3 Results

3.1 Range of BMI of the Participants

The patients were randomly assigned to either intervention Group (using Tens received by GNEEZAP during the treatment, in addition to wearing a knee sleeve during the post-treatment tests) or control group (using Tens received by conventional electrodes during the treatment, in addition to wearing a knee sleeve during

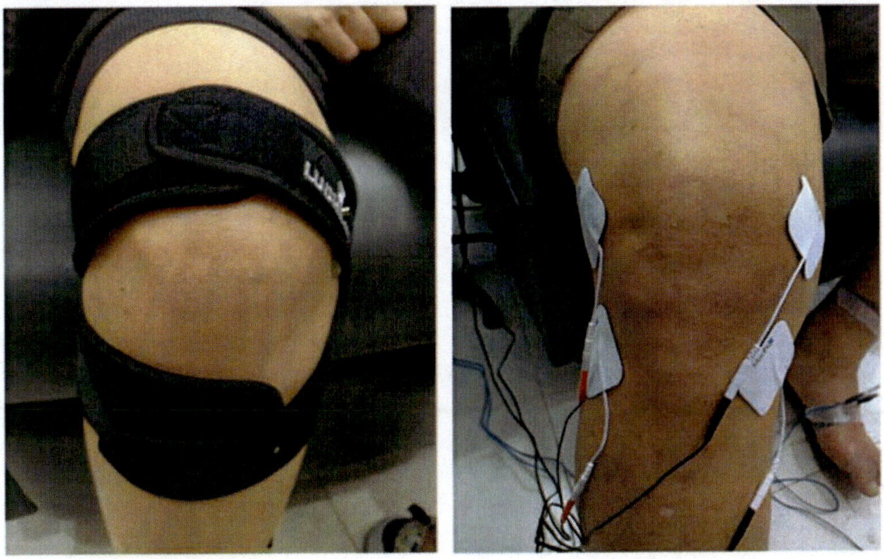

Fig. 1 GNEEZAP (left) versus conventional electrodes (right)

Table 1 Range of BMI of the participants

Range of BMI	No. of participants	
	Intervention group	Control group
< 18.5 (underweight)	0	0
18.5–24.9 (normal weight)	3	2
25.0–29.9 (overweight)	4	3
> 30.0 (obese)	2	4

the post-treatment tests). The BMI of the participants from each group is shown in Table 1.

This table indicates that most of the participants from each group were above the normal weight, where the intervention group encompassed four overweight participants and two obese participants, and the control group encompassed three overweight participants and four obese participants.

3.2 *Paired Sample T-Test*

A paired sample t-test was conducted to test whether the treatments combinations can improve the knee OA patients' condition. Data were collected both before and after the eight treatment sessions among the participants by the pre- and post-treatment

Table 2 Paired-samples T-test for 6MWT

Group	Pre-treatment		Post-treatment		*df*	t	Sig
	Mean	SD	Mean	SD			
Intervention group	242.17	40.5	280.33	37.7	8	3.0	0.016*
Control group	221.00	52.2	249.67	47.3	8	2.3	0.052*

tests where all patients were required to wear knee sleeves during the post-treatment tests.

6 Minute Walk Test

Table 2 shows the paired-sample t-test for 6MWT which compared the distance walked by the patients (in meters) for 6 min before and after all treatment sessions for both groups. The results denoted that the mean distance walked by the control group patients during the post-treatment 6MWT (M = 249.7, SD = 47.3) was significantly higher than the mean distance walked by them during the pre-treatment 6MWT (M = 221.0, SD = 52.2), t(8) = 2.28, $p = 0.052$. And that the mean distance walked by the intervention group patients during the post-treatment 6MWT (M = 280.3, SD = 37.7) was significantly higher than the mean distance walked by them during the pre-treatment 6MWT (M = 242.2, SD = 40.5), t(8) = 2.04, $p = 0.016$. Therefore, both treatments show effectiveness in improving the patients' condition since the patients walked a longer distance after the treatment. The results also showed that the difference between means of pre- and post-treatment test scores for the intervention group (38.17) is higher than the control group (28.67).

Stairs Climbing Test

The paired-sample t-test for the stairs climbing test compared the time taken (in seconds) by patients of both groups to climb up and down the stairs before and after all treatment sessions as shown in Table 3. The results indicated that the mean time taken by the control group patients during the post-treatment test (M = 11.8, SD = 2.36) was significantly lower than the mean time taken by them during the pre-treatment test (M = 15.1, SD = 3.61), t(8) = −4.25, $p = 0.003$. And that the mean time taken by the intervention group patients during the post-treatment test (M = 12.5, SD = 5.297) was significantly lower than the mean time taken by them during the pre-treatment test (M = 16.1, SD = 4.28), t(8) = −4.84, $p = 0.001$. Thus, the results support the conclusion that both treatments are effective in improving the

Table 3 Paired-samples T-test for stairs climbing test

Group	Pre-treatment		Post- treatment		*df*	t	Sig
	Mean	SD	Mean	SD			
Intervention group	16.06	4.3	12.49	5.3	8	4.8	0.001*
Control group	15.13	3.6	11.75	2.4	8	4.2	0.003*

Table 4 Paired-samples T-test for TUG test

Group	Pre-treatment		Post-treatment		*df*	t	Sig
	Mean	SD	Mean	SD			
Intervention group	9.85	1.1	7.56	0.8	8	6.5	0.000*
Control group	11.02	2.7	8.76	1.9	8	4.8	0.001*

patients' condition since the patients spent a shorter time conducting the test after treatment. The results also denoted that the difference between means of pre- and post-treatment test scores is slightly more in the intervention group (3.57) than the control (3.37) group.

Timed Up and Go test

Table 4 showed the paired-sample t-test for the TUG test that compared the time taken by patients of both groups to complete the test before and after all treatment sessions. The results elucidated that the mean time taken by the control group patients during the post-treatment test (M = 8.8, SD = 1.90) was significantly lower than mean time taken by them during the pre-treatment test (M = 11.0, SD = 2.67), t(8) $= -4.76, p = 0.001$. And that the mean time taken by the intervention group patients during the post-treatment test (M = 7.6, SD = 0.76) was significantly lower than mean time taken by them during the pre-treatment test (M = 9.9, SD = 1.06), t(8) = $-6.54, p = 0.000$. This proves the effectiveness of both interventions. It is also seen in the tables that the difference between means of pre- and post-treatment test scores is slightly more in the intervention group (2.29) than the control group (2.26).

4 Discussion

This experiment aimed to compare the effectiveness of improving knee OA patients' pain condition by conventional TENS electrode versus GNEEZAP; in the state of wearing a knee sleeve.

The results section showed and compared the effectiveness of both treatment combinations by comparing the results of 18 patients before applying any treatment or wearing a knee sleeve, and after four weeks of treatment with all patients wearing a knee sleeve during the post-treatment tests, where the control group received electrical stimulation by conventional TENS electrodes and the intervention group received electrical stimulation by GNEEZAP.

The range of BMI of the participants listed in Table 1 supports the previous studies that indicated the presence of a link between overweight and the risk of knee osteoarthritis since 13 out of 18 patients were overweight. This occurs due to the increased weight that the body needs to withstand and results in a larger load and stress that could lead to the breakage of the hyaline cartilage [14].

Many physical functioning and performance tests, such as range-of-motion and strength, have been used as a proxy for objective pain measurement [7]. Such as the timed "Up and Go" test for osteoarthritis [18]. Where the outcomes of the functional tests indicate the pain felt during the performance.

The results displayed in Tables 2, 3, and 4 demonstrated that both treatment combinations improve the patients' pain condition, this was caused by an increase in the pressure pain threshold which occurred in the form of a reduction of time taken to perform the tests (during the TUG test and the stairs climbing test) and an increase of distance walked (during the 6MWT), where the pain felt by the patients while performing the functional tests decreased since their pain tolerance was improved.

Since the difference in results before and after treatment was larger in the intervention group than the control group, the GNEEZAP and knee sleeve combination is proven to have a larger effect than the traditional TENS and knee sleeve combination.

Some factors affected the functional test results, such as the patients' physical activity in addition to the knee condition and symptoms. Some patients do minimal physical activities in their daily life, a decreased physical activity will cause an increase in knee stiffness which will lead to worsening the knee OA case [15]. Moreover, the intensity of the clinical symptoms may differ from one patient to another [8]. For instance, some patients couldn't bend their knee properly; this affected their results in some tests that involved knee bending such as the stairs climbing test.

5 Conclusion

To sum up, this pre-post study aimed at evaluating and comparing the effects of two combinations of physical non-operative modalities in managing the knee OA pain condition. The objective of this study was to evaluate and compare the efficiency of GNEEZAP TENS combined with knee sleeves, and conventional TENS combined with knee sleeves.

The main objective of this study was achieved by carrying out the assessment methods mentioned in the methodology on 18 patients divided into two groups. The data presented in the results section indicated that both intervention combinations are effective in managing knee OA pain condition. Moreover, it stated that GNEEZAP and knee sleeve make a better combination in managing knee OA pain and improving the knee OA patient's condition.

Acknowledgements This study received financial support from the Malaysian Ministry of Higher Education's Fundamental Research Grant Scheme (FRGS No: FP130-2019A) and Universiti Malaya's Faculty Research Grant (RF009A-2018). GNEEZAP (Patent number: 2018704119) by Nalika Ventures Sdn Bhd.

Conflict of Interest The authors hereby believe and declare there is no any conflict of interest from this work.

References

1. Charlesworth, J., Fitzpatrick, J., Perera, N.K.P., Orchard, J.: Osteoarthritis—a systematic review of long-term safety implications for osteoarthritis of the knee. BMC Musculoskelet. Disord. **20**(1), 151 (2019). https://doi.org/10.1186/s12891-019-2525-0
2. Cherian, J.J., Harrison, P.E., Benjamin, S.A., Bhave, A., Harwin, S.F., Mont, M.A.: Do the effects of transcutaneous electrical nerve stimulation on knee osteoarthritis pain and function last? J. Knee Surg. **29**(06), 497–501 (2016)
3. Chuang, S.H., Huang, M.H., Chen, T.W., Weng, M.C., Liu, C.W., Chen, C.H.: Effect of knee sleeve on static and dynamic balance in patients with knee osteoarthritis. Kaohsiung J. Med. Sci. **23**(8), 405–411 (2007)
4. Collins, A., Blackburn, J.T., Olcott, C., Yu, B., Weinhold, P.: The impact of stochastic resonance electrical stimulation and knee sleeve on impulsive loading and muscle co-contraction during gait in knee osteoarthritis. Clin. Biomech. **26**(8), 853–858 (2011). https://doi.org/10.1016/j.clinbiomech.2011.04.011
5. Dobson, F., Hinman, R.S., Roos, E.M., Abbott, J.H., Stratford, P., Davis, A.M., Bennell, K.L.: OARSI recommended performance-based tests to assess physical function in people diagnosed with hip or knee osteoarthritis. Osteoarthr. Cartil. **21**(8), 1042–1052 (2013). https://doi.org/10.1016/j.joca.2013.05.002
6. Erdem, D., Yesilpinar, S., Senol, Y., Karadibak, D., Akkan, T.: Design of TENS electrodes using conductive yarn. Int. J. Cloth. Sci. Technol. **28**(3), 311–318 (2016). https://doi.org/10.1108/IJCST-03-2016-0030
7. Harding, V.R., de C Williams, A.C., Richardson, P.H., Nicholas, M.K., Jackson, J.L., Richardson, I.H., Pither, C.E.: The development of a battery of measures for assessing physical functioning of chronic pain patients. Pain **58**(3), 367–375 (1994)
8. Hsu, H., Siwiec, R.M.: Knee osteoarthritis. StatPearls Publishing, Treasure Island (FL)
9. Li, L., Man, W., Li, Y., Wan, K., Wan, S., Wong, K.: Design of intelligent garment with transcutaneous electrical nerve stimulation function based on the intarsia knitting technique. Text. Res. J. **80**, 279–286 (2010). https://doi.org/10.1177/0040517509105276
10. Liebano, R.E., Rakel, B., Vance, C.G.T., Walsh, D.M., Sluka, K.A.: An investigation of the development of analgesic tolerance to TENS in humans. PAIN **152**(2), 335–342 (2011). https://doi.org/10.1016/j.pain.2010.10.040
11. Lohmander, L.S., Gerhardsson de Verdier, M., Rollof, J., Nilsson, P.M., Engström, G.: Incidence of severe knee and hip osteoarthritis in relation to different measures of body mass: a population-based prospective cohort study. Ann. Rheum. Dis. **68**(4), 490 (2009). https://doi.org/10.1136/ard.2008.089748
12. Manninen, P., Riihimäki, H., Heliövaara, M., Mäkelä, P.: Overweight, gender and knee osteoarthritis. Int. J. Obes. Relat. Metab. Disord. **20**(6), 595–597 (1996)
13. Marino, K., Lee, R., Lee, P.: Effect of germanium-embedded knee sleeve on osteoarthritis of the knee. Orthop. J. Sports Med. **7**(10), 2325967119879124 (2019). https://doi.org/10.1177/2325967119879124
14. Mh, H.: Arthrosen. Georg Thieme Verlag (2002)
15. Michael, J.W.P., Schlüter-Brust, K.U., Eysel, P.: The epidemiology, etiology, diagnosis, and treatment of osteoarthritis of the knee. Deutsches Arzteblatt International **107**(9), 152–162 (2010). https://doi.org/10.3238/arztebl.2010.0152
16. Osiri, M., Welch, V., Brosseau, L., Shea, B., McGowan, J., Tugwell, P., Wells, G.: Transcutaneous electrical nerve stimulation for knee osteoarthritis (Cochrane review). Cochrane Database Syst. Rev. **4** (2000)
17. Schween, R., Gehring, D., Gollhofer, A.: Immediate effects of an elastic knee sleeve on frontal plane gait biomechanics in knee osteoarthritis. PLoS ONE **10**(1), e0115782 (2015). https://doi.org/10.1371/journal.pone.0115782
18. Stratford, P.W., Kennedy, D.M., Woodhouse, L.J.: Performance measures provide assessments of pain and function in people with advanced osteoarthritis of the hip or knee. Phys. Ther. **86**(11), 1489–1496 (2006)

Biosensors, Biosignals, and Biomedical Imaging

Infant-Wrap (*InfaWrap*) Device as Pediatric Technology Tool: The Heart Rate and SpO^2 Monitoring for Neonates

Mohd Hanafi Abdul Rahim, Mohd Azrul Hisham Mohd Adib, Mohamad Zairi Baharom, and Nur Hazreen Mohd Hasni

Abstract Today, advances in science and technology may contribute to the resolution of medical devices for pediatric. This research focused on the development of the *InfaWrap* device; a tool to monitor neonate's heart rate and SpO^2. *InfaWrap* is designed to help the clinicians and parents to observe the baby's heart rate and oxygen saturation. The *InfaWrap* device uses a pro mini Arduino as a microcontroller, a MAX30100 oximeter sensor to measure SpO^2 and heart rate, and an LM35 to measure body temperature. Besides, we focus on the design and convenience wear criteria, including design characteristics, and structures to ensure the device is lightweight and more comfortable. The proposed *InfaWrap* device embedded an advanced wireless network sensor system. The data will be appeared in the mobile application installed on the doctor's or parent's mobile phone via Bluetooth module. Overall, based on three different babies as a subject in this study, we obtained that the *InfaWrap* device accuracy results reach the average of 96% for SpO^2, 81 bpm for baby heart rate, and 36.4 °C for baby body temperature.

Keywords Neonates · Medical device · Mobile application · InfaWrap · Pediatrics · Oximeter

---

M. H. A. Rahim · M. A. H. M. Adib (✉)
Medical Engineering & Health Intervention Team (MedEHiT), Department of Mechanical Engineering, College of Engineering, Universiti Malaysia Pahang, 26300 Lebuhraya Tun Abdul Razak, Kuantan, Pahang, Malaysia
e-mail: azrul@ump.edu.my

M. Z. Baharom
Human Engineering Group (HEG), Faculty of Mechanical & Automotive Engineering Technology, Universiti Malaysia Pahang, 26600 Pekan, Pahang, Malaysia

N. H. M. Hasni
Human Family Health Unit Pahang State Health Department, Jalan IM 4, 25582 Bandar Indera Mahkota, Kuantan, Pahang, Malaysia

J. Usman et al. (eds.), *6th Kuala Lumpur International Conference on Biomedical Engineering 2021*, IFMBE Proceedings 86,
https://doi.org/10.1007/978-3-030-90724-2_36

1 Introduction

Newborns are monitored for oxygen saturation from the first life until six months of age because of its possible adverse effects on brain development [1–4]. The American Academy of Pediatrics (AAP) and the American Heart Association (AHA) in 2010 [5] determined the SpO^2 objectives for the first 10 min after birth, establishing the arterial oxygen saturation that a baby must-have in the first minutes after birth [5]. The SpO^2 objectives table has assisted in the assessment of recovery and in avoiding the unnecessary administration of oxygen in newborns [5].

A study was performed in which 90% of babies with congenital cyanotic heart disease [6, 7] were detected using a pulse oximeter for use of screening within a few hours of birth. According to the evidence, infants with cyanotic heart disease is a critical sudden infant death syndrome (SIDS) may also be linked genetically to congenital coronary cyanotic diseases. It may be difficult to identify the major causes of SIDS [8, 9] most parents are making an extraordinary effort for their baby's health. By using the wireless healthcare technology, People who use sensing devices can move freely openly without being hindered by complicated wires [10, 11], and doctors at a remote care center can keep a close watch on the patient's health and thus offer patient recovery advice and long-term care in real time [12, 13].

This paper discusses the intelligent baby wrap model framework, *InfaWrap*, developed together with an accuracy test. One of the special aspects of the *InfaWrap* device features uses a wireless sensor to reduce clinicians and parents' load. This system is assembled and bundled in a compact, micro and Android smartphone using Bluetooth connectivity. This device is often fitted with battery charging cards, so that it can be refilled without changing the battery once the power runs out. It is easy to use this measurement device by connecting one of the foot sole to the specified sensor, then the three parameters of the scale would conveniently show on the LCD and Android mobile.

2 Methodology

2.1 Design Specification

The *InfaWrap* prototypes were designed using SolidWorks 2019 software and then shaped directly using 3D printing technology. For convenient wear of the *InfaWrap* device, the structure's design consequently had to be smaller, more comfortable to wear, and user-friendly. *InfaWrap* device is designed to monitor SpO^2, heart rate, and neonatal temperature through a cable-free wrapping concept.

This device is designed to have a small screen to prevent too many electronic parts inside the device. *InfaWrap* device is so lightweight with maximum total weight is 44.36 g. Figure 1 shows the final product of the *InfaWrap* device. By using the

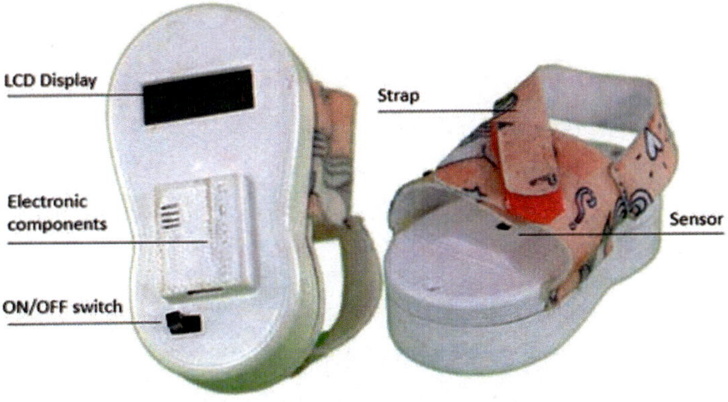

Fig. 1 Final product of *InfaWrap* device

Arduino board, all the measured values were monitored, analyzed, and displayed on the LCD screen. The results will be sent to an android application.

2.2 Device Components

Two sensors were used to measure three different conditions using this device. Figure 2 shows the complete system and electronic components of *InfaWrap*. The Arduino microcontroller is utilized to control the whole system. The SpO^2 and heart rate are measured using the MAX30100 sensor. Meanwhile, for LM35 sensor is used to measure of temperature [14, 15]. The HC-05 Bluetooth module is used to transfers measurement data from device to MyI-Wrap application or mobile app.

Figure 3b shows the development of the MyI-Wrap mobile app, which allows parents or doctors to monitor their baby's health status from anywhere, in a quick

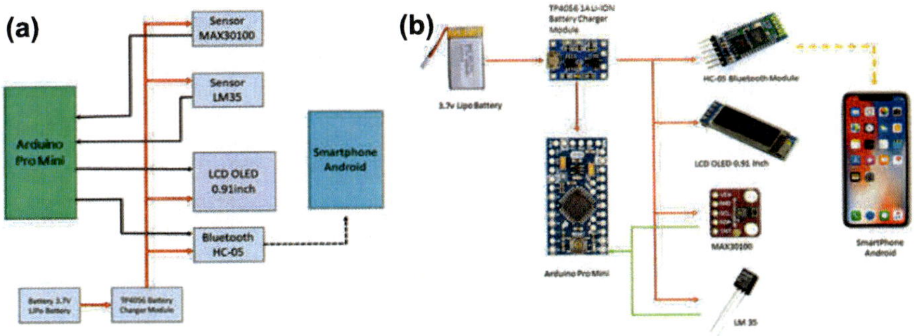

Fig. 2 Represented the; **a** block diagram of system; and **b** the electronic components of the *InfaWrap* device

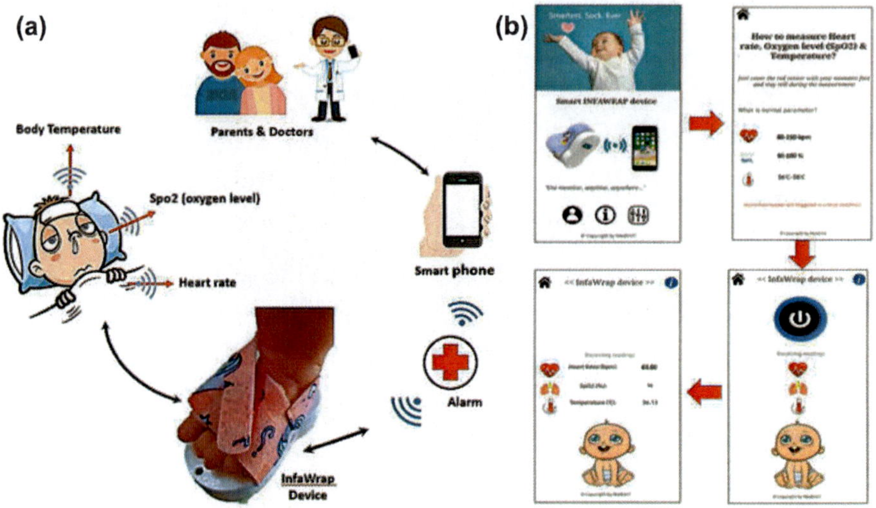

Fig. 3 **a** *InfaWrap* working; **b** *My*I-Wrap mobile application

and efficient manner. This software is available free through Google Play. Parents may also monitor their children's health while they sleep with this MyI-Wrap. As illustrated in Fig. 3a, the monitoring process is split into two steps; (1) data from the sensor was gathered; (2) data will be shown on the device and mobile phone via Bluetooth connection [16].

3 Results and Discussions

The *InfaWrap* device is specifically designed for newborns to assist clinicians and parents in monitoring their baby's heart rate, SpO^2 and temperature. Besides, this device needs several criteria requirements, such as small [17], light-weight, ergonomics, and low power consumption (or long battery life) that shows in Fig. 4. This section discusses the functionality of the *InfaWrap* device [18], standard operation how to wear the *InfaWrap*, and the sensor's accuracy based on three participants with differences in demographic data [19].

3.1 Accuracy Test

The participants involved in this study were two baby girls and one baby boy. All of them are the Malaysian citizens. The participants were volunteer for their contribution. Details about the participants as shows in Table 1.

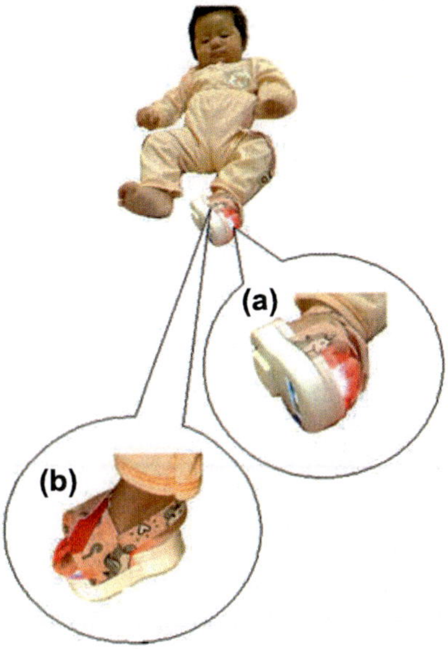

Fig. 4 The process of wearing the *InfaWrap* device to the baby; **a** bottom view with LDC monitor; and **b** top view wrapping or attach the device on baby foot sole

Table 1 Demographics information

Criteria	Subject 1	Subject 2	Subject 1
Gender	Female	Female	Male
Age (days)	97	102	91
Height (cm)	56.2	55.1	58.2
Weight (kg)	6.3	5.4	5.8

A reliability test is conducted to measure the *InfaWrap* device performances by repeated the measurement in 10 times. Table 2 shows the heart rate values obtained in 10 min' duration. Figure 5 clearly shows the trend of heart rate in 10 min reading. In the starting evaluation, subject 3 shows higher in heart rate. This is due to the situation where this baby a bit afraid and he cried during wearing the *InfaWrap* device.

Table 3 shows the SpO^2 of the babies in 10-time reading. Figure 6 shows the normal percentage of the SpO^2 for the baby is around 98–100%. We observed the trend of the SpO^2 for the three babies are good and acceptable which is around 97–99% [20]. For the resuscitation, stabilization and continuing treatment of the extremely low birth weight baby the optimum oxygen saturation values remain mostly undefined. We examined existing evidence for the usage of clinical oxygen in newborns. Median SpO^2 in babies delivered vaginally was 3% greater than for those born in the first 10 min of life in the previous research than in infants born with cesarean delivery.

Table 2 Heart rate reading in 10 min

Time (s)	Heart rate (bpm)		
	Subject 1	Subject 2	Subject 3
60	80	80	91
120	79	79	83
180	81	81	81
240	84	83	84
300	82	84	82
360	85	85	85
420	83	83	86
480	79	78	85
540	80	80	80
600	79	75	81

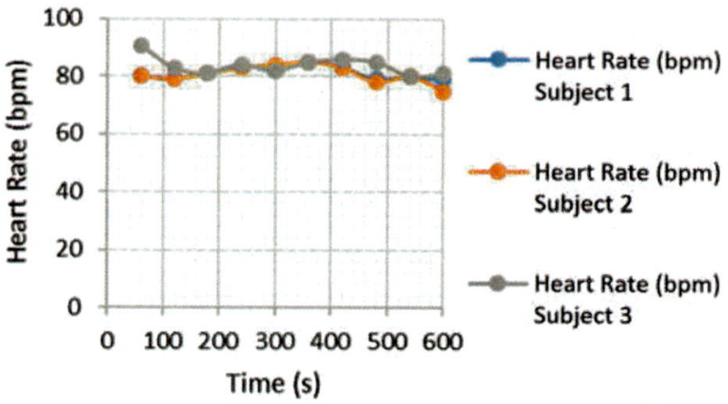

Fig. 5 Trend of the heart rate on difference participants. The values obtained in the morning session

Table 3 SpO^2 reading in 10 min

Time (s)	SpO^2 (%)		
	Subject 1	Subject 2	Subject 3
60	97	98	98
120	97	98	99
180	96	97	97
240	96	96	98
300	97	96	97
360	98	96	98
420	98	97	98
480	98	97	99
540	98	98	98
600	98	98	98

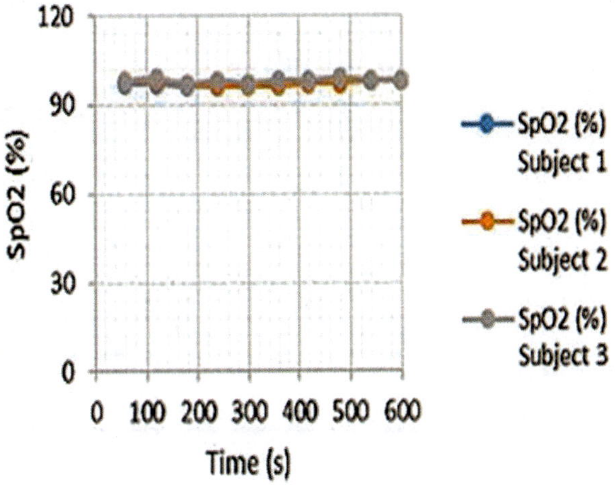

Fig. 6 Trend of the SpO^2 on difference participants. The values obtained in the morning session

Term infants had considerably greater saturation and saturation than preterm infants amounted to 90% quicker namely 4.7 min versus 6.5 min.

Table 4 shows the temperature level of the baby. Temperature is essentially important to know the condition of the baby especially during daily activities. Figure 7 shows the three babies' healthy condition without fever. The temperature value also presented good in detected the baby body temperature. A normal temperature for your baby is defined as a rectal reading between 36.5 and 37.0 °C; a temperature of 37.7 °C or higher is called a fever.

Table 4 Temperature reading in 10 min

Time (s)	Temperature (°C)		
	Subject 1	Subject 2	Subject 3
60	35	35	36
120	35	36	36
180	36	36	36
240	37	37	35
300	36	37	35
360	34	36	36
420	36	36	36
480	35	37	36
540	36	36	36
600	36	37	36
60	35	35	36
120	35	36	36

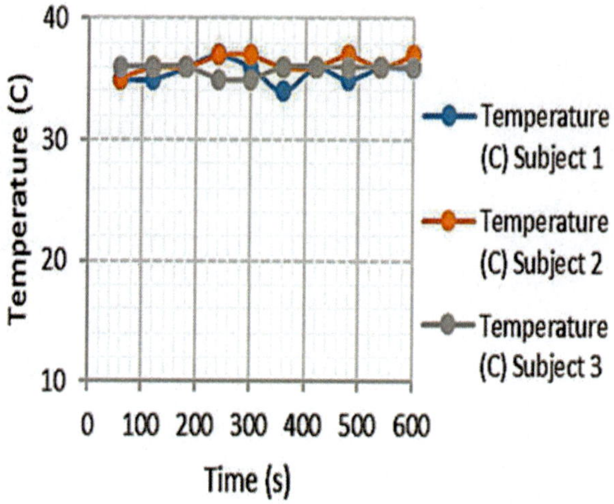

Fig. 7 Trend of the temperature on difference participants. The values obtained in the morning session

When a baby's temperature is abnormally high, it can indicate infection and it is better to meet a pediatrician, particularly if other symptoms such as a stuffy nose, sore throat, or cough continue. Based on the observation of the heart rate, SpO^2 and temperature values, the *InfaWrap* device's performance shows good and acceptable value especially in the accuracy of the data analysis.

4 Conclusion

This paper presented the product of the *InfaWrap* device that has successfully developed. The studies were focused on the functionality of the *InfaWrap* device, standard operation of wearing the *InfaWrap* device, and the sensor's accuracy based on three participants with differences in demographic data. The *InfaWrap* device is designed to monitor oxygen saturation SpO^2, heart rate, and temperature neonatal through a cable-free wrapping concept. Besides the measured value, it can analyze the health status for warning indicators are sent through mobile applications via Bluetooth to be stored and shared with the parents and clinicians. Besides, the *InfaWrap* device also has been developed to provide patients with the necessary support.

Acknowledgements Thank you to Universiti Malaysia Pahang (UMP) and Medical Engineering & Health Intervention Team (MedEHiT) for providing us with excellent facilities to complete these research activities under grant PDU203205 and PGR2003200.

References

1. Saugstad, O.: Oxygen saturations immediately after birth. J. Pediatr. **148**, 569–570 (2006)
2. Dawson, J.A., Davis, P.G., O'Donnell, C.F., Kamlin, C.O., Morley, C.J.: Pulse oximetry for monitoring infants in the delivery room: a review. Arch. Dis. Child Fetal Neonatal Ed. **92**, F4–F7 (2007)
3. Kamlin, O., Colm, P., O'Donnell, C., Davis, P.G., Morley, C.J.: Oxygen saturation in healthy infants immediately after birth. J. Pediatr. **148**, 585–589 (2006)
4. Toth, B., Becker, A., Seelbach-Gobel, B.: Oxygen saturation in healthy newborn infants immediately after birth measured by pulse oximetry. Arch. Gynecol. Obstet. **266**, 105–107 (2002)
5. Kattwinkel, J., Perlmann, J.M., Aziz, K.: Neonatal "Resuscitation 2010 American Heart Association Guidelines for Cardiopulmonary Resuscitation and Emergency Cardiovascular Care. Circulation **122**, S909–S919 (2010)
6. Limaye, D.: Development of medical devices. Curr. Ther. Res. **78**, S9 (2016)
7. Mathur, N.B., Gupta, A., Kurien, S.: Pulse oximetry screening to detect cyanotic congenital heart disease in sick neonates in a neonatal intensive care unit. Indian Pediatr. **52**(9) (2015)
8. Jortveit, J., et al.: Sudden unexpected death in children with congenital heart defects. Eur. Heart J. **37**(7), 621–626 (2016). https://doi.org/10.1093/eurheartj/ehv478
9. Miladinia, M., Baraz, S., Nouri, E.M.: Sudden infant death syndrome: risk factors and the relationship between them. Int. J. Pediatr. **3**(6), 1103–1110 (2015)
10. Sola, A., et al.: Safe oxygen saturation targeting and monitoring in preterm infants: can we avoid hypoxia and hyperoxia? Acta Paediatr. Int. J. Paediatr. **103**(10), 1009–1018 (2014). https://doi.org/10.1111/apa.12692
11. Seifi, S., Khatony, A., Moradi, G., Abdi, A., Najafi, F.: Accuracy of pulse oximetry in detection of oxygen saturation in patients admitted to the intensive care unit of heart surgery: comparison of finger, toe, forehead and earlobe probes. BMC Nurs. 1–7 (2018)
12. Chen, B., Varkey, J.P., Pompili, D., Li, J.K., Marsic, I.: Patient vital signs monitoring using wireless body area networks. In: Proceedings of the 2010 IEEE 36th Annual Northeast Bioengineering Conference (NEBEC) 2010, April 2010. https://doi.org/10.1109/NEBC.2010.5458139
13. Ajith, S., Praveen, K., Ibrahim, S.I., Nagaraj, M.: Wireless monitoring of patients by IoT through pulse-OX & heart rate sensor. Int. J. Pure Appl. Math. **119**(15), 973–979 (2018)
14. Adib, M.A.H.M., Rashid, M.A.A., Hasni, N.H.M.: Development of smart Infant-Wrap (*InfaWrap*) device for neonates. Proc. Mech. Eng. Res. Day **2019**, 186–187 (2019)
15. Suprayitno, E.A., Marlianto, M.R., Mauliana, M.I.: Measurement device for detecting oxygen saturation in blood, heart rate, and temperature of human body. J. Phys. Conf. Ser. **1402**(3), 6 (2019). https://doi.org/10.1088/1742-6596/1402/3/033110
16. Nakib Ul Hasan, M., Negulescu, I.I.: Wearable technology for baby monitoring: a review. J. Text. Eng. Fash. Technol. **6**(4), 112–120 (2020). https://doi.org/10.15406/jteft.2020.06.00239
17. Rahim, M.H.A., Adib, M.A.H.M., Hasni, N.H.M.: The comprehensive study of product criteria on Infant-Wrap (*InfaWrap*) device: engineering perspective. J. Phys. Conf. Ser. **1529**(5) (2020). https://doi.org/10.1088/1742-6596/1529/5/052082
18. Dangerfield, M.I., Ward, K., Davidson, L., Adamian, M.: Initial experience and usage patterns with the owlet smart sock monitor in 47,495 newborns. Glob. Pediatr. Health **4**, 2333794X1774275 (2017). https://doi.org/10.1177/2333794x17742751
19. Rahim, M.H.A., Adib, M.A.H.M., Baharom, M.Z., Hasni, N.H.M.: Improving the Infant-Wrap (*InfaWrap*) device for neonates using *MyI-Wrap* mobile application. In: The 3rd Symposium on Intelligent Manufacturing & Mechatronics (SIMM 2020). The Lecture Notes in Mechanical Engineering (2020)
20. Rahim, M.H.A., Adib, M.A.H.M., Baharom, M.Z., Sahat, I.M., Hasni, N.H.M.: Non-invasive study: monitoring the heart rate and SpO2 of the new born using InfaWrap device. In: 2020 IEEE-EMBS Conference on Biomedical Engineering and Sciences (IECBES), 2021, pp. 212–217.https://doi.org/10.1109/IECBES48179.2021.9398749

Optimization and Performance Evaluation of Apodization Function for Fiber Bragg Grating as Vital Sign Sensor

Ramya Arumugam, Ramamoorthy Kumar, and Samiappan Dhanalakshmi

Abstract Sensing is the recent and most widely executed implementation of Fiber Bragg Grating (FBG). In this paper, a comprehensive investigation of various apodization functions based on Reflectivity, Maximum side lobe (MSL), Side lobe suppression ratio (SLSR), Full width Half maximum (FWHM), Sensitivity, Detection Accuracy and Quality parameter are evaluated and a novel apodization function was proposed which can be implemented in FBG to use it as vital sign sensor for measuring temperature and heart rate. The simulations were carried out for the grating parameters of L = 10 mm and $\Delta n = 0.0001$. From the results, peak reflectivity of −0.564754 dB was achieved in Uniform apodization function but it also has larger side lobe level and less sensitivity. The highest side lobe suppression ratio was achieved by Gaussian function which is −32.58601 dB. Based on the sensing characteristics, the proposed apodization function has lower FWHM of 0.06 nm and the highest sensitivity of 5.9698AU/RIU, thus having a better detection accuracy of 26,114. Higher sensitivity and narrow FWHM, leads to greater quality parameter of 99.49667 AU/nm-RIU which is a desirable characteristics of sensor. Also the proposed function proved to have better wavelength shift for the measurement of heart rate and temperature compared to other apodizations with 1.3 pm/$\mu\varepsilon$ and 13 pm/°C.

Keywords Apodization · Fiber Bragg grating · Optical sensor · Sensitivity · Strain · Temperature

R. Arumugam (✉) · R. Kumar · S. Dhanalakshmi
Department of Electronics and Communication Engineering, College of Engineering and Technology, SRM Institute of Science and Technology, SRM Nagar, Kancheepuram, Chengalpattu Dt., Tamil Nadu 603203, India
e-mail: ramyaa@srmist.edu.in

J. Usman et al. (eds.), *6th Kuala Lumpur International Conference on Biomedical Engineering 2021*, IFMBE Proceedings 86,
https://doi.org/10.1007/978-3-030-90724-2_37

1 Introduction

Fiber Bragg Gratings (FBGs) was first presented by Hill in 1978. These grating based sensors have advantages of smaller weight, linearity in output, immune to electromagnetic waves, robust in nature, enables remote sensing, small size, very stable, long durability, easy fabrication, easy installation, low maintenance etc. [1–3]. It is used widely used in photonics field such as lasers [4, 5], buffers [6], filters [7], multiplexers [8], sensing applications like structural health monitoring, medical field, aerospace based on strain and temperature [9]. FBG is an optical fiber with induced periodic variation of refractive index in the core region in the direction of fiber axis for a length called grating length. This periodic grating results in reflection of particular wavelength called as Bragg wavelength (λ_B). The modulation of index (Δn), length of the grating (L) and periodicity of the grating (Λ) determines and controls the optical characteristics of FBG [10–12].

The reflection spectrum of uniform FBG has main lobe corresponding to reflected wavelength along with many side lobes adjacent to it. For sensing applications, the presence of these side lobes interfere in detection of reflected peak, making it as undesirable characteristics. Applying proper truncating or apodization functions suppresses the side lobes in optical response of FBG. Many literatures [13–18], have proposed new apodization functions for enhancing the sensing characters, simultaneous measurements of temperature and strain, Dispersion compensation etc. These are achieved by narrow full width half maximum (FWHM), greater side lobe suppression ratio, better leakage factor, highest detection accuracy etc. In this work, we have proposed a novel apodization function for increasing the sensing characteristics such as sensitivity, detection accuracy and quality parameter to enable the application of FBG as vital sign sensor. We have considered two vital signs, heart rate (measured as strain) and temperature and proved the increase in wavelength shift in the sensing signal. In few literatures they have increased the sensitivity by using coating materials [21, 22]. The present work is organized as follows: Sect. 2 explains the theoretical formulation of FBG and various apodization profiles and in Sect. 3, the results obtained are analysed and discussed. It is followed by the conclusion and references.

2 Background and Theory

2.1 Fiber Bragg Grating

The schematic of the principle of operation of the FBG with uniform apodization is shown in Fig. 1. The periodic variation is along the fiber axis. The refractive index variation of the grating is given as [19]

$$n(z) = n_{core} + \Delta n \cos\left(\frac{2\pi z}{\Lambda}\right) \quad (1)$$

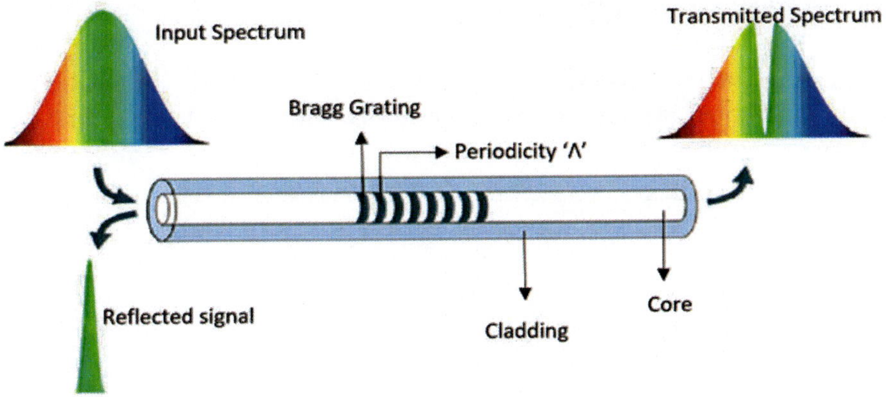

Fig. 1 Principle of fiber Bragg grating

where n_{core} is the refractive index of the core region and Δn is the refractive index modulation, Λ is the periodicity of the grating and z is the direction of propagation. The reflected Bragg wavelength is defined as

$$\lambda_B = 2n_{eff}\Lambda \quad (2)$$

n_{eff} is the effective refractive index of fiber core. The reflectivity of FBG is given as

$$R(L, \lambda_B) = \frac{k^2 \sinh^2(sL)}{\Delta\beta^2 \sinh^2(sL) + s^2 \cosh^2(sL)} \quad (3)$$

where k is the coupling coefficient, Δβ is the detuning wave vector and is given as β-Π/Λ and s2 = $k^2 - \beta^2$. The shift in Bragg wavelength due to strain and temperature is given as [20]

$$\Delta\lambda_B = \lambda_B(1 - p_e)\Delta\varepsilon \quad (4)$$

$$p_e = n[p_{11} - v_f(p_{11} + p_{12})]/2 \quad (5)$$

where p_e is the effective photoelastic coefficient and v_f is the poisson ratio.

$$\Delta\lambda_B = \lambda_B(\alpha_f + \alpha_n)\Delta T \quad (6)$$

where α_f is thermal expansion coefficient and α_n is thermo optic coefficient.

2.2 Apodization Profiles

Apodization index at various boundaries. It is one of the powerful methodology that reduces side lobes. Few such functions compared in this work are given below. The functions are chosed based on the literature [13–18].

1. Uniform Function

$$g(x) = 1 \quad \text{for } 0 \le x \le L \tag{7}$$

2. Gaussian Function

$$g(x) = \exp\left(-\ln\left(2\frac{2(x-(\frac{L}{2})}{0.5L}\right)^2\right) \quad \text{for } 0 \le x \le L \tag{8}$$

3. Bessel Function [15]

$$g(x) = J_0\left[\cos\left(\frac{3x}{L}\right)\right]^8\left[\cos\left(\frac{2x}{L}-1\right)\right]^4 \quad \text{for } 0 \le x \le L \tag{9}$$

4. Proposed Function

$$g(x) = J_0\left[\cos\left(\frac{2\Pi x}{L}\right)\right]^8\left[\cos\left(\frac{2x}{L-1}\right)\right]^4 \quad \text{for } 0 \le x \le L \tag{10}$$

J_0 is the Bessel function of first kind of zero order.

The performance of these apodization functions can be analyzed using parameters such as maximum side lobe (reflectivity level of dominating side lobe), Side lobe suppression ratio (Difference between peak reflectivity and MSL), Sensitivity, Detection Accuracy and Quality parameter [14].

$$\text{Sensitivity} = \frac{\text{Change in reflectivity of sensing signal}}{\partial \Delta n} \tag{11}$$

$$\text{Detection accuracy} = \frac{\text{wavelength of resonance peak}}{\text{FWHM}} \tag{12}$$

$$\text{Quality Parameter} = \frac{\text{Sensitivity}}{\text{FWHM}} \tag{13}$$

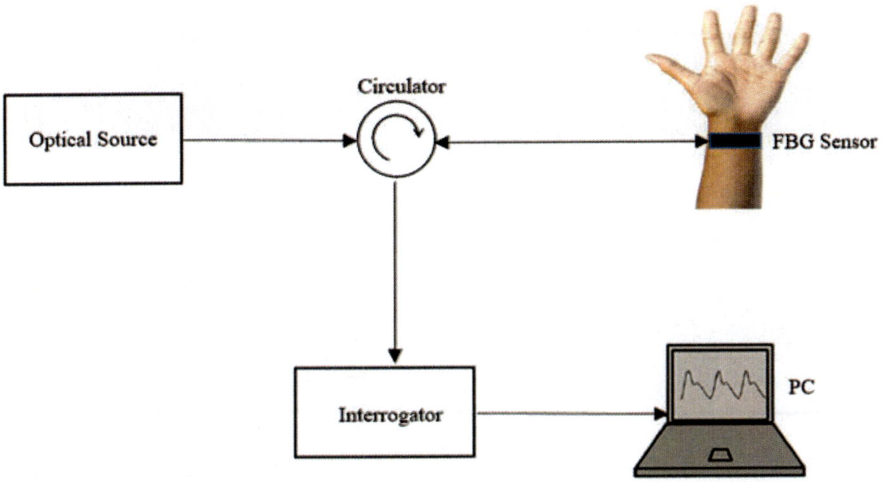

Fig. 2 Schematic diagram of sensor system

2.3 FBG Sensing System

The schematic of the FBG based vital sign monitoring sensor system is shown in Fig. 2. The main components are optical source, 3 port circulator, FBG sensor, Optical interrogator and data acquisition system. The sensor is placed in wrist using a medical self-adhesive tape. The reflected signal from the sensor positioned in the wrist is measured by FBG interrogator and PC. The applied strain and temperature introduces the wavelength shift in the peak resonance.

3 Results and Discussion

The comparison of the performance of various apodization functions are done by considering silica based single mode fiber with 1.46 as core refractive index and 1.45 as cladding refractive index. The designed wavelength is 1550 nm and the periodicity of the grating is 0.5380287 μm. The radius of core and cladding is taken as 4 μm and 8 μm respectively. For performance evaluation the grating length is varied from 5 to 15 mm and index change is varied from 1×10^{-4} to 2.5×10^{-4}. Simulations are performed using Optigrating software. Figure 3 shows the profile of various apodization considered and the proposed apodization function.

Figure 4 shows the change in peak reflectivity with respect to increasing grating length (keeping index change as 0.0001) and index change (keeping L = 10 mm). It shows that with increase in index modulation and grating length, the peak reflectivity of main lobe increases. But as a tradeoff reflectivity level of side lobe also increases. Table 1 shows the optical characteristics of various apodization. Gaussian

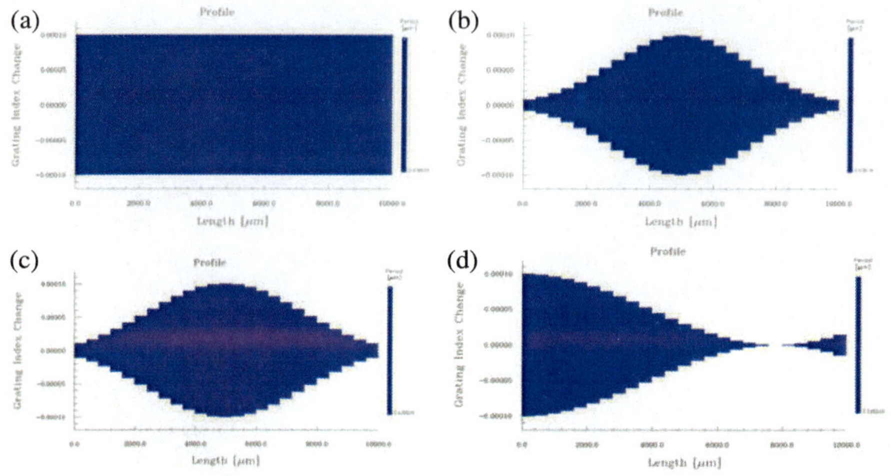

Fig. 3 Profile of various apodizations **a** uniform; **b** Gaussian; **c** Bessel; **d** proposed

and proposed function has the lowest full width half maximum of **0.06 nm** which determines the detection accuracy. Lower the FWHM, better the detection accuracy. The highest side lobe suppression of **−35.4861 dB** is provided by Gaussian and poorest is for uniform apodization **(−14.1033 dB)**. Proposed function has moderate side lobe level (**−22.5521 dB**) but it performs better in other aspects.

Table 2 shows the evaluation parameters such as sensitivity, Detection accuracy and Quality parameter. The proposed apodization function has highest sensitivity of **5.9698 AU/RIU** and lowest sensitivity of **1.6783 AU/RIU** is for Uniform apodization. Highest detection accuracy of **26,114** is achieved by Gaussian and proposed apodization function. Thus the optimized Bessel function has the highest quality parameter of **99.4967 AU/nm-RIU.** All the evaluations were carried out for L = 10 mm and $\Delta n = 0.0001$.

Figure 5a shows the wavelength shift for the applied strain in steps of 50 $\mu\varepsilon$. Better shift of 1.3 pm/$\mu\varepsilon$ was achieved with proposed apodization function when compared to other functions. Likewise Fig. 5b shows the variation in reflected wavelength corresponding to variation in temperature in steps of 10 °C. It is proved that the proposed function has better wavelength shift of 13 pm/°C when compared with other functions.

4 Conclusion

Apodization has the ability to suppress side lobes and control FWHM. Thus it is most significantly used to enhance performance of sensors. Apodization profile also improves the spectral response. The novel proposed apodization function is proved to have most desirable performance parameters to implement in the field of FBG as

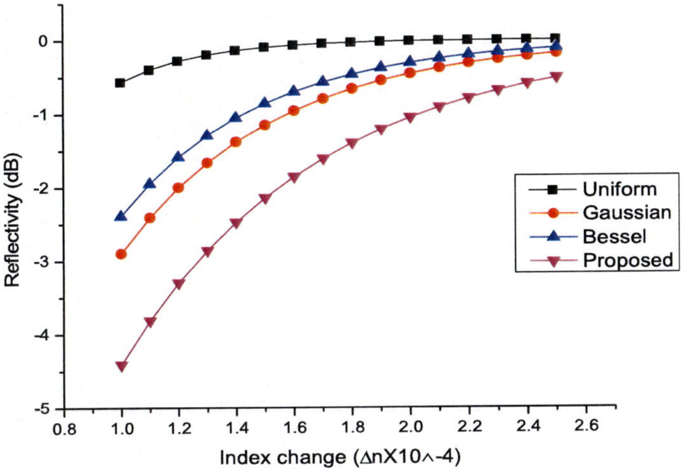

(a)

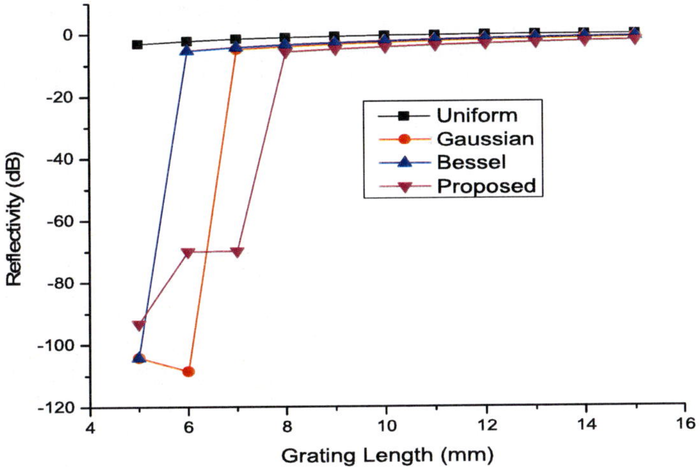

(b)

Fig. 4 Reflectivity level of mainlobe of various apodization for **a** change in index change; **b** change in grating length

Table 1 Optical characteristics of apodization profiles

Type of apodization	FWHM (nm)	Reflectivity (dB)	MSL (dB)	SLSR (dB)	Slope (dB/nm)
Uniform	0.12	−0.56475	−14.0133	−17.7356	−125.82
Gaussian	0.06	−2.90009	−35.4861	−32.5860	−67.4465
Bessel	0.12	−2.38807	−34.9419	−32.5538	186.9966
Proposed	0.06	−4.41083	−22.5521	−18.1413	15.5365

Table 2 Performance parameters of apodization profiles

Type of apodization	Sensitivity (AU/RIU)	Detection accuracy	Quality parameter (AU/nm-RIU)	Wavelength shift $(\Delta\lambda_B)/\mu\varepsilon$ (pm)	Wavelength shift $(\Delta\lambda_B)/°C$ (pm)
Uniform	1.6783	13,057	13.9858	1.2	12
Gaussian	4.8888	26,114	81.4667	1.2	12
Bessel	4.4017	13,057	36.6808	1.2	12
Proposed	5.9698	26,114	99.4967	1.3	13

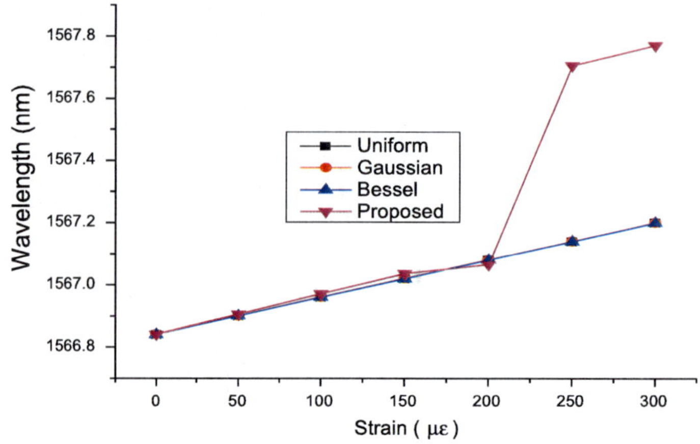

(a)

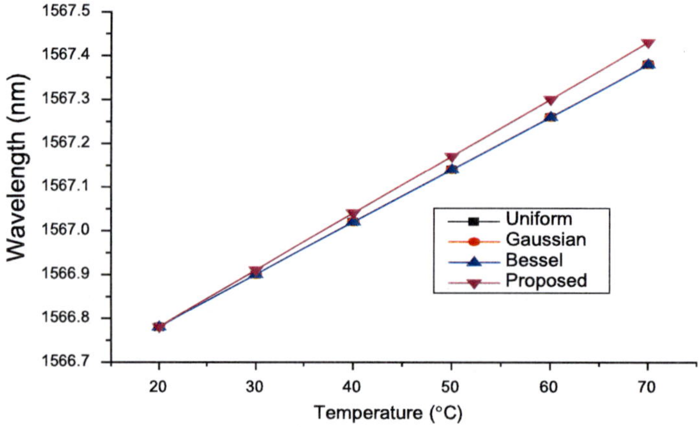

(b)

Fig. 5 Wavelength shift for **a** change in strain; **b** change in temperature sensors. It has smaller FWHM, highest sensitivity (5.9698 AU/RIU) and detection accuracy of 26,114 which makes it better choice for sensing applications in medical field. FBG based strain and temperature sensor with proposed apodization function, shows improvement in sensitivity as 1.3 pm/ $\mu\varepsilon$ and 13 pm/°C respectively.

References

1. R. Kashyap, Fiber Bragg Gratings, Academic (2010)
2. Othonos, A., Kalli, K.: Fiber Bragg Gratings: Fundamentals and Applications in Telecommunications and Sensing. Artech House (1999)
3. Nicolas, M.J., Sullivan, R.W., Richards, W.L.: Large scale applications using FBG sensors: determination of in-flight loads and shape of a composite aircraft wing. Aerospace **3**(3), 18 (2016)
4. Lecourt, J.-B., Duterte, C., Narbonneau, F., Kinet, D., Hernandez, Y., Giannone, D.: All-normal dispersion, all-fibered PM laser mode-locked by SESAM. Opt. Express **20**, 11918–11923 (2012)
5. Keshk, M.M., Ashry, I.A., Aly, M.H., Okaz, A.M.: Analysis of different fiber Bragg gratings for use in a multi-wavelength Erbium doped fiber laser. In: Proceedings of the IEEE Conference on Radio Science, Cairo, pp. 1–13 (2007)
6. Ashry, I., Shalaby, H.M.H.: All-optical variable delay buffer for next generation optical networks. In: Proceedings of the IEEE Conference on Transparent Optical Network, Munich, pp. 1–3 (2010)
7. Ashry, I., Shalaby, H.M.H.: Tunable Fabry-Perot interferometer based on fiber Bragg gratings. In: Proceedings of the IEEE Conference on Telecommunications (ICT), Doha, pp. 543–537 (2010)
8. Orr, P., Niewczas, P.: High-speed, solid state, interferometric, interrogator and multiplexer for fiber Bragg grating sensors. J. Lightwave Technol. **29**, 3387–3392 (2011)
9. Goncalves, A.F., Ferreira, L.A., Araujo, F.M.M., Mendes, P.M., Correia, J.H.: A smart skin PVC foil based on FBG sensors for monitoring strain and temperature. IEEE Trans. Ind. Electron. **58**, 2728–2735 (2011)
10. Yu, Q., Zhang, Y., Dong, Y., Li, Y.P., Wang, C., Chen, H.: Study on optical fiber Bragg grating temperature sensors for human body temperature monitoring. In: Symposium Photonics Optoelectron SOPO (2012)
11. Liu, L., Zhang, H., Zhao, Q., Liu, Y., Li, F.: Temperature independent FBG pressure sensor with high sensitivity. Opt. Fiber Technol. **13**, 78–80 (2007)
12. Campanella, C.E., Cuccovillo, A., Campanella, C., Yurt, A., Passaro, V.M.N.: Fibre Bragg grating based strain sensors: review of technology and applications. Sensors (2018)
13. Naguib, B.A., Ata, M.M., Alzalabani, M.M., Yousif, B.B.: Performance evaluation and enhancement of apodized fiber Bragg grating for dispersion compensation. AIP Adv. **11**, 015231 (2021)
14. Maiti, S., Singh, V.: Performance analysis of apodized fiber Bragg gratings for sensing applications. Silicon (2020)
15. Dwivedi, K.M., Trivedi, G., Khijwania, S.K.: Theoretical Study and Optimization of Apodized Fiber Bragg Grating for Single and Quasi-distributed Structural Health Monitoring Applications. IEEE Xplore (2020)
16. Mohammed, N.A., Ali, T.A., Aly, M.H.: Evaluation and performance enhancement for accurate FBG temperature sensor measurement with different apodization profiles in single and quasidistributed DWDM systems. Opt. Lasers Eng. **58**, 22–34 (2014)
17. Toba, M., Mustafa, F.M., Barakat, T.M.: New simulation and analysis fiber Bragg grating: narrow bandwidth without side lobes. J. Phys. Commun. (2019)

18. Ashik T.J., Kachare, N., Kalyani bai, K., Sriram Kumar, D.: Analysis of simultaneous measurement of temperature and strain using different combinations of FBG. AIP Conf. Proc. **1849**, 020031 (2017)
19. Ugale, S.P., Mishra, V.: Fiber Bragg grating modeling, characterization and optimization with different index profiles. Int. J. Eng. Sci. Technol. **2**, 4463–4468 (2010)
20. Shan-chao, J., Jing, W., Qing-mei, S., Qing-lin, Y., Li-jun, W.: Study of three-component FBG vibration sensor for simultaneous measurement of vibration, temperature, and verticality. J. Sens. (2015)
21. Chakravartula, V., Samiappan, D., Kumar, R.: Sensitivity enhancement analysis due to different coating materials of Fibre Bragg Grating-based depth sensor for underwater applications. Opt. Quantum Electron. **52**(1), 1–15 (2020)
22. Samiappan, D., Kesarikiran, A.V.S., Chakravartula, V.: Enhancing sensitivity of fiber Bragg grating-based temperature sensors through Teflon coating. Wirel. Pers. Commun. **110**, 593–604 (2020)

Analysis of Heart Rate and Heart Rate Variability for Stress Evaluation

Li Ann Lim, Jee Hou Ho, Jong Chern Lim, Einly Lim, and Bee Ting Chan

Abstract Heart rate (HR) and Heart rate variability (HRV) have been proposed as useful indicators for stress evaluation. The reliability and ultra-short-term analysis of these parameters require further investigation. This study aims to: (1) identify the reliable parameters for stress evaluation and (2) determine the surrogacy of ultra-short-term HR and HRV for conventional recording using the recommended standardised tests. Electrocardiograms (ECG) from the WESAD database consisting of 15 subjects were processed and analysed. Individual response to stress was evaluated. The reliability of ultra-short-term recording was examined by evaluating both the correlation and limits-of-agreement of ultra-short (1-min) and conventional short-term (5-min) recording. Our results showed that *mean RRi* and the *mean HR* were reliable in identifying stress condition. In the ultra-short-term analysis, most of the parameters showed significantly high correlation ($r > 0.7$, $p < 0.05$) with only the *mean RRi* and *mean HR* having good agreement ($PE < 30\%$) and were statistically consistent between the 1-min and 5-min recordings. In conclusion, the ultra-short *mean RRi* and *mean HR* from 1-min recording could be potential surrogates for the standard 5-min recording.

Keywords HRV · Ultra-short · Stress

L. A. Lim · J. H. Ho · B. T. Chan (✉)
Department of Mechanical, Materials and Manufacturing Engineering, Faculty of Science and Engineering, University of Nottingham Malaysia, Semenyih, Malaysia
e-mail: BeeTing.Chan@nottingham.edu.my

J. C. Lim
Realta Solutions Sdn. Bhd., Kuala Lumpur, Malaysia

E. Lim
Department of Biomedical Engineering, Faculty of Engineering, Universiti Malaya, Kuala Lumpur, Malaysia

J. Usman et al. (eds.), *6th Kuala Lumpur International Conference on Biomedical Engineering 2021*, IFMBE Proceedings 86,
https://doi.org/10.1007/978-3-030-90724-2_38

1 Introduction

Mental health cases are increasing at a worrying rate. Early recognition of stress may prevent its detrimental impact and proper stress management may reduce the risk of being afflicted by its related diseases [1]. With its simplicity and non-invasive approach, heart rate (HR) and heart rate variability (HRV) have been proposed as practical indicators for stress evaluation through the use of wearable sensors e.g. chest-strap detectors with electrocardiogram (ECG) electrodes, or finger or wrist-worn photoplethysmography devices [2–4]. HRV is the measure of the difference between two consecutive heartbeats or R-R interval (interval between two R waves in the ECG signal), which reflects the interactions between heart and brain and balance of parasympathetic and sympathetic reactions of autonomic nervous system (ANS). During stressful moments, the sympathetic nervous system will stimulate the release of hormones that cause the "flight-or-fight" reaction, increasing HR and affecting HRV [5]. Numerous parameters have been proposed to evaluate stress based on a group analysis [2, 3, 5]. However, HR and HRV in response to stress may vary between individuals, thus the significant parameter differences between stress and baseline conditions in the subject group may not truly reflect a unique response in individuals.

The HR and HRV in response to stress are usually measured in the short term (conventionally 5 min) and long term. However, real-time requirement restricts the use of conventional short-term HRV in routine medical practice, brief experimental tasks and the sports industry [6]. Thus, this has led to an interest in developing ultra-short-term metrics, in which HR and HRV analyses are obtained from recordings at a shorter duration [7]. Studies have attempted to establish the correlation between ultra-short-term and short-term recordings to identify reliable parameters [8–10]. However, the validity and reliability of practised techniques and tests are questionable [6]. Therefore, a standardised guideline has been proposed to determine reliable parameters are to be determined using the validation tests [7].

This study aims to identify reliable HR and HRV parameters for stress conditions by implementing the recommended standardised guideline [7]. The surrogacy of ultra-short-term recording for conventional short-term recording in stress evaluation is also investigated.

2 Methodology

2.1 Dataset

The WESAD dataset [11] was used to perform HRV analysis. The data was collected from 15 subjects (mean age 27 ± 2, 12 males). Exclusion criteria included pregnant women, heavy smokers, mental health patients, and those with chronic and cardio-vascular diseases. This dataset contained physiological and acceleration signals in

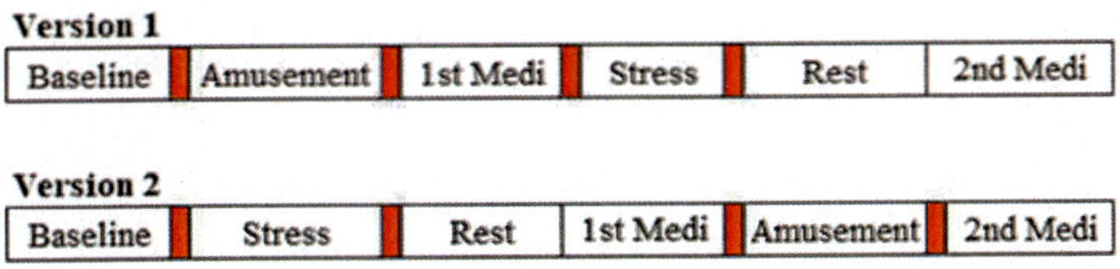

Fig. 1 Two versions of event sequences used in data collection. The red boxes indicate a pause where participants fill in self-reported questionnaires after a stimulation session [11]

three conditions—baseline (control), amused and stressed. Participants were asked to undergo a guided meditation to allow their heart rate activities return to baseline level after amusement and stress stimulation. The entire process of data collection took about two hours with interchanging arrangement of conditions to avoid event sequence effects (Fig. 1).

For this study, only the baseline and stress conditions were evaluated. In the baseline condition, a 20-min recording was obtained from subjects who were given neutral reading materials (magazines). In stress condition, the Trier Social Stress Test (TSST), which is a test to stimulate moderate mental stress in a laboratory setting, was performed. The TSST had been proven to be able to stimulate cortisol secretion, which was a stress hormone related to the "flight or fight" reaction [11]. To obtain this dataset, subjects were asked to give speech in public speaking for five minutes, and followed by arithmetic task of counting down from 2023 to zero with steps of 17 for the next five minutes. Participants were required to start over if mistakes were made. The total duration of TSST was 10 min. The data was sampled at 700 Hz and recorded using a *RespiBAN Professional* chest device (Wireless Biosignals S.A., Lisbon, Portugal). Only the ECG signals were used in the analysis.

2.2 Data Analysis

The ECG data was extracted using MATLAB R2020b (The Mathworks Inc, Natick, MA, USA) and imported into SinusCor for HRV analysis [12]. Table 1 shows all parameters that were extracted and analysed in this study.

The ECG signals were visually inspected and manual peak corrections were performed (Fig. 2). The moving median filter was applied to eliminate noise while the quotient filter was employed to remove abnormal beats. The incorrect beats were identified if the changes between two successive R-R interval values were exceeded by 20 percent [14]. The comparison of raw and filtered ECG signals is illustrated in Fig. 3. The R-R interval was then extracted from the processed ECG signal. In baseline condition, the 10 min of the R-R intervals were segmented from the middle of the full 20-min recording, while the full 10 min duration of the stress condition was analysed. These ECG signals were used to obtain the parameters for stress evaluation.

Table 1 HR and HRV parameters based on Camm et al. [13]

Parameters	Unit	Description
Mean RR	ms	Mean R-R interval
Mean HR	bpm	Mean heart rate
RMSSD	ms	Root mean square of successive R-R interval differences
SDNN	ms	Standard deviation of N-N intervals
pNN50	%	Percentage of consecutive R-R intervals that diverge by more than 50 ms
VLF	ms^2	Absolute power of the very-low-frequency band (0.0033–0.04 Hz)
LF	ms^2	Absolute power of the low-frequency band (0.04–0.15 Hz)
HF	ms^2	Absolute power of the high-frequency band (0.15–0.4 Hz)
LF/HF		Ratio of LF-to-HF power
LFnu	nu	Relative power of the low-frequency band (0.04–0.15 Hz) in normal units
HFnu	nu	Relative power of the high-frequency band (0.15–0.4 Hz) in normal units
SD1	ms	Poincaré plot standard deviation perpendicular to the line of identity
SD2	ms	Poincaré plot standard deviation along the line of identity

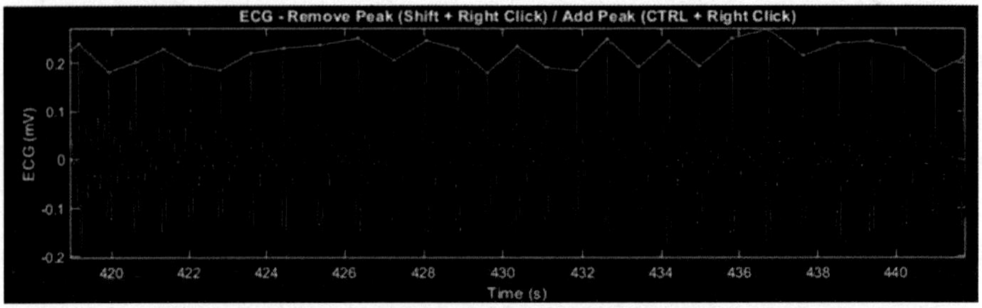

Fig. 2 A fragment of raw ECG data obtained under baseline condition

The HRV was analysed in time and frequency domains. The time domain measurements were evaluated for every successive 30 s segments without overlapping, while Welch's method was implemented to estimate the frequency domain measurements with a segment size of 256 with 50% overlap. Hanning window was used with a linear polynomial fit for signal de-trending to control spectral leakage [14]. To investigate the reliability of ultra-short HRV, the 10-min segments of the filtered ECG signal under baseline and stress conditions were truncated into 5-min and 1-min segments (Fig. 4).

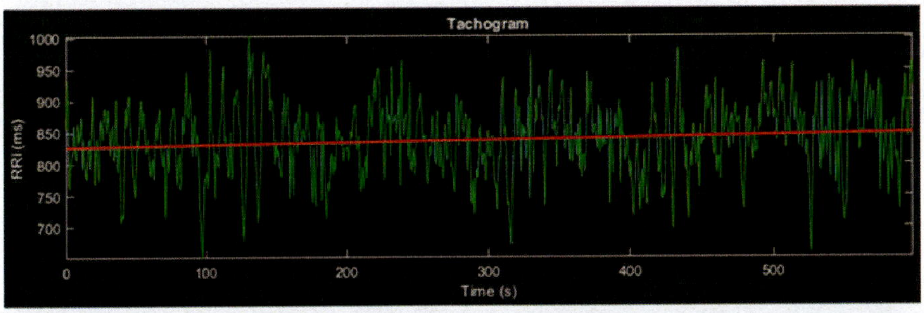

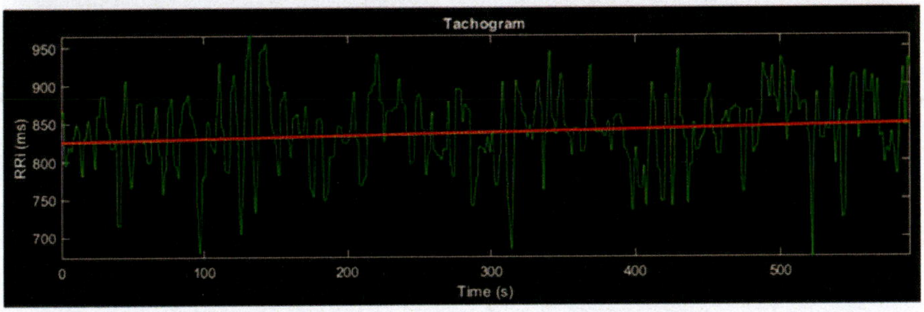

Fig. 3 The raw ECG signal (top) and the filtered R-R tachogram (bottom)

Fig. 4 Illustration of 1-min and 5-min segment extraction

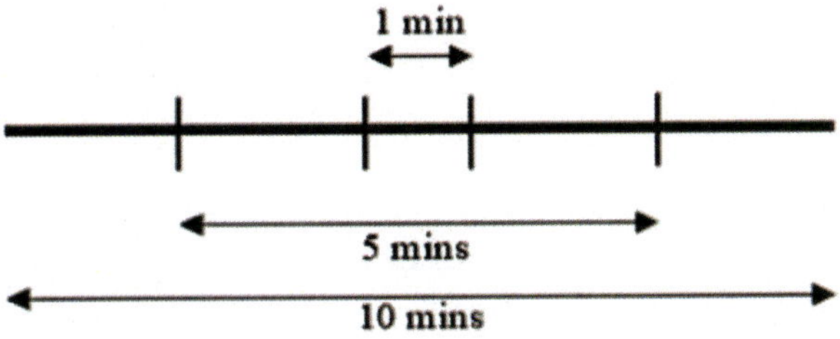

2.3 *Statistical Analysis*

Statistical analysis was performed using GNU PSPP V1.4.1 (GNU Project, Boston, USA) and Microsoft Excel (Microsoft Corporation, Redmond, USA). Figure 5 shows the flowchart of analysis implemented in this study. The data normality was examined by using Shapiro–Wilk test. For normally distributed data, independent t-test was used to compare the significant differences between the baseline and stress measurements, while data with non-normal distribution was tested using Mann–Whitney U test. Levene's test and two-sample Kolmogorov–Smirnov test were applied to assess the equality of variances and distribution of data, respectively, to find out whether the assumptions of the Mann–Whitney U test was met by the datasets.

The reliability of ultra-short-term parameters was examined using the algorithm proposed by Pecchia et al. [7]. All the appropriate tests (Levene's test and two-sample

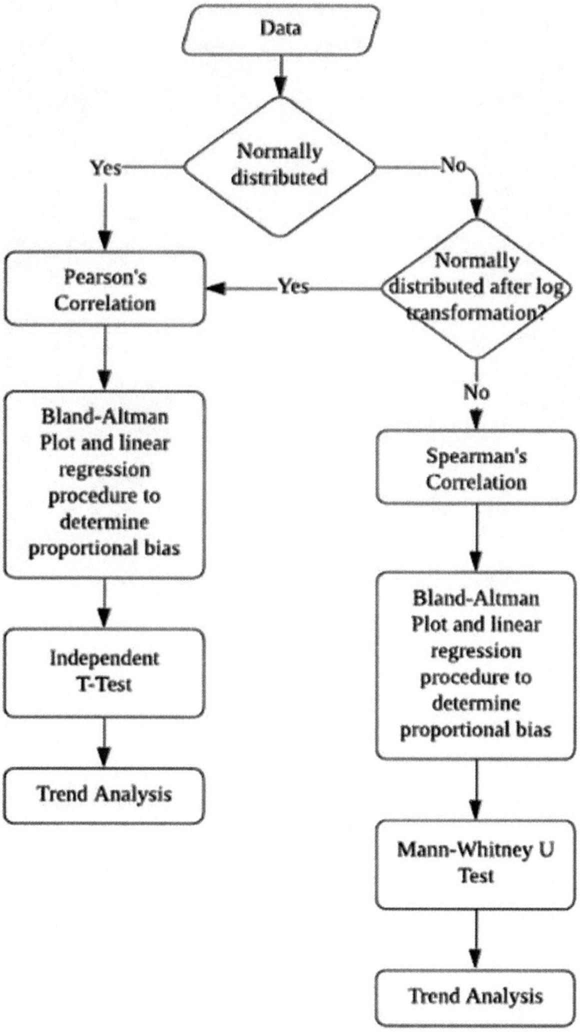

Fig. 5 Flowchart of the procedure carried out in this study

Kolmogorov–Smirnov test) were applied on the dataset to confirm that they met the assumptions of statistical tests used to compare the significant differences. Parametric and non-parametric tests like Pearson's correlation and Spearman's correlation were used to identify the correlation. The Bland–Altman plot and linear regression procedure were used to verify the data's agreement. Once all steps were performed, the ultra-short HR and HRV could be presumed to be good surrogates if the parameters preserved the same behaviour between the 5-min and 1-min recordings, and showed significantly high correlation ($r > 0.7$ and $p < 0.05$) for both 5-min and 1-min recordings. All significant thresholds were set at 0.05, and the correlation coefficient threshold was set at 0.7.

3 Results and Discussion

3.1 HR and HRV for Stress Evaluation

HR and HRV in response to stress condition could vary between individuals, thus individual stress response was evaluated based on the significant difference between stress and baseline condition (Table 2: Individual analysis). The parameters with resulting high frequency indicate good potential to identify stress from majority of the subjects. To show the results trend, the comparison between baseline and stress condition was shown as mean ± standard error across the subjects (Table 2: Group analysis). From the results, all 15 subjects under stress demonstrated a significantly lower *mean RRi*, while 14 showed significantly higher *mean HR* under stress. This was followed by 13 subjects with lower *RMSSD, SD1* and *HF*, whereas 12 subjects showed greater *LF/HF* and *LFnu* in stress condition ($p < 0.05$). Only the *mean RRi* and *mean HR* classified stress condition in the group analysis.

From the analysis, most of the parameters were non-normaly distributed and heteroscedastic and thus requires logarithmic transformation. There was a certain degree of fluctuation in these parameters, with the least changes in *mean RRi* and *mean HR*. When the subjects were under stress, the HRV parameters of *RMSSD, SDNN, pNN50, SD1, mean RRi, VLF, HF*, and *HFnu* were lower than the baseline condition, while *SD2, mean HR, LF, LF/HF*, and *LFnu* increased. These findings

Table 2 Comparison between baseline and stress conditions based on individual (left) and group analysis (right)

Parameters	Individual analysis	Group analysis	
	Frequency ($p < 0.05$)	Baseline	Stress
Mean RRi (ms)	15	853.11 ± 33.12*	662.29 ± 29.45*
Mean HR (bpm)	14	72.05 ± 2.97*	94.12 ± 4.72*
RMSSD (ms)	13	50.45 ± 7.50	38.66 ± 6.27
SDNN (ms)	8	60.86 ± 5.25	59.58 ± 6.42
pNN50 (%)	10	25.56 ± 5.08	14.66 ± 3.14
SD1 (ms)	13	36.18 ± 5.41	27.62 ± 4.49
SD2 (ms)	9	76.91 ± 5.72	78.92 ± 8.01
VLF (ms^2)	5	370.28 ± 68.29	344.50 ± 73.19
LF (ms^2)	8	1645.34 ± 230.48	1980.67 ± 361.08
HF (ms^2)	13	1174.31 ± 319.59	1064.16 ± 319.05
LF/HF	12	2.89 ± 0.51	5.11 ± 1.46
LFnu	12	60.00 ± 3.91	69.60 ± 3.48
HFnu	11	40.00 ± 3.91	30.40 ± 3.48

Group analysis was expressed as mean ± standard error with * indicates significant difference ($p < 0.05$)

followed the expected trend, where when mean HR increases, the duration between successive R-R would decrease. The ANS was activated, suppressing the parasympathetic nervous system (PNS), and activating the sympathetic nervous system (SNS). The SNS sustained homeostasis through sweating, heat dissipation and increased cardiac output. Once the stress had subsided, the PNS would facilitate the return of the body to equilibrium, countering the SNS effects [15]. SNS activity could be reflected by *LF* while *HF* denoted PNS activity [15]. From the results, an increase in *LF* and *LF/HF* during stress condition confirmed the SNS ascendancy.

3.2 Ultra-Short-Term Analysis

In the ultra-short-term analysis, all parameters demonstrated significant correlations ($r > 0.6$), with majority showing a very high correlation ($r > 0.7, p < 0.05$) between the 5-min and 1-min recordings (Table 3). Nevertheless, the good correlation did not imply good agreement as the data could be widely spread. As such, the Bland–Altman plot was used to identify the agreement between 5-min and the 1-min measurements. The linear regression was used to determine whether the existence of proportional bias. This bias was observed to exist ($q < 0.05$) in *LF*, *LF/HF*, *LFnu*, and *HFnu* under both conditions, and *VLF* under stress only. The limits of agreement (LOA) values varied greatly due to the widespread of values between parameters (Table 3). The percentage error (PE) was calculated because the information presented from the LOA was unclear, and no significant visual differences between all parameters in the Bland–Altman plots (Fig. 6). The PE presented a more context-sensitive value, in which the LOA was divided by the mean of the measurements with a threshold of $\pm$ 30% [16]. Based on this, all parameters with PE > 30% in both conditions were disregarded and the accepted parameters were *mean RRi*, *mean HR*, *VLF*, *LF*, and *HF* (Table 3).

The reliable ultra-short parameters should exhibit a significantly high correlation and portray the same trend for baseline and stress conditions between 1-min and 5-min recordings. Most of the parameters preserve the same trend of comparison between baseline and stress conditions in 1-min and 5-min recordings, except for *SDNN* and *HF* (Table 4), in which the *SDNN* increased during stress condition for the 1-min recording, whereas a decrease was observed in the 5-min analysis. The same went for *HF*. From this analysis, *mean RRi* and *mean HR* not only preserved the resulting trend, but also significantly reflected the stress condition in both 1-min and 5-min recordings.

Our results were generally concurred with Salahuddin et al. [8], who also reported the *mean HR* and *mean RR* as among the reliable parameters for ultra-short 50 s recording. Esco and Flatt [10] found that the 1-min segment showed the strongest correlation and considered the natural log of RMSSD as promising, while Baek et al. [9] accepted *RMSSD* and *HF* as good surrogates. However, there were no standardised tests used in those studies. Other studies did not justify the reliability of ultra-short-term HRV [17]. Although some studies made valuable comparisons

Table 3 Significant correlation (r) and proportional bias (q) between the 1-min and 5-min recordings during baseline and stress conditions

		MeanRRi (ms)	*MeanHR* (bpm)	*RMSSD* (ms)	*SDNN* (ms)	*pNN50* (%)	*SD1* (ms)	*SD2* (ms)	*VLF* (ms^2)	*LF* (ms^2)	*HF* (ms^2)	*LF/HF*	*LFnu*	*HFnu*
Baseline	*r*	0.980	0.989	0.953	0.796	0.958	0.953	0.775	0.752	0.894$^{\#}$	0.891	0.695$^{\#}$	0.731$^{\#}$	0.731$^{\#}$
	LOA	50.513	3.413	0.131	33.659	11.244	0.131	0.195	0.470	0.339	0.372	2.344	17.580	17.580
	PE (%)	5.929**	4.747**	7.848	47.492	41.451	8.591	10.089	16.797**	10.835**	12.500**	133.900	30.487	41.537
Stress	*r*	0.982	0.968	0.923	0.880	0.938	0.923	0.853	0.848$^{\#}$	0.914$^{\#}$	0.862	0.666$^{\#}$	0.684$^{\#}$	0.684$^{\#}$
	LOA	60.135	10.348	25.344	29.142	10.183	18.113	41.481	0.521	0.431	0.588	0.478	18.833	18.833
	PE (%)	8.791**	11.241**	59.860	40.457	62.755	60.297	42.934	18.541**	13.808**	20.598**	180.523	29.804	51.160

All the correlation, r is significant ($p < 0.05$), $^{\#}q < 0.05$ indicates proportional bias exists, $^{**}PE < 30\%$ in both baseline and stress conditions

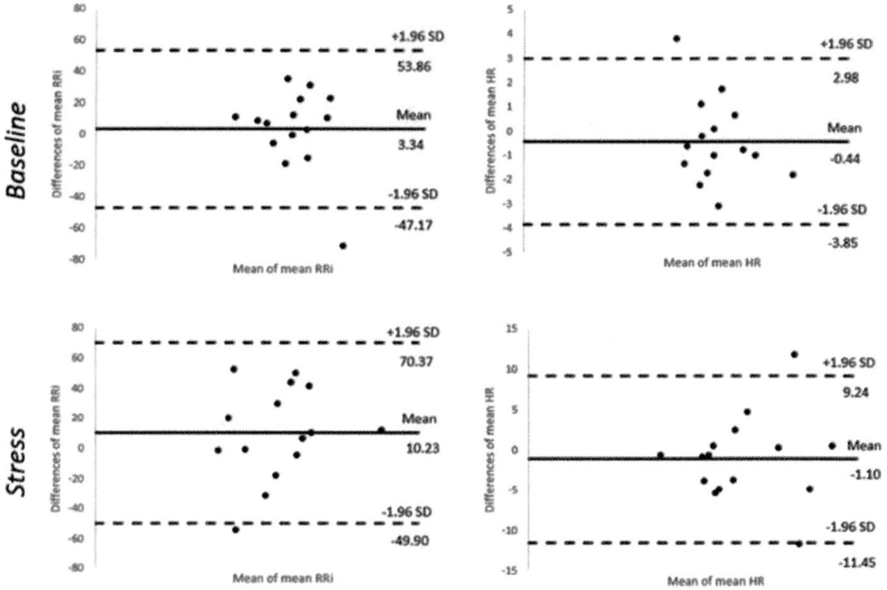

Fig. 6 Bland–Altman plot of *mean RRi* (left) and *mean HR* (right) during baseline (top row) and stress conditions (bottom row)

Table 4 Comparison of HR and HRV parameters during baseline and stress conditions for 1-min and 5-min recordings

HRV parameters	1-min		5-min	
	Baseline	Stress	Baseline	Stress
***Mean RRi* (ms)**	**853.66 ± 118.16***	**689.16 ± 161.12***	**850.32 ± 125.62***	**678.92 ± 154.47***
***Mean HR* (bpm)**	**71.68 ± 10.96***	**91.51 ± 21.06***	**72.12 ± 11.51***	**92.61 ± 20.70***
RMSSD (ms)	54.45 ± 30.22	42.12 ± 32.33	52.10 ± 29.72	42.56 ± 26.21
SDNN (ms)	72.12 ± 26.27	75.41 ± 29.22	69.63 ± 33.95	68.65 ± 30.96
pNN50 (%)	27.65 ± 19.06	16.51 ± 18.12	26.60 ± 19.99*	15.95 ± 16.78*
SD1 (ms)	38.78 ± 21.57	29.95 ± 23.03	36.90 ± 21.05	30.13 ± 18.56
SD2 (ms)	89.78 ± 44.51	91.48 ± 39.49	94.55 ± 32.35	101.75 ± 38.53
VLF (ms^2)	538.45 ± 604.30	597.25 ± 637.28	1352.55 ± 1047.02	1606.67 ± 1679.35
LF (ms^2)	1575.75 ± 1724.08	1784.63 ± 1971.17	1968.00 ± 1376.95	2326.29 ± 2091.03
HF (ms^2)	1619.04 ± 1648.63	1725.63 ± 2099.44	1226.31 ± 1434.38	1138.14 ± 1158.88
LF/HF	0.98 ± 0.32*	1.27 ± 0.38*	2.52 ± 1.40	3.60 ± 3.19
LFnu	48.35 ± 8.26*	54.77 ± 7.20*	67.00 ± 13.02	71.60 ± 12.97
HFnu	51.65 ± 3.26*	45.23 ± 7.20*	33.00 ± 13.02	28.40 ± 12.97

Data are expressed as mean ± standard deviation
* $p < 0.05$ indicates significant different pairs
Bold text indicates the significant pairs (baseline vs. stress) in both 1-min and 5-min recordings

between various time intervals [8–10], there was no comparison made between control and the ultra-short-term measurements for the parameter's capability in preserving information (result trend and significant pairs) [8–10, 17, 18].

It is commonly mistaken to corroborate a surrogate measure based on the correlation alone because this was insufficient as validating tool. Our results showed that only *mean RRi* and *mean HR* were able to preserve the information (showing same result trend and significant pairs), although most of the parameters demonstrated a good correlation. Another misconception for accepting a marker as good surrogate was when the null hypothesis of the statistical test between the standard and the marker was accepted [7]. Measurements for at least one minute would be required to avoid result inaccuracies when it involved *LF* and *HF* power spectra. The bandwidth of the *LF* power spectrum was 25 s and a minimum of 250 s of HRV signals were required to completely measure the full *LF* power spectrum. At least one minute was required for the *HF* power spectrum [13].

The limitations of this study included a small sample size and uneven gender distribution. Future studies should gather a larger sample with equal gender participation to investigate the influence of different activity levels and breathing pace to better reflect the behaviours of HR and HRV parameters [19].

4 Conclusion

The *mean RRi, mean HR, RMSSD, SD1, HF, LF/HF* and *LFnu* could reflect individual stress level in majority of subjects. With the implementation of recommended standardised tests, the *mean RRi* and *mean HR* could be the potential indicators to identify stress condition. Consistent trends were found in ultra-short analysis and the 1-min *mean RRi* and *mean HR* could become possible surrogates for conventional short-term analysis.

References

1. McCraty, R., Shaffer, F.: Heart rate variability: new perspectives on physiological mechanisms, assessment of self-regulatory capacity, and health risk. Glob. Adv. Health Med. **4**(1), 46–61 (2015). https://doi.org/10.7453/gahmj.2014.073
2. Stahl, S.E., An, H.-S., Dinkel, D.M., Noble, J.M., Lee, J.-M.: How accurate are the wrist-based heart rate monitors during walking and running activities? Are they accurate enough? BMJ Open Sport Exerc. Med. **2**(1), e000106 (2016). https://doi.org/10.1136/bmjsem-2015-000106
3. Speer, K.E., Semple, S., Naumovski, N., McKune, A.J.: Measuring heart rate variability using commercially available devices in healthy children: a validity and reliability study. Eur. J. Investig. Heal. Psychol. Educ. **10**(1), 390–404 (2020). https://doi.org/10.3390/ejihpe10010029
4. Gilgen-Ammann, R., Schweizer, T., Wyss, T.: RR interval signal quality of a heart rate monitor and an ECG Holter at rest and during exercise. Eur. J. Appl. Physiol. **119**(7), 1525–1532 (2019). https://doi.org/10.1007/s00421-019-04142-5

5. Taelman, J., Vandeput, S., Spaepen, A., Van Huffel, S.: Influence of mental stress on heart rate and heart rate variability. IFMBE Proc. **22**, 1366–1369 (2008). https://doi.org/10.1007/978-3-540-89208-3_324
6. Shaffer, F., Meehan, Z.M., Zerr, C.L.: A critical review of ultra-short-term heart rate variability norms research. Front. Neurosci. **14**, 1–11 (2020). https://doi.org/10.3389/fnins.2020.594880
7. Pecchia, L., Castaldo, R., Montesinos, L., Melillo, P.: Are ultra-short heart rate variability features good surrogates of short-term ones? State-of-the-art review and recommendations. Healthc. Technol. Lett. **5**(3), 94–100 (2018). https://doi.org/10.1049/htl.2017.0090
8. Salahuddin, L., Cho, J., Jeong, M.G., Kim, D.: Ultra short term analysis of heart rate variability for monitoring mental stress in mobile settings. Annual International Conference of the IEEE Engineering in Medicine and Biology Society—Proceedings, pp. 4656–4659 (2007). https://doi.org/10.1109/IEMBS.2007.4353378
9. Baek, H.J., Cho, C.H., Cho, J., Woo, J.M.: Reliability of ultra-short-term analysis as a surrogate of standard 5-min analysis of heart rate variability. Telemed. e-Health **21**(5), 404–414 (2015). https://doi.org/10.1089/tmj.2014.0104
10. Esco, M.R., Flatt, A.A.: Ultra-short-term heart rate variability indexes at rest and post-exercise in athletes: evaluating the agreement with accepted recommendations. J. Sport Sci. Med. **13**(3), 535–541 (2014)
11. Schmidt, P., Reiss, A., Duerichen, R., Marberger, C., Van Laerhoven, K.: Introducing Wesad, a multimodal dataset for wearable stress and affect detection. In: Proceedings of the 20th ACM International Conference on Multimodal Interaction, 2018, pp. 400–408
12. Bartels, R., Neumamm, L., Peçanha, T., Carvalho, A.R.S.: SinusCor: an advanced tool for heart rate variability analysis. Biomed. Eng. Online **16**(1), 1–15 (2017)
13. Camm, A., et al.: Heart rate variability: standards of measurement, physiological interpretation, and clinical use. Circulation **93**(5), 1043–1065 (1996). https://doi.org/10.1161/01.CIR.93.5.1043
14. Piskorski, J., Guzik, P.: Filtering Poincare plots. Comput. Methods Sci. Technol. **11**(1), 39–48 (2005)
15. Kim, H.G., Cheon, E.J., Bai, D.S., Lee, Y.H., Koo, B.H.: Stress and heart rate variability: a meta-analysis and review of the literature. Psychiatry Investig. **15**(3), 235–245 (2018). https://doi.org/10.30773/pi.2017.08.17
16. Odor, P.M., Bampoe, S., Cecconi, M.: Cardiac output monitoring: validation studies—how results should be presented. Curr. Anesthesiol. Rep. **7**(4), 410–415 (2017)
17. Papousek, I., Nauschnegg, K., Paechter, M., Lackner, H.K., Goswami, N., Schulter, G.: Trait and state positive affect and cardiovascular recovery from experimental academic stress. Biol. Psychol. **83**(2), 108–115 (2010)
18. Arza, A., Garzón, J.M., Hemando, A., Aguiló, J., Bailón, R.: Towards an objective measurement of emotional stress: preliminary analysis based on heart rate variability. In: 2015 37th Annual International Conference of the IEEE Engineering in Medicine and Biology Society (EMBC), 2015, pp. 3331–3334
19. Sammito, S., Böckelmann, I.: Factors influencing heart rate variability. Int. Cardiovasc. Forum J. **6**, 18–22 (2016)

Fabrication of Carbon Nanofibers Using MEMS Technique for Future Electrochemical Biosensors

Elyana Kosri, Fatimah Ibrahim, and Marc Madou

Abstract This paper presents the fabrication of the inter-porosity carbon nanofibers (CNFs) obtained by the Carbon Microelectromechanical Systems (C-MEMS) method using electrospinning of SU-8 2100 photoresist polymer, photolithography, and pyrolysis techniques. The optimized electrospinning parameters identified in this research produced smooth inter-porosity CNFs with an average fibre diameter range between 167 ± 58 nm and 197 ± 104 nm. The CNFs samples were subsequently investigated using the cyclic voltammetry (CV) technique at sweep rate 50 mV s^{-1} with Zobell's solution as a redox probe in three-electrode configuration [CNFs as working electrode (WE), counter electrode (CE), and reference electrode (RE) from the screen-printed electrode (SPE)]. Based on CV analysis, the inter-porosity CNFs showed that the CV curve obtained at high sweep rates proved that the consumption of redox species rate at the electrode surface is very high. Additionally, the high surface area of our developed CNFs has the potential to be used as massive regions for bacteria detection with further modification of electrode configuration; leading to an increase in the detection sensitivity.

Keywords Carbon nanofibres · Carbon MEMS · Electrospinning · Cyclic voltammetry · Screen-printed electrode

E. Kosri · F. Ibrahim (✉)
Department of Biomedical Engineering, Faculty of Engineering, Universiti Malaya, 50603 Kuala Lumpur, Malaysia
e-mail: fatimah@um.edu.my

E. Kosri · F. Ibrahim · M. Madou
Centre For Innovation in Medical Engineering, Faculty of Engineering, Universiti Malaya, 50603 Kuala Lumpur, Malaysia

F. Ibrahim
Centre of Printable Electronics, Universiti Malaya, 50603 Kuala Lumpur, Malaysia

M. Madou
Department of Biomedical Engineering, University of California, Irvine, USA

Department of Mechanical and Aerospace Engineering, University of California, Irvine, USA

J. Usman et al. (eds.), *6th Kuala Lumpur International Conference on Biomedical Engineering 2021*, IFMBE Proceedings 86,
https://doi.org/10.1007/978-3-030-90724-2_39

1 Introduction

Carbon-Microelectromechanical Systems (C-MEMS) and Carbon-Nanoelectromechanical Systems (C-NEMS) [1] fabrication techniques allow the production of the high aspect ratio of carbon structures via patterning desired shapes of photoresist polymers by a photolithography process and subsequently pyrolysis process which results in the carbonization of resultants pattern structures [2, 3]. Carbon material can be easily obtained from the carbonization of certain precursor polymers e.g. negative photoresist [4]. Silicon (Si) wafer is used as the substrate platform for most MEMS techniques [5]. Pyrolytic carbon shows high biocompatibility [6] and promotes cell adhesion if treated with oxygen plasma [7]. Fabrication techniques of carbon-based MEMS are low cost, biocompatibility, ease of manufacturing processes, the surface properties can be adjusted based on its application [8], allow good control of resistivity and mechanical properties of carbon by controlling the temperature of pyrolysis, for porosity by varying the temperature ramp rates, and high reproducibility [9]. Carbon obtained via C-MEMS or C-NEMS techniques features an excellent physicochemical of glassy carbon with good stability of chemical and electrochemical stability.

The electrospinning of polymer precursors easily produces high aspect ratio CNFs through optimizing the electrospinning, photolithography and pyrolysis parameters [10, 11]. The advantages of the SU-8 derived CNFs are biocompatible [12], with tunable hydrophilicity based on the surface texture of the CNFs [13]. Furthermore, the electrical properties of carbon films derived from SU-8 polymer are thickness-dependent [14]. Interestingly, the CNFs obtained from electrospinning enable the production of fibres with diameters ranging from 2 nm to several micrometres (μm) by employing the effect of generated electrical forces on polymer solutions [15]. Hence, this paper presents an inter-porosity, high surface area of three-dimensional carbon nanofibres via pyrolysis of patterned electrospun SU-8 polymer fibres.

This paper reports a method to increase the surface area of CNFs using the MEMS technique and convenient electrospinning to yield an inter-porosity nanofibers (NFs) structure. The electrospinning parameters were optimized to produce smooth inter-porosity NFs using SU-8 2100 photoresist polymer. Standard photolithography and pyrolysis were used to produce the final inter-porosity CNFs film. The results showed smooth, inter-porosity of CNFs with an average fibre diameter range between 167 $\pm$ 58 nm and 197 $\pm$ 104 nm. Finally, the morphology and electrochemical properties of inter-porosity CNFs as a WE were investigated. The CV single-mode was performed to study the redox reaction that occured between CNFs, RE and CE from screen-printed electrode (SPE), and using Zobell's solution as a redox probe. The redox reaction that occurred between CNFs, RE, and CE showed the CV curve achieved at high sweep rates (50 mV s^{-1}) demonstrating that the consumption of redox species rate at the electrode surface is high. Thus, the potential application of CNFs as a future electrochemical biosensing platform for bacteria detection can be further enhanced by integrating modification of CNFs electrode design.

2 Methodologies

The SU-8 2100 negative photoresist polymers and SU-8 developer (1-methoxy-2-propyl acetate) were purchased from MicroChem (USA). Cyclopentanone, acetone, and isopropyl alcohol were obtained from Sigma-Aldrich (USA). The ink solution used is SU-8 2100 diluted with cyclopentanone (wt. 75%:25%), as the high viscosity of SU-8 2100 requires a dilution process to facilitate electrospinning. The ink solution (SU-8 2100) was stirred for 48 h at room temperature to ensure a homogenous solution. Following this, the solution was drawn into the syringe and placed vertically to remove all air bubbles trapped inside the syringe before electrospinning. The NFs were fabricated on Silicon (Si) wafer substrates (University Wafers, USA). The Si wafer was successively rinsed in acetone, isopropyl alcohol, and distilled water, dried under compressed nitrogen gas flow, and kept in the constant temperature oven (DKM410C, Japan) for twelve hours at 120 °C to ensure the surface was fully dehydrated before electrospinning.

The electrospinning apparatus included a high voltage power supply (ULTRAVOLT., USA), syringe pump (kdScientific, USA), Si wafer, aluminium foil (Al foil), syringe and needle (Terumo, Philippines), positively and negatively charged cable, and ground collector. The high voltage power supply was customized with a voltage supply ranging from 8.5 to 10 kV and a syringe pump to control the flow rate of the ink solution. 2 cm^2 Si wafer was used as the collector attached to a grounded copper tape on Al foil. The positively charged cable was attached to the needle and the negatively charged cable was attached to the Al foil using crocodile clips, respectively. The applied voltage, flow rate, and distance from tip-to-collector were optimized and listed in Table 1. Four samples were electrospun using SU-8 2100 ink solution for 4 min on Si wafer substrate according to specified parameters. The humidity of the electrospinning setup area was controlled between 42% to 60% r.h. to avoid the formation of beads. The electrospinning experiment was completed under yellow light to avoid crosslinking of SU-8 solutions.

Four samples of inter-porosity NFs were exposed to UV irradiation for 20 s using a mask aligner system (MIDAS MDA-400M, Korea). Then, these samples underwent post-exposure baking at 75 °C in the constant temperature oven for 10 min and cooled

Table 1 Summary of the electrospinning parameters, an average diameter of NFs and CNFs, % shrinkage, and resistance of CNFs

Sample No.	D (cm)	FR (mL min^{-1})	V (kV)	Average fiber diameter (nm)		%S	R (kΩ)
				NFs	CNFs		
1	15	0.005	8.5	258 ± 112	174 ± 63	32.8	53.3
2	15	0.005	9.0	241 ± 137	180 ± 52	23.3	80.8
3	15	0.005	9.5	257 ± 135	167 ± 58	35.2	29.8
4	15	0.008	10.0	304 ± 151	197 ± 104	34.6	27.1

D Distance, *FR* Flow rate, *V* Voltage, *S* Shrinkage, *R* Resistance to room temperature before the pyrolysis process. Subsequently, all samples were developed using SU-8 developer solution, rinsed with isopropyl alcohol, and dried in nitrogen gas flow.

The patterned SU-8 polymer samples of inter-porosity NFs were converted to electrically conductive CNFs electrodes by pyrolyzing in inert atmosphere N_2 (99.9995%) conditions. The pyrolysis process was carried out in a tubular furnace (Nabertherm, Germany) following a previously reported method with some modifications to the heating rate [5, 16]. The samples were first heated to 300 °C for 30 min with a heating rate of 20 °C min^{-1}. Subsequently, the temperature was increased to 900 °C at a heating rate of 10 °C min^{-1} and maintained at 900 °C for 1 h. The samples were allowed to cool to room temperature under continuous N_2 flow before taking it out from the furnace and storing it under ambient conditions. The pyrolyzed inter-porosity nanofibers are referred to as carbon nanofibers (CNFs).

Resistance of all sample CNFs electrodes was measured using a multimeter (Sanwa CD800A Digital Multimeter (ORG), Japan) on a 1 cm^2 sample area. The resistance measurement was repeated 3 times to obtain the average for each sample. All CNFs samples were tested for electrochemical analysis using CV. CV was performed using Zobell's solution (0.1 M KCl, 0.005 M $K_4Fe(CN)_6 \cdot 3H_2O$, and 0.005 M $K_3Fe(CN)_6$) as electrolyte at 50 mV s^{-1} sweep rate. Field Emission Scanning Electron Microscope (FESEM) (AURIGA, Carl Zeiss, S.E.Asia) with Energy Dispersive X-Ray Spectroscopy (EDX) (EDAX, AMETEK, USA) were used to characterize the morphology of the inter-porosity NFs, CNFs, and the elemental composition of CNFs.

3 Results and Discussions

Fabrication of CNFs was optimized by varying the following electrospinning parameters: flow rate, voltage, and distance from tip-to-collector. Four samples of CNFs electrodes labelled as Sample 1, 2, 3, and 4 were prepared using electrospinning parameters mentioned in Table 1. Table 1 summarizes the optimization of electrospinning parameters, NFs and CNFs average fiber diameter obtained, % shrinkage and resistance of each sample. FESEM was used to characterize the surface morphology of nanofibers before and after pyrolysis. An accelerating voltage of 1 kV was used to reduce the surface charging of the samples during beam scanning. 100 diameter measurements were recorded to determine the average fibre diameter. The NFs and CNFs diameter was measured using the public domain ImageJ software [17].

Figure 1 showed FESEM images of inter-porosity NFs and CNFs. Based on the results from Fig. 1, all samples showed smooth and continuous inter-porosity NFs with minimal beaded NFs. From all samples, Sample 3 achieved the smallest average fibre diameter of CNFs 167 ± 58 nm at flow rate 0.005 mL min^{-1} and voltage 9.5 kV. The smaller diameter of NFs was obtained when the voltage applied increased and caused stretching of the polymer solution in correlation with the charge repulsion within the polymer jet [15, 18]. At 8.5 kV and 0.005 mL min^{-1}, the average diameter

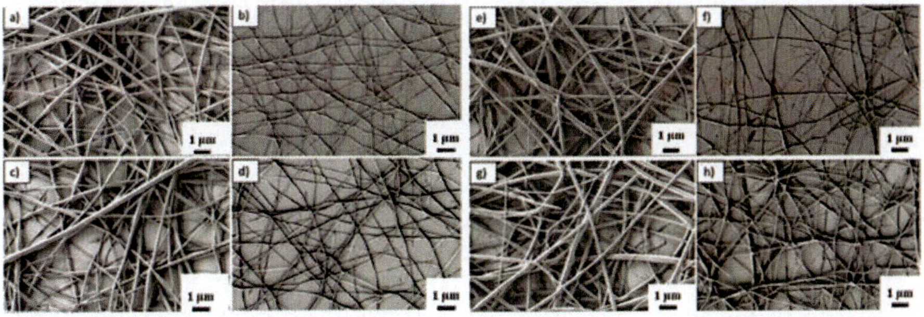

Fig. 1 FESEM micrographs of inter-porosity NFs **a** sample 1, **c** sample 2, **e** sample 3, **g** sample 4 and CNFs **b** sample 1, **d** sample 2, **f** sample 3, **h** sample 4

of NFs shrunk from 258 ± 112 nm to 174 ± 63 nm (CNFs) for Sample 1. The average diameter of CNFs for Sample 2 recorded 180 ± 52 nm when 9 kV voltage was applied and the flow rate remained unchanged, 0.005 mL min^{-1}. Sample 4 showed the average diameter of NFs reduced from 304 ± 151 nm to 197 ± 104 nm (CNFs) when 10 kV voltage was applied and flow rate increased to 0.008 mL min^{-1}. The shrinkage of NFs occurs due to the carbonization of SU-8 structures during pyrolysis [19]. Shrinkage percentage was calculated using the formula [16]:

$$\%\ \text{Shrinkage} = \frac{\text{Initial dimension} - \text{Final dimension}}{\text{Initial dimension}} \times 100 \quad (1)$$

Shrinkage for Samples 1, 2, 3 and 4 were calculated as 32.8%, 23.3%, 35.2% and 34.6% respectively. The shrinkage of Sample 2 is the lowest (23.3%) compared to other samples' shrinkage percentage. The pyrolysis step affected the polymer to shrink in size and volume (Fig. 1b, d, f, h). The reason shrinkage happened is because the temperature ramp is controlled during the process so that temperature in the oven is always lower than the temperature of glass transition of the material at any given temperature of carbon/photoresist [16, 19, 20]. Furthermore, Park et al. mentioned that temperatures above 600 °C cause slight shrinkage for the SU-8 films [19].

The flow rate was increased for Sample 4 due to results from our previous experiment (unpublished data) proved that a higher percentage of beaded fibres were obtained when voltage increases while flow rate remained at 0.005 mL min^{-1}. This verified that flow rate affected the diameter of nanofibers [15]. Steach et al. reported that 75% SU-8 concentration was tested at the flow rate of 0.005, 0.01, 0.02, 0.05, 0.1, and 0.2 mL min^{-1} while the distance between needle tip to the collector was held at 10 cm and voltage was constant at 9 kV and they found that when the flow rate was 0.2 mL min^{-1}, the fibre diameter increased to 635 ± 379 nm [21]. Thus, a higher flow rate assisted to produce a smaller fibre diameter. However, beaded nanofibers could be formed if the flow rate increases above critical value [22].

We conducted a trial electrospinning experiment by maintaining the humidity of the experiment area above 60% r.h. and obtained beaded fibres and beads for all electrospinning parameters listed in Table 1. The morphology and diameter of electrospun NFs are affected by environmental (ambient) factors such as relativhumidity and temperature. From the trial experiment results, we conclude that humidity also played an essential part that affecting the nanofibers' architecture. Humidity controls the solidification process of the charged jet that leads to a change in the diameter of the NFs [23]. Hence, we controlled the humidity level between 42% to 60% r.h. for all samples fabrication to obtain smooth inter-porosity NFs.

The resistance values of CNFs are shown in Table 1. All samples of CNFs present high resistance value due to the uneven layer of inter-porosity three-dimensional shape and the long, inter-connected CNFs were cut-off or over shrunk during pyrolysis that making it less covering or disconnected on some area of Si wafer. Despite high resistance recorded in whole samples, Samples 3 and 4 recorded low resistance 29.8 kΩ and 27.1 kΩ respectively among all samples. Both Sample 1 (53.3 kΩ) and Sample 2 (80.8 kΩ) electrodes indicate higher resistance value. From the results, we conclude that increasing the electrospinning time by more than four minutes to several hours will develop a thicker layer of inter-connected three-dimensional CNFs and improve the performance of the CNFs to be utilized as an electrode.

The electrochemical properties of all electrodes were analyzed using the CV technique in the 3-electrode configuration setup. The CNFs electrodes are used as WE, while for CE and RE from the SPE respectively. CV was carried out in Zobell's solution as the redox probe. The CV curve was obtained by applying a voltage range of -1.0 to $+1.0$ V vs SPE reference and a counter electrode at a sweep rate of 50 mV s^{-1} and the current density output was recorded. Figure 2a illustrates the CV curves obtained for CNFs samples. CV analysis indicated that all samples are electrochemically active. The graph showed that the typical CV curve for all samples was obtained with Sample 4 obtaining the highest current density compared

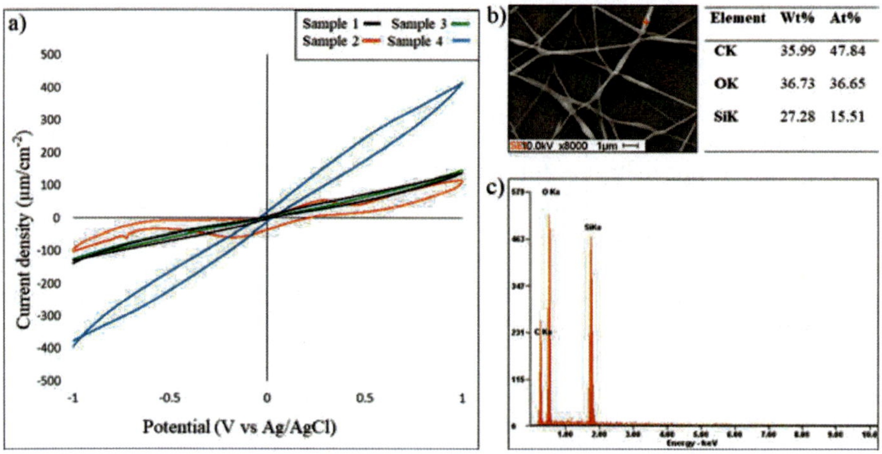

Fig. 2 a CV of CNFs in Zobell's solution at 50 mV s^{-1} sweep rate. **b** FESEM of CNFs morphology (10 kV, 8000× magnification) and **c** EDX elemental composition

to Samples 1, 2, and 3. The CV curve obtained at high sweep rates (50 mV s^{-1}) proved that the consumption of redox species rate at the electrode surface is very high. Moreover, the bulk diffusion cannot offer adequate mass transport to reach a steady-state condition. Thus, the insufficient mass transport affected the current to reach the peak [4]. Furthermore, from Fig. 1, the inter-porosity CNFs covered the substrate unevenly which remained some substrate area uncovered with CNFs. Consequently, these affected the CV curves as well due to the uncovered substrate area hindering better anodic and cathodic peak potential and current in redox cycling performances. Thus, modification of the CNFs electrode is prominent to increase electrochemical sensitivity.

Figure 2b shows the CNFs area (red mark) chosen to identify the elemental composition and Fig. 2c illustrates the EDX elemental composition of the red mark point in Fig. 2b. Figure 2c shows the elemental composition for the CNFs WE contain C, O, and Si elements. Si and O elements recorded higher readings together with C because the substrate used is SiO_2 wafer. The wt% of C element is 35.99%, O element recorded 36.73% and Si element is 27.28% respectively. Hence, the CNFs based MEMS contained a high percentage of carbon has been proven despite short electrospinning time.

4 Conclusion

A high surface area, electroconductive CNFs platform as WE has been fabricated using convenient electrospinning of SU-8 2100, photolithography, and pyrolysis techniques (C-MEMS). The optimized electrospinning parameters of SU-8 2100 achieved an average CNFs diameter from 167 ± 58 nm to 197 ± 104 nm. The CNFs were electrochemically active and able to support redox reactions on their surface. These have been proved by the single-mode CV in a three-electrode configuration setup. For the future experiment, the modification of the CNFs electrode is necessary to increase signal amplification and the electrochemically active surface area interacting with the analyte if to be used as a bacteria sensor. This study shows that the high surface area of the CNFs is a promising platform for investigation in future electrochemical biosensing applications.

Acknowledgements The authors would like to thank the Ministry of Higher Education (MOHE) Prototype Research Grant Scheme (PRGS) (PR005-2019A) : (Development of Rapid Point-of-Care (POC) Salmonella Detection Prototype Device For Food Safety Application) and Universiti Malaya Impact-Oriented Interdisciplinary Research Grant Program (IIRG007A-19HWB) : (Enchanced Microporous Carbon-nased MEMS Bioscaffolds for Stem Cells Growth).

References

1. Madou, M.J.B.R.: Fundamentals of Microfabrication: The Science of Miniaturization. CRC (2002)
2. Madou, M. et al.: Carbon micromachining (C-MEMS). In: Proceedings of the Symposium on Chemical and Biological Sensors and Analytical Electrochemical Methods, 1997, vol. 97, no. 19, pp. 61–69. The Electrochemical Society, Inc., Pennington, NJ
3. Wang, C., Jia, G., Taherabadi, L.H., Madou, M.J.: A novel method for the fabrication of high-aspect ratio C-MEMS structures. J. Microelectromech. Syst. **14**(2), 348–358 (2005)
4. Kamath, R.R., Madou, M.J.: Three-dimensional carbon interdigitated electrode arrays for redox-amplification. Anal. Chem. **86**(6), 2963–2971 (2014)
5. Thiha, A., et al.: All-carbon suspended nanowire sensors as a rapid highly-sensitive label-free chemiresistive biosensing platform. Biosens. Bioelectron. **107**, 145–152 (2018)
6. Cook, S.D., Beckenbaugh, R.D., Redondo, J., Popich, L.S., Klawitter, J.J., Linscheid, R.L.: Long-term follow-up of pyrolytic carbon metacarpophalangeal implants. JBJS **81**(5), 635–648 (1999)
7. Teixidor, G.T. et al.: Carbon microelectromechanical systems as a substratum for cell growth. Biomed. Mater. **3**(3), 034116 (2008)
8. Sharma, S., Madou, M.: Micro and nano patterning of carbon electrodes for bioMEMS. Bioinspired Biomim. Nanobiomater. **1**(4), 252–265 (2012)
9. Kim, J., Song, X., Kinoshita, K., Madou, M., White, R.: Electrochemical studies of carbon films from pyrolyzed photoresist. J. Electrochem. Soc. **145**(7), 2314–2319 (1998)
10. Heo, J.I., Shim, D.S., Teixidor, G.T., Oh, S., Madou, M.J., Shin, H.: Carbon interdigitated array nanoelectrodes for electrochemical applications. J. Electrochem. Soc. **158**(3), J76 (2011)
11. Kakunuri, M., Kaushik, S., Saini, A., Sharma, C.S.: SU-8 photoresist-derived electrospun carbon nanofibres as high-capacity anode material for lithium ion battery. Bull. Mater. Sci. **40**(3), 435–439 (2017)
12. Jao, P.F., Franca, E.W., Fang, S.-P., Wheeler, B.C., Yoon, Y.-K.: Immersion lithographic patterning of electrospun nanofibers for carbon nanofibrous microelectrode arrays. J. Microelectromech. Syst. **24**(3), 703–715 (2015)
13. Sharma, C.S., Sharma, A., Madou, M.: Multiscale carbon structures fabricated by direct micropatterning of electrospun mats of SU-8 photoresist nanofibers. Langmuir **26**(4), 2218–2222 (2010)
14. Singh, A., Jayaram, J., Madou, M., Akbar, S.: Pyrolysis of negative photoresists to fabricate carbon structures for microelectromechanical systems and electrochemical applications. J. Electrochem. Soc. **149**(3), E78–E83 (2002)
15. Bhardwaj, N., Kundu, S.C.: Electrospinning: a fascinating fiber fabrication technique. Biotechnol. Adv. **28**(3), 325–47 (2010)
16. Natu, R., Islam, M., Martinez-Duarte, R.: Shrinkage analysis of carbon micro structures derived from SU-8 photoresist. ECS Trans. **72**(1), 27–33 (2016)
17. Schneider, C.A., Rasband, W.S., Eliceiri, K.W.: NIH image to ImageJ: 25 years of image analysis. Nat. Methods **9**(7), 671 (2012)
18. Baumgarten, P.K.: Electrostatic spinning of acrylic microfibers. J. Colloid Interface Sci. **36**(1), 71–79 (1971)
19. Park, B.Y., Taherabadi, L., Wang, C., Zoval, J., Madou, M.J.: Electrical properties and shrinkage of carbonized photoresist films and the implications for carbon micro electromechanical systems devices in conductive media. **152**(12), J136–J143 (2005)
20. Martinez-Duarte, R., Renaud, P., Madou, M.J.: A novel approach to dielectrophoresis using carbon electrodes. Electrophoresis **32**(17), 2385–2392 (2011)
21. Steach, J.K., Clark, J.E., Olesik, S.V.: Optimization of electrospinning an SU-8 negative photoresist to create patterned carbon nanofibers and nanobeads. J. Appl. Polym. Sci. **118**(1), 405–412 (2010)

22. Haider, A., Haider, S., Kang, I.K.: A comprehensive review summarizing the effect of electrospinning parameters and potential applications of nanofibers in biomedical and biotechnology. Arab J Chem **11**(8), 1165–1188 (2018)
23. Li, D., Xia, Y.: Electrospinning of nanofibers: reinventing the wheel? Adv. Mater. **16**(14), 1151–1170 (2004)

The Study of Polarization Properties of Agarose Gel in Normal Line of Light Transmission

Siti Nurainie Tukimin, Salmah Binti Karman, Wan Safwani Wan Kamarul Zaman, and Mohd Yazed Ahmad

Abstract Most conventional techniques utilize the degree of polarization (DOP) feature for quantitative analysis rather than the angle of polarization (AOP). There are very limited journals constantly publishing and reporting both AOP and DOP as reliable and significant parameters for imaging or detection approach in current biomedical technologies. Hence, such an approach is highlighted in this paper for the fundamental concept to understand light polarization manners for future research and applications in the development of new imaging technologies in the medical field. This study highlights important parameters of both light polarization features (DOP and AOP) in the development of high-performance medical imaging abilities for a successful diagnostic or prognostic approach in medical applications. Hence, the main objective of this study is to propose a fundamental basis of light polarization manners for monochromatic light as a framework for successful future research, especially for cancer research and the development of new imaging technologies.

Keywords Light polarization · Polarized angle · Orientation angle · Tissue phantom · Agarose gel and agar-based phantom

1 Introduction

Polarization can be explained as a fundamental property of light with a powerful sensing tool in numerous applications of biomedical research. Light polarization occurs when an electromagnetic wave of light rays interacts with matters of different refractive indices. Polarization occurs as a beam passes through a medium or material of a certain refractive index, resulting in birefringence effects [1–4]. Diagram 1 shows the fundamental properties of light polarization that interact and penetrate a medium with known refractive index. The objective of this paper is to study the polarization properties (optical activeness) of agarose gel when light is transmitted in normal line.

S. N. Tukimin · S. B. Karman (✉) · W. S. W. K. Zaman · M. Y. Ahmad
Biomedical Department, Faculty of Engineering, Universiti Malaya, 50603 Kuala Lumpur, Malaysia
e-mail: salmah_karman@um.edu.my

J. Usman et al. (eds.), *6th Kuala Lumpur International Conference on Biomedical Engineering 2021*, IFMBE Proceedings 86,
https://doi.org/10.1007/978-3-030-90724-2_40

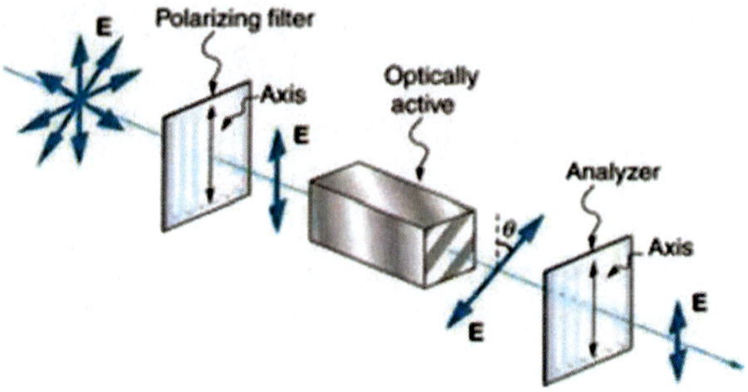

Diagram 1 Fundamental polarization of light that interact with optical material (Adapted from http://www.fiberoptics4sale.com/blogs/wave-optics/103704710-what-are-optically-active-materials)

2 Polarization of Light: A Reliable and Significant Feature

From biomedical point of view, the polarization of turbid media or bulk tissues occurs due to optical properties owing to cell or tissue refractive indices. Different characteristics of tissue, cell, or biological material surfaces are major contributors resulting in a wide range of polarization state of different wavelengths [5].

The relationship between these characteristics and light polarization has been extensively explored for medical imaging technologies or spectroscopy devices [6–8], like reflectance spectroscopy, autofluorescence, Raman spectroscopy, optical coherence tomography, magnetic resonance spectroscopy, polarized light microscopy, and Mueller polarimetry. These technologies have demonstrated and proved that the degree of polarization (DOP) has a significant level of accuracy. However, instead of DOP, angle of polarization (AOP) is rarely reported with high performance or similar achievement. Hence, this study proposed and proved that AOP is a reliable and significant feature for future research in the development of high-performance medical imaging technologies.

3 Research Methodology

3.1 Agarose Gel Preparaion

According to previous studies, gelatin, agar, and agarose powder have been intensively studied on tissue mimicking phantom. Different concentrations or weight percentages of such materials indicate similar compositions and characteristics of real tissues. Generally, the weight percentage of agar powder of less than 4 wt% in concentration is a pure healthy and normal soft tissue phantom, whereas agar powder with the weight percentage of higher than 4 wt% in concentration indicates a hard tissue that is possibly close to cancer or tumor tissue phantom. The procedures for preparing agar with certain concentrations are presented here in detail. The experiment started with the preparation of all materials or samples involved, such as agarose

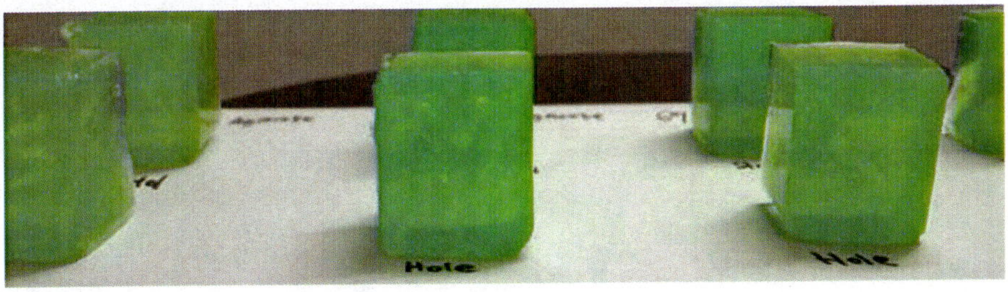

Fig. 1 Agarose gel for tissue mimicking phantom

powder. The powder was obtained from a local supplier in Universiti Malaya. Agar powder with different mass concentrations was diluted separately with 100 mL of hot, degassed distilled water. Once the mixture of agarose powder and distilled water had completely dissolved, the solution was poured into a cube mold to allow the solution to turn into a cooled gel. The gel was ready for further experiment once the solution completely solidified. The image of the prepared agarose gel was shown in Fig. 1. The steps involved were repeated for different mass concentrations of 3, 6, 8, and 10 g for 3%, 6%, 8%, and 10% (w/w) of agarose gel, respectively.

3.2 *Setting Up Normal Plane of Light Polarization*

Light polarization setup was prepared following Diagram 2 (for top view) and Diagram 3 (for side view). In this experiment, the items required for calibrating

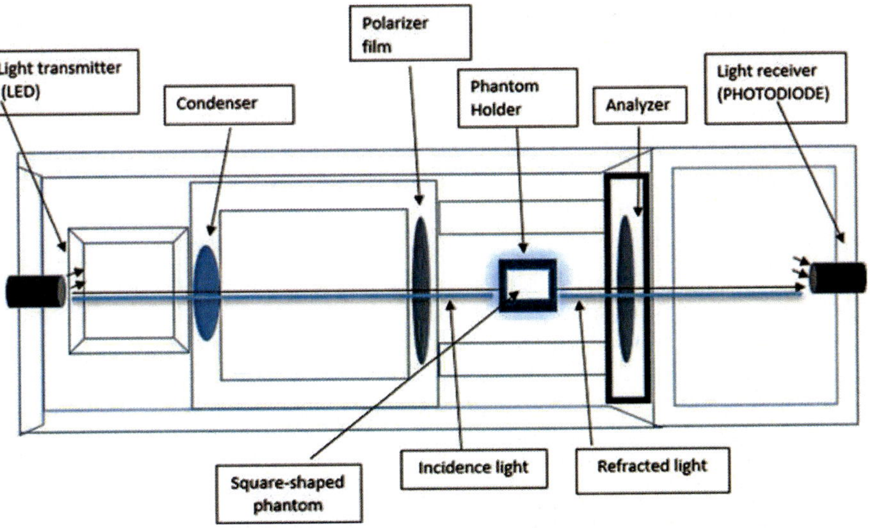

Diagram 2 Light polarization setup from top view (normal line transmission)

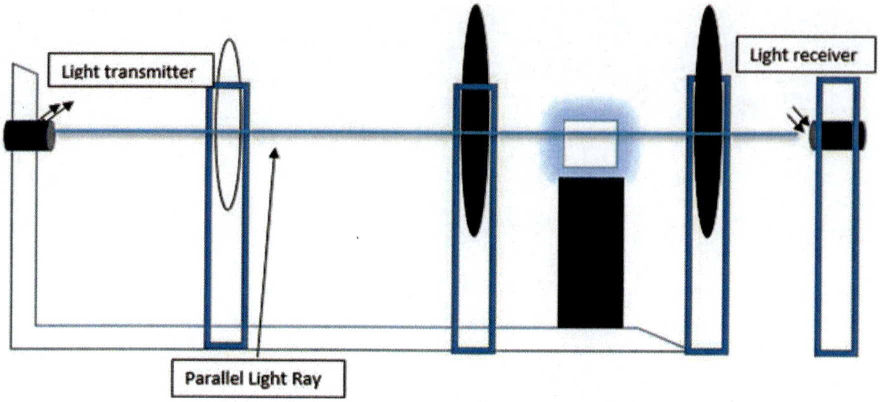

Diagram 3 Light polarization setup from side view (normal line transmission)

polarization properties were a double convex lens (at the focal point of 10 cm), a light polarization film that consists of a linear polarization filter as the polarizer and analyzer films, light-emitting diodes (LED) as the monochromatic light source, a photodiode as a light receiver, a power supply, and a voltage regulator. Once all components and materials had been set up, the experiment was conducted in a dark room and the measurements taken were divided into two parts.

3.3 Measurement

The first measurement was taken to obtain the highest voltage relevant to the highest intensity of light and the second measurement was taken to obtain the orientation angle relevant to the highest voltage and the highest intensity by the photodiode or light receiver. Both measurements were tested for all prepared agarose gel with different weight percentages (3, 6, and 8% (w/w)). However, before the agarose gel was tested in the normal plane of light polarization setup as shown in Diagrams 2 and 3, the highest voltage with no phantom was recorded at the polarizer film and the analyzer film for the calibration of all wavelengths, including blue (460 nm), green (520 nm), yellow (590 nm), and red (625 nm) light. The experiment was then calibrated for different distances (3, 6, and 9 cm) for complete data or measurement.

4 Result

According to Table 1, the red light intensity relevant to the recorded voltage increased as the density of agarose gel increased from 3% (w/w) to 8% (w/w), but slightly dropped when the density of agarose gel reached 10% (w/w). A similar pattern was

Table 1 Voltage readings for all prepared agarose gel for red (R), yellow (Y), and green (G) LEDs at the distance of 3 cm

Density of agarose	3%	6%	8%	10%
R	0.003	0.005	0.009	0.005
Y	0.004	0.007	0.008	0.006
G	0.044	0.059	0.065	0.056

Table 2 Voltage readings for red, yellow, and green LEDs at the distance of 3, 6, and 9 cm for agarose density of 3% (w/w)

Density of agarose	3 cm	6 cm	9 cm
R	0.003	0.003	0.004
Y	0.004	0.004	0.005
G	0.044	0.05	0.048

also observed for yellow and green light. Among all light, green was noted with the highest light intensity based on the highest voltage obtained.

Table 2 presents complete data of voltage (light intensity) specifically for 3% (w/w) of agarose gel by considering all wavelengths and distances involved. The values of light intensity varied with the distance of agarose gel from the polarizer. For all the wavelengths considered, green was again recorded as the highest light intensity relevant to the highest voltage.

5 Discussion

See Table 3.

The angle of polarized light was obtained by simply calculating the difference of orientation angle before and after agarose gel was implemented onto the setup. However, all light wavelengths showed 0° of polarized light for three consecutive trials. The agarose gel showed consistency in increasing the voltage as the density of agarose gel increased for all wavelengths involved in a completed experiment. Like as shown in 3%, 6% and 8% (w/w) of agarose gel for respective 0.003, 0.005 and 0.009 in red wavelength, as well as 0.004, 0.007 and 0.008 in yellow LED and 0.044, 0.059 and 0.065 respectively in green wavelength. For this outcome, Beer-Lambert

Table 3 Average calculated polarized light angle for agarose density of 3% (w/w) at all distances

Distance	3			6			9		
LED/wavelength	R	Y	G	R	Y	G	R	Y	G
Polarization angle without agarose	30	55	50	30	55	50	30	55	50
orientation angle with agarose	30	55	50	30	55	50	30	55	50
Polarized degree	0	0	0	0	0	0	0	0	0

law relates the attenuation of light to the properties of the materials to which the light is traveling [9, 10]. Nevertheless, when the agarose gel reached 10% (w/w), which is the highest of all, the voltage readings slightly dropped instead of increased for all wavelength involved like as shown in Table 3. Again, the law itself stated that they tend to break down at very high concentrations of materials, especially if the materials involved are highly scattered [11]. Thus, this hypothesis has proved that agarose gels own the scattering property, one of the main optical property of light. However, the result could not prove the polarization properties of agarose gel as the polarized angle obtained remained at 0° for all wavelengths within all distances involved. Nevertheless, this outcome obeys the fundamental principle of parallel light at normal plane. No attenuation or polarization of light was observed in the agarose gel if the reflected light ray is vertically parallel to the incident light ray, which interacted with the agarose gel. Hence, this experiment is insufficient to prove the agarose gel-based phantom as a good optical depolarizing agent. This is because the experiment was limited only to normal plane of light transmission. Further investigation of light polarization on the agarose gel-based phantom should be enhanced and emphasized, especially on planes other than normal line of light transmission.

6 Conclusion

In conclusion, the light polarization setup is a reliable and relevant setup for studying light polarization properties in agarose gel-based phantom. Meanwhile, the agarose gel-based phantom should be emphasized for further research as it obeys the Beer-Lambert law. There is no significant light attenuation observed in the perspective of the angle of polarized light after known polarized incident light interacted onto agarose gel with different mass concentrations at normal plane of light transmission.

7 Outlook

If continuous research of light polarization at different planes of light transmission is further emphasized, the outcome of the study could probably be reliable features that can be implemented in current medical imaging technologies for detection or diagnostic approach. This study highlights important parameters of both light polarization features (DOP and AOP) for great qualitative and quantitative optical measurement in new medical imaging devices, and thus, would be a major contributor in medical applications, especially in cancer research.

Acknowledgements We would like to thanks to University of Malaya for providing fund in this project under grant no. BK088-2017, IIRG002B-19SAH and FP114-2020. Special thanks also to reviewers and associate editor for their comments which improved this manuscript.

References

1. Martin, L., Le Brun, G., Le Jeune, B.: Mueller matrix decomposition for biological tissue analysis. Opt. Commun. **293**, 4–9 (2013)
2. Ortega-Quijano, N., Fanjul-Vélez, F., De Cos-Pérez, J., Arce-Diego, J.L.: Analysis of the depolarizing properties of normal and adenomatous polyps in colon mucosa for the early diagnosis of precancerous lesions. Opt. Commun. **284**(19), 4852–4856 (2011)
3. Das, N.K., Dey, R., Chakraborty, S., Panigrahi, P.K., Meglinski, I., Ghosh, N.: Quantitative assessment of submicron scale anisotropy in tissue multifractality by scattering Mueller matrix in the framework of Born approximation. Opt. Commun. **413**(Dec 2017), 172–178 (2018)
4. Borovkova, M., et al.: Complementary analysis of Mueller-matrix images of optically anisotropic highly scattering biological tissues. J. Eur. Opt. Soc. Publ. **14**(1), 1–8 (2018)
5. Jacques, S.L., Roman, J.R., Lee, K.: Imaging of superficial tissues with polarized light. Ann. Biomed. Eng. **28**(Suppl. 1), 119–129 (2000)
6. Mackanos, M.A., Contag, C.H.: Fiber-optic probes enable cancer detection with FTIR spectroscopy. Trends Biotechnol. **28**(6), 317–323 (2010)
7. Huser, T., Chan, J.: Raman spectroscopy for physiological investigations of tissues and cells. Adv. Drug Deliv. Rev. **89**, 57–70 (2015)
8. Liang, L., et al.: Identification of breast cancer through spectroscopic analysis of cell-membrane sialic acid expression. Anal. Chim. Acta **1033**, 148–155 (2018)
9. Onorato, P., Gratton, L.M., Polesello, M., Salmoiraghi, A., Oss, S.: The Beer Lambert law measurement made easy. Phys. Educ. **53**(3), 35033 (2018)
10. Gobrecht, A., Bendoula, R., Roger, J.-M., Bellon-Maurel, V.: Combining linear polarization spectroscopy and the representative layer theory to measure the Beer-Lambert law absorbance of highly scattering materials. Anal. Chim. Acta **853**, 486–494 (2015)
11. Gobrecht, A., Bendoula, R., Roger, J.-M., Maurel, V.B.: Retrieving Beer-Lambert law absorbance of highly scattering materials by combining light polarization spectroscopy and the representative layer theory. In: 17th International Conference on Near Infrared Spectroscopy (NIR 2015), p. 1 (2015)

Design of Rectifier Circuit to Harvest the RF Energy for Wearable Medical Devices

Hussein Yahya Alkhalaf, Mohd Yazed Ahmad, and Harikrishnan Ramiah

Abstract This paper focused on the essential part of the RF energy harvesting system by designing a rectifier circuit capable of harvesting the ambient RF energy to power the wearable medical devices. The bridge rectifier, along with the impedance matching network, has been developed. The simulated results show that conversion efficiencies of 38, 69.22 and 78.77% for the input power of −10, 0 and 5 dBm consecutively at 2.45 GHz. The maximum RF-DC conversion efficiency of 84.63% has been accomplished when the input power was 10 dBm at 1.5 kΩ load resistance. The Simulated DC output voltage of this rectifier is 3.563 V which is adequate to energize low-power medical devices.

Keywords Wearable medical devices · Rectifier circuit · Bridge rectifier

1 Introduction

Nowadays, most wearable medical devices are powered by batteries. The main issue with the battery is that it powers these devices for a limited time. The lifetime of batteries depends on the power consumption of the whole system with batteries' size and energy density. Consequently, the battery of these devices required regular replacement. On the other hand, recycling batteries is complicated and negatively affects the environment. The voltages needed for wearable medical devices such as Combo Insulin Pump, Pulse Oximeter, and Dia II BTE Hearing Aid are 1.5 V,4.2 V, and 1.5 V, respectively [1]. Radiofrequency RF energy harvesting is considered a suitable alternative to batteries by providing the required energy to operate the low power device with an unlimited lifespan. The approach of RF energy harvesting involves converting the ambient RF signals to electrical energy utilizing an antenna. The RF energy harvesting system circuit encompasses an antenna, matching network, rectifier, and power management system, as seen in Fig. 1. The rectifier circuit is the core of the harvesting system for the RF energy; a rectifier circuit converts

H. Y. Alkhalaf · M. Y. Ahmad (✉) · H. Ramiah
Universiti Malaya, 50603 Kuala Lumpur, Malaysia
e-mail: myaz@um.edu.my

J. Usman et al. (eds.), *6th Kuala Lumpur International Conference on Biomedical Engineering 2021*, IFMBE Proceedings 86,
https://doi.org/10.1007/978-3-030-90724-2_41

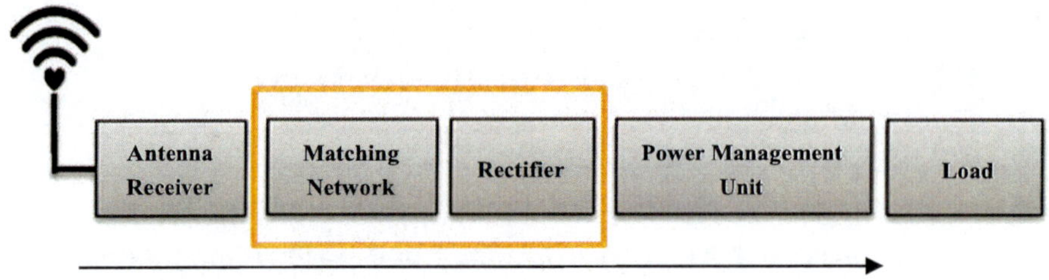

Fig. 1 Block diagram of RF energy harvesting system

the collected RF energy to dc power. An impedance matching network is essential for the efficient transmission of the received power to the rectifier stage. Multiple researches have been conducted to harvest the RF energy for low power devices using numerous topologies of the rectifier circuits. For instance, the study by [2] presented a single stage Cockcroft Walton rectifier that operated at 2.45 GHz; the impedance-matching network of this system is L-shaped, and the DC output voltage is 3.24 V. The system achieved a peak conversion efficiency value of 75.5%. Another study presented two stages rectifier circuits operated at the ISM band. The DC output voltage of this rectifier is 5.2 V with a maximum efficiency of 64%. A single-stage full-wave Greinacher rectifier was designed in [3]. The output voltage of this rectifier 2.2 V with a power conversion efficiency of 17%.

Furthermore, multi section impedance matching with a Series diode rectifier at 2.45 GHz has been proposed [4]. The simulated results of this work obtain 62 and 52% RF to DC conversion efficiency, achieving an output voltage of 3.2 V. The aforementioned related researches show the need to design an efficient rectifier with high output voltage to meet the requirements of common applications for power. Therefore, in this paper, a simulation of an efficient bridge rectifier with an impedance matching network has been designed to absorb the RF energy from the ambient environment at 2.45 GHz frequency.

1.1 Rectifier Circuit Topologies

The rectifier circuit is the vital element of a wireless energy harvesting system. Thus, the development of efficient and compact rectifier circuits has become a critical research issue lately. Rectifiers are classified into two categories diode-based rectifier and metal–oxide–semiconductor field-effect transistor MOSFET based. The diode-based rectifier has a low forward voltage drop compared with Complementary Metal Oxide Semiconductor CMOS circuits which make it used more. Many rectifier topologies have been designed, as shown in Fig. 2. For the half-wave rectifier design, only 50% of the passing AC waveform remains, which means half of the positive or negative AC voltage cycle will be blocked, and the other half of the cycle will pass. The full-wave rectifier topology is mainly used when a half-wave rectifier may not

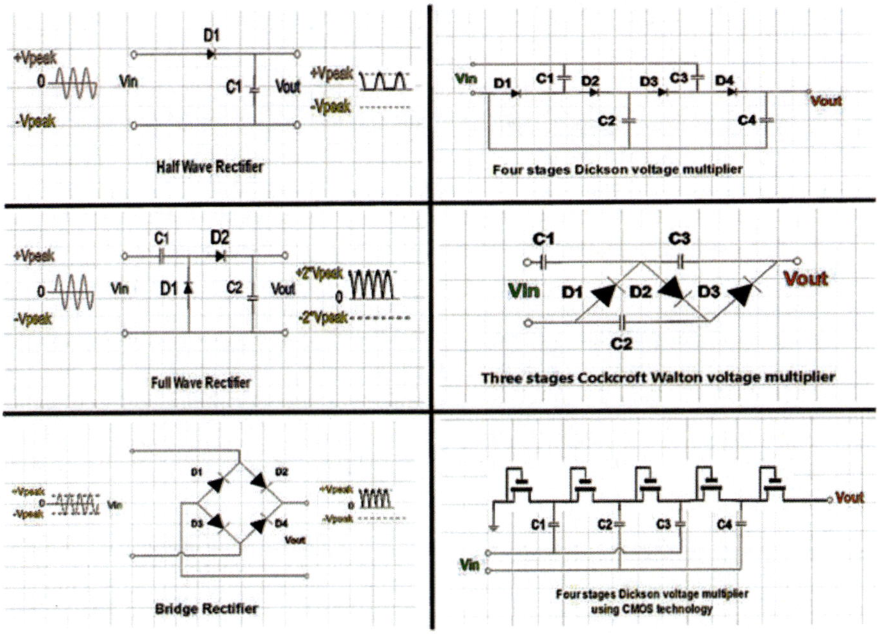

Fig. 2 Various topologies of the rectifier circuits

serve efficiently in common applications. During the first negative cycle of the input AC in the full-wave rectifier, the first diode D1 is fully conductive. At the same time, the capacitor C1 is charged to a similar level as the input peak voltage, Vpeak. After that, at the positive cycle, D2 is conductive, D1 is blocked to charge the capacitor C2. As a result, two capacitors store the Vpeak in the output voltage, becoming double the VPeak. Thus, a full-wave rectifier is considered more efficient than a half-wave rectifier. Bridge rectifier differs from half and full-wave rectifiers by rectifying both negative and positive cycles, keeping the output voltage equal to the peak voltage by blocking 2 diodes pairs D1, D4, and D2, D3. A particular type of rectifier design known as voltage multiplier is used due to more power for some applications; it is used to transform and boost the AC to DC. The voltage multiplier is comprised of several single rectifiers that are assembled in series [5]. Cockcroft–Walton voltage multiplier is the most common topology of the voltage multiplier. This rectifier is comparable to a full-wave rectifier with more stages to get higher voltage gains. On the other hand, MOSFET-based diode features a fast-switching speed but suffers from electromagnetic interference and thermal runaway; a high threshold voltage is also required, limiting EH circuits' performance [6]. Dickson multiplier is a rectifier suitable for small voltage applications used by MOSFET technology; it can be combined with the integrated circuit by changing the diode with a negative channel metal oxide semiconductor NMOS.

2 Design and Analysis of the Proposed Rectifier

A rectifier circuit designed with the impedance matching network ensures efficient energy transfer avoiding power leakage. The source is the receiver antenna which considers operating at 2.45 GHz with 50 Ω. The developed matching circuit involves two microstrip lines. The proposed rectifier circuit is a bridge rectifier and consists of Schottky diodes HSMS-2850 with a low for-ward voltage bias of 0.15 V; it achieves fast switching at high frequencies, making it suitable for use applications with low RF input power. The proposed rectifier operates at the 2.45 GHz ISM band. After the rectification process, the voltage is stored in the load capacitor. Figure 3 shows the rectifier's schematic diagram. Table 1 illustrates the values of the parameters of the rectifier and impedance matching network.

The components of the simulation of the rectifier are as follows: C1 represents the storing capacitor; R1 refers to the load resistance; W1, L1, W2, and L2 are the width and the length of the microstrip lines, and they are used in the simulation of the matching circuit.

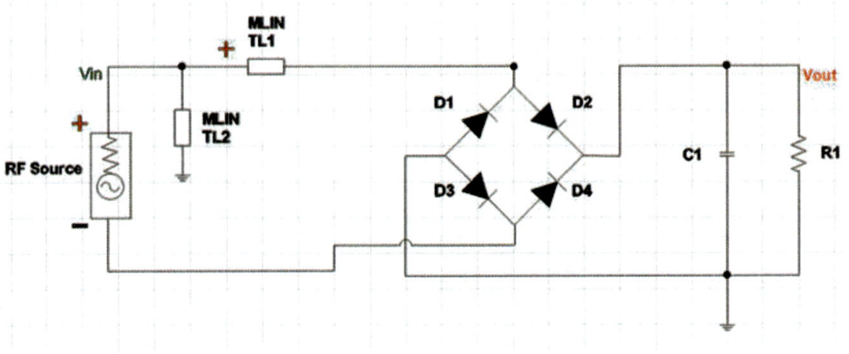

Fig. 3 Schematic diagram of the proposed rectifier circuit

Table 1 The simulation parameters of the impedance matching network and the rectifier

Parameters	Value
W1	0.257045 mm
L1	4.944530 mm
W2	0.257045 mm
L2	15.6250 mm
C1	0.5 PF
R1	1.5 KΩ

3 Results and Discussion

Figure 4 illustrated the S11 characteristic of the Impedance matching network when we tested three different Agilent's Schottky diodes HSMS family to choose the perfect diode for the proposed bridge rectifier. The simulation results demonstrate that the reflection coefficient of the rectifier based on diode HSMS-2850 is −23 dB at 2.45 GHz, which shows that the system is well matched. On the other hand, applying the diodes of HSMS-2860 and HSMS-2820 in the design will decrease the reflection coefficient to −3.5 at 2.45 GHz and −1.4 at 2.2 GHz, respectively, which is not identical with the circuit. Therefore, the HSMS-2850 diode was selected for this design to enable the rectifier to supply load efficiently from the antenna.

Figure 5 shows the response of the rectifier circuit when we keep increasing the input power (which will raise the output voltage level). The output voltage of the proposed rectifier circuit for the input power of −40, −30, −20, −10, 0, 5, 10 dBm were 0.005, 0.016, 0.057, 0.239, 1.019, 1.933, 3.563 V respectively, at load resistance of 1.5 kΩ and frequency band of 2.45 GHz (Table 2).

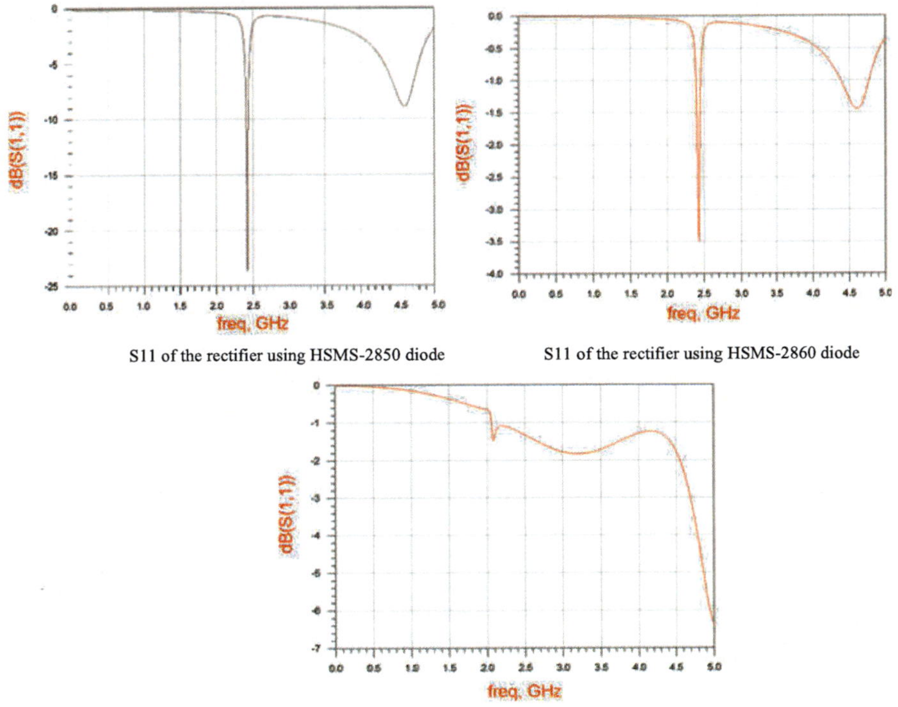

S11 of the rectifier using HSMS-2850 diode

S11 of the rectifier using HSMS-2860 diode

S11 of the rectifier using HSMS-2820 diode

Fig. 4 Reflection coefficient (S11) Effect for different diodes at 2.45 GHz

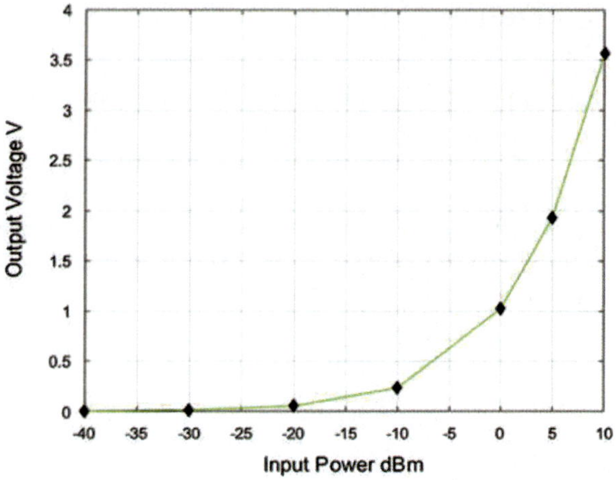

Fig. 5 Output voltage versus input power at 1 kΩ

Table 2 Comparison of the proposed rectifier with related published works

References	Rectifier	Frequency (GHz)	Input power range (dBm)	Output voltage (V)	Diode	Conversion Efficiency %
[7]	Half wave rectifier	2.45	−20 to 0	–	HSMS-286C	61.4
[8]	Bridge rectifier	0.9–2.45	−30 to 30	6.5	HSMS-2850	78
[9]	Grienarcher voltage multiplier	0.9, 1.8, 2.1, 2.45	−30 to 15	1.5	HSMS-2852	55
[10]	Bridge rectifier	2.4	−20 to 20	0.19	HSMS-2850	96
Proposed rectifier	Bridge rectifier	2.45	−40 to 10	3.563	HSMS-2850	84.63

3.1 Conversion Efficiency of the Proposed Rectifier Circuit

The most crucial factor to consider when evaluating the performance of a rectifier circuit is efficiency. The conversion efficiency of the suggested rectifier was calculated thus:

$$\eta = \frac{(V_{DC})^2/R_L}{P_{IN}} \quad (1)$$

V_{DC} represents the direct current output voltage, R_L refers to the load resistance, and P_{in} indicates the input power.

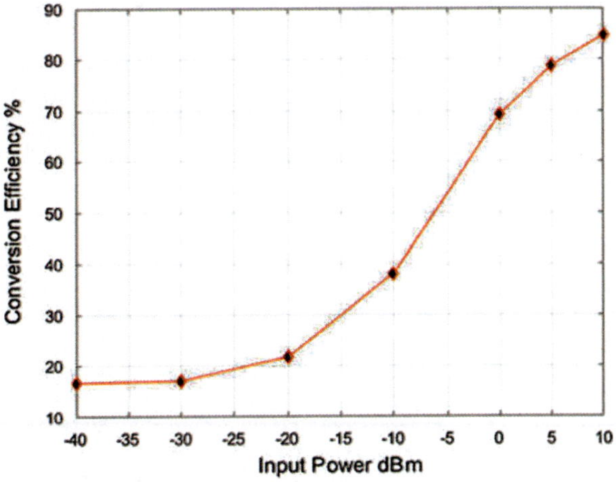

Fig. 6 Conversion efficiencies of the rectifier at a various input power level

Figure 6 shows the fluctuations in the rectifier efficiency as a result of the variations in input power. The conversion efficiencies of the projected rectifier at −40 dBm, −30 dBm, −20 dBm, -10 dBm, 0 dBm, 5 dBm,10 dBm are 16.6%, 17%, 21.66%, 38%, 69.22%, 78.77%, and 84.63 respectively.

4 Conclusion

In this paper, the rectifier circuit topologies of the RF energy harvesting system have been investigated with the design of an efficient rectifier to harvest the RF energy for wearable medical devices. The proposed bridge rectifier circuit designed based on Schottky diode HSMS-2850 tested at 2.45 GHz. The peak efficiency was 84.63% at 10 dBm input power when the load resistance is 1.5 kΩ. The rectifier simulation result showed an output voltage of 3.563 V, which is suitable to power most low-power wearable medical devices.

Acknowledgements This work was supported by the Ministry of Higher Education of Malaysia (MOHE), grants codes No. FP124-2020, GPF001A-2019, GPF06A-2018.

References

1. Khan, N.U., Khan, F.U.: RF energy harvesting for portable biomedical devices. In: 2019 22nd International Multitopic Conference (INMIC). IEEE (2019)
2. Awais, Q., et al.: A compact rectenna system with high conversion efficiency for wireless energy harvesting. IEEE Access **6**, 35857–35866 (2018)

3. Lin, C.-H., Chiu, C.-W., Gong, J.-Y.: A wearable rectenna to harvest low-power RF energy for wireless healthcare applications. In: 2018 11th International Congress on Image and Signal Processing, BioMedical Engineering and Informatics (CISP-BMEI). IEEE (2018)
4. Gupta, A., Pattapu, U., Das, S.: High efficiency low power series diode rectifier design. In: 2018 3rd International Conference on Microwave and Photonics (ICMAP). IEEE (2018)
5. Gosset, G., Flandre, D.: Fully-automated and portable design methodology for optimal sizing of energy-efficient CMOS voltage rectifiers. IEEE J. Emerg. Sel. Top. Circ. Syst. **1**(2), 141–149 (2011)
6. Kailuke, A.C., Agrawal, P., Kshirsagar, R.: Design and implementation of low power Dickson charge pump in 0.18 μm. CMOS Process **15**, 3 (2013)
7. Chen, Y.-S., Chiu, C.-W.: Maximum achievable power conversion efficiency obtained through an optimized rectenna structure for RF energy harvesting. IEEE Trans. Antennas Propag. **65**(5), 2305–2317 (2017)
8. Marian, V., et al.: Strategy for microwave energy harvesting from ambient field or a feeding source. IEEE Trans. Power Electron. **27**(11), 4481–4491 (2012)
9. Sun, H., et al.: Design of a high-efficiency 2.45-GHz rectenna for low-input-power energy harvesting. IEEE Antennas Wirel. Propag. Lett. **11**, 929–932
10. Hamzi, I., et al.: Conversion efficiency study of the bridge rectifier at 2.4 GHz. Procedia Manuf. **46**, 771–776 (2020)

Assessing Clinical Usefulness of Readmission Risk Prediction Model

Kareen Teo, Ching Wai Yong, Joon Huang Chuah, Khairunnisa Hasikin, Maheza Irna Mohd Salim, Yan Chai Hum, and Khin Wee Lai

Abstract Readmission manifests signs of degraded quality of care and increased healthcare cost. Such adverse event may be attributed to premature discharge, unsuccessful treatments, or worsening comorbidities. Predictive modeling provides useful information to identify patients at a higher risk for readmission for targeted interventions. Though many studies have proposed readmission risk predictive models and validated their discriminative ability with performance metrics, few examined the net benefit realized by a predictive model. We compared traditional logistic regression against modern neural network to predict unplanned readmission. An added value of 7% on discriminative ability is observed for modern machine learning model compared to regression. A cost analysis is provided to assist physicians and hospital management for translating the theoretical value into real cost and resource allocation after model implementation. The neural network model is projected to contribute 15× more savings by reducing readmissions. Aside from constructing better performing models, the results of our study demonstrate the potential of a clinically helpful prediction tool in terms of strategies to reduce cost associated with readmission.

Keywords Cost saving · Predictive modeling · Readmission

K. Teo · C. W. Yong · K. Hasikin · K. W. Lai (✉)
Faculty of Engineering, Department of Biomedical Engineering, Universiti Malaya, Kuala Lumpur, Malaysia
e-mail: lai.khinwee@um.edu.my

J. H. Chuah
Faculty of Engineering, Department of Electrical Engineering, Universiti Malaya, Kuala Lumpur, Malaysia

M. I. M. Salim
Faculty of Engineering, School of Biomedical Engineering, Universiti Teknologi Malaysia, Johor Bahru, Malaysia

Y. C. Hum
Department of Mechatronics and Biomedical Engineering, Universiti Tunku Abdul Rahman, 43000 Sungai Long, Malaysia

J. Usman et al. (eds.), *6th Kuala Lumpur International Conference on Biomedical Engineering 2021*, IFMBE Proceedings 86,
https://doi.org/10.1007/978-3-030-90724-2_42

1 Introduction

Precision medicine refers to a more personalized and targeted care that aims to ensure every patient receive treatment and care tailored to individual precise needs throughout not only during the inpatient stay, but also recovery phases of a disease. Unplanned readmission is a popular indicator to determine quality of care. From a hospital perspective, high readmission rates can result in negative financial and reputational ramifications.

Improving the quality-of-care delivery is challenging. It requires close coordination between different stakeholders in health system to deliver low-cost and high-quality care to patients. As an attempt to reduce readmission rate, lower healthcare cost, and thus improving overall quality of care, healthcare regulatory agencies have proposed the Hospital Readmission Reduction Program (HRRP) [1]. Under the HRRP, readmission is defined as a readmission episode that is unplanned and happen within 30 days of discharge from the index admission. Penalties are levied on hospitals depending on their performance with respect to readmission rate. The total fines cost healthcare providers an amount of over $500 million annually, or $200 k per hospital [2, 3]. Thus, identifying patients at high-risk of readmission is crucial to allow early interventions.

The recent availability of large amount of clinical data and emergence of machine learning (ML) methods offer the potential to predict high-risk readmission accurately. ML-based tools have been proven to be able to achieve at least or above prognostic and diagnostic capabilities of human [4–6]. This success is driven by newer and better prediction algorithms, such as random forests, gradient boosting, neural networks, and other methods. Unlike traditional statistical approaches, these models can leverage large-scale clinical data to discover predictive variables regardless of parametric or nonparametric nature of data [7, 8].

A predictive model estimates the risk of readmission for an individual based on the values of multiple predictors (risk factors) such as age, comorbidity, and other biomarkers. A large number of readmission risk prediction models have been published in medical literature. For example, Allam et al. [9] explored the predictability of readmission with neural network-based models versus logistic regression using administrative data. Min et al. [10] developed various ML models (e.g., regression, random forest, support vector machines and multi-layer perceptron (MLP)) to predict readmission risk from patients' claims data. Recently, deep learning, a type of neural network model with multiple hidden layers is gaining popularity because it mimics the way human brain works, where more informative features are obtained at each layer. The potential of such architecture has also been explored in readmission literature. Wang et al. [11] proposed the use of convolutional neural networks (CNN) to automatically learn time series vital sign and encode statistical features via embedding. Both features are fed into MLP for prediction. Rajkomar et al. [12] leveraged patients' entire raw electronic medical records (EMR), including free text notes for prediction with the ensemble of three deep learning models.

Despite promising results shown by neural networks, a recent review confirmed that regression was the main prediction method utilized in most of the studies [13].

Theoretically, a model should have good discriminative performance, often measured using area under receiver operating characteristic curve (AUC). However, this metrics may be less meaningful and end users might find it to be unclear on how to translate these performance benefits into cost and resource allocation. Specifically, implementation of cost-effective interventions is critical to mitigate the risk of readmission, and thus reducing direct costs incurred by readmission. The goal of this paper is to assess the clinical usefulness of readmission prediction model with cost analysis. We comprehensively examined the cost on post-model implementation. This should guide decision making on planning and optimizing hospital resources. The focus of research is therefore shifting from conventional attempts to optimize performance of models to studying models' impacts on outcomes in real-world intervention.

2 Data and Methods

In this paper, we aim to (1) explore the application of logistic regression versus neural networks for predicting readmission and (2) examine the value of such predictive models in clinical adoption. The output of model is the estimated probability of each patient being readmitted within 30 days of a prior hospital discharge. Such prediction is made on the day of discharge.

2.1 *Dataset*

The patient records were acquired from a publicly available real-world electronic health record repository of ICU cohort known as the Multiparameter Intelligent Monitoring in Intensive Care (MIMIC-III) dataset [14]. MIMIC-III consists of the EMR data of 58,976 unique hospital admissions from 46,520 patients in the Beth Israel Deaconess Medical Center between 2001 and 2012. ADMISSIONS and NOTEEVENTS tables of MIMIC-III database were retrieved to obtain discharge summaries as predictor variables.

2.2 *Predictors and Model*

Preparing clinical notes to be analyzable and predictable requires a combination of text representation and prediction model. We composed logistic regression as the baseline model. Representation method, i.e., bag of words (BoW) creates vector representations of document-based features. These features were fed into regression for prediction in Scikit-learn. For the neural networks, word embed-ding model was trained to capture semantic relationship within text data via Word2Vec. After identification of word vector, we applied CNN to predict readmission with clinical notes. After exploring several architectures, we composed these models with a 1D shallow network structure that achieved the highest AUC. Therefore, the final model consists of an embedding layer initialized with pre-trained Word2vec, a convolutional (CNN) layer with 256 hidden units, and a dense output label sigmoid. The filter size of 5 produces the best result for CNN with a max pooling layer right after the convolution structure. CNN was trained for 25 epochs with a batch size of 64 in Keras. All models were trained on 80% of data and remaining 20% were withheld for validation and testing, respectively.

2.3 Experimental Pipeline

The experimental pipeline comprised two major parts. The first one was examining the performance of predictive models. The set of models was evaluated with ability to detect readmission (proportion of readmission predicted as True), and the AUC. The second part was validating the clinical usefulness of models on entire MIMIC-III dataset with cost analysis. The procedure for the experimental pipeline is illustrated in Fig. 1.

After readmission prediction, models were evaluated for their clinical usefulness via cost-saving analysis. There are 3 factors associated with the effort to maximize cost savings with optimal intervention threshold: (1) readmission cost, (2) expected intervention cost, and (3) effectiveness of intervention (intervention might not be effective to prevent readmission). Given a set of N patients, the net saving can be calculated using the following equation:

$$Netsavings : C_r N_{TP} \delta - (N_{TP} + N_{FP}) C_i \tag{1}$$

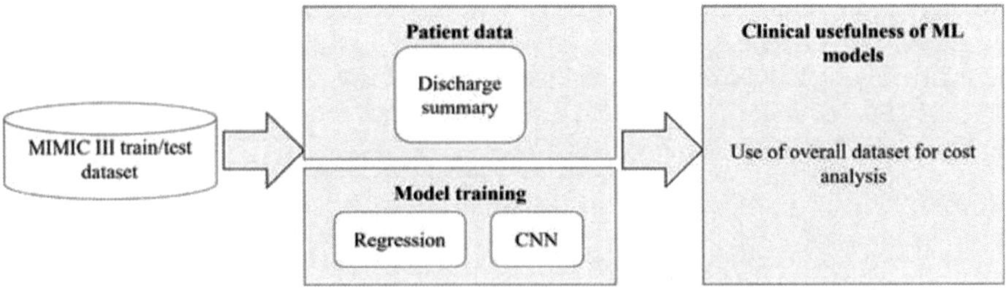

Fig. 1 Readmission prediction uses models trained with balanced patient data comprises clinical notes contained in EMR. The models then tested on the entire database for cost analysis

Table 1 Performance of models on test dataset for the detection of readmission during discharge

Models	Readmissions detected (%)	AUC
Regression	66	0.67
CNN	84	0.72

Table 2 Percentage change of TP, TN, FP, FN readmissions due to implementation of predictive models upon discharge on entire patient population

Models	TP, %	TN, %	FP, %	FN, %	Discriminative ability
Regression	0.37	92.53	0.85	6.25	0.52
CNN	5.70	81.21	12.17	0.92	0.87

where C_r is the average readmission cost per patient; N_{TP} is the number of true positive; δ is the intervention success rate; $N_{TP} + N_{FP}$ is the number of predicted positives; and C_i represents intervention cost.

3 Results

3.1 Predictive Performance

Table 1 depicts the performance of models on the prediction of readmission made upon discharge. For classifying readmission instances, neural network model substantially outperformed predictions mapped from traditional statistical regression.

For each model, we then evaluated the performance outcome for entire patient database. 0.8 threshold was employed to label readmission as high-risk. This is due to it is impossible to target all high-risk patients for interventions. We report in Table 2 the percentage of True Positive (TP), True Negative (TN), False Positive (FP), and False Negative (FN) predictions in the overall dataset, defined as the ratio of respective number of patients over the entire base. Discrimination ability was reported in comparison with these numbers. As compared to evaluation on test set, CNN generalizes prediction much better than regression model on entire base.

3.2 Cost Analysis

After identifying high-risk patients accurately, healthcare providers need to plan on the cost-effective interventions to prevent readmission. Intervention success rate is important here as it indicates the rate of successfully preventing a readmission after applying intervention to a patient predicted as high-risk. For example, the rate of 50% means another 50% of patients who underwent interventions would still be

Table 3 Net savings from readmission reduction by selecting patients for intervention at different success rate

Intervention success rate (%)	Regression net saving, $	CNN net saving, $
10	−645,658	−9,346,354
20	−487,316	−6,929,707
30	−328,974	−4,513,061
40	−170,632	−2,096,414
50	−12,290	320,233
60	146,052	2,736,879
70	304,394	5,153,526
80	462,736	7,570,172
90	621,078	9,986,819
100	779,420	12,403,465

readmitted within 30 days. For this cost saving analysis, the estimation of actual values might be difficult, we then used the followings values established in past literature for calculation [15]: Readmission cost per patient: $9655, Intervention cost per patient: $1500. Table 3 shows the maximum net savings from readmission reduction considering the intervention success rate from 10 to 100%.

As depicted in Table 3, if healthcare providers were able to prevent as much readmission through interventions, the more savings can be generated, provided a minimum response rate of 50% is achieved. For CNN, every incremental in the success rate by 10%, extra 2.5 mil of saving can be projected. On the other hand, regression model does not bring significant economic benefits, due to its poor discriminative ability. When comparing both models at positive saving (60% response rate and above), at least 15 times more saving could potentially be generated by CNN over regression approach.

4 Discussion

This was a study which applied regression baseline and neural network model on unstructured clinical prose to construct a risk prediction model for 30-day readmission. While almost all studies used AUC to measure how well a model performs, the main issue is the absent of a clear translation from making ML solutions to creating real clinical impact [16]. Therefore, we studied model's impact on the financial performance to offer an analysis metric that is more meaningful to hospital management.

We found that word embedding methods like Word2Vec paired with neural networks improved overall predictive ability of models, when compared to simpler BOW/logistic regression. Considering evaluation made on test set which consists of balanced positive/negative label, the highest AUC was observed at 0.72 using model built with CNN, which is 7% improvement over regression. While the exact number of preventable readmission episode is unclear, our paper shows that the cost saving for all-cause readmission could exceed $12 million dollars if all readmission events could be prevented with early interventions.

With these observations, we found that predicting readmission remains challenging. Unlike other domains such as computer vision where ML/deep learning models have been proved to have achieved very high accuracy, medical prognosis is much more complicated. In addition, less training samples are available due to the sensitivity of patient information. In this case, domain knowledge could play a vital role in model building process so that we could train a good model without 'sufficiently large' patient dataset. Because neural network are less interpretable, simpler model built from identifying factors contributing to performance could be potentially more helpful.

5 Conclusion

We conducted a study on 30-day readmission predictive modeling based on unstructured clinical notes with the combination of natural language processing and classification algorithms, considering both traditional and modern machine learning models. Our results also provide an insight for identifying the economic benefits that could be generated by selecting intervention enrollees based on predicted readmission risk. This financial impact assessment is necessary so that policymakers and regulators are more confident with the integration of such predictive tool into care provider workflow.

Acknowledgements This work was supported by the 2020 APT EBC-C (Extra-Budgetary Contributions from China) Project on Promoting the Use of ICT for Achievement of Sustainable Development Goals, and University Malaya under grant IF015-2021.

References

1. McIlvennan, C.K., Eapen, Z.J., Allen, L.A.: Hospital readmissions reduction program. Circulation **131**(20), 1796–1803 (2015)
2. Boccuti, C., Casillas, G.: Aiming for fewer hospital U-turns: the Medicare hospital readmission reduction program. Policy Brief (2015)
3. Hoffman, G.J., Yakusheva, O.: Association between financial incentives in medicare's hospital readmissions reduction program and hospital readmission performance. JAMA Netw. Open **3**(4), e202044–e202044 (2020)
4. Topol, E.J.: High-performance medicine: the convergence of human and artificial intelligence. Nat. Med. **25**(1), 44–56 (2019)
5. Yong, C.W., et al.: Knee osteoarthritis severity classification with ordinal regression module. Multimedia Tools and Applications (2021)

6. Yong, C.W., et al.: Comparative study of encoder-decoder-based convolutional neural networks in cartilage delineation from knee magnetic resonance images. Curr Med Imaging (2020)
7. Teo, K., et al.: Discovering the predictive value of clinical notes: machine learning analysis with text representation. J Med Imag Health Inform **10**(12), 2869–2875 (2020)
8. Teo, K., et al.: Early detection of readmission risk for decision support based on clinical notes. J. Med. Imag. Health Inform. **11**(2), 529–534 (2021)
9. Allam, A., et al.: Neural networks versus Logistic regression for 30 days all-cause readmission prediction. Sci. Rep. **9**(1), 9277 (2019)
10. Min, X., Yu, B., Wang, F.: Predictive modeling of the hospital readmission risk from patients' claims data using machine learning: a case study on COPD. Sci. Rep. **9**(1), 2362 (2019)
11. Wang, H., et al.: Predicting hospital readmission via cost-sensitive deep learning. IEEE/ACM Trans. Comput. Biol. Bioinf. **15**(6), 1968–1978 (2018)
12. Rajkomar, A., et al.: Scalable and accurate deep learning with electronic health records. npj Digital Medicine **1**(1), 18 (2018)
13. Artetxe, A., Beristain, A., Graña, M.: Predictive models for hospital readmission risk: a systematic review of methods. Comput. Methods Programs Biomed. **164**, 49–64 (2018)
14. Johnson, A.E.W., et al.: MIMIC-III, a freely accessible critical care database. Sci. Data **3**(1), 160035 (2016)
15. Golas, S.B., et al.: A machine learning model to predict the risk of 30-day readmissions in patients with heart failure: a retrospective analysis of electronic medical records data. BMC Med Inform Decis Mak **18**(1), 44 (2018)
16. Mateen, B.A., et al.: Improving the quality of machine learning in health applications and clinical research. Nat. Mach. Intell. **2**(10), 554–556 (2020)

Prediction of Spine Decompression Post-surgery Outcome Through Transcranial Motor Evoked Potential Using Linear Discriminant Analysis Algorithm

Mohd Redzuan Jamaludin, Saw Lim Beng, Joon Huang Chuah, Khairunnisa Hasikin, Maheza Irna Mohd Salim, Yan Chai Hum, and Khin Wee Lai

Abstract Transcranial motor evoked potential (TcMEP) is one of the modalities in intraoperative neuromonitoring (IONM) which has been used in spine surgeries to prevent motor function injuries. Studies have shown that improvement to TcMEP could be a potential prognostic information on the actual improvement to the patient after surgery. There is no objective way currently to identify which TcMEP signal is significant to indicate actual positive relief of symptoms. The proposed method utilized linear discriminant analysis (LDA) machine learning algorithm to predict the TcMEP response that correlates to relieve of symptoms post-surgery. TcMEP data were obtained from four patients that had pre surgery symptoms with post-surgery actual relief of symptoms, and six patients that had no pre surgery and post-surgery symptoms which were divided into training and prediction test. The result of the proposed method produced 87.5% of accuracy in prediction capabilities.

M. R. Jamaludin · K. Hasikin · K. W. Lai (✉)
Faculty of Engineering, Department of Biomedical Engineering, Universiti Malaya, Kuala Lumpur, Malaysia
e-mail: lai.khinwee@um.edu.my

J. H. Chuah
Faculty of Engineering, Department of Electrical Engineering,, Universiti Malaya, Kuala Lumpur, Malaysia

M. I. M. Salim
Faculty of Engineering, School of Biomedical Engineering, Universiti Teknologi Malaysia, Johor Bahru, Malaysia

Y. C. Hum
Department of Mechatronics and Biomedical Engineering, Universiti Tunku Abdul Rahman, 43000 Sungai Long, Malaysia

S. L. Beng
Spine Surgery Department, Sunway Medical Centre, Petaling Jaya, Selangor, Malaysia

J. Usman et al. (eds.), *6th Kuala Lumpur International Conference on Biomedical Engineering 2021*, IFMBE Proceedings 86,
https://doi.org/10.1007/978-3-030-90724-2_43

Keywords Transcranial motor evoked potential · TcMEP · Intraoperative neuromonitoring · IONM · TcMEP improvement · Prognostic information · Linear discriminant analysis · Machine learning

1 Introduction

1.1 Background Information

Intraoperative neuromonitoring (IONM) has been used in spine surgeries to assist in preventing nerve injury during the procedures [1]. It has different modalities to cater different nerve pathways and locations depending on which structures that are in risk during the procedures.

Transcranial motor evoked potential (TcMEP) is one of the modalities in IONM which is used to monitor the integrity of the patient's motor pathway [2]. The method of TcMEP monitoring is by applying external stimulus onto the motor cortex of the brain through cranial [3]. Once the stimulus is applied to the motor cortex, it will trigger the neurons along the motor pathways towards the nerve roots and finally will evoke action potentials that causes contraction on the muscles while the patient is asleep under anaesthesia. The action potentials can then be captured via electrodes placed on the muscles.

1.2 Problem Statement

TcMEP has been used mainly as indicator to warn any nerve damages during surgery by comparing the TcMEP response from time to time with the baseline reading [2]. The warning can help the surgeons and the surgical teams to decide on what could have happened to the surgical site and try to reverse the situation before the damage becomes significant and permanent.

There has been a new approach of using the TcMEP as an indicator to show if neurological improvement is achieved after the surgical procedure has been done. The use of TcMEP as a valued prognostic information can help the surgeon to decide whether the surgical maneuver such as decompression during discectomy is enough to suggest symptoms elevations and the surgery time can be shortened and reduces risk to the nerves [4].

But there are multiple ways or indicators used in the literatures to show which TcMEP response is significant to predict positive outcome in terms of patient's relief of symptoms after surgery. The challenge is to determine an objective single indicator also come from the high variability of TcMEP from one response to another, which leads to the difficulty in making assumptions that the final TcMEP response has significant improvement compare to the baseline reading.

This paper is proposing a method to determine a significant improved TcMEP response that indicates actual positive functional outcome of patient's relief of symptoms by using linear discriminant analysis machine learning algorithm.

2 Literature Review

There are no fixed amplitude improvement criteria throughout the literatures. A study from [5] used 50% of amplitude increment as the significant improvement criteria, while another study by [6] used 200% of amplitude increment to be significant in order to overcome the effect of anaesthesia which could have affected the baseline reading. Meanwhile other studies only mentioned that TcMEP improvement indicated patient's improvement of symptoms post-surgery without mentioning what features from the signal used as the indicator [6–12].

The TcMEP response improvement were compared with post-surgery patients' clinical evaluation consisted of various methods in the form of pain perception [5], questionnaire [13], sensory and motor function assessment [14], and several researchers did not mentioned the method that they used for patients' symptoms improvement assessments [7–9, 12]. There were correlation between the two in the studioes which implying that TcMEP could predict patients' symptoms relief post-surgery.

3 Methodology

3.1 Equipment Setup

The MEP were stimulated by using corkscrew electrodes placed at the C3 and C4 over the motor cortex on the scalp according to the International 10–20 System scalp electrode placements. The electrode placement for monitoring by using dual subdermal needle electrodes were placed at different muscles bilaterally according to the spine level where the surgery was performed. Each muscle is called channel. The monitoring was done by using NIM Eclipse E4 Medtronic machine. The muscles and the spine levels that they are associated with are listed as in Table 1.

The stimulus intensity varied from 250 to 600 V. Train pulse stimulus of three to five pulses was applied to most of the patients to overcome the response variability or inconsistency. Sometimes, double train stimulation of five pulses and three pulses was used if it was difficult to elicit MEP response. Interstimuli interval was set to be either at 5 or 10 ms which was based on which produced the better MEP response. Overall, the ideal MEP stimulation would be to elicit the response of more than 20 μV for each channel with minimal patient movement.

Table 1 Muscles that are used for MEP and EMG monitoring and their nerve root levels

Spine level	Muscles
C8–T1	(upper limb as reference) Abductor digiti minimi (ADM)
L2–L4	Vastus lateralis (VL)
L5	Tibialis anterior (TA)
S1–S2	Abductor hallucis (AH)

3.2 Data Acquisitions and Patients Selection

The TcMEP data were obtained and selected from patients that underwent various types of thoracolumbar surgeries from September 2018 until April 2021 that had IONM assistance at Sunway Medical Centre. The data were separated into two groups, Group 1 (G1) consisted of four patients that had one or more of the following symptoms such as motor weakness, back and leg pain, and leg numbness that were confirmed through surgeons' consultations and clinical reports. The patients had decompression surgeries such as endoscopic discectomy or microendoscopic discectomy, and thoracolumbar interbody fusion (TLIF).

Group 2 (G2) consisted of six patients without any symptoms described before and most of their operations involved instrumentations and pedicle screws fixations and corrections such as scoliosis surgery, and minimally invasive surgery (MIS) screws fixation. Consultations were done with the surgeons to know what is the outcome of each surgery whether patients really had relief of symptoms or not.

3.3 Features Extraction

Features for the machine learning model were extracted from two channels of the TcMEP data which were from tibialis anterior (TA) and abductor hallucis (AH) bilateral channels. The features were obtained through MATLAB programming language are peak-to-peak amplitude, area under the curve (AUC), maximum amplitude, minimum amplitude, standard deviation, and zero crossing rate (ZCR).

The features' parameters were obtained from the baseline TcMEP reading, and the percentage of difference with the values obtained from the final TcMEP reading were calculated and recorded. These differences of percentages were the features used to feed the linear discriminant analysis classifier by using MATLAB embedded classification learner application.

The training data consisted of two patients from G1 and four patients from G2. While the prediction accuracy test was done with two patients from G1 and two patients from G2.

3.4 Performance Evaluation

The performance of the classifier was evaluated by using the commonly used evaluation for classification algorithms which are [15]:

$$Accuracy = \frac{TP + TN}{TP + FN + FP + TN} \tag{1}$$

$$Sensitivity = \frac{TP}{TP + FN} \tag{2}$$

$$Specificity = \frac{TN}{TN + FP} \tag{3}$$

$$Precision = \frac{TP}{TP + FP} \tag{4}$$

$$f\ measures = 2 \times \frac{Precision \times sensitivity}{Precision + sensitivity} \tag{5}$$

where TP stands for true positive where patient with improvement is correctly identified as having post-surgery improvement, TN is true negative value that indicates patients with no improvement is correctly predicted to have no post-surgery improvement, FP is false positive indicating patients with improvement falsely predicted as having no post-surgery improvement, and FN is false negative that indicates patients with no improvement as having post-surgery improvement.

4 Results and Discussion

For training of the algorithm, a total of 12 samples were used taken from six patient's left and right legs. There were 144 values of features used for LDA algorithm training. As much as four patients' data used which makes a total of eight samples from bilateral legs used for algorithm accuracy test. This leads to a total 96 features used for testing of the algorithm. The results showed that 100% of TP, 75% of TN, 0% of FP rate and 25% of FN rates were achieved. These results to 87.5% of system accuracy, with 80% sensitivity, 100% specificity, and 100% of precision. The f measures resulted as 0.8889. Table 2 summarizes the results through confusion matrix:

One instance of TcMEP in one of the patients were predicted to be improved even though there is no actual improvement post-surgery. This happened because of the percentage difference for TA amplitude, TA AUC, and TA standard deviation were too large with the values 476.63%, 657.4%, and 538.07% respectively causing the algorithm to make false prediction.

Table 2 Confusion matrix of the results obtained from 4 samples of patients with actual improvement and 4 samples of patients with no improvement clinically

	Positive clinical improvement	No clinical improvement
Positive (predict improvement)	4	1
No improvement predicted	0	3

The false prediction could be caused by anaesthesia protocol. At Sunway Medical Centre, most of the anaesthetists used muscle relaxant and/or inhalational agents during intubation which suppresses the TcMEP response [16]. This will affect the baseline reading, that is if the TcMEP is suppressed during the baseline establishment, the response could be thought as having weakness and the final outcome could be thought as improved even though it is just the effect after all of the suppressing anaesthesia agents have worn off which can lead to the proposed algorithm error.

The baseline establishment could be further improved by doing stimulation from time to time before the decompression procedure is done. The baseline reading needs to be renewed until the best reading is achieved so that it could be compared effectively with the final TcMEP response.

5 Conclusion

The proposed method of predicting the post-surgery improvement through intraoperative TcMEP by using LDA achieved 87.5% of accuracy. Though more improvement needs to be done, such as the number of samples to train and to test the algorithm, and the features that could be extracted from the TcMEP response.

Predicting patients to have a relief of symptoms during surgeries could help the surgeons to decide on the depth of spine decompressions that is needed. Once the TcMEP could be reliable to identify the patients' improvement, the length of surgeries duration can be cut down and will benefit in terms of risk of injury and infection, and cost can be reduced.

Acknowledgements This work was supported by the Fundamental Research Grant Scheme (FRGS)

FRGS/1/2019/TK04/UM/01/2 (FP046-2019A), Ministry of Education, Malaysia

References

1. Gonzalez, A.A., Jeyanandarajan, D., Hansen, C., Zada, G., Hsieh, P.C.: Intraoperative neurophysiological monitoring during spine surgery: a review. Neurosurg Focus **27**(4), E6 (2009)

2. Agrawal, G., Iyer, S., All, A.H.: A comparative study of recording procedures for motor evoked potential signals. In: Proceedings of IEEE Engineeing in Medicine and Biology Society (2009)
3. MacDonald, D.B., Skinner, S., Shils, J., Yingling, C.: Intraoperative motor evoked potential monitoring—a position statement by the American Society of Neurophysiological Monitoring. Clin. Neurophysiol. **124**(12), 2291–2316 (2013)
4. Tanaka, S., Hirao, J., Oka, H., Akimoto, J., Takanashi, J., Yamada, J.: Intraoperative monitoring during decompression of the spinal cord and spinal nerves using transcranial motor-evoked potentials: the law of twenty percent. J. Clin. Neurosci. **22**(9), 1403–1407 (2015)
5. Voulgaris, S., Karagiorgiadis, D., Alexiou, G.A., Mihos, E., Zigouris, A., Fotakopoulos, G., Drosos, D., Pahaturidis, D.: Continuous intraoperative electromyographic and transcranial motor evoked potential recordings in spinal stenosis surgery. J. Clin. Neurosci. **17**(2), 274–276 (2010)
6. Visser, J., Verra, W.C., Kuijlen, J.M., Horsting, P.P., Journee, H.L.: Recovery of TES-MEPs during surgical decompression of the spine: a case series of eight patients. J Clin. Neurophysiol. **31**(6), 568–574 (2014)
7. Barley, J.L., Mooney, J.F., Glazier, S.S., Johnson, T., Kornegay, A.L., Turner, R.P., Edwards, J.C.: Sudden appearance of new upper extremity motor function while performing neurophysiologic intraoperative monitoring during tethered cord release: a case report. J. Pediatr. Orthop. **30**(6), 624–628 (2010)
8. Rodrigues, L.M., Rosa, F.W., Ferreira, R.J., Ueno, F., Milani, C.: Herniated lumbar disc surgery in triathlon athletes with intraoperative neurophysiologic monitoring. Einstein (Sao Paulo) **9**(4), 530–533 (2011)
9. Raynor, B.L., Bright, J.D., Lenke, L.G., Rahman, R.K., Bridwell, K.H., Riew, K.D., Buchowski, J.M., Luhmann, S.J., Padberg, A.M.: Significant change or loss of intraoperative monitoring data: a 25-year experience in 12,375 spinal surgeries. Spine (Phila Pa 1976) **38**(2), E101-8 (2013).
10. Wang, S., Tian, Y., Wang, C., Lu, X., Zhuang, Q., Peng, H., Hu, J., Zhao, Y., Shen, J., Weng, X.: Prognostic value of intraoperative MEP signal improvement during surgical treatment of cervical compressive myelopathy. Eur. Spine J. **25**(6), 1875–1880 (2016)
11. Wi, S., Lee, H.-J., Kang, T., Chang, S.Y., Kim, S.-M., Chang, B.-S., Lee, C.-H., Kim, H.: Clinical significance of improved intraoperative neurophysiological monitoring signal during spine surgery: a retrospective study of a single-institution prospective cohort. Asian Spine J. **14** (2019)
12. He, S., Ren, Z., Zhang, X., Li, J.: Neurophysiologic monitoring for treatment of upper lumbar disc herniation with percutaneous endoscopic lumbar discectomy: a case report on the significance of an increase in the amplitude of motor evoked potential responses after decompression and literature review. Int. J. Surg. Case Rep. **67**, 271–276
13. Piasecki, K., Kulik, G., Pierzchala, K., Pralong, E., Rao, P.J., Schizas, C.: Do intra-operative neurophysiological changes predict functional outcome following decompressive surgery for lumbar spinal stenosis? A prospective study. J. Spine Surg. **4**(1), 86–92 (2018)
14. Dhall, S.S., Haefeli, J., Talbott, J.F., Ferguson, A.R., Readdy, W.J., Bresnahan, J.C., Beattie, M.S., Pan, J.Z., Manley, G.T., Whetstone, W.D.: Motor evoked potentials correlate with magnetic resonance imaging and early recovery after acute spinal cord injury. Neurosurgery **82**(6), 870–876 (2017)
15. Altay, O., Ulas, M.: Prediction of the autism spectrum disorder diagnosis with linear discriminant analysis classifier and K-nearest neighbor in children. In 2018 6th International Symposium on Digital Forensic and Security (ISDFS) (2018)
16. Malcharek, M.J., Loeffler, S., Schiefer, D., Manceur, M.A., Sablotzki, A., Gille, J., Pilge, S., Schneider, G.: Transcranial motor evoked potentials during anesthesia with desflurane versus propofol—a prospective randomized trial. Clin. Neurophysiol. **126**(9), 1825–1832 (2015)

Restoring Lesions in Low-Dose Computed Tomography Images of COVID-19 Using Deep Learning

K. A. Saneera Hemantha Kulathilake, Nor Aniza Abdullah, Abhishek Shivanand Lachyan, A. M. Randitha Ravimal Bandara, Dhrumil Deveshkumar Patel, and Khin Wee Lai

Abstract The use of Low-dose Computed Tomography (LDCT) in clinical medicine for diagnosis and treatment planning is widespread due to the minimal exposure of patients to radiation. Also, recent studies have confirmed that LDCT is a feasible medical imaging modality for diagnosing COVID-19 cases. In general, X-ray tube current is being reduced to acquire the LDCT images. Reduction of the X-ray flux introduces the Quantum noise into the generated LDCT images and, as a result, it produces visually low-quality CT images. Therefore, it is challenging to differentiate the lesions in the diagnosis of COVID-19 patients using the LDCT images due to low contrast and failure to preserve the subtle structures. Therefore, in this study, we proposed a Deep Learning (DL) model based on the Generative Adversarial Network (GAN) for post-processing the LDCT images to enhance their visual quality. In this proposed model, the generator network is designed as a U-net to generate the restored CT images by filter out the noise. Also, the discriminator network follows a patch-GAN model to discriminate the real and generated images while preserving the texture details. The quantitative and qualitative results demonstrated the effectiveness of noise suppression and structure preservation of the proposed DL method. Hence,

K. A. S. H. Kulathilake · N. A. Abdullah (✉)
Faculty of Computer Science and Information Technology, Department of Computer System and Technology, Universiti Malaya, 50603 Kuala Lumpur, Malaysia
e-mail: noraniza@um.edu.my

A. S. Lachyan
Faculty of Medicine, Department of Social and Preventive Medicine, Universiti Malaya, 50603 Kuala Lumpur, Malaysia

A. M. R. R. Bandara
Faculty of Applied Sciences, Department of Computer Science, University of Sri Jayewardenepura, Nugegoda, Sri Lanka

D. D. Patel
Department of Radiology, Seth GS Medical College, King Edward Memorial Hospital, Acharya Donde Marg, Parel East, Parel, Mumbai, Maharastra 400012, India

K. W. Lai
Faculty of Engineering, Department of Biomedical Engineering, Universiti Malaya, 50603 Kuala Lumpur, Malaysia

J. Usman et al. (eds.), *6th Kuala Lumpur International Conference on Biomedical Engineering 2021*, IFMBE Proceedings 86,
https://doi.org/10.1007/978-3-030-90724-2_44

it provides an acceptable quality improvement for LDCT images to discriminate the lesions for diagnosing the COVID-19 positive cases.

Keywords Low-dose computed tomography · Generative adversarial network · Lesion discrimination · LDCT denoising

1 Introduction

The severe acute respiratory syndrome coronavirus 2 (COVID-19) has emerged in December 2019 in Wuhan, China, and presently, it has become a major global pandemic. According to current medical statistics to date, it has caused death to more than a 3.9 million human lives worldwide [1]. It is an infectious disease that affects the respiratory system and causes mild or severe respiratory disorders, including pneumonia. The usage of Low-dose Computed Tomography (LDCT) images has become widespread in recent diagnosing of COVID-19 cases [2]. The reliability obtained compared to the polymerase chain reaction technique and the minimal exposure of patients to radiation were the main reasons for using LDCT in the diagnosis.

In clinical procedures, X-ray flux is being reduced to obtain the LDCT images. Lowering the X-ray flux introduces the quantum noise to the acquired images. As a result, the visual quality of the LDCT images is degraded and causes obstructions in detecting some lesions. Sometimes, in ultra-low-dose cases, the retaining noise within the LDCT images formulates as a lesion (false-lesion artifact). Therefore, proposing a solution for reducing the noise and restoring the fine structural details for LDCT-based COVID-19 diagnosis is crucial.

To improve the visual quality of the low-dose COVID-19 CT images, in this study, we proposed a Deep Learning (DL) model based on the Generative Adversarial Network (GAN) [3]. The proposed model has gained noise reduction through a U-net-based generator. Experimental results have proven its ability to structure preservation and noise reduction. Thus, this proposed DL model provides a baseline for improving the visual quality of LDCT images to obtain a reliable diagnosis.

2 Literature Review

Recently, DL has gained attention in implementing the LDCT restoration algorithms due to its data-driven execution and high performance in noise suppression, structure fidelity, and lesion discrimination [4]. Accordingly, various Convolutional Neural Network (CNN) models have been proposed to obtain clinically significant Computed Tomography images using LDCT image processing [5, 6]. However, the deeper the network increases the vanishing gradient problem. However, the residual network proposed by He et al. [7] has overcome the vanishing gradient issue. Shiri et al. [8] recently used this concept and proposed a DL model for enhancing the

COVID-19 LDCT images. However, this proposed model fails to separate lesions such as Ground-Glass Opacities (GGO) and consolidation (CS), required to detect COVID-19 cases. Besides, the non-uniform distribution of noise and mixing of the texture and the geometric shapes of LDCT images make CNN-based LDCT denoising methods inefficient to preserve various structural information [9].

Recently, GAN [3] has gained much attention in medical imaging and is widely applied in LDCT denoising. Data generation without explicit modeling of the probability density function, ability to enforce custom objective functions, and the adversarial learning mechanism encouraged to apply GAN for denoising LDCT images. Wolterink et al. [10] have proposed the first GAN model for solving the limitation of voxel-wise regression in denoising LDCT. After that, various LDCT denoising applications have been proposed based on GAN models [11]. In addition to that, the image-to-image translation model published in [12] has contributed significantly to LDCT denoising. Moreover, this image-to-image translation implements a mapping function that transforms the LDCT images to expected Routing-dose Computed Tomography (RDCT) images via the adversarial learning mechanism.

3 Research Methodology

3.1 GAN Architecture

The proposed conditional GAN architecture is depicted in Fig. 1. Accordingly, the objective of generator G is to synthesize the denoised images (I_G) from the input LDCT images (I_{LD}), and the Discriminator D attempts to distinguish these synthesized images and RDCT images (I_{RD}). The generator is designed based on U-net model due to its ability to capture subtle details in input LDCT images [13]. Discriminator D is designed as a patch-GAN model mentioned in [12]. The effective receptive field of the model is 190×190. It accepts the input feature map (I_G and I_{RD}) of size 256×256 and outputs a feature map of size 16×16. The objective function of this proposed GAN is given in Eq. (1).

$$G^* = \arg\min_G \max_D \left[\lambda_1(\mathcal{L}_{cGAN}(G, D)) + \lambda_2\left(\mathcal{L}_{L_1}(G)\right)\right] \tag{1}$$

$$\mathcal{L}_{cGAN}(G, D) = E_{x,y}\left[\log D(x, y)\right] + E_{x,z}\left[\log(1 - D(x, G(x, z))\right] \tag{2}$$

$$\mathcal{L}_{L_1}(G) = E_{x,y,z}[||y - G(x, z)||_1] \tag{3}$$

where E is the expectation of the entropy of the generator G and the discriminator D. Variables x, y, and z represent LDCT, RDCT, and the random noise vector, respectively. However, z is replaced with data distribution of the LDCT images in the image-to-image translation model [12] and performs direct mapping between x and

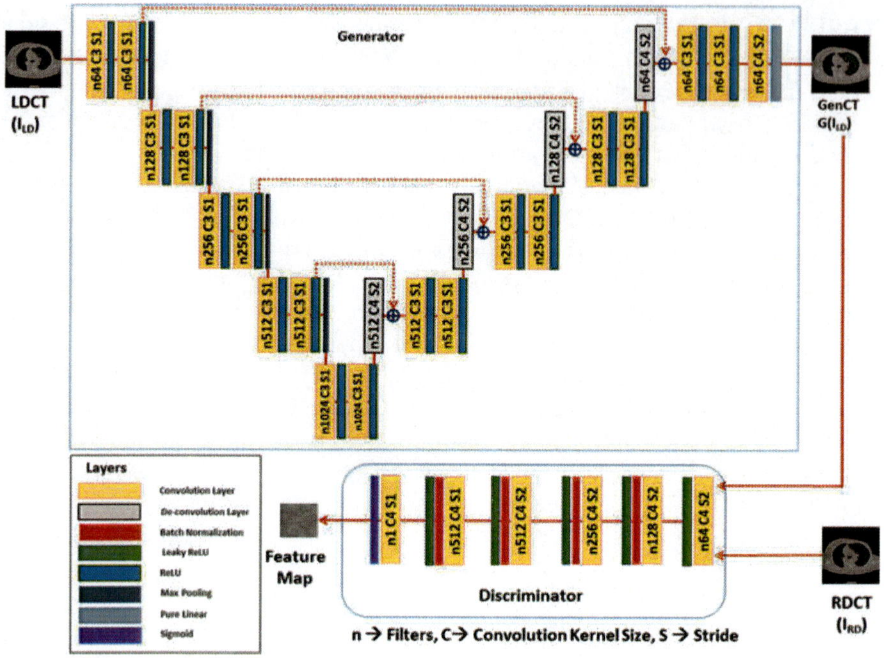

Fig. 1 The proposed GAN architecture

y. λ_1 and λ_2 are the respective weights assigned for adversarial loss and *L*1 loss to balance the training process. In this study, the λ_1 and λ_2 are initialized empirically to 0.05 and 0.99, respectively.

3.2 Network Training and Implementation

Adam with learning rate 1×10^{-4} and $\beta = 0.5$ was used as the optimization method. All the kernels were initialized with random Gaussian distribution with 0 mean and standard deviation of 0.001. The slope of the LeakyReLU activation function is set to 0.2. The network was trained for 200 epochs with a mini-batch size of 10. Also, the proposed model was programmed using Python with Keras platform. All experiments were executed on a workstation (Intel Core I7 10750H 2.6 GHz with 32 GB ram) with NVIDIA RTX 2070 (8 GB) Graphic Processing Unit.

3.3 Data Preparation

The official simulated clinical data were extracted from "the 2016 NH-AAPM-Mayo Clinic Low Dose Grand Challenge" dataset for training the proposed model [14]. The data set consists of 3255 pairs of routing-dose and quarter-dose CT images from 10 anonymous patients with 512 × 512 sizes. Later, the image patches of size 256 × 256 (stride = 256) were extracted from the AAPM-Mayo dataset to train the proposed network. Test data were extracted from RSNA International COVID-19 Open Radiology Database (RICORD) [15]. The dataset consists of randomly selected 40 non-contrast enhanced chest CT images of 10 anonymous patients. All the extracted images were in.png format and 512 × 512 of size. Low-dose CT data is simulated based on the method mentioned in [16]. Accordingly, there were two LDCT datasets with scan incident flux I_0 = 100,000 and I_0 = 500,000. Before training and testing, all the images were normalized to [-1,1].

3.4 Evaluation Metric

To evaluate the proposed LDCT denoising method, the results were quantitatively evaluated using three evaluation metrics; Peak Signal to Noise Ratio (PSNR), Mean Squared Error (MSE), and Structured Similarity Index Matrix (SSIM). The results of the proposed method were compared with BM3D and CNN200 algorithms. BM3D is a well-known conventional denoising algorithm, and CNN200 is a CNN-based LDCT denoising method [6].

4 Results and Discussion

4.1 Visual Performance

Figure 2 depicts a visual performance of the denoised results obtained from the various algorithms under the two different noise levels. According to the results, BM3D has smoothed the fine details and formed streaking artifacts over the denoised results. Usage of the MSE-based loss function in the CNN200 method has caused over smoothing and blurring edges in processed LDCT images. The proposed method has performed well compared to the results of the comparative algorithms and preserved the subtle structures while suppressing the noise. Intensity profile analysis depicts in Fig. 3 has also aligned with these facts and shown the effectiveness of noise reduction in the proposed method. Additionally, Fig. 4 depicts the ability of lesion discrimination of the proposed method. Accordingly, it has acceptably enhanced the visualization of the GGO and CD lesions of COVID-19 positive cases that are considered challenging in ultra- LDCT images [8].

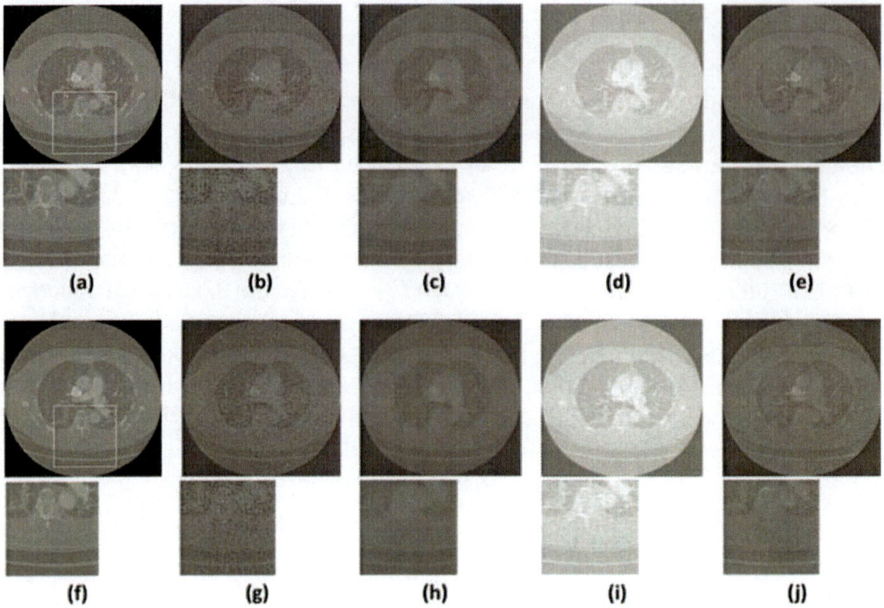

Fig. 2 Denoised results of the LDCT images to compare the effectiveness of the proposed method. The top row depicts the images recorded under $I_0 = 500{,}000$, and the bottom row depicts the images recorded under $I_0 = 100{,}000$. **a** and **f** RDCT, **b** and **g** LDCT, **c** and **h** BM3D, **d** and **i** CNN200, **e** and **j** Proposed method. The region of interest is marked in the RDCT image and extracted to emphasize the enhanced results

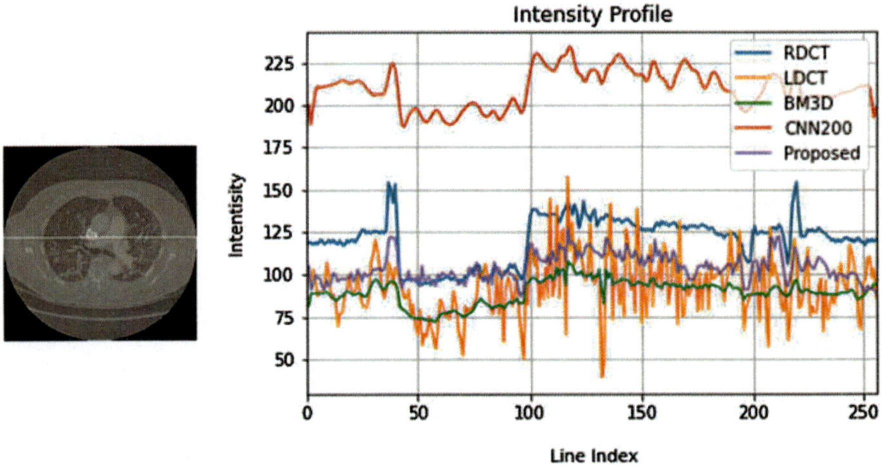

Fig. 3 Analysis of intensity profile

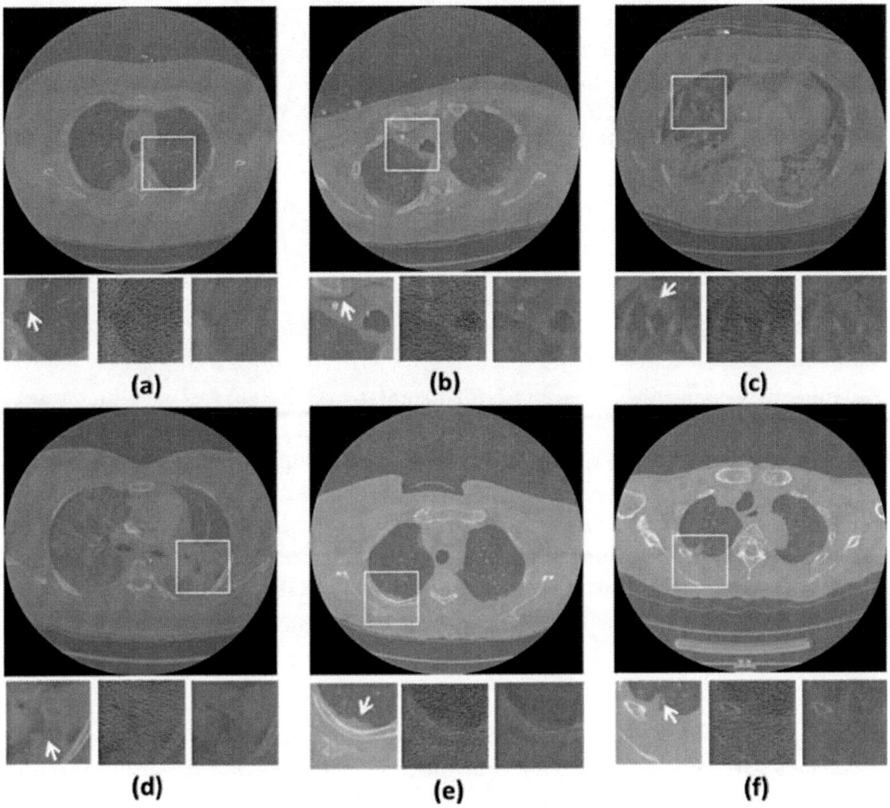

Fig. 4 Lesion discrimination, **a**–**f** top image represents the COVID-19 positive RDCT image, and the three sub-images depict the enlarged ROIs of respective RDCT, LDCT, and generated CT images. The marked region in the RDCT image represents different lesion types. Arrowheads indicate the following lesions, **a** peripheral GGO, **b** pneumo-mediastinum, **c** peripheral GGOs with fine reticulations, (d) CD patch, **e** pleural plaque, **f** peripheral CD patch

4.2 Quantitative Analysis

Table 1 presents the quantitative results of the study. It has clearly emphasized that the proposed method has gained acceptable signal quality and structure preservation compared to the BM3D and CNN200 methods. However, in $I_0 = 1 \times 10^5$

Table 1 Quantitative analysis results

Test dataset—RDCT	$I_0 = 1 \times 10^5$			$I_0 = 5 \times 10^5$		
	PSNR	MSE	SSIM	PSNR	MSE	SSIM
LDCT-RDCT	27.12	1546.16	0.30	26.76	1470.57	0.33
BM3D- RDCT	27.42	1435.70	0.60	26.94	1387.55	0.61
CNN200-RDCT	**28.35**	766.64	0.57	27.50	863.99	0.57
Proposed-RDCT	27.86	**733.82**	**0.63**	**28.09**	**771.23**	**0.64**

noise level CNN200 performed high PSNR due to its' the MSE based loss function. According to the intensity correlation (MSE) and structure similarity (SSIM) measures our proposed method has reported highest value compared to the other two tested methods. The adversarial learning of the GAN model preserves structures in LDCT images. Unlike the MSE-based loss functions of CNN 200, the L1 loss in the loss function of the proposed model minimizes the adverse smoothing of the structures.

5 Conclusion

This study proposed a GAN-based LDCT denoising method to facilitate diagnosing the COVID-19 positive cases. The generator of the proposed model consists of U-net-based architecture. It filters out the noise embedded in the input LDCT images. The discriminator is designed based on patch-GAN architecture. The empirical results showed that the proposed GAN model has effectively enhanced the subtle structure details of the LDCT images while suppressing the noise. As a consequence of that, it facilitates detecting the lesions to diagnose the COVID-19 positive cases reliably. Modifying the proposed network for capturing the visual attention facilitates improving the structural similarity of the processed CT images and it will be done as the future extension of this study.

Acknowledgements This work was supported by the 2020 EBC-C (Extra-Budgetary Contributions from China) Project on Promoting the Use of ICT for Achievement of Sustainable Development Goals and Universiti Malaya (IF015-2021), and the World Bank-funded Accelerating Higher Education Expansion and Development Operation, Sri Lanka [Grant number: AHEAD/PhD/R1-PART-2/ENG&TECH/105].

References

1. Huang, Y.,Yang, L., Dai, H.,Tian, F.,Chen, K.: Epidemic situation and forecasting of COVID-19 in and outside China. Bulleting World Health Organization (2020)
2. Xu, B., Xing, Y., Peng, J., Zheng, Z., Tang, W., Sun, Y., Xu, C., Peng, F.: Chest CT for detecting COVID-19: a systematic review and meta-analysis of diagnostic accuracy. Eur. Radiol. **30**, 5720–5727 (2020)
3. Goodfellow, I., Pouget-Abadie, J., Mirza, M., Xu, B., Warde-Farley, D., Ozair, S., Courville, A., Bengio, Y.: Generative adversarial nets. In: Advances in Neural Information Processing Systems, pp. 2672–2680. MIT Press Cambridge (2014)
4. Shan, H., Padole, A., Homayounieh, F., Kruger, U., Khera, R.D., Nitiwarangkul, C., Kalra, M.K., Wang, G.: Competitive performance of a modularized deep neural network compared to commercial algorithms for low-dose CT image reconstruction. Nat. Mach. Intell. **1**(6), 269–276 (2019)
5. Kang, E., Min, J., Ye, J.C.: A deep convolutional neural network using directional wavelets for low-dose X-ray CT reconstruction. Med. Phys. **44**(10), e360–e375 (2017)

6. Chen, H., Zhang, Y., Zhang, W., Liao, P., Li, K., Zhou, J., Wang, G.: Low-dose CT via convolutional neural network. Biomed. Opt. Express **8**(2), 679–694 (2017)
7. He, K., Zhang, X., Ren, S., Sun, J.: Deep residual learning for image recognition. In: Proceedings of the IEEE Conference on Computer Vision and Pattern Recognition, pp. 770–778 (2016)
8. Shiri, I., Akhavanallaf, A., Sanaat, A., Salimi, Y., Askari, D., Mansouri, Z., Shayesteh, S.P., Hasanian, M., Rezaei-Kalantari, K., Salahshour, A.: Ultra-low-dose chest CT imaging of COVID-19 patients using a deep residual neural network. Eur. Radiol. **31**(3), 1420–1431 (2020)
9. Li, M., Hsu, W., Xie, X., Cong, J., Gao, W.: SACNN: self-attention convolutional neural network for low-dose CT denoising with self-supervised perceptual loss network. IEEE Trans. Med. Imaging **39**(7), 2289–2301 (2020)
10. Wolterink, J.M., Leiner, T., Viergever, M.A., Išgum, I.: Generative adversarial networks for noise reduction in low-dose CT. IEEE Trans. Med. Imaging **36**(12), 2536–2545 (2017)
11. Sorin, V., Barash, Y., Konen, E., Klang, E.: Creating artificial images for radiology applications using generative adversarial networks (GANs)—a systematic review. Acad. Radiol. **27**(8), 1175–1185 (2020)
12. Isola, P., Zhu, J. –Y., Zhou, T., Efros, A.A.: Image-to-image translation with conditional adversarial networks. In: Proceedings of the IEEE Conference on Computer Vision and Pattern Recognition, pp. 1125–1134 (2017)
13. Ronneberger, O., Fischer, P., Brox, T.: U-net: Convolutional networks for biomedical image segmentation. In: International Conference on Medical Image Computing and Computer-Assisted Intervention, pp. 234–241. Springer (2015)
14. AAPM, https://www.aapm.org/GrandChallenge/lowdosect/. Last accessed 05 Mar 2021
15. TCIA, https://www.cancerimagingarchive.net/. Last accessed 10 Feb 2021
16. Gholizadeh-Ansari, M., Alirezaie, J., Babyn, P.: Deep learning for low-dose CT denoising using perceptual loss and edge detection layer. J. Digit. Imaging **33**(2), 504–515 (2019)

Detection of COVID-19 on Chest X-Ray Using Neural Networks

Anis Shazia, Tan Zi Xuan, Joon Huang Chuah, Hamidreza Mohafez, and Khin Wee Lai

Abstract Coronavirus of 2019 is an ongoing pandemic that has infected millions of people and costed the life of more than three million people. It is a highly transmitting disease that has exhausted all the healthcare facilities trying to contain its spread. It has exposed the need for more health facilities and experts to cope with this pandemic without impacting on the safety of healthcare workers. The hardworking and struggling healthcare sector is in need of automated diagnostic devices that could lift the burden off the limited practitioners and also ensure their safety from coming in direct contact with the infection. This pandemic has made the world realize the need of automation for an infectious disease like COVID-19. Deep learning in radiology is an extensively researched topic over the last decade and has the potential to provide the much-needed automation required for COVID-19 diagnosis. In this paper we have fine-tuned three deep learning models—ResNet50, DenseNet121 and InceptionV3—for classification of COVID-19 CXR from regular pneumonia cases. Our models achieved an accuracy of 99.45, 99.50 and 98.55 respectively.

Keywords Coronavirus of 2019 · Transfer learning · ResNet50 · DenseNet121 · InceptionV3

1 Introduction

Severe Acute Respiratory Syndrome Coronavirus 2 (SARS-CoV-2) also known as the Coronavirus Disease of 2019 or COVID-19 is a novel coronavirus that has infected people globally since its origin. It has resulted into a global pandemic that has affected millions of people globally since its emergence in Wuhan City of Hubei Province of China towards the end of 2019. Its symptoms vary from person to person; however, the

A. Shazia · T. Z. Xuan · H. Mohafez · K. W. Lai (✉)
Department of Biomedical Engineering, Universiti Malaya, 50603 Kuala Lumpur, Malaysia
e-mail: lai.khinwee@um.edu.my

J. H. Chuah
Department of Electrical Engineering, Universiti Malaya, 50603 Kuala Lumpur, Malaysia

J. Usman et al. (eds.), *6th Kuala Lumpur International Conference on Biomedical Engineering 2021*, IFMBE Proceedings 86,
https://doi.org/10.1007/978-3-030-90724-2_45

common symptoms include cough, fever, fatigue, body pain, loss of smell and taste, diarrhea etc. [1]. In extreme cases it leads to shortness of breath, severe pneumonia, multiple organ failure and death. The virus has the tendency to mutate and transmit from person to person in the form of respiratory droplets or aerosols.

While the vaccinations are made available to help combat the severity of COVID-19, the existing measure to fight its spread include early diagnosis and isolation. To diagnose COVID-19 diagnostic test such as reverse transcription polymerase chain reaction (RT_PCR) is used. RT-PCR uses nasopharyngeal swab to detect the presence of viral RNA and results are available within few hours. However, with the large influx of cases these results get delayed up to 48 h [2]. Chest computed tomographs (CT) scans and chest radiographs (CXR) have also been useful in diagnosing COVID-19 in early stages and as it progresses [3]. It indicates the presence of virus with ground-glass opacities, consolidations and nodular shadowing visible on the scan [4]. However, X-ray is more commonly available and used in a medical facility when compare with CT; and it is also faster and cheaper alternative in this case [5].

With the availability of digital data and high computing power, several computing techniques are implemented in the current healthcare sector [6, 7]. One of the recent interventions is the application of artificial intelligence and deep learning in radiology [5]. These advancement has the capability to perform similar to a radiologist or better when trained properly [8]. To meet the extensive demand of Covd-19 detection and diagnosis these AI based automated radiological tool could lift the burden off the physicians and also help in keeping the healthcare worker safe by reducing the contact with infected patients.

2 Literature Review

Since the rise of this pandemic researchers have started testing various neural networks that works best with COVID-19 diagnosis [9–12] and classification from regular pneumonia [13–15]. Since CXR's is the cheapest and fastest diagnostic tool various researches are done in this field [16]. Studies have shown deep neural networks has successfully identified pneumonia from X-rays also performing better than radiologists [8]. Hence its only wise to apply DNN in identification of COVID-19 on CXR. COVID-Net a deep network designed by Wang and Wong [16], achieved an accuracy of 92.6% on chest radiographs in detecting of COVID-19. Apostolopoulos and Mpesiana [17] implemented a combination of transfer learning technique with VGG 19 and achieved and accuracy of 98.75%. Similarly Asif et al. [18] achieved 98% accuracy in distinguishing COVID-19 cases from viral pneumonia and normal CXR using Inception-V3. DarkCOVIDNet designed by Ozturk et al. [19] achieved 98.08% for binary classes and 87.02% for multi-class classification. Shelke et al. [20] trained and tested DenseNet161 for binary class classification and achieved 98.9% accuracy. Minaee et al. [21] modified and compared four pretrained networks -DenseNet121, SqueezNet, ResNet18 and ResNey50- with different thresholds for

Table 1 CXR images used for training, validation and testing

	Raw data	Testing data (10%)	Augmented data	Training data (80%)	Validation data (20%)
COVID-19	307	30	1662	1329	333
Pneumonia	5629	3969	–	1328	332

probability score and observed SueezNet to outperform the rest with 98% sensitivity and 92.9% specificity.

3 Methodology

3.1 Data Collection and Image Preprocessing

For this study a total of 307 COVID-19 and 5629 pneumonia images were used from three different opensource databases; namely COVID_Data_GradientCresent [22], COVID-chestxray-dataset [23], and COVID-19 Radiography Database [24] Version 1. Common images from these databases were eliminated from this study. 10% of raw data were randomly selected and separated initially itself for testing the model in the end. Due to limited available COVID-19 images the rest of the images are augmented to have sufficient images for training [25]. Different techniques such as flip, rotation, translation, shearing and noise were added using scikit-image library. Hence a total of 1662 COVID-19 images was generated for this study. From these COVID-19 and pneumonia images, 80% images were randomly selected for training and the remaining 20% was used for validation. Preprocessing techniques such as resize, rescale and normalization was done to obtain a uniform dataset for training the models (Table 1).

3.2 Transfer Learning and Training

All three models were modified and finetuned on TensorFlow 2.4 with Keras API and were trained on a 12 GB NVIDIA Tesla K80 GPU. This study aimed at binary classification of COVID-19 and Pneumonia cases. Due to limited COVID-19 data available, transfer learning was the preferred technique to develop our models. This study has modified the existing pretrained models such as ResNet50, DenseNet121 and InceptionV3 to study its performance on COVID-19 data. All the models were instantiated with pretrained weights of ImageNet dataset providing feature extraction benefit for small datasets. However, to adapt to binary classification for this study the last layer of the models was fine-tuned. The last fully-connected layer along with softmax activation function was removed. The processed input from the previous layers is passed through a flatten layer—to transform the data into 1 dimensional tensor- and a dense layer with 0.5 dropout to avoid overfitting. A softmax activation is added to give the two probable outcomes—COVID-19 and Pneumonia. Figures 1, 2 and 3 shows our fined-tuned models. Model was compiled using categorical_crossentropy as loss function and Adam optimizer with learning rate 0.0001 was used. All three models were trained up till 100 epochs, with batch size 23.

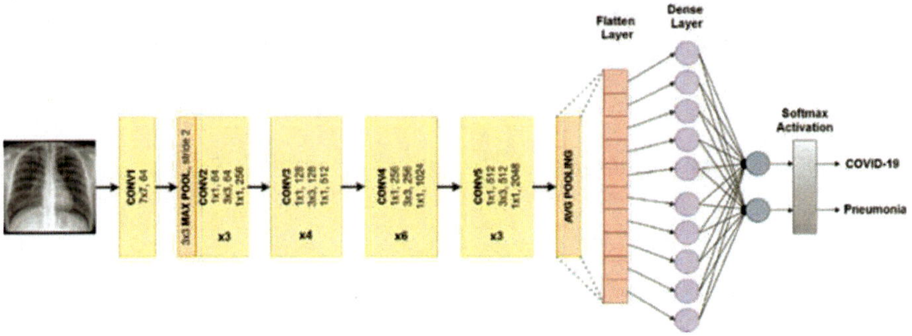

Fig. 1 ResNet50 architecture

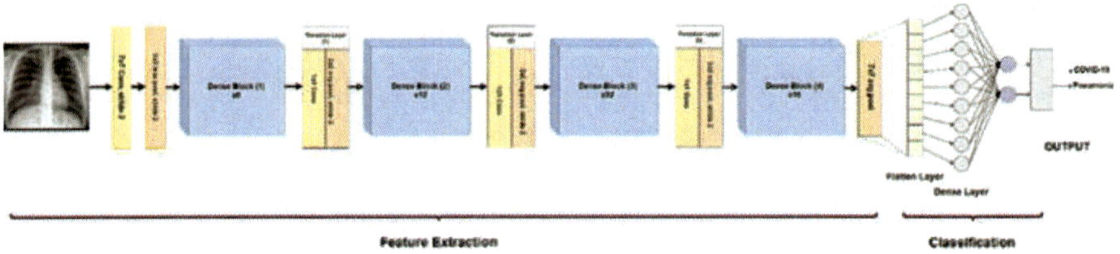

Fig. 2 DenseNet121 architecture

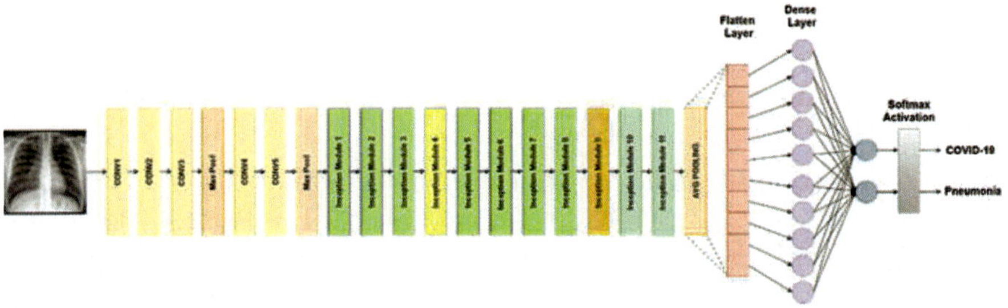

Fig. 3 InceptionV3 architecture

3.3 Prediction and Performance Metrics

Once the model was trained and validated, it was tested on 30 COVID-19 and 3969 Pneumonia raw images. To analyze the models, multiple evaluation metrics were used. These metrics included accuracy (ACC), precision (PRE), recall (REC) and F1-score (F1). They are defined as follows:

$$\text{ACC} = (TP + TN)/(TP + TN + FP + FN) \tag{1}$$

$$\text{PRE} = TP/(TP + FP) \tag{2}$$

$$\text{REC} = TP/(TP + FN) \tag{3}$$

$$\text{F1} = 2 \times (REC \times PRE)/(REC + PRE) \tag{4}$$

where

TP stands for True Positive i.e., COVID-19 image correctly identified

TN stands for True Negative i.e., Pneumonia image correctly identified

FP stands for False Positive i.e., Pneumonia image wrongly identified as COVID-19

FN stands for False Negative i.e., COVID-19 image wrongly identified as Pneumonia.

4 Result and Discussion

4.1 Accuracy and Loss During Training and Validation

The accuracy and loss values in training and validation process at the end of 100th epoch is listed in the Table 2 and shown in Figs. 4, 5 and 6. Throughout the training it was observed that all three models achieved high training accuracy and stabilized after 20 epoch itself, whereas the training loss reached zero and stabilized after 10 epochs only. Indicating that training until 100 epochs was not necessary, the models are capable to learn the distinctive features in few epochs only. When taking into

Table 2 Accuracy and loss during training and validation

	Training loss	Training accuracy	Validation loss	Validation accuracy
ResNet50	5.1596e−07	1.0000	0.0320	0.9969
DenseNet121	1.3700e−04	1.0000	0.0269	0.9984
InceptionV3	1.1694e−06	1.0000	0.0449	0.9953

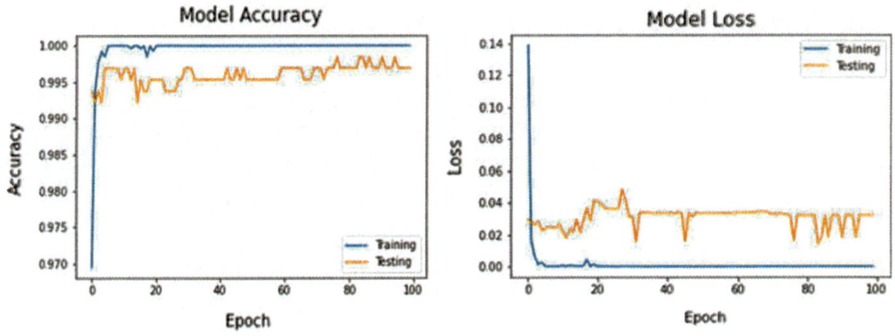

Fig. 4 ResNet50 accuracy loss plot

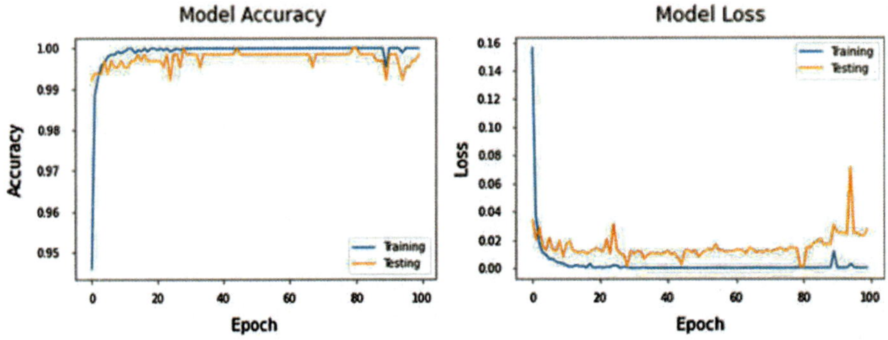

Fig. 5 DenseNet121 accuracy loss plot

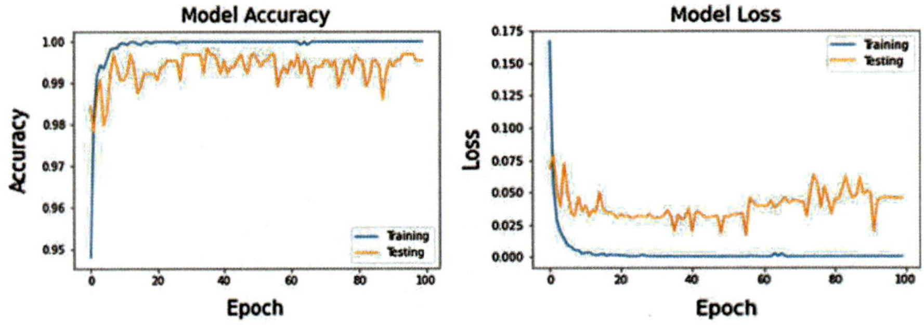

Fig. 6 InceptionV3 accuracy loss plot

consideration the values for training loss and accuracy for these three models it is observed that training accuracy is same for all whereas training loss is lowest for ResNet50. However, during validation DenseNet121 outperformed the other models.

Table 3 Confusion Matrix

TP COVID-19 identified correctly	FN COVID-19 identified as Pneumonia
FP Pneumonia identified as COVID-19	TN Pneumonia identified correctly

Table 4 Summarized confusion matrix of validation and test set

Model	Validation				Testing			
	TP	TN	FP	FN	TP	TN	FP	FN
ResNet50	332	331	1	1	30	3947	22	0
DenseNet121	333	331	1	0	30	3949	20	0
InceptionV3	332	330	2	1	30	3911	58	0

Also, it was observed that loss during validation was higher than that of training, which could be the result of model overfitting.

4.2 Confusion Matrix

The confusion matrix displays numbers of images identified correctly and incorrectly by the model. Confusion matrix (Table 3) was generated for both validation dataset and test dataset. Table 4 shows the summarized confusion matrix of validation and test data of each model. Validation set consisted of 333 COVID-19 image and 332 Pneumonia images and the test set comprised of 30 COVID-19 images and 3969 Pneumonia images. From the confusion matrices it was observed that models correctly identified COVID-19 images even with the limited data available. However, the models faced slight confusion with few pneumonia cases and identified it as COVID-19. Of the three models, DenseNet121 had lowest false positive, so therefore it is derived that DenseNet121 has performed better in terms of having least error.

4.3 Performance Metrics

This section compares modified ResNet50, DenseNet121 and InceptionV3 based on their performance metrics such as accuracy, precision, recall, F1-score, training time and testing time taken by each model. The results are tabulated in Table 5. indicating all the three models have done remarkably well. Though DenseNet121 has highest score when compared with the rest. However, when training and testing

Table 5 Performance metrics

Model	ACC (%)	PRE (%)	REC (%)	F1 (%)	Training time (s)	Testing time (s)
ResNet50	99.45	99.68	99.45	99.52	4963	1043
DenseNet121	99.50	99.70	99.50	99.56	5790	1913
InceptionV3	98.55	99.51	98.55	98.90	4540	1580

time is observed DenseNet121 has taken the longest time to give result with highest accuracy and precision.

5 Conclusion

Coronavirus of 2019 is a fast transmitting and mutating virus which has the tendency to affect the public for a long time to come. The best that can be done minimize its impact on the patient and people surrounding them is to reform the diagnosis process to be able to stop its spread at early stages and get vaccinated quickly. Though CXR's provide a faster diagnosis but with the huge number cases every day, it is over burdening the physicians to read so many scans. This issue could be made easier with the intervention of deep learning in identifying lung anomalies. In this study we have tested three models to COVID-19 cases from the regular Pneumonia cases. DenseNet121 has shown to the best model with 99.5% accuracy to identify COVID-19 images. However, if a faster model is required to perform the same task, ResNet50 could be used.

Acknowledgements This work was supported by the 2020 APT EBC-C (Extra-Budgetary Contributions from China) Project on Promoting the Use of ICT for Achievement of Sustainable Development Goals, and University Malaya under grant IF015-2021.

References

1. Vaira, L.A., et al.: Anosmia and ageusia: Common findings in COVID-19 patients. Laryngoscope **130**(7), 1787–1787 (2020)
2. Durrani, M., et al.: Chest X-rays findings in COVID 19 patients at a University Teaching Hospital—a descriptive study. Pak. J. Med. Sci. **36**(COVID19-S4), S22–S26 (2020)
3. Khalil, A., et al.: Multimodality registration of two-dimensional echocardiography and cardiac CT for mitral valve diagnosis and surgical planning. J. Med. Imaging (Bellingham) **4**(3), 037001 (2017)
4. Oh, Y., Park, S., Ye, J.C.: Deep learning COVID-19 features on CXR using limited training data sets. IEEE Trans. Med. Imaging **39**(8), 2688–2700 (2020)
5. Anis, S., et al.: An overview of deep learning approaches in chest radiograph. IEEE Access **8**, 182347–182354 (2020)
6. Yong, C.W., et al.: Knee osteoarthritis severity classification with ordinal regression module. Multimedia Tools Appl. (2021)

7. Teo, K., Yong, C.W., Lai, K.W., Murphy, B.P., Chuah, J.H.: Discovering predictive value of clinical notes: a machine learning analysis with text representation. J. Med. Imag. Health Inform. **10**(12), 2869–2875
8. Rajpurkar, P., et al.: Deep learning for chest radiograph diagnosis: A retrospective comparison of the CheXNeXt algorithm to practicing radiologists. PLOS Med. **15**(11), e1002686 (2018)
9. Jamshidi, M., et al.: Artificial intelligence and COVID-19: deep learning approaches for diagnosis and treatment. IEEE Access **8**, 109581–109595 (2020)
10. Song, Y., et al.: Deep learning enables accurate diagnosis of novel coronavirus (COVID-19) with CT images. IEEE/ACM Trans. Comput. Biol. Bioinform. 1 (2021)
11. Wang, S., et al.: A fully automatic deep learning system for COVID-19 diagnostic and prognostic analysis. Eur. Respir. J. **56**(2), 2000775 (2020)
12. Halgurd, S.M., et al.: *D*iagnosing COVID-19 pneumonia from x-ray and CT images using deep learning and transfer learning algorithms. In: Proceedings of SPIE (2021)
13. Karar, M.E., Hemdan, E.E.-D., Shouman, M.A.: Cascaded deep learning classifiers for computer-aided diagnosis of COVID-19 and pneumonia diseases in X-ray scans. Complex Intell. Syst. **7**(1), 235–247 (2021)
14. Li, L., et al.: Using artificial intelligence to detect COVID-19 and community-acquired pneumonia based on pulmonary CT: evaluation of the diagnostic accuracy. Radiology **296**(2), E65–E71 (2020)
15. Yong, C.W., et al.: Comparative study of encoder-decoder-based convolutional neural networks in cartilage delineation from knee magnetic resonance images. Curr. Med. Imag. (2020)
16. Wang, L., Lin, Z.Q., Wong, A.: COVID-Net: a tailored deep convolutional neural network design for detection of COVID-19 cases from chest X-ray images. Sci. Rep. **10**(1), 19549 (2020)
17. Apostolopoulos, I.D., Mpesiana, T.A.: COVID-19: automatic detection from X-ray images utilizing transfer learning with convolutional neural networks. Phys. Eng. Sci. Med. **43**(2), 635–640 (2020)
18. Asif, S., et al.: Classification of COVID-19 from chest X-ray images using deep convolutional neural networks. medRxiv (2020)
19. Ozturk, T., et al.: Automated detection of COVID-19 cases using deep neural networks with X-ray images. Comput. Biol. Med. **121**, 103792–103792 (2020)
20. Shelke, A., et al., *Chest X-ray classification using Deep learning for automated COVID-19 screening*. medRxiv, 2020: p. 2020.06.21.20136598.
21. Minaee, S., et al.: Deep-COVID: predicting COVID-19 from chest X-ray images using deep transfer learning. Med. Image Anal. **65**, 101794 (2020)
22. Li, Z.: Run some COVID-19 lung X-Ray classification and CT detection demo (2020)
23. Cohen, J.P.: COVID-chestxray-dataset. GitHub (2020)
24. Rahman, T., Chowdhury, M., Khandakar, A.: COVID-19 Radiography Database. Kaggle (2020)
25. Muhammad Ali, S., et al.: Speckle noise diffusion in knee articular cartilage ultrasound images. Curr. Med. Imag. **16**(6), 739–751 (2020)

Assessment of LV Myocardial Function in Aortic Stenosis Using Personalized 3D+ Time Cardiac MRI Modelling

Shoon Hui Chuah, Wen Dee Thong, Nor Ashikin Md Sari, Li Kuo Tan, Khairunnisa Hasikin, and Yih Miin Liew

Abstract Left ventricular hypertrophy (LVH) in aortic stenosis (AS) is known as an adaptive response affected by pressure overload as a result of the progressive narrowing of the aortic valve orifice. Both systolic and diastolic function of the left ventricular (LV) could be affected due to the structural remodelling as a sequel of AS. Therefore, this study utilized 3D+ time personalized LV modelling algorithm which was developed in-house to evaluate the LV function throughout the 20 cardiac phases of short- and long-axis cine MRI in different severity of AS patients. A total of 9 healthy cohorts and 13 AS patients with different degrees of severity were analyzed. This study demonstrated that majority of the AS patients have systolic dysfunction accompanied by deterioration of radial strain (RS) and longitudinal strain (LS) when compared against healthy cohorts ($p < 0.05$). Only those with concomitant concentric LVH (i.e. 38% of the AS patients) exhibited normal systolic and diastolic functions with a couple of exceptions observed. LVH was found developed in those with moderate and severe AS. No clear correlation was found between diastolic dysfunction and the severity of AS.

Keywords Aortic stenosis · LVH · Cardiac modelling

S. H. Chuah · W. D. Thong · K. Hasikin · Y. M. Liew (✉)
Faculty of Engineering, Department of Biomedical Engineering, Universiti Malaya, Kuala Lumpur, Malaysia
e-mail: liewym@um.edu.my

N. A. M. Sari
Faculty of Medicine, Department of Medicine, Universiti Malaya, Kuala Lumpur, Malaysia

L. K. Tan
Faculty of Medicine, Department of Biomedical Imaging, Universiti Malaya, Kuala Lumpur, Malaysia

J. Usman et al. (eds.), *6th Kuala Lumpur International Conference on Biomedical Engineering 2021*, IFMBE Proceedings 86,
https://doi.org/10.1007/978-3-030-90724-2_46

1 Introduction

Aortic stenosis (AS) is known as the most common native valvular heart disease that correlated with ageing condition [1]. The cause of AS is primarily due to the progressive calcification and thickening of the aortic leaflets. The progression of this disease tends to inhibit the leaflet movement and reduce the valve area causing restriction in blood flow. Consequently, overload pressure condition encountered by the left ventricle (LV) results in wall hypertrophy and structural remodelling which helps to sustain end-systolic stress and preserve adequate cardiac output [2, 3]. Up to now, the clinical diagnostic method for AS still mainly depends on echocardiograms. Practically, this noninvasive methods for the prognosis of AS were implemented to evaluate the severity based on aortic valve area (AVA), aortic velocity and mean gradient to determine the treatment decision such as transcatheter (TAVR) or aortic valve replacement (AVR). However, such assessment often suffers from errors due to geometric assumptions. In addition, studies on LV diastolic dysfunction in AS were predominantly discussed as the aftermath of surgical treatment and such analysis in AS without surgical treatment is still uncommon. Early detection and treatment of diastolic dysfunction would allow the prevention of irreversible structural alteration and systolic dysfunction [4]. Therefore this study aims to provide a more accurate visualization and quantitative assessment using 3D+ time analysis of MRI to overcome limitations of echocardiography especially in the presence of hypertrophy. The is the first implementation of personalized assessment using 3D+ time LV modelling and registration techniques for the whole cardiac cycle on AS cases. This study also intended to determine both systolic and diastolic functions across the full cardiac cycle in AS patients of different severities prior to surgical treatment using the developed framework.

2 Literature Review

Pressure overload is the consequence of the development of AS. According to Lamb, et al. [5], AS and aortic regurgitation are often accompanied by an elevation in pressure overload and LV volume, causing either concentric or eccentric LVH/remodelling. Correspondingly, this adaptive hypertrophic response provokes myocardial impairment which can be a risk element for cardiac mortality [6]. LV diastolic dysfunction is incurred when ventricular filling pressure is increased due to relaxation deficiency as well as increased ventricular stiffness [7]. LV systolic dysfunction, by contrast, manifests as depreciated contractility and inadequate hypertrophic process of the LV.

A recent study by Steine et al. [8] have proposed a new insight for the prognostic factor of AS besides the conventional parameters. They suggested that both LV systolic and diastolic dysfunction could emerge simultaneously in AS patients. Nevertheless, this findings was obtained from 2D analysis for moderate AS using tissue Doppler imaging which is lacking of 3D regional details. So far, only LV systolic dysfunction has been practically used as the clinical prognostic factor in diagnosing AS, and diastolic dysfunction is rarely considered during the assessment. Majority of the published researches Gjertsson et al. [9], Stewart et al. [10], Koifman et al. [11] emphasized on the assessment of LV systolic dysfunction for the recommendation of aortic valve replacement or transcatheter techniques to treat AS. Klein et al. [12] had suggested that pre-operative diastolic dysfunction represents a novel indicator for the investigation of myocardial function in AS groups. However, they focused on severe AS alone which is lacking of mild and moderate cases that considered the degree of severity of AS while diastolic dysfunction varies among patients, and the causes are often multifactorial.

LV filling pressures was determined mainly by LV compliance and elasticity. The increased LV filling pressures above normal leads to diastolic dysfunction which is often compensated by the contraction of the atrium to overcome the lack of early diastolic filling. According to Lund, et al. [13] diastolic dysfunction develops ahead of reduced EF and can remain asymptotic in AS patients for quite some time. Advanced diastolic dysfunction is likely in progress when EF starts to decrease as characterized by elevated end-diastolic pressure and diminished diastolic filling. Early detection of diastolic dysfunction can be managed with medical drugs without demanding critical strategies such as surgical treatment. Therefore, a more refined approach with the inclusion of diastolic dysfunction assessment may aid diagnosis and assist in better treatment management for AS patients. Findings regarding the behavior of diastolic function in AS, however, has not been thoroughly explored and warrant further investigation.

3 Research Methodology

3.1 Data Acquisition and Segmentation

Cardiac MRI scans of 13 AS patients and 9 healthy cohorts were retrieved from PACS in the University of Malaya Medical Centre (UMMC). The scans consisted of standard short-axis (SA) cine stacks covering from base to apex, as well as 2-chamber and 4-chamber long-axis cine (LA) scans. A 1.5 T MRI system (Signa HDxt 1.5 T, GE Healthcare, WI, U.S.A) was utilized in obtaining the MRI scans. In SA scans, multi-breath-hold SSFP scans with FOV of 350 × 350 mm, 256 × 256 image matrix, pixel size of 1.37 × 1.37 mm, slice thickness of 8 mm, 0 mm slice gap, TE/TR of 1.6/3.7 ms, flip angle of 55°, number of slices of 10–15, 20 cardiac time frames, and end-expiration breath-hold time of 15 s were applied. The same acquisition parameters were used for LA cine scans (2- and 4-chamber) acquisition. As for controls, 9 age-matched healthy subjects with normal cardiac functions and no cardiovascular disease as determined by echocardiography were recruited separately with prior informed consent. The standard clinical cine scanning protocol was used and the study was approved by the Institutional Ethics Committee (989.75). Segment software (Medviso AB; Version 3.1 R8215) were utilized [14] to semi-automatically delineate endocardial and epicardial contours on both SA and LA cine scans.

3.2 Reconstruction and Assessment of the Global and Regional Functions from 3D+ Time LV Models

3D+ time personalized models of each AS patients were reconstructed from the endocardial and epicardial contours over a full cardiac cycle as shown in Fig. 1 with an in-house algorithm [15]. A multi-slice rigid image registration was applied to reduce motion artifacts of the sequential MRI scans Liew et al. [16]. Global and regional indices such as end-systolic volume (ESV), end-diastolic volume (EDV), LV mass (LVM), Max EDWT (maximum end-diastolic wall thickness), absolute wall thickening (AWT), stroke-volume (SV), ejection fraction (EF), mass-to-volume ratio (M/V ratio), heart rate (HR), cardiac output (CO) and myocardial strain (i.e., radial (RS), circumferential (CS), and longitudinal strains (LS)) were extracted automatically from the models. The regional parameters were spatially mapped to a bulls eye diagram to aid visual and quantitative assessment. The aortic valve area (AVA) was retrieved from the MR report and the AS severity was stratified according to the reference guideline [7], where AVA > 1.5 cm^2 is categorized as mild, 1.0 $cm^2 \leq$ AVA $\leq$ 1.5 cm^2 as moderate and AVA < 1.0 cm^2 as severe AS. The blood flow rate was computed from the gradient of blood volume, from which the diastolic function of the LV was assessed through the mitral E velocity and E/A Ratio [8, 11]. E wave represents the peak velocity blood flow from LV relaxation in early diastole, whereas A wave represents peak velocity flow in late diastole caused by atrial contraction.

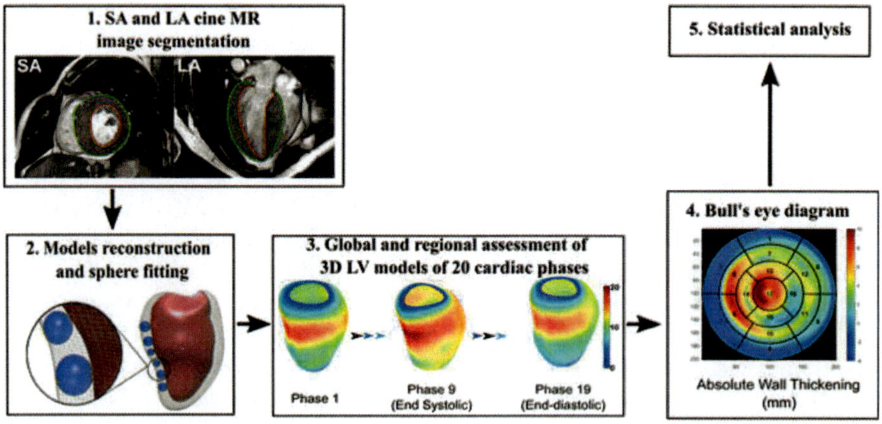

Fig. 1 The 3D+ time personalized LV modeling framework for the assessment of AS patients using cine MRI scans

Table 1 The demographic variables and LV functional parameters of the healthy cohorts and AS patients present in median (IQR). The significant differences between the healthy and AS cohort were made bold, while significant difference between different severities of AS (mild, moderate and severe) against healthy cohorts were marked with symbols alongside the variables

Variables	Healthy (n = 9)	Aortic Stenosis (n = 13)	*p-value*
Gender (male:female)	7:2	10:3	–
EDV (ml)	124.5 (20.1)	133.4 (40.4)	0.491
ESV (ml)	46.3 (16.8)	66.9 (45.2)	**0.046**
SV (ml)	80.0 (6.8)	64.5 (20.3)	**0.039**
LVM (g)[b]	87.6 (24.1)	112.7 (61.3)	**0.02**
MaxEDWT (mm)[b]	10.2 (2.2)	12.9 (2.2)	**0.004**
AWT (mm)	3.6 (0.7)	2.1 (2.5)	0.123
HR (bpm)[c]	72.0 (7.0)	85.0 (15.0)	**0.013**
CO (ml/min)	5889.5 (780.0)	5232.2 (2729.1)	0.246
EF (%)	62.8 (3.9)	40.7 (20.4)	**0.009**
M/V ratio[b]	10.2 (2.2)	0.8 (0.3)	**0.002**
RS (%)[a,b,c]	80.0 (17.6)	33.4 (32.4)	**0.001**
CS (%)	−28.2 (14.6)	−19.3 (14.6)	0.097
LS (%)[b,c]	−14.2 (3.3)	−7.3 (4.4)	**< 0.0001**
AVA (cm^2)[d,e,f]	–	1.3 (0.3)	–
E peak (ml/s)[a]	296.6 (77.8)	284.0 (202.5)	**0.048**
A peak (ml/s)	225.0 (49.4)	163.7 (98.6)	0.110
E/A ratio	1.3 (0.3)	1.0 (1.2)	0.277

[a] healthy versus mild AS; [b] healthy versus moderate AS, [c] healthy versus severe AS; [d] mild vs moderate AS; [e] mild versus severe AS; [f]moderate versus severe AS

3.3 Statistical Analysis

Statistical analysis was executed using the IBM SPSS Statistics (Version 22) statistical software. Data was tested to be not normally distributed for 2/17 parameters using the Kolmogorov–Smirnov test. Therefore, all results were reported in median (IQR) and the non-parametric Kruskal–Wallis test was used to compare the parameters between AS (as well as different severity) and control subjects as presented in Table 1. A significance level of $p < 0.05$ was utilized as the threshold for statistical significance.

4 Results and Discussion

Table 1 shows the demographic data and LV functional parameters of both healthy and AS cohorts. We found that ESV, LV mass, Max EDWT, M/V ratio and HR of the

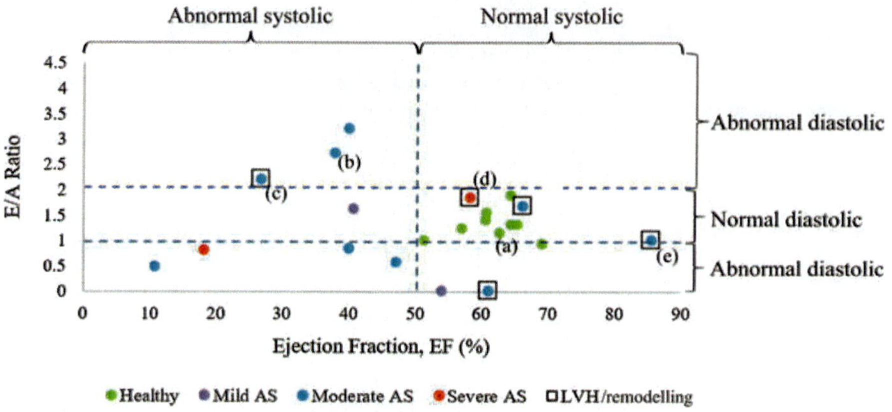

Fig. 2 The scatter plot of E/A ratio versus EF for different severities of AS groups (mild, moderate, severe) and healthy cohorts (as the reference). The dotted line represents the reference boundary of EF = 50% (vertical) as a cutoff to decide systolic abnormality whereas E/A ratio = 1 and 2 (horizontal) as a cutoff to decide diastolic abnormality. AS patients with LVH are indicated by square icon. The patients labeled with alphabets (a)–(e) are further explored in Table 2 in the form of bulls eye diagram

AS cohort showed significantly greater values as compared against healthy cohort. Generally, AS cohort with reduced EF were often observed with increased myocardial mass and significant degradation of myocardial strain (i.e. RS and LS). For diastolic function, there was a significant reduction ($p = 0.048$) of E peak (284.0(202.5) ml/s) compared with healthy cohort (296.6 (77.8) ml/s). The AVA of severe, moderate, and mild AS was 0.7(0.3) cm^2, 1.3(0.1) cm^2 and 1.9(0.1) cm^2, respectively. Overall, significant difference was observed when mild AS have lower E peak; moderate AS have relatively greater LVM, Max EDWT and M/V ratio as well as deterioration of RS and LS; severe AS have higher HR and deterioration of RS and LS compared against healthy cohort.

Additionally, 38% (n = 5) AS patients were identified to have LVH. Figure 2. illustrates the correlation between E/A ratio versus EF of the study population. A threshold line was plotted on x-axis indicating 50% EF to separate patients with normal (EF > 50%) and abnormal (EF < 50%) systolic function [7]. Another threshold line (y = 1, y = 2) was plotted for E/A ratio to distinguish diastolic dysfunction. 7/8 of the AS patients without LVH have reduced EF (<50%). Generally, 8/13 AS patients were determined with diastolic dysfunction (i.e. E/A ratio < 1 or ≥ 2). One of the AS case had missing A wave and their diastolic dysfunction could not be determined, therefore indicated by E/A ratio = 0. For AS with LVH, 3/5 have preserved EF > 50%; one with moderate AS had abnormal EF < 50% (Fig. 2c) and one with hyperdynamic LV had EF > 75% (Fig. 2e).

The regional end-diastolic wall thickness and absolute wall thickening of some of these patients (with and without LVH) were further explored through a bulls eye diagram and other related functional parameters as depicted in Table 2. Many

Table 2 The bulls eye diagram of the healthy and AS cohort with and without LVH

	Healthy	Aortic stenosis				
		No LVH/remodelling		LVH/remodelling		
EDWT Bulls Eye Diagram (Max EDWT (mm))	(a) 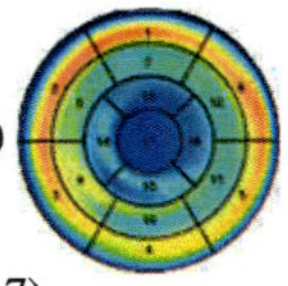 (9.7)	(b) 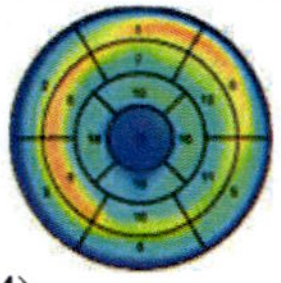 (9.4)	(c) 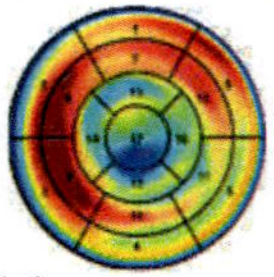 (16.5)	(d) 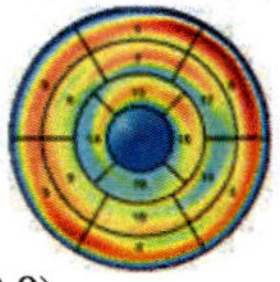 (12.9)	(e) 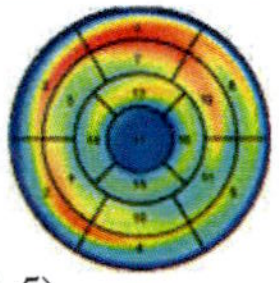 (11.5)	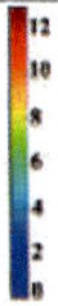
AWT Bulls Eye Diagram (Mean AWT (mm))	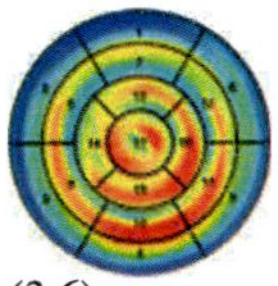 (3.6)	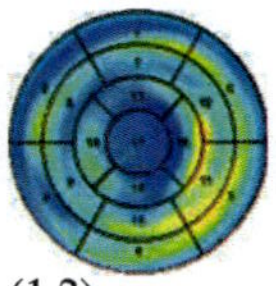 (1.2)	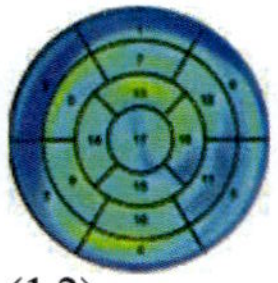 (1.2)	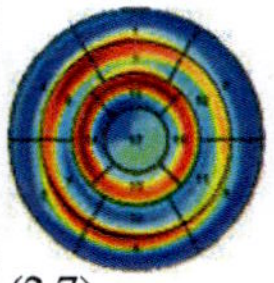 (2.7)	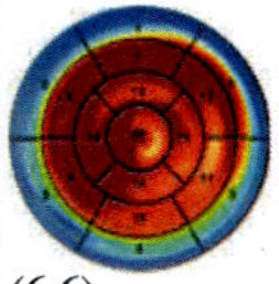 (6.6)	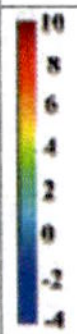
Severity	Healthy	Moderate	Moderate	Severe	Moderate	
EF (%)	62.8	37.8	27.0	58.2	85.4	
EDV (ml)	124.5	133.4	239.1	160.0	77.8	
LVM (g)	88.8	92.9	201.0	145.4	94.2	

(continued)

Table 2 (continued)

	Healthy	Aortic stenosis				
		No LVH/remodelling		LVH/remodelling		
SV (ml)	78.2	50.4	64.5	93.1	66.4	
HR (bpm)	66	126	82	96	92	
CO (ml/min)	5554.3	6347.8	5285.3	8936.7	6108.4	
RS (%)	95.0	20.2	21.6	54.0	137.4	
CS (%)	−19.6	−18.1	−10.0	−33.2	−52.6	
LS (%)	−13.7	−6.8	−5.4	−9.8	−7.8	
E/A ratio	1.2	2.7	2.2	1.8	1.0	

variations were observed among AS patients in terms of their LV structures and functions. AS with LVH were characterized by maximum EDWT $\geq$ 11 mm. Different variations of EF (reduced, preserved and hyperdynamic) in AS with LVH were shown in (c), (d) and (e) of Table 2. Abnormalities in LV systolic function was observed in both moderate AS patients with and without LVH as determined from their low EF of 37.8% and 27.0% (Table 2 (b) & (c)). The deterioration of AWT, RS and LS were noted in these patients resulting in reduced EF. These AS groups had E/A ratio $\geq$ 2 which indicates the presence of Grade III diastolic dysfunction/restrictive filling phase [11]. Restriction in filling of the heart is the characteristics in this severe form of diastolic dysfunction that could lead to heart failure. Additionally, the moderate AS patient without LVH (b) was also found to have tachycardia (high HR = 126BPM). In contrast, severe AS patient (d) had concentric LVH, showing preserved EF with increased max EDWT, EDV and LVM that is believed to be due to adaptive response of myocardial hypertrophy. Comparing patients (c) and (d), we observe extreme difference in their functional measurements. Patient (c) showed low wall thickening (majority blue colour segments) with concomitant enlargement of EDV, asymmetrical EDWT and high LVM that likely indicates eccentric LVH with LV wall hypokinesia and dilatation. Patient (e), on the other hand, shows intense wall thickening (red colour about the apical and apex region in AWT bulls eye diagram), leading to extremely high EF values of 85.4%. This particular patient exhibits concentric remodelling characteristics with small LV chamber (i.e. small EDV), hyperkinetic LV wall and normal diastolic function.

This study demonstrates that deterioration of myocardial strain (especially RS and LS) were significant in AS patients (with and without LVH) while compared against the healthy cohorts (RS: 33.4(32.4)% vs. 80.0(17.6)% and LS: −7.3(4.4)% vs. −14.2(3.3)%). These condition causes reduction of EF contributing to LV systolic dysfunction. The results were consistent with Lamb et al. [5] findings of impaired radial and longitudinal functions that reduced EF (<50%) in AS patients. Diastolic dysfunction in AS characterized by E/A ratio < 1 or $\geq$ 2 was verified in most moderate cases. Although concentric hypertrophy is the most common form of remodelling developed by cardiac structure in response to elevated pressure afterload in AS, eccentric hypertrophy could also develop due to volume overload resulting in LV dilation [1]. Eccentric hypertrophy was spotted in a moderate AS case in our study which is known as one of the major contributing factors of severe diastolic dysfunction that goes along with Lamb, et al. [5] findings.

Besides this, the present study indicates that LV systolic and diastolic functions are independent of severity which is in agreement with Steine et al. [12] although both LV dysfunctions can develop simultaneously in AS patients. The inability of the myocardium to contract (systolic) and relax (diastolic) would lead to heart failure in the former, and passive filling of the LV, causing angina, dyspnea, and pulmonary congestion in the latter if left untreated [1]. The present study also shows that all AS patients have relatively higher HR and LVM as compared to the healthy cohort. However, no correlation was observed between E/A ratio and the severity of AS cohort and not all AS patients develop LVH. This is in line with the recent findings of Rader et al. [3] and Kupari et al. [6] that the compensatory effect of hypertrophy is independent of the severity of AS. Majority of AS with LVH was identified in moderate and severe AS patients in this study. The presence of LVH/remodelling in AS comes with benefits and drawbacks which is supported by several studies, suggesting that LVH may not necessarily an adaptive response but in fact could be maladaptive to AS [4, 7].

5 Conclusion

Present study developed an in-house 3D + time personalized LV model assessment with the implementation of registration technique to facilitate visual and quantitative analysis on AS patients using cardiac MRI imaging. In this trail, AS patients demonstrates that diastolic dysfunction does not correlate with the severity of AS. Majority of the AS patients can be differentiated from healthy cohort by reduced EF as well as increased LVM apart from narrowed aortic valve area.

Acknowledgements This study was supported by Universiti Malaya Faculty Research Grant (GPF053B-2020).

References

1. Elahi, M.M., Chuang, A., Ewing, M.J., Choi, C.H., Grant, P.W., Matata, B.M.: One problem two issues! Left ventricular systolic and diastolic dysfunction in aortic stenosis. Ann. Transl. Med. **2**(1) (2014)
2. Shah, S., et al.: Left ventricular hypertrophy with strain and aortic stenosis. Circulation **130**(18), 1607–1616 (2014)
3. Rader, F., Sachdev, E., Arsanjani, R., Siegel, R.J.: Left ventricular hypertrophy in valvular aortic stenosis: mechanisms and clinical implications. Am. J. Med. **128**(4), 344–352 (2015)
4. Satpathy, C., Mishra, T.K., Satpathy, R., Satpathy, H.K., Barone, E.J.: Diagnosis and management of diastolic dysfunction and heart failure. Am. Fam. Physician **73**(5), 841–846 (2006)
5. Lamb, H.J., et al.: Left ventricular remodeling early after aortic valve replacement: differential effects on diastolic function in aortic valve stenosis and aortic regurgitation. J. Am. Coll. Cardiol. **40**(12), 2182–2188 (2002)
6. Kupari, M., Turto, H., Lommi, J.: Left ventricular hypertrophy in aortic valve stenosis: preventive or promotive of systolic dysfunction and heart failure? Eur. Heart J. **26**(17), 1790–1796 (2005)
7. Nagueh, S.F., et al.: Recommendations for the evaluation of left ventricular diastolic function by echocardiography: an update from the American Society of Echocardiography and the European Association of Cardiovascular Imaging. Eur. J. Echocardiogr. **17**(12), 1321–1360 (2016)
8. Steine, K., Rossebø, A.B., Stugaard, M., Pedersen, T.R.: Left ventricular systolic and diastolic function in asymptomatic patients with moderate aortic stenosis. Am. J. Cardiol. **102**(7), 897–901 (2008)

9. Gjertsson, P., Caidahl, K., Farasati, M., Odén, A., Bech-Hanssen, O.: Preoperative moderate to severe diastolic dysfunction: a novel Doppler echocardiographic long-term prognostic factor in patients with severe aortic stenosis. J. Thorac. Cardiovasc. Surg. **129**(4), 890–896 (2005)
10. Stewart, R.A., et al.: Left ventricular systolic and diastolic function assessed by tissue Doppler imaging and outcome in asymptomatic aortic stenosis. Eur Heart J **31**(18), 2216–2222 (2010). https://doi.org/10.1093/eurheartj/ehq159
11. Koifman, E., et al.: Impact of baseline left ventricular diastolic dysfunction in patients with severe aortic stenosis undergoing transcatheter aortic valve implantation. Am. J. Cardiol. **125**(2), 258–263 (2020)
12. Klein, L., Ramchand, J., Nagueh, S.F.: Aortic Stenosis and Diastolic Dysfunction: Partners in Crime. American College of Cardiology Foundation Washington DC (2020)
13. Lund, O., et al.: Left ventricular systolic and diastolic function in aortic stenosis: prognostic value after valve replacement and underlying mechanisms. Eur. Heart J. **18**(12), 1977–1987 (1997). https://doi.org/10.1093/oxfordjournals.eurheartj.a015209
14. Heiberg, E., Sjögren, J., Ugander, M., Carlsson, M., Engblom, H., Arheden, H.: Design and validation of segment-freely available software for cardiovascular image analysis. BMC Med. Imaging **10**(1), 1–13 (2010)
15. Chuah, S.H., et al.: Phenotyping of hypertensive heart disease and hypertrophic cardiomyopathy using personalized 3D modelling and cardiac cine MRI. Physica Med. **78**, 137–149 (2020)
16. Liew, Y.M., et al.: Motion corrected LV quantification based on 3D modelling for improved functional assessment in cardiac MRI. Phys. Med. Biol. **60**(7), 2715 (2015)

Development of Automated Segmentation of the Thigh Muscles from Dixon MRI for Fat Fraction Quantification

Ashrani Aizzuddin Abd. Rahni, Mohd Izuan Ibrahim, Devinder Kaur Ajit Singh, Noor Ibrahim Mohamed Sakian, and Suzana Shahar

Abstract Sarcopenia, an age related condition is associated with decreased in lean muscle mass and increased in muscle fat. As a result, there is a decline in muscle strength and function in older adults. Diagnosis can be performed using bio-electrical impedance analysis (BIA) though accuracy is influenced by factors such as age, gender, hydration and ethnicity. Image based biomarkers have emerged as potentially more objective for diagnosis and from several possible modalities, MRI is considered a reference. In particular multiecho sequences for chemical shift imaging such as the Dixon method can be used to enhance muscle and fat contrast and calculate intramuscular fat (IMF) infiltration. In image based analysis, there is a need for automation, specifically in the segmentation of the muscles. In this work, we propose an automatic segmentation pipeline for a multipoint Dixon sequence. We evaluated the method with a publicly available dataset and compared it with the ground truth. We also demonstrated the method using local data from an MRI scan of the thigh muscles of an older person. The results showed that the mean PDFF of the right thigh muscle segmented by the proposed method correlates well with the mean PDFF from the ground truth segmentation, with a correlation value of 0.877. Qualitatively, the proposed method also produced a good segmentation of our local data. This suggests that the proposed method of muscle fat quantification can be used in future studies.

Keywords Automated · Segmentation · Thigh muscles · Dixon · MRI · Fat fraction · Sarcopenia

A. A. Abd. Rahni (✉)
Department of Electrical, Electronic and Systems Engineering, Faculty of Engineering and Built Environment, Universiti Kebangsaan Malaysia, 43600 Bangi, Malaysia
e-mail: ashrani@ukm.edu.my

M. I. Ibrahim · D. K. A. Singh · N. I. M. Sakian · S. Shahar
Centre for Healthy Ageing and Wellness, Faculty of Health Science, Universiti Kebangsaan Malaysia, 50300 Kuala Lumpur, Malaysia

J. Usman et al. (eds.), *6th Kuala Lumpur International Conference on Biomedical Engineering 2021*, IFMBE Proceedings 86,
https://doi.org/10.1007/978-3-030-90724-2_47

1 Introduction

There is an increased interest in research related to sarcopenia due to the increased number of older people worldwide. Sarcopenia is defined by the European Working Group on Sarcopenia in Older People (EWGSOP) as a muscle disease rooted in adverse muscle changes that accrue across a lifetime [1]. It has an impact on the activities of daily living and may lead to further negative consequences in older adults [2].

One of the criteria for the diagnosis of sarcopenia is low lean mass or low percentage of muscle mass in the body. This can be measured clinically using bio-electrical impedance analysis (BIA) that estimates the body's fat and muscle mass based on its' resistance (impedance) of a weak electric current. However, this estimate is influenced by several factors such as age, gender, hydration and ethnicity [2]. This together with the variability of definitions of sarcopenia can affect its' diagnosis. Hence several imaging biomarkers have been researched which are more objective. The imaging modalities that can be used are dual-energy X-ray absorptiometry (DXA), computed tomography (CT), ultrasound and magnetic resonance imaging (MRI). DXA can be used for evaluating body composition (BC) more objectively than BIA though it is limited in assessing muscle quality (muscle fat infiltration) and can still be influenced by the individual's hydration status.

For lean mass estimation of certain muscles, from the other modalities, the cross-sectional areas (CSA) of the muscles can be found. CSA can still be an indication of body composition [1, 3]. Between those three cross-sectional imaging modalities, MRI is considered to be the reference for non-invasive assessment [2, 4]. Using a multiecho sequence for chemical shift imaging such as the Dixon method, muscle and fat contrast can be enhanced in imaging and hence intramuscular fat (IMF) infiltration can be quantified.

In image based diagnosis, there is a need for automation, in particular for the segmentation of the muscles and other tissue from the images [5]. In this work, we propose an automatic segmentation pipeline for a multipoint Dixon sequence. The proposed method only requires a selected image slice and no subsequent interaction as it is automated. Section 2 describes the proposed method in more detail and the evaluation methodology. We present the results and discussion in Sect. 3. Finally, we conclude with suggestions for future directions in Sect. 4.

2 Methodology

Our proposed segmentation methodology is intended to be used on a mid-thigh image slice from a multipoint Dixon sequence. As the scanning protocol at Universiti Kebangsaan Malaysia Medical Centre (UKMMC) is to perform an MRI scan of the right thigh, we only apply the proposed method on the right thigh. We describe this in more detail in Sect. 2.1 and the evaluation in Sect. 2.2.

2.1 Processing Pipeline

From a multipoint Dixon sequence, we use both the derived water ($\boldsymbol{I}_W$) and fat ($\boldsymbol{I}_F$) images for muscle segmentation. The Otsu method [6] was use to automatically define a threshold for each image. Connected component analysis was then used on the thresholded image to select the two largest components corresponding to each thigh. The resulting initial segmentations are as shown in Fig. 1.

The water image segmentation ($\boldsymbol{W}$) may still not isolate the thigh muscles accurately as it may include high intensity pixels which corresponds to the skin surface. Therefore we remove the pixels which from the fat image segmentation ($\boldsymbol{F}$) to get a resultant muscle segmentation ($\boldsymbol{M}$). This can be represented by Boolean operations as in Eq. (1) below:

$$\boldsymbol{M} = \boldsymbol{W}\&(!\boldsymbol{F}) \tag{1}$$

Connected component analysis is then applied to the resultant muscle segmentation ($\boldsymbol{M}$) to obtain two largest components corresponding to each thigh. This muscle segmentation is shown in Fig. 2.

The last step is to calculate the intramuscular fat (IMF) infiltration which is represented by the proton density fat fraction (PDFF) within the segmented thigh muscle region of interest (ROI). For each pixel i, the PDFF image ($\boldsymbol{I}_{PDFF}$) is obtained according to Eq. (2) below:

$$\boldsymbol{I}_{PDFF}(i) = \boldsymbol{I}_F(i)/(\boldsymbol{I}_W(i) + \boldsymbol{I}_F(i)) \tag{2}$$

where $\boldsymbol{I}_W$ and $\boldsymbol{I}_F$ are the corresponding water and fat images (i.e. their intensities). As our assessment is only done on the right thigh, from the segmentation in Fig. 2 we only select the right thigh muscles as the ROI. This ROI displayed in the PDFF

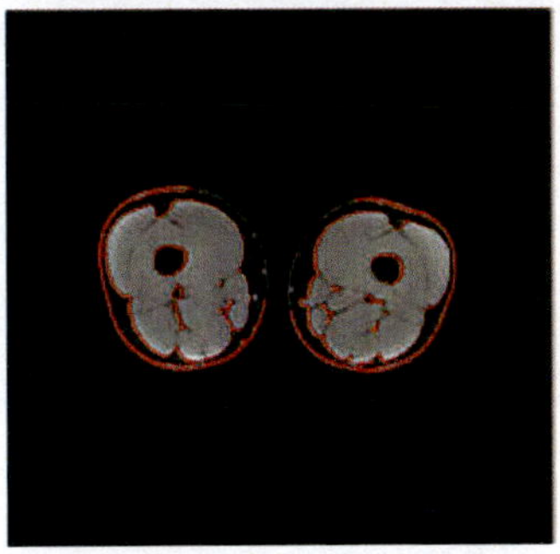

(a) Water image segmentation

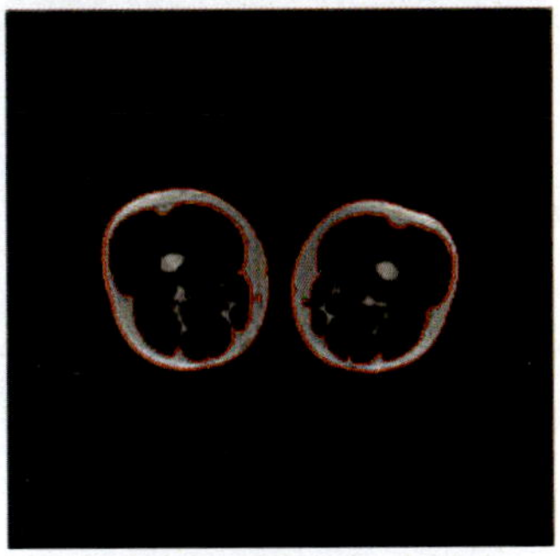

(b) Fat image segmentation

Fig. 1 Initial segmentations of corresponding **a** water and **b** fat image slices. The segmentations are indicated by the red outlines and correspond to high intensity regions in the images

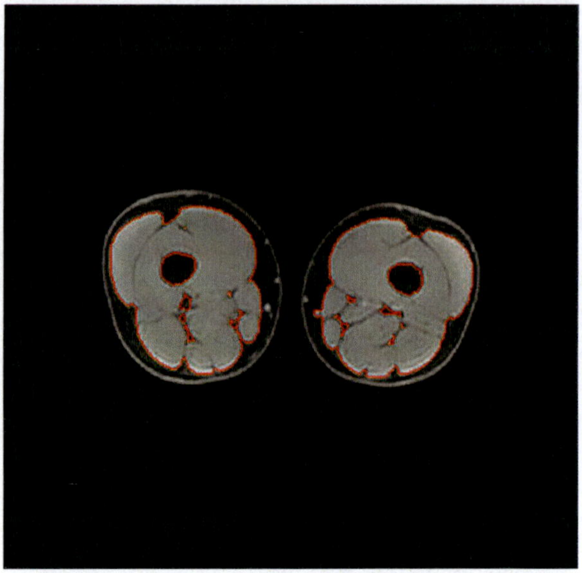

Fig. 2 Final muscle segmentation shown as a red outline on top of a water image slice

image is as shown in Fig. 3. The mean and standard deviation of the PDFF is then calculated within this ROI.

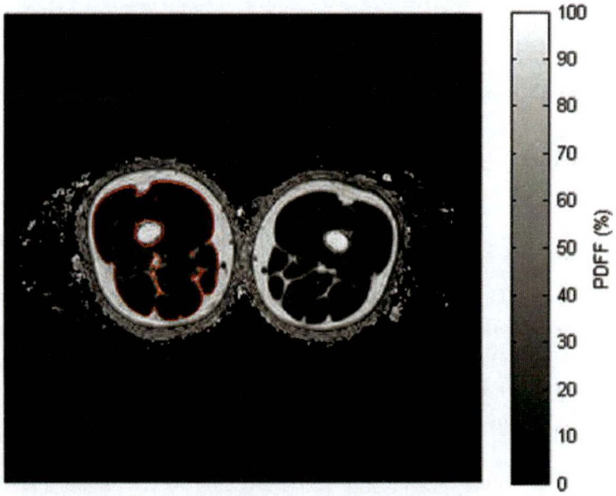

Fig. 3 Right thigh muscle ROI shown as a red outline on top of the corresponding PDFF image

2.2 Evaluation

For evaluation, we used our proposed methods on all the images from the MyoSegmenTUM reference dataset [7]. In brief, this dataset consists of Dixon MRI of 15 volunteers and 4 patients. Three of the volunteers underwent three repeated scans each, hence in total there are 25 scans. 6-point Dixon was acquired for each scan with various values of $TR/TE_{min}/\Delta TE$ and field of view. The voxel size used for our analysis is $1 \times 1 \times 4$ mm^3. The MyoSegmenTUM dataset includes manual segmentations of the Quadricepts ($\boldsymbol{Q}$), Sartorius ($\boldsymbol{S}$), Gracilis ($\boldsymbol{G}$) and Hamstrings ($\boldsymbol{H}$). Since our proposed method considers the thigh muscles as a whole, we combine the manual segmentations into a single ground truth ($\boldsymbol{T}$) for each subject. The ground truth is thus represented by the Boolean operations in Eq. (3) below:

$$\boldsymbol{T} = \boldsymbol{Q} + \boldsymbol{S} + \boldsymbol{G} + \boldsymbol{H} \quad (3)$$

We thus compare the PDFF calculated within our segmented ROI (Fig. 3) with the PDFF from the same slice within the ground truth. As mentioned in Sect. 2.1 above, we focus on the right thigh for our work.

As a proof of concept, we also apply the proposed method to an acquisition from a participant at Universiti Kebangsaan Malaysia Medical Centre (UKMMC). The acquisition protocol consists of a T1 scan with a reconstructed voxel size of $0.6875 \times 0.6875 \times 6.75$ mm^3 and a multipoint Dixon scan with a reconstructed voxel size of $0.9375 \times 0.9375 \times 6.75$ mm^3. The T1 image was rigidly registered to the Dixon image using NiftyReg [8]. Only the right thigh was scanned.

3 Results and Discussion

Following the evaluation methodology as outlined in Sect. 2.2 above, for a selected slice in each scan from the MyoSegmenTUM dataset, we automatically segment the thigh muscles and find the mean PDFF within the segmented ROI. We the compare this against the mean PDFF of the same slice within an ROI defined by the combined ground truth segmentation ($\boldsymbol{T}$) as defined in Eq. (3) above. Figure 4 shows a scatter plot of both quantities with the mean PDFF from the proposed method along the x-axis against the mean PDFF from the ground truth segmentation along the y-axis. A linear fit is also shown as a green line.

Despite the difference in the segmentation methodology (whole thigh vs four compartments of the thigh with the exclusion of Adductor muscles), from Fig. 4 we can still see a linear correlation between the mean PDFF from the ROI segmented by the proposed method with the mean PDFF from the ground truth segmentation. Quantitatively, the correlation has a value of 0.877 as measured by the Pearson correlation coefficient.

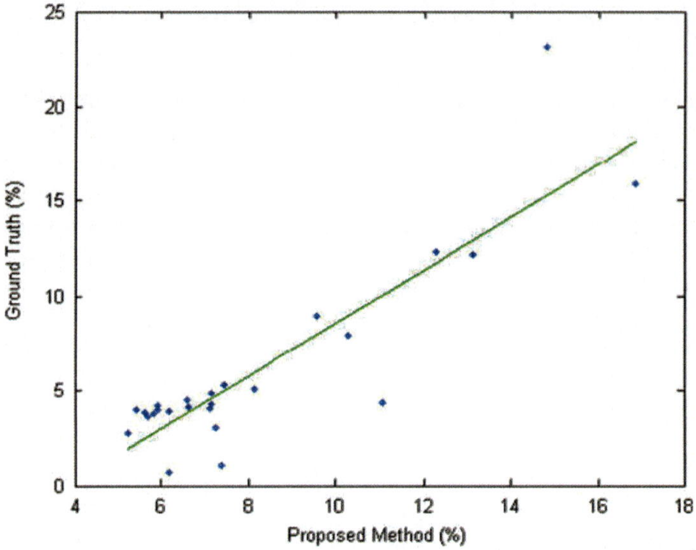

Fig. 4 Mean PDFF of the right thigh muscle ROI segmented by the proposed method against the mean PDFF from the ground truth segmentation of the same slice for all 25 scans. A linear fit is shown as a green line

As mentioned in Sect. 2.2 above, we applied the proposed method on imaging data from a volunteer at UKMMC. The segmentation results of the water and fat images are as shown in Fig. 5. Qualitatively, it can be seen that they are well segmented. In this case, there is no further processing needed for the water image segmentation, though the fat image segmentation can be used to delineate the thighs.

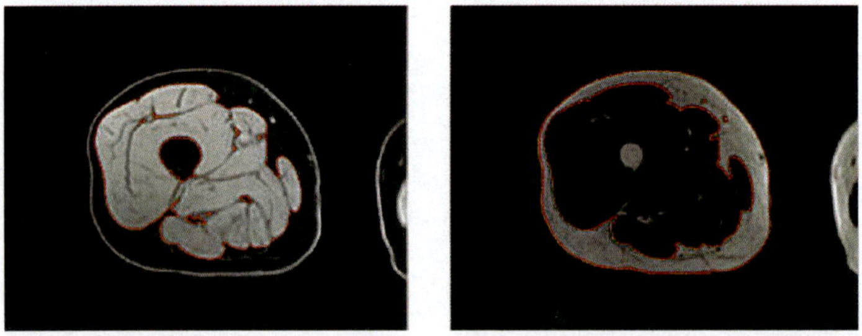

(a) Water image segmentation (b) Fat image segmentation

Fig. 5 Segmentations of corresponding **a** water and **b** fat image slices of the volunteer. The segmentations are indicated by the red outlines and correspond to high intensity regions in the images

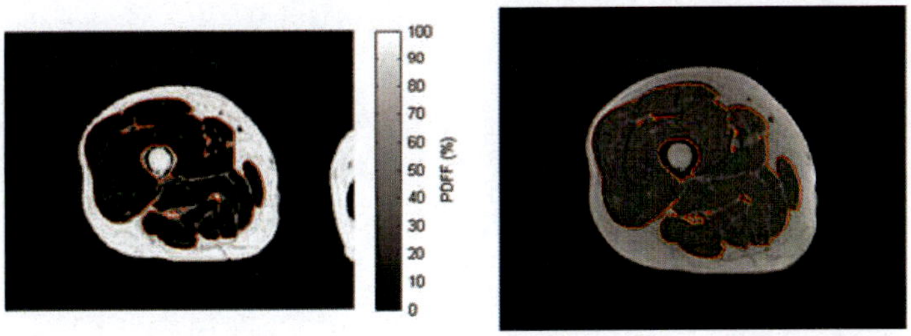

(a) PDFF image (b) T1 image

Fig. 6 The thigh muscle ROI shown as a red outline on the corresponding **a** PDFF and **b** registered T1 image slices of the volunteer

Figure 6 on the other hand shows the segmented muscles on top of the PDFF and registered T1 image slices. For the PDFF image, we use the thigh segmentation to remove noise outside of the thighs.

From Fig. 6, the mean PDFF within the ROI is calculated to be 8% which is within the normal range. On the other hand, Fig. 6b shows that the T1 image is well registered, although this can be improved with deformable image registration.

4 Conclusion and Future Work

We have evaluated the proposed method on the publicly available MyoSegmenTUM dataset and achieved a high correlation of mean PDFF from our segmented ROI with the mean PDFF of the ground truth segmentation. We have also demonstrated the method on a participant's imaging dataset with good segmentation of the thigh muscles. We intend to use this proposed method for muscle fat quantification in older adults with sarcopenia in future studies.

Acknowledgements This study is supported under grant no. NN-2019-098.

References

1. Albano, D., Messina, C., Vitale, J., Sconfienza, L.M.: Imaging of sarcopenia: Old evidence and new insights. Eur. Radiol. **30**, 2199–2208 (2019)
2. Sanz-Requena, R., Martínez-Arnau, F.M., Pablos, A., Flor-Rufino, C., Barrachina-Igual, J., García-Martí, G., Martí-Bonmatí, L., Pérez-Ros, P.: The role of imaging biomarkers in the assessment of sarcopenia. Diagnostics **10** (2020)
3. Yang, Y.X., Chong, M.S., Lim, W.S., Tay, L., Yew, S., Yeo, A., Tan, C.H.: Validity of estimating muscle and fat volume from a single MRI section in older adults with sarcopenia and sarcopenic obesity. Clin. Radiol. **72**, 427.e9–427.e14 (2017)

4. Codari, M., Zanardo, M., di Sabato, M.E., Nocerino, E., Messina, C., Sconfienza, L.M., Sardanelli, F.: MRI-derived biomarkers related to sarcopenia: a systematic review. J. Magn. Reson. Imag. **51**(4), 1117–1127 (2019)
5. Chaudry, O., Friedberger, A., Grimm, A., Uder, M., Nagel, A.M., Kemmler, W., Engelke, K.: Segmentation of the fascia lata and reproducible quantification of intermuscular adipose tissue (IMAT) of the thigh. Magn. Reson. Mater. Phys. Biol. Med. **34**, 367–376 (2020)
6. Otsu, N.: A threshold selection method from Gray-level histograms. IEEE Trans. Syst. Man Cybern. **9**(1), 62–66 (1979)
7. Schlaeger, S., Freitag, F., Klupp, E., Dieckmeyer, M., Weidlich, D., Inhuber, S., Deschauer, M., Schoser, B., Bublitz, S., Montagnese, F., Zimmer, C., Rummeny, E.J., Karampinos, D.C., Kirschke, J.S., Thomas Baum, T.: Thigh muscle segmentation of chemical shift encoding-based water-fat magnetic resonance images: the reference database MyoSegmenTUM. PLoS One **13**(6) (2018)
8. Modat, M., Cash, D.M., Daga, P., Winston, G.P., Duncan, J.S., Ourselin, S.: Global image registration using a symmetric block-matching approach. J. Med. Imag. **1**(2) (2014)

Longitudinal Assessment of Optical Properties in Early Demineralization of Enamel Using pH Cycling Model

Fatin Najwa, Yih Miin Liew, Ngie Min Ung, and Prema Sukumaran

Abstract Over the decades, examination of caries lesion has been performed conventionally by visual assessment where assessment methods such as ICDAS, and Nyvad Criteria were used as a reference to determine the severity of the caries. However, the conventional dental diagnosis was unable to detect early demineralization accurately due to the indistinct physical appearance of caries lesions at early stage. The objective of this research is to study the ability of optical coherence tomography (OCT) in diagnosing early demineralization of enamel layer without involving ionizing radiation. Sound human molar teeth samples were subjected to pH cycling for 3, 7, 14, 21 and 28 days to induce caries at the region of interest. Samples were scanned using OCT to assess the progression of demineralization, whereby the optical mean attenuation coefficient for each of the samples were extracted and compared. We found that the normalized mean attenuation of samples increased with the length of pH cycling, i.e. 1.33, 1.52 and 1.79 for 3, 7, and 14 days of pH cycling. The changes could be due to the increase of porosity in enamel layer. Irregular trend started to occur after 14 days, where to the normalized attenuation coefficient decreased on day 21 and then increased again on day 28, i.e. 1.46 and 1.65 respectively. Hypermineralization was suspected to happen after 14 days of pH cycling, causing irregular mineral concentration on the tooth surface. This study shows the potential use of optical properties from OCT system to detect early demineralization of the tooth.

Keywords Optical coherence tomography · Human teeth · Attenuation coefficient · pH cycling · Demineralization

F. Najwa · Y. M. Liew (✉)
Faculty of Engineering, Department of Biomedical Engineering, Universiti Malaya, Kuala Lumpur, Malaysia
e-mail: liewym@um.edu.my

N. M. Ung
Faculty of Medicine, Clinical Oncology Unit, 50603 Kuala Lumpur, Malaysia

P. Sukumaran
Faculty of Dentistry, Department of Restorative Dentistry, Universiti Malaya, Kuala Lumpur, Malaysia
e-mail: prema@um.edu.my

J. Usman et al. (eds.), *6th Kuala Lumpur International Conference on Biomedical Engineering 2021*, IFMBE Proceedings 86,
https://doi.org/10.1007/978-3-030-90724-2_48

1 Introduction

Microstructures and mineral composition of human teeth vary with the intraoral condition and are influenced by food intake, hygiene measures, and health condition. Consumption of food with excessive acid and sugar content, and xerostomia condition (low salivary flow in the intraoral) can lead to the formation of caries lesions on teeth. Caries lesions occur when demineralization process is initiated on the enamel or dentin layer by acids produced by cariogenic bacteria during metabolism of fermentable carbohydrates. Demineralization is supported by conditions such as low pH value and reduced salivary buffering capacity which is conducive for the growth of cariogenic bacteria. This condition eventually results in an imbalanced growth of cariostatic and cariogenic bacteria and leads to a shift in the equilibrium to initiate demineralization on the outer surface of teeth [1]. Demineralization is an irreversible process of removing some of the mineral in the enamel or dentin layer of the tooth and is mainly due to the lack of oral hygiene measures. In the clinical diagnosis of the severity of caries lesion, the conventional method based on visual assessment seems to be quite unreliable and perhaps even ambiguous due to the subjective nature of the measure and different opinions from clinicians of varying experience levels.

Caries lesions occur when demineralization is initiated on enamel by acids produced by cariogenic bacteria during metabolism of fermentable carbohydrates. If left undetected, the lesions can extend from enamel to dentine, which is the second layer of tooth structure. It is clinically challenging to detect or monitor early caries lesions on enamel using visual inspection. Optical coherence tomography (OCT) has seen broad applications in dentistry and has been used to image both dental hard and soft tissues. OCT is a non-destructive imaging system that can utilize near-infrared (NIR) light to produce depth-resolved images in dental enamel. Demineralization in enamel cause significant scatter of NIR light, and OCT measures this increase in backscatter intensity. It can therefore be utilized in an objective manner to detect and quantify early caries lesions in enamel and monitor the progress of these lesions.

2 Literature Review

Early caries is defined as the start of demineralization on the surface of enamel. Severity of this lesion can be determined using two visual assessment methods, known as ICDAS and Nyvad [2–4]. However, visual assessment of caries has a high inter-rater variability as the physical appearances of early carious lesions are subtle and can easily lead to misclassification. Thus, a new efficient and effective method is desired for a better lesion diagnosis at all levels of severity.

One of the non-invasive technologies that is proposed as a diagnosis tool in caries assessment is optical coherence tomography (OCT). OCT is an optical imaging modality which uses low-coherence near infrared light to obtain real-time images of tissue sample with excellent spatial resolution in microns. Low-coherence light that is generated by a laser or superluminescent diode is split at the beam splitter to incident on the two arms (sample and reference arms), which are then recombined as interference fringe patterns at the beam splitter. The reflected signal gathered from a raster scan of the specimens are used to form cross-sectional and 3D images [5]. Different sample compositions and surfaces result in different images due to the different light scattering properties of the samples.

The purpose of this study, which is part of a larger study, is to use OCT to track progression of early enamel caries, induced using the pH cycling model. Although there are previous studies [6] which have documented the optical changes in early caries lesions, the present study specifically tracks longitudinal changes in mean attenuation of early caries lesions over different time points. OCT was applied to early caries lesions, mainly demineralization in enamel which could potentially pave for more evidenced-based diagnosis and treatment management.

3 Materials and Method

3.1 Sample Preparation and Caries Induction

Three sound molar teeth used in this study were obtained from dental clinics around Klang Valley, Kuala Lumpur, Malaysia. The teeth were sectioned into half using the Micracut machine and subjected to pH cycling. Each sample was colored using red nail polish (Revlon) except for a window of 4 mm $\times$ 4 mm square which was treated as region of interest (ROI) for OCT scanning. Only this window was exposed for the induction of artificial lesion. The exposed window was induced with artificial caries lesion and subsequent OCT scanning for tracking of caries lesion (Fig. 1).

The artificial caries lesion was induced using pH cycling method to mimic the intraoral condition which involves demineralization and remineralization processes alternately. The pH cycling model used in this research, referred to as modified Featherstone model [7] involved immersing all samples in a demineralization solution containing 2.0 mM calcium nitrate tetrahydrate, 2.0 mM monopotassium phosphate, 75.0 mM acetic acid and sodium hydroxide which was maintained at pH 4.5 for 6 h. After demineralization, all samples were immersed in remineralization solution containing 1.5 mM calcium nitrate tetrahydrate, 0.9 mM monopotassium phosphate, 130.0 mM potassium chloride, 20.0 mM sodium cacodylate and hydrochloric acid, which was maintained at pH 7.0 for 17.5 h. The demineralization and remineralization procedures were alternated and repeated up to 14 days. In between, half an hour was allocated to change the solution and to scan the samples using OCT. The OCT scans were performed prior to pH cycling (to obtain baseline measurement) and at days 3, 7 and 14 of pH cycling.

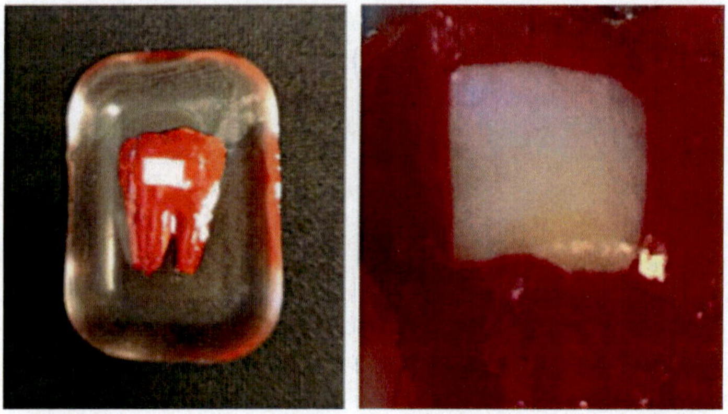

Fig. 1 Tooth sample was colored with red nail polish leaving a 4 mm × 4 mm square window (right). The tooth sample was molded into epoxy resin for positioning, inducing of caries and scanning under the OCT (left)

3.2 OCT System and Image Acquisition

OCT images over the ROI were acquired using Thorlabs OCS1300SS swept-source OCT (SS-OCT) system (Thorlabs, USA). The OCT system used superluminescent laser diode (SLD) with central wavelength at 1300 nm, and 10mW output power. The axial scan rate was 16 kHz with the imaging speed of 25fps, and maximum imaging depth of 3 mm. Images of 800 × 800 × 512 pixels over an area of 4 mm × 4 mm were generated with transverse resolution of 25 μm, and axial resolution in air and water of 12 μm and 9 μm, respectively.

3.3 Extraction of Optical Properties

Optical attenuation coefficient of each tooth sample was extracted computationally (Fig. 2). Specifically, the OCT images in linear scale were converted into logarithmic scale, covering signal intensity from 5 dB to −40 dB. Surface of the tooth samples was detected using Canny edge detector and median filtering was used to remove erroneous spikes. B-scan of the OCT images was subsequently smoothened by averaging every 5 adjacent A-scans using a sliding window. Least square fitting was performed on each average A-scan at 100 μm to extract regional attenuation coefficient μ of the samples z using Beer-Lambert Law equation (Eq. 1) [8] as follows:

$$InI(z) = -2z + C \tag{1}$$

where I(z) represented the depth dependent backscattered signal intensity and C is the initial value of reflection or incident signal intensity (surface peak). The fitting

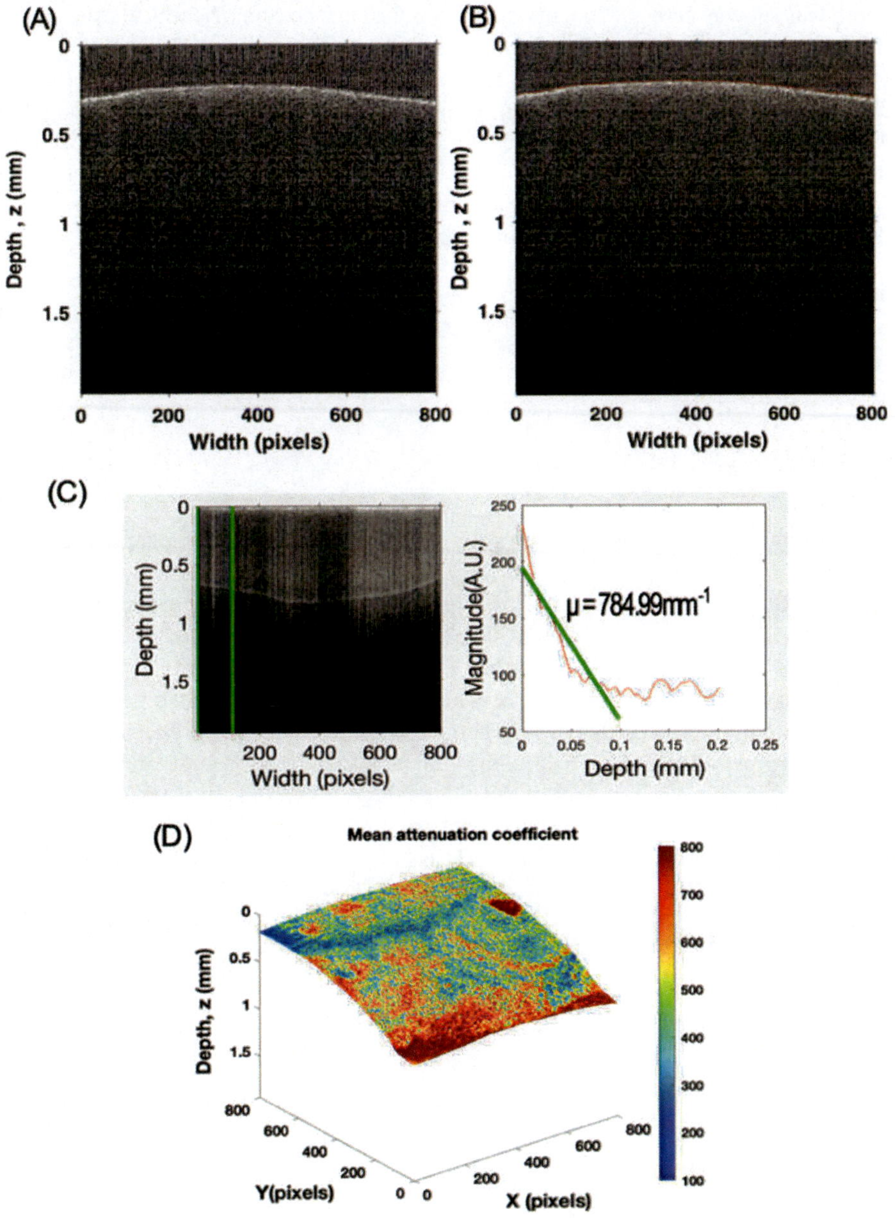

Fig. 2 **a** The OCT B-scan of a tooth, **b** surface of the tooth was detected using Canny edge detector and filtered with median filtering to remove erroneous spikes, **c** least square fitting was performed on each average A-scan to extract regional attenuation coefficient μ of the samples z. The fitting was indicated by the green line in both OCT image and the graph. **d** Surface map of mean attenuation coefficient. Colorbar represent the mean attenuation coefficient (mm^{-1}). A.U. stands for arbitrary unit

depth was set was across 100 μm depth from the surface (empirically determined as the depth of enamel layer). The fitting was performed on all A-scans within the 3D volume to produce surface maps color-coded with regional attenuation coefficient for each sample. The mean attenuation coefficient was then computed across the ROI for each duration of pH cycling. Since each tooth sample may have different demineralization conditions before pH cycling, the relative changes of this coefficient (μ_R) with respect to baseline attenuation (Eq. 2) were therefore reported to reflect the changes that have occurred longitudinally with caries induction.

$$\mu_R = \frac{\mu_{\text{pH cycling}}}{\mu_{baseline}}. \quad (2)$$

4 Results and Discussion

Figure 3 illustrates that the average ratio of mean attenuation coefficient to the baseline, μ_R for all samples showed an increasing trend from day 0 to day 14 of pH cycling. Attenuation coefficient of the signal before pH cycling process was lower compared to days 3, 7, and 14 of pH cycling, and this is consistent with the results obtained by Ueno et al. 2016 and Chan et al. 2015 [9, 10], whom have shown the increase of sample scattering with the progression of caries. The changes in the scattering properties could be due to the changes in the porosity of the enamel layer as a result of the loss of mineral density during the demineralization and remineralization process [10]. When the porosity of the enamel layer increases, the microstructure of the enamel layer is altered, producing distant gaps and larger opening of transverse rods in between from significant mineral loss [11, 12]. Larger opening rods may have

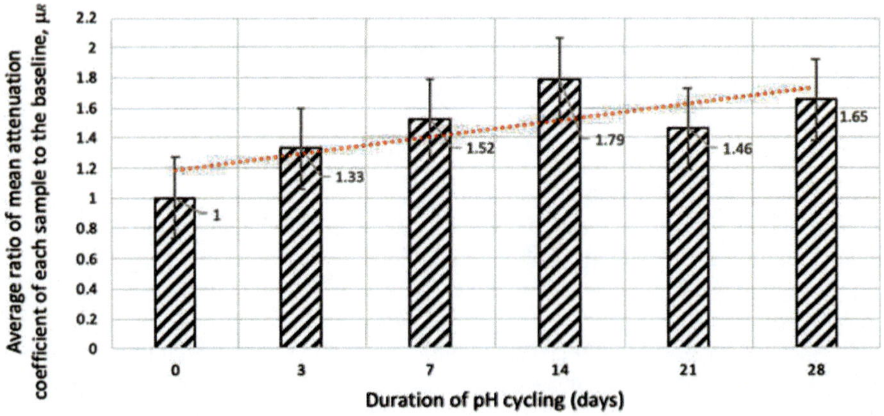

Fig. 3 Graph of average ratio of mean attenuation coefficient of each sample to the baseline, μ_R against the duration of pH cycling

increased multiple scattering of incident light, which causes more signal attenuation (less penetration depth) in the enamel layer, therefore the detection of higher attenuation coefficients through the system [13–15]. The demineralized region was shown as the region with higher signal intensity and therefore can be distinguished as the whitish region in the OCT images. However, an irregular trend was shown after day 14 of pH cycling where the μ_R started to decrease on day 21 and increase again on day 28 of pH cycling.

Hypermineralization was suspected to happen after 14 days of pH cycling where a complex structure was formed on the tooth surface. Mineral composition started to build up from the outmost layer towards the dentin-enamel junction (DEJ) with the inner part remained porous. As the teeth samples undergo a continuous cycle of demineralization and remineralization in a controlled environment, it formed a layer of hypermineralized enamel at the surface. The hypermineralized layer at the surface can serve to prevent further diffusion of acidic solution into the body of the carious lesion and thereby preventing further demineralization of body of lesion. This explains how caries lesions are arrested intraorally. However, as the samples were subjected to further demineralization, the hypermineralized layer tend to be dissolved, leading to increased porosity and easier pathway of diffusion of acidic solution. Under such circumstances, there will be advancement of demineralization of body of lesion and increased porosity. OCT signal could still travel through part of the porous region but attenuated more at hypermineralized region. This phenomenon could potentially explain the reduction in signal attenuation between day 14 and 21, postulating the formation of hypermineralized layer at the surface of the enamel. With the further immersion of samples in remin-demin solution, progression of caries in body of lesion can be reflected from the increase in signal attenuation between day 21 and 28.

Albeit the increasing trend, the changes of attenuation coefficient are small from one time point to another, showing that the caries induction through pH cycling occurs at a slow rate [13].

5 Conclusion

During pH cycling, demineralization and remineralization processes took place alternately which results in mineral composition alteration in the enamel layer. The average ratio of mean attenuation coefficient to the baseline for each sample increases from day 0 to day 14 of pH cycling. The changes in signal attenuation could be due to the increment in porosity level resulted from the demineralization process during pH cycling. Thus, it is shown that OCT system has the potential to be used for the detection and follow-up assessment of early tooth demineralization by assessing the optical properties of the tooth.

Acknowledgements This research was funded by the University of Malaya Faculty Research Grant (GPF010C-2019).

References

1. Gupta, N., et al.: Radiation-induced dental caries, prevention and treatment—a systematic review. Nat. J. Maxillofacial Surg. **6**(2), 160 (2015)
2. Ismail, A.I., et al.: The international caries detection and assessment system (ICDAS): an integrated system for measuring dental caries. Commun. Dent. Oral Epidemiol. **35**(3), 170–178 (2007)
3. ICDAS I: International Caries Detection and Assessment System (ICDAS) Coordinating Committee. ICDAS II International Caries Assessment and Detection System (2008)
4. Gugnani, N., et al.: International caries detection and assessment system (ICDAS): a new concept. Int. J. Clin. Pediatric Dentistry **4**(2), 93 (2011)
5. Huang, D., et al.: Optical coherence tomography. Science **254**(5035), 1178–1181 (1991)
6. de Cara, A.C.B., et al.: Comparative analysis of optical coherence tomography signal and micro-hardness for demineralization evaluation of human tooth enamel. In: Biophotonics: Photonic Solutions for Better Health Care III. International Society for Optics and Photonics (2012)
7. Stookey, G.K.: The Featherstone laboratory pH cycling model: a prospective, multi-site validation exercise. Am. J. Dent. **24**(5), 322 (2011)
8. Schmitt, J.M., et al.: Optical-coherence tomography of a dense tissue: statistics of attenuation and backscattering. Phys. Med. Biol. **39**(10), 1705 (1994)
9. Ueno, T., et al.: Optical analysis of enamel and dentin caries in relation to mineral density using swept-source optical coherence tomography. J. Med. Imag. **3**(3), 035507 (2016)
10. Chan, K.H., et al.: Use of 2D images of depth and integrated reflectivity to represent the severity of demineralization in cross-polarization optical coherence tomography. J. Biophotonics **8**(1–2), 36–45 (2015)
11. Damato, F., Strang, R., Stephen, K.: Comparison of solution-and gel-prepared enamel lesions-an in vitro pH-cycling study. J. Dent. Res. **67**(8), 1122–1125 (1988)
12. Ten Cate, J., Duijsters, P.: Alternating demineralization and remineralization of artificial enamel lesions. Caries Res. **16**(3), 201–210 (1982)
13. Marquezan, M., et al.: Artificial methods of dentine caries induction: a hardness and morphological comparative study. Arch. Oral Biol. **54**(12), 1111–1117 (2009)
14. Amaechi, B., et al.: Use of optical coherence tomography for assessment of dental caries: quantitative procedure. J. Oral Rehabil. **28**(12), 1092–1093 (2001)
15. Damodaran, V., Vasa, N.J.: Imaging artificially induced dental caries using optical coherence tomography near 800 and 1300 nm region. In: 2015 Workshop on Recent Advances in Photonics (WRAP). IEEE (2015)

Investigate the Velocity Difference Between MRI Measurement and CFD Simulation on Patient-Specific Blood Flow Analysis

Sheh Hong Lim, Mohd Azrul Hisham Mohd Adib, Mohd Shafie Abdullah, Nur Hartini Mohd Taib, Radhiana Hassan, and Azian Abd Aziz

Abstract This paper tends to investigate the velocity difference between magnetic resonance imaging (MRI) measurement and computational fluid dynamics (CFD) simulation on patient-specific blood flow analysis. Three patients diagnosed with particular cerebral aneurysms are involved in the current investigation. The raw image data from patients have been processed through image segmentation for model reconstruction using several threshold coefficients, C_{thres} from 0.2 to 0.6 according to the threshold value determined using threshold determination method. Besides, the velocity profile is extracted from the MRI measurement and applied in the inlet boundary condition setup. Meanwhile, pressure-fixed (P-fixed) approach is applied at all the outlets prior to CFD simulation. Based on the comparison made between the MRI measurement and CFD results, the model geometries reconstructed with threshold coefficients, C_{thres} of 0.3, 0.4, and 0.5 are considered to be the optimized model geometries which have shown significantly small velocity difference between 0.3% and 12%, in term of average velocity among the model geometries of respective patient. The results also depict that the artery branch and the bifurcation regions, which are subjected to high velocity concentration could be the hemodynamics factor contributing to cerebral aneurysm growing and rupturing.

Keywords Cerebral aneurysm · Threshold determination · Image processing · Segmentation · Hemodynamics

---

S. H. Lim (✉) · M. A. H. Mohd Adib (✉)
Medical Engineering and Health Intervention Team (MedEHiT), Department of Mechanical Engineering, College of Engineering, Universiti Malaysia Pahang, Lebuhraya Tun Razak, 26300 Kuantan, Pahang, Malaysia
e-mail: azrul@ump.edu.my

M. S. Abdullah · N. H. Mohd Taib
Department of Radiology, School of Medical Sciences, Universiti Sains Malaysia, Health Campus, 16150 Kubang Kerian, Kelantan, Malaysia

Hospital Universiti Sains Malaysia, Health Campus, 16150 Kubang Kerian, Kelantan, Malaysia

R. Hassan · A. Abd Aziz
Department of Radiology, Kulliyyah of Medicine, International Islamic University Malaysia, 25200 Kuantan, Pahang, Malaysia

J. Usman et al. (eds.), *6th Kuala Lumpur International Conference on Biomedical Engineering 2021*, IFMBE Proceedings 86,
https://doi.org/10.1007/978-3-030-90724-2_49

1 Introduction

Based on the advancement of medical imaging technique, magnetic resonance imaging (MRI) has been extensively applied in the current trend due to its unrestricted three-dimensional (3D) anatomical coverage image. Furthermore, MRI can provide the image of velocity flow field noninvasively. The flow velocity of blood, particularly within the blood vessel can be extracted from MRI measurement for qualitative analysis concerning physiological blood flow pattern on particular subject [1, 2]. From the PC-MRI images, it is possible to calculate velocity from the extracted data, however it produces high error in measurement during the image smoothing process as the images are usually produced in low resolutions [3–5].

However, the limited spatial and temporal resolutions of MRI image data make the hemodynamics analysis less accurate [2, 6, 7]. Thus, computational fluid dynamics (CFD) simulation is recognized as an alternative in predicting behaviour or physiological blood flow patterns in various vascular models, especially in cardiovascular models [4, 8] and cerebrovascular models [7, 9–15]. The research frameworks available nowadays infuse the velocity profiles from MRI measurement in the CFD simulation [5, 13] and the studies concluded that this approach is effective in obtaining physiological blood flow pattern in determining hemodynamics factors contributing to cerebral aneurysm growing and rupturing.

The current study aims to present the differential percentage, in term of velocity among MRI measurement and CFD simulation through the model geometry reconstructed with systematic image segmentation procedure on patient-specific cerebral aneurysm. The optimized model geometries which best represent the blood flow pattern and hemodynamics factor contributing to the cerebral aneurysm growing and rupturing have been identified, this approach tends to provide evidence to the medical industry in targeting the diagnosis and treatment of patient-specific cerebral aneurysm as well as to alleviate the cases of cerebrovascular diseases.

2 Methodology

2.1 Model Geometry Reconstruction

The present investigation constitutes of three male patients of 48, 58, and 65 years old diagnosed with cerebral aneurysms. All the patients had undergone both biplane digital subtraction angiography (DSA) and magnetic resonance imaging (MRI) screening at radiology department, Hospital Universiti Sains Malaysia (HUSM), Health Campus, Kubang Kerian, Kelantan. The DSA images were captured using Siemens Artis Zee Angiography Biplane (Siemens Healthineers, Erlangen, Germany) with image projection voxel matrix of 512 $\times$ 512 and voxel size of 0.48 mm^3, however the MRI images were captured using Philips Achieva 3.0 T MRI system (Philips Healthcare, Best, The Netherland) with image projection voxel matrix of 512 × 512 and voxel size of 1.0 mm^3. The details of the acquired medical image data are listed in Table 1.

The model reconstruction was performed on DSA image data through image segmentation with several threshold coefficients, C_{thres} such as 0.2, 0.3, 0.4, 0.5, and 0.6 using threshold determination method [2, 16, 17]. There were five patient-specific cerebral aneurysm model geometries reconstructed from each patient model using AMIRA™ 2019.3. In other words, 15 model geometries were reconstructed in total and smoothing procedure was performed on the model geometries with standardized smoothing factor of 0.5 without compromising the local or global geometry configuration. The reconstructed cerebral aneurysm model geometries of each patient are illustrated in Fig. 1. The model geometry from Patient 1 at threshold coefficient, C_{thres} of 0.6 is excluded from the current investigation as the geometry configuration is out of shape and there is branch dislocation [2, 18] as indicated at the circle.

Table 1 Details of acquired image data with respective patient

Patient	Age (years old)	Aneurysm location	Aneurysm size (mm)
1	48	MCA	3.0 (AP) × 4.0 (W)
2	58	ICA	4.2 (AP) × 4.1 (W)
3	65	IC-PC	5.1 (AP) × 1.1 (W)

MCA middle cerebral artery, *ICA* internal carotid artery, *IC-PC* internal carotid-posterior communicating, *AP* anteroposterior, *W* width

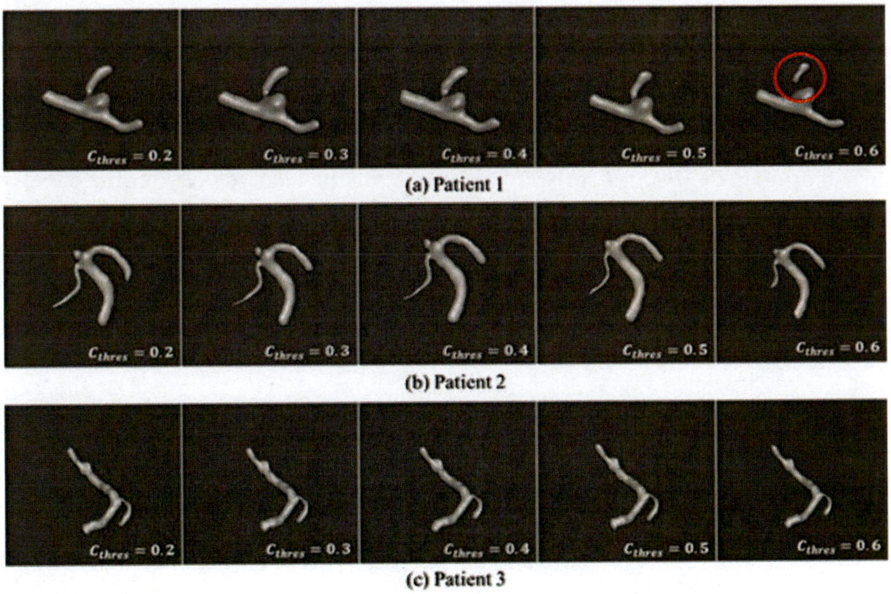

Fig. 1 Model geometries of patients with respective threshold coefficient, C_{thres}

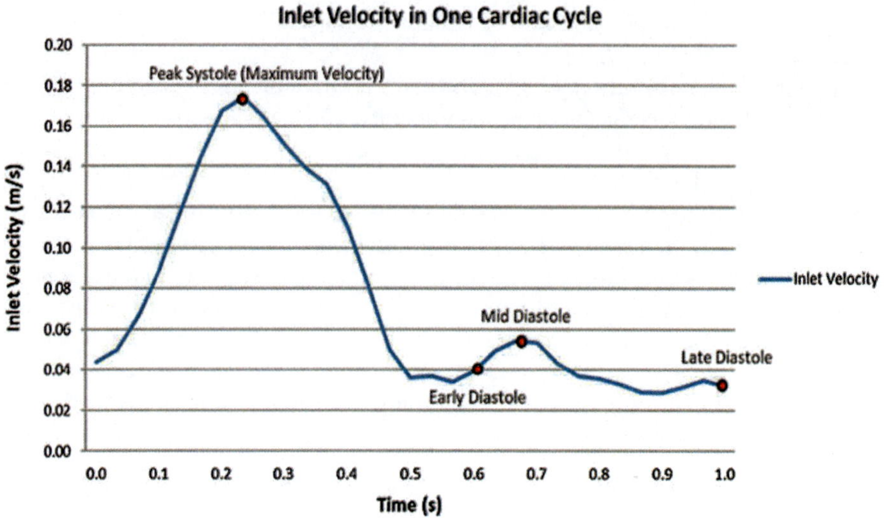

Fig. 2 Velocity profile curve in one cardiac cycle

Table 2 Inlet velocity extracted from MRI measurement in one cardiac cycle

Patient	1	2	3
V_{inlet} (m/s)	0.2117	0.1723	0.2511

2.2 Velocity Profile Extraction

The velocity profile was extracted from MRI medical image data of each patient using *ImageJ* software. MRI image data was inputted at the multivolume explorer, which is an extension in the *ImageJ* software for extracting the inlet velocity profile curve in one cardiac cycle. Figure 2 shows an example of the velocity profile curve extracted in one cardiac cycle while Table 2 presents the inlet velocity, V_{inlet} extracted from the MRI measurement. It is noted that the inlet velocity, V_{inlet} at the peak systole is taken into account for inlet boundary condition setup as it is the maximum velocity which tends to cause the rupture of cerebral aneurysm [19–21].

2.3 Computational Fluid Dynamics (CFD) Simulation

The present simulation was performed at CFD solver, *ANSYS Fluent 16.2*. The continuity and Navier–Stokes equations [2] were employed at computational domain, $\acute{\Omega}$ as follows:

Table 3 Parameters for blood flow [2]

Parameter	Viscosity (Pa s)	Density (kg/m^3)	Temperature (K)	Specific heat (J/kg K)	Thermal conductivity (W/m K)
Value	0.0035	1060	310	3513	0.44

$$\frac{\partial u_i}{\partial x_i} = 0 \tag{1}$$

$$\rho\left(\frac{\partial u_i}{\partial t} + u_j\frac{\partial u_i}{\partial x_i}\right) = -\frac{\partial P}{\partial x_j} + \mu\frac{\partial^2 u_i}{\partial x_j \partial x_j} + f_i \tag{2}$$

in which u_i, P, f_i, ρ, μ, and ∂_{ij} refers to the velocity in the ith direction, pressure, body force, density, viscosity, and Kronecker delta, respectively.

The blood was treated as incompressible, laminar, and Newtonian fluid with the parameters as listed in Table 3. The present simulation was performed in steady-state and the only specific boundary condition set at the inlet was the inlet velocity, V_{inlet} of respective patient as listed in Table 2 while for the outlet, the outlet pressure was set according to pressure-fixed (P-fixed) approach, in which all the outlet pressures were set to zero [19, 22] as follows:

$$p^{(i)} = 0 \quad \text{for } i \in [1, I] \tag{3}$$

where I refers to the quantity of outlet in total and $p^{(i)}$ is the corresponding outlet pressure [19].

3 Results and Discussion

Figure 3 illustrates the MRI measurement and the results generated from the CFD simulation of all patients in the current study. From the CFD simulation results, the velocity flow fields have shown consistent agreement with the MRI measurement qualitatively. There are certain parts (as indicated at the circle) of the velocity flow fields are invisible or unclear from the MRI measurement as compared to the CFD simulation results. This might be due to low spatial and temporal resolutions of the MRI image data which tend to diminish the velocity flow field visualization [2, 17, 23].

Moreover, in the perspective of quantitative comparison, the average velocity obtained from the CFD simulation results, $V_{CFD,avg}$ has good agreement with the average velocity obtained from the MRI measurement, $V_{MRI,avg}$. The lowest and highest differential percentage of approximately 0.3% and 12%, respectively do exist among the MRI measurement and CFD simulation results from respective patient as tabulated in Table 4. The differential percentage might be arisen from the model

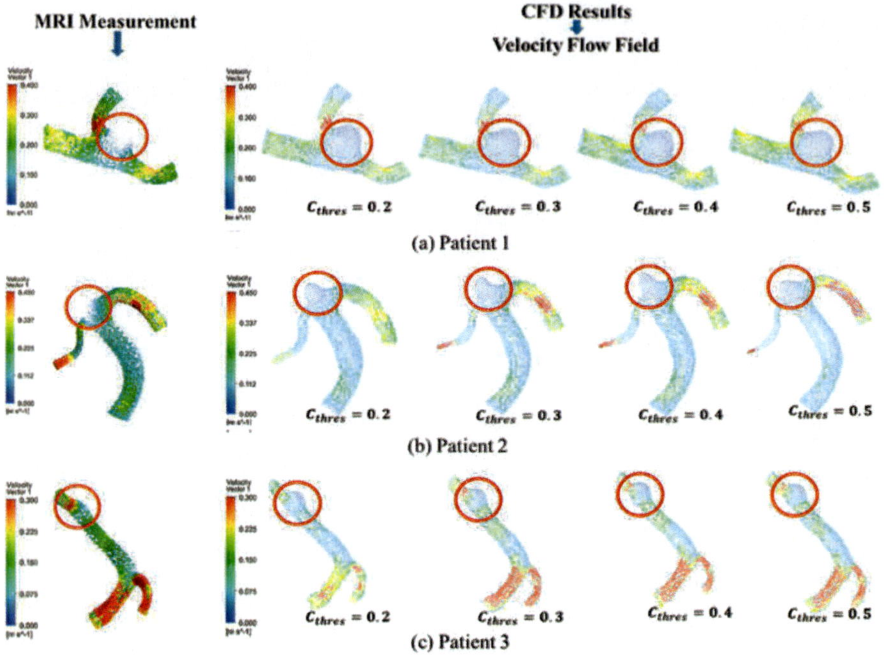

Fig. 3 MRI measurement and CFD simulation results from each patient

Table 4 Quantitative comparison on respective average velocity obtained from MRI, $V_{MRI,avg}$ and CFD simulation result, $V_{CFD,avg}$

Patient	$V_{MRI,avg}$ (m/s)	$V_{CFD,avg}$ (m/s)	Percentage difference (%)
1	0.1886	0.1678 ($C_{thres} = 0.4$)	11.6723
2	0.1886	0.1891 ($C_{thres} = 0.5$)	0.2648
3	0.1971	0.1839 ($C_{thres} = 0.3$)	6.9291

geometry reconstruction techniques [24–27] and image data resolution [23], in terms of human and parallax errors.

It is noted that the magnitude of average velocity obtained from the MRI measurement and CFD simulation results does have correlation with the threshold coefficient, C_{thres}. Upon the validation between the model geometries among the same patient, the optimized model geometries which have smallest differential percentage, high visualization, and high consistency of hemodynamics flow pattern for Patient 1, Patient 2, and Patient 3 are at threshold coefficient, C_{thres} of 0.4, 0.5, and 0.3, respectively as compared between MRI measurement and CFD simulation results. Besides, the artery branch and the bifurcation regions are cultivated with high velocity concentration, which have the tendency contributing to the cerebral aneurysm growing and rupturing. These findings have linear consensus as the previous research frameworks concerning the infused approach of MRI measurement into CFD simulation [5, 16, 19].

4 Conclusion

The present research work shows that the differential percentage, in term of average velocity among MRI measurement and CFD simulation is still significant, in which there is still approximately 12% of differential percentage found in the current research framework. The optimized model geometries are found to be available at threshold coefficient, C_{thres} of 0.3–0.5. Moreover, the artery branch and the bifurcation regions have the tendency contributing to the cerebral aneurysm growing and rupturing.

Acknowledgements The support from Ministry of Higher Education under FRGS grant FRGS/1/2018/TK03/UMP/02/23, UMP under grant RDU190153 and PGRS2003201, and Medical Engineering & Health Intervention Team (MedEHiT) are gratefully acknowledged.

References

1. Pelc, N.J., Herfkens, R.J., Shimakawa, A., Enzmann, D.R.: Phase contrast cine magnetic resonance imaging. Magn. Reson. Q. **7**, 229–254 (1991)
2. Lim, S.H., Mohd Adib, M.A.H., Abdullah, M.S., Mohd Taib, N.H., Hassan, R., Abd Aziz, A.: Study of extracted geometry effect on patient-specific cerebral aneurysm model with different threshold coefficient (Cthres). CFD Lett. **12**, 1–14 (2020)
3. Markl, M., Chan, F.P., Alley, M.T., Wedding, K.L., Draney, M.T., Elkins, C.J., Parker, D.W., Wicker, R., Taylor, C.A., Herfkens, R.J., Pelc, N.J.: Time-resolved three-dimensional phase-contrast MRI. J. Magn. Reson. Imag. **17**, 499–506 (2003)
4. Juffermans, J.F., Westenberg, J.J.M., Palen, R.L.F., Van Der Boogaard, P.J., Van Den, Lamb. H.J.: Geometrically induced wall shear stress variability in CFD-MRI coupled simulations of blood flow in the thoracic aortas. Comput. Biol. Med. **133** (2021)
5. Ngo, M.T., Lee, U.Y., Ha, H., Jin, N., Chung, G.H., Kwak, Y.G., Jung, J., Kwak, H.S.: Comparison of hemodynamic visualization in cerebral arteries: can magnetic resonance imaging replace computational fluid dynamics? J. Pers. Med. **11**, 253 (2021)
6. Harloff, A., Nußbaumer, A., Bauer, S., Stalder, A.F., Frydrychowicz, A., Weiller, C., Hennig, J., Markl, M.: In vivo assessment of wall shear stress in the atherosclerotic aorta using flow-sensitive 4D MRI. Magn. Reson. Med. **63**, 1529–1536 (2010)
7. Abdul Kadir, M.R., Taib, I., Osman, K., Abdul Hamid, M.H.: Blood flow simulation of stented aneurysm model. In: IFMBE Proceedings, vol. 21, pp. 398–402. IFMBE (2008)
8. Canstein, C., Cachot, P., Faust, A., Stalder, A.F., Bock, J., Frydrychowicz, A., Küffer, J., Hennig, J., Markl, M.: 3D MR flow analysis in realistic rapid-prototyping model systems of the thoracic aorta: comparison with in vivo data and computational fluid dynamics in identical vessel geometries. Magn. Reson. Med. **59**, 535–546 (2008)
9. Naito, T., Miyachi, S., Matsubara, N.: Magnetic resonance fluid dynamics for intracranial aneurysms—comparison with computed fluid dynamics, pp. 993–1001 (2012)

10. Lim, S.H., Mohd Adib, M.A.H., Matalif, M.U., Abdullah, M.S., Mohd Taib, N.H., Hassan, R.: Modeling and simulation of blood flow analysis on simplified aneurysm models. IOP Conf. Ser. Mater. Sci. Eng. **917**, 012067 (2020)
11. Cebral, J.R., Putman, C.M., Alley, M.T., Hope, T., Bammer, R., Calamante, F.: Hemodynamics in normal cerebral arteries: qualitative comparison of 4D phase-contrast magnetic resonance and image-based computational fluid dynamics, pp. 367–378 (2009)
12. Szajer, J., Ho-shon, K.: A comparison of 4D flow MRI-derived wall shear stress with computational fluid dynamics methods for intracranial aneurysms and carotid bifurcations—a review. Magn. Reson. Imag. **48**, 62–69 (2018)
13. Marshall, I., Zhao, S., Papathanasopoulou, P., Hoskins, P., Xu, X.Y.: MRI and CFD studies of pulsatile flow in healthy and stenosed carotid bifurcation models. J. Biomech. **37**, 679–687 (2004)
14. Tan, F.P.P., Soloperto, G., Wood, N.B., Thom, S., Hughes, A., Xu, X.Y.: Advanced computational models for disturbed and turbulent flow in stenosed human carotid artery bifurcation. In: IFMBE Proceedings, vol. 21, pp. 390–394. IFMBE (2008)
15. Mohd Adib, M.A.H., Lim, S.H., Abdullah, M.S., Hassan, R., Wada, S.: A perspective review: technical study of combining phase contrast magnetic resonance imaging and computational fluid dynamics for blood flow on carotid bifurcation artery. J. Mech. Eng. Sci. **14**, (2020)
16. Omodaka, S., Inoue, T., Funamoto, K., Sugiyama, S.I., Shimizu, H., Hayase, T., Takahashi, A., Tominaga, T.: Influence of surface model extraction parameter on computational fluid dynamics modeling of cerebral aneurysms. J. Biomech. **45**, 2355–2361 (2012)
17. Lim, S.H., Mohd Adib, M.A.H., Abdullah, M.S., Mohd Taib, N.H., Hassan, R., Abd Aziz, A.: Investigation into physical and pathophysiological changes of hemodynamics on segmented patient-specific cerebral aneurysm models through computational analysis. In: 2020 IEEE-EMBS Conference on Biomedical Engineering and Sciences (IECBES), pp. 136–141 (2021)
18. Lim, S.H., Mohd Adib, M.A.H., Abdullah, M.S., Mohd Taib, N.H., Hassan, R., Abd Aziz, A.: Reconstruction of patient-specific cerebral aneurysm model through image segmentation BT. Presented at the Intelligent Manufacturing and Mechatronics (2021)
19. Adib, M.A.H.M., Ii, S., Watanabe, Y., Wada, S.: Minimizing the blood velocity differences between phase-contrast magnetic resonance imaging and computational fluid dynamics simulation in cerebral arteries and aneurysms. Med. Biol. Eng. Comput. **55**, 1605–1619 (2017)
20. Rispoli, V.C., Nielsen, J.F., Nayak, K.S., Carvalho, J.L.A.: Computational fluid dynamics simulations of blood flow regularized by 3D phase contrast. MRI Biomed. Eng. Online, 1–23 (2015)
21. Akshaya, B., Atchaya, G., Barakath Nisha, A., Hemalatha, K., Tamilarasan, T., Shanmugavalli, M.: Blood Flow Analysis in Thoracic Aorta During Aneurysm, vol. 8, pp. 40–44 (2020)
22. Wang, Z., Mhd, H., Alargha, H.: A new concept of data assimilation method between PC-MRI measurement and CFD simulation of blood flow analysis on patient-specific cerebral aneurysm (2009)
23. Lim, S.H., Mohd Adib, M.A.H., Abdullah, M.S., Hassan, R.: Qualitative and quantitative comparison of hemodynamics between MRI measurement and CFD simulation on patient-specific cerebral aneurysm—a review J. Adv. Res. Fluid Mech. Therm. Sci. **68**, 112–123 (2020)
24. Yasiran, S.S., Ibrahim, A., Rahman, W.E.Z.W.A., Mahmud, R.: Efficiency of enhanced distance active contour (EDAC) for microcalcifications segmentation BT. In: Presented at the 5th Kuala Lumpur International Conference on Biomedical Engineering (2011)
25. Harun, N.H., Mashor, M.Y., Rosline, H.: Cluster approach for auto segmentation of blast in acute Leukimia blood slide images BT. In: Presented at the 5th Kuala Lumpur International Conference on Biomedical Engineering (2011)
26. Sasikala, M., Kumaravel, N.: Wavelet based automatic segmentation of brain tumors using optimal texture features. In: IFMBE Proceedings. vol. 21, pp. 637–640. IFMBE (2008)
27. Saad, N.M., Abu-Bakar, S.A.R., Muda, S., Mokji, M.: Segmentation of brain lesions in diffusion-weighted MRI using thresholding technique. In: 2011 IEEE International Conference on Signal Image Processing Application (ICSIPA 2011), pp. 249–254 (2011)

A Preliminary Assessment of Neuro-Salutogenic Landscape Stimuli in Neighbourhood Parks: Theory-Based Model for Stress Mitigation

Sharifah Khalizah Syed Othman Thani, Ng Siew Cheok, and Hazreena Hussein

Abstract Salutogenesis works on a prospective basis by considering creating, enhancing, and improving physical, mental, and social well-being. This research aims to identify the best landscape stimuli that comply with the criteria of both cognitive and salutogenic aspects for reducing stress. This research was conducted by first developing the theory-based model and assessment checklist, followed by preliminary studies that assessed18 parks in Klang Valley based on a neuro-salutogenic landscape checklist. The results indicated that Taman Aman, Petaling Jaya recorded the best neuro-salutogenic landscape stimuli with the highest score for all three aspects of adaptive, restorative, and assertive elements. This research concludes an interesting theory for design professionals about how neural potentials could explains the specific human response to different design settings.

Keywords Salutogenic · Cognitive · Stress mitigation · Landscape stimuli

1 Introduction

Good community health is important for a resilient urban environment, and it is quite clear that urban design plays a role in achieving this. The hustle-bustle of the city lifestyle exposed city dwellers to the risk of developing stress, depression, and major psychological issues compared to people who live in the countryside. Psychological issues are worrisome especially in urban areas where it is possibly the more important

S. K. S. O. Thani · H. Hussein (✉)
Centre of Sustainable Urban Planning and Real Estate, Faculty of Built Environment, Universiti Malaya, 50603 Kuala Lumpur, Malaysia
e-mail: reenalambina@um.edu.my

N. S. Cheok
Department of Biomedical Engineering, Faculty of Engineering, Universiti Malaya, 50603 Kuala Lumpur, Malaysia

S. K. S. O. Thani
Centre of Studies for Landscape Architecture, Faculty of Architecture, Planning and Surveying, Universiti Teknologi MARA, Puncak Alam, 42300 Selangor, Malaysia

J. Usman et al. (eds.), *6th Kuala Lumpur International Conference on Biomedical Engineering 2021*, IFMBE Proceedings 86,
https://doi.org/10.1007/978-3-030-90724-2_50

source of a rising depression rate, and researchers believe that there must be notable factors that relate mental states with quality of urban planning and design [1, 2].

Neuroscience is a branch of biological and scientific study that focuses on brain function, including studying emotions and human behaviour that arises from the brain and nervous system [3]. The study on neuroscience is widely associated with experimental psychology and for areas such as mental health where cognitive and neural data are necessary to examine brain-body-environment interactions. Specific neural signals are observable according to what we are doing or feeling. Scientists believe that there are five different types of human brainwaves where it changes depending on what activities and emotional feeling we are having. The brainwaves move at different speeds which comprises Gamma (>30 Hz), Beta (15–30 Hz), Alpha (8–15 Hz), Theta (3–8 Hz), and Delta (0.5–3 Hz) [4]. Stress is positively correlated with the Beta brainwave at the anterior temporal lobe of the brain [5]. Prolonged exposure to a stressful environment could result in a high increased of spectral power in all brain areas, which remained even in a rest mode [6]. Anxiety, sleep deprived, impulsive behavior, and over-arousal brain areas usually cause anger whereas insomnia, attention discrepancy, and depression are usually linked to under-arousal of brain areas. Therefore, for stress reduction the brain wave needs to be appropriate in a state of arousal, where it is generally associated with the alpha band (resting state of the brain).

Linking neuroscience to design practice will explain how their practitioners view these two fields and how neuroscience studies can offer new knowledge for landscape architects in creating restorative environments. This will foster a broader understanding of whether the aesthetics of landscape design is scientifically valuable and to what extent it could stimulate positive brain functioning for stress mitigation.

2 Literature Review

2.1 Theorizing Salutogenesis Concept into Landscape Environment

Aaron Antonovsky, a sociologist whose work concerned with stress, health and well-being has come out with the term salutogenesis. His works looked into health enhancing or creating health benefits [7, 8]. Antonovsky first introduced the salutogenic term and concept of Sense of Coherence (SOC) to the scientific world in 1979. He describes the SOC as a person's reflection of life and corresponds to stressful circumstances [9].

The concept of salutogenesis was expanded further in the architectural and design field by Dilani [10]. He developed the theory of salutogenic design, and his works focused on design typologies of healthcare infrastructure globally. The salutogenic design emphasized the strategies to promote the health and well-being of all users [10, 11]. Therefore, the design usually more universal and inclusive of all age levels.

Salutogenic design principles create a pleasant environment that stimulates the mind towards enjoyment, satisfaction, and creativity to keep the inhabitants operate at their greatest intensity. Maikov [12, 13] further expanded the salutogenic design concept into the landscape perspectives by introducing the Emotional Character Line Method (ECLM). The ECLM presented eight 'garden rooms as a journey of therapy'. Each garden room comprises elements and characteristics that match the concept of salutogenic design and SOC theory. The salutogenic landscape properties in each garden room include visual stimuli, sensory stimuli, natural elements, cultural elements, and social spaces.

2.2 How Landscape Design Affect the Brain Activity

Research has identified that brainwave patterns are associated with all sorts of emotional and neurological conditions. Several studies observed the association of brain regions and mental processes with mindfulness and positive external stimuli [14, 15]. The physical elements found in our surroundings strongly influence how our brain operating the stimuli and correspond with the environment. Several studies have observed that specific landscape designs could induce alpha and theta brainwaves associated with mindfulness and mental recovery [16–18]. This could assist professionals' designers further in discovering the healing potential of those designed spaces. Figure 1 shows how landscape design characteristics are associated with the positive effect of brain activity.

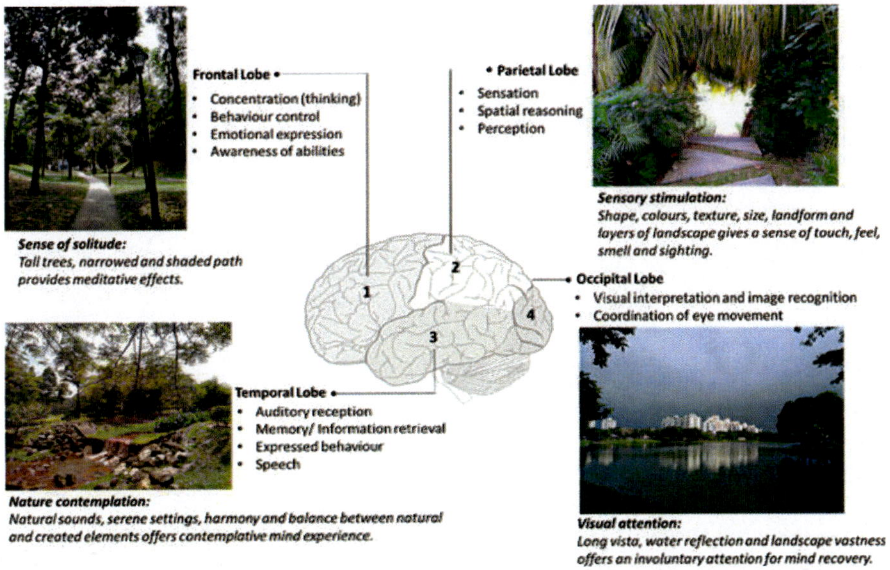

Fig. 1 Characteristics of landscape that induce positive brain activity towards stress reduction. (*Source* Authors)

3 Research Methodology

This research was conducted in two steps. The first step involved desk study of theoretical sources, secondary data from local authorities, and expert validation on typologies of neighbourhood parks. They were used to propose a checklist of neuro-salutogenic criteria for neighbourhood parks. The second step was site assessments to identify neuro-salutogenic landscape stimuli at selected neighbourhood parks in Klang Valley. Finally, the obtained data were analyzed using descriptive statistics.

3.1 Development of Theory-Based Model

A systematic literature review was conducted by searching four databases such as SCOPUS, Web of Science, PubMed, and APA PsycINFO to develop the theory-based model for neuro-salutogenic criteria. The systematic review helps identify the landscape attributes that potentially stimulate cognitive function, the key aspects of salutogenesis, and the characteristics of neuro-salutogenic stimulus in reducing stress. The formation of the theory-based model was established on two aspects. Firstly, the salutogenesis aspects and how it is being conceptualized in salutogenic design. Secondly, the neurological aspects and how the cognitive function is attributed with the theory of SOC and landscape design.

A theoretical foundation based on literature findings proposed a theory-based model of neuro-salutogenic landscape with three main mechanisms for stress mitigation: adaptive, restorative, and assertive (refer Fig. 2). The adaptive mechanism

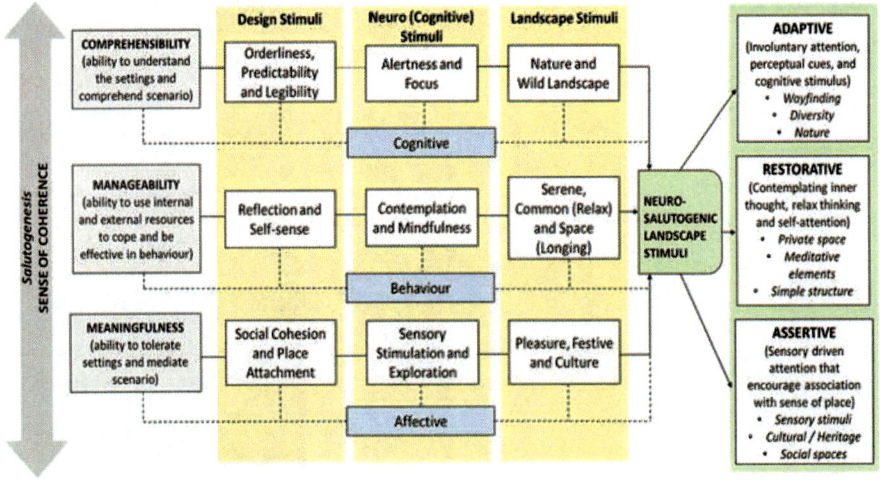

Fig. 2 Theory-based model of neuro-salutogenic landscape stimuli in designing restorative environment for stress mitigation. (*Source* Authors)

highlights cognitive development as an essential aspect of adaptation. Through the adaptive process, people would be able to adopt new behaviours that make them better prepared to cope with the world. Restorative mechanism focuses on returning a mentally exhausted person with heightened negative affect to a state in which this response is reduced. The assertive mechanism is a balanced response that is neither defensive nor offensive, and it relies heavily on self-confidence. Elements that promote stimuli-driven attention could encourage the sensation and feelings of a person and associate them with a sense of place.

3.2 Preliminary Site Assessment

The assessment checklist for site preliminary studies was developed based on the aspects of the neuro-salutogenic landscape as proposed in the theory-based model. The key landscape elements were categorized accordingly to meet the criteria of adaptive, restorative, and assertive mechanism, and to follow the quality of neighbourhood parks criteria [19]. The assessment checklist was scaled based on a five-level Likert-type scale (Very Poor (1), Poor (2), Fair (3), Good (4) and Excellent (5)) for each factor. Five experts from local authorities and practice landscape architects validated the typologies of neighbourhood parks and their characteristics. A representative sample of 18 parks was assessed using the proposed checklist at selected neighbourhood parks in this research. The preliminary site assessments were conducted between 10 September and 12 October 2020.

4 Results and Discussion

4.1 Distribution of Neuro-Salutogenic Landscape Stimuli

The results presented that Taman Aman, Petaling Jaya recorded the highest scores with 81 scores. This indicates that Taman Aman has the best neuro-salutogenic landscape stimuli compared to other neighbourhood parks. Taman Western Park in Setia Alam recorded the lowest score with only 45 scores. Other neighbourhood parks recorded an average total of 60 accumulative scores based on three aspects of adaptive, restorative, and assertive elements. In general, most neighbourhood parks recorded the highest scores for adaptive features with an average of 23 scores, followed by restorative elements with an average of 20 scores. Assertive elements recorded the least score, with an average of 17 scores. This indicates that our neighbourhood parks are highly adaptive, where the design emphasized the importance of wayfinding and legibility to make people aware of their surroundings. These findings support the study of Golembiewski [20], where it was observed that readable

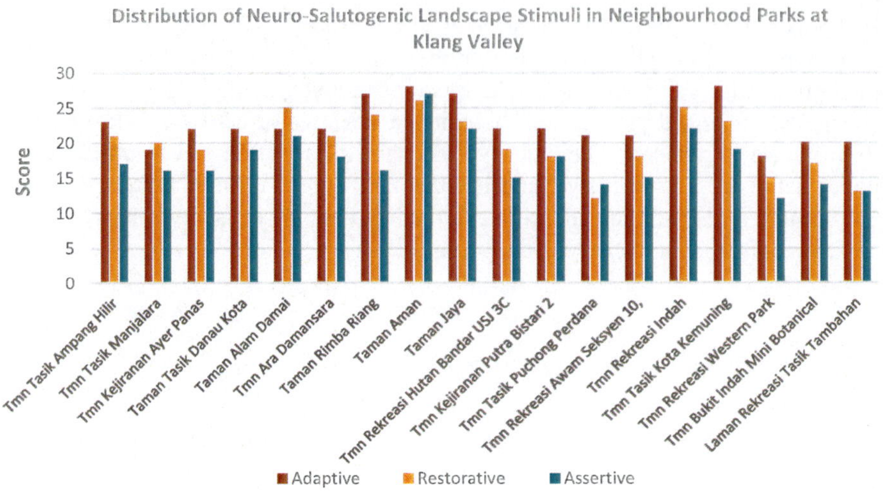

Fig. 3 Bar graph shows the distribution of neuro-salutogenic landscape scores for all neighbourhood parks

space and a clear sense of direction aid the capacity of mental process to screen out distractions, hence promote fascination to cognitive memory.

The results revealed that only Taman Alam Damai, Cheras recorded higher restorative scores than the two elements compared to other neighbourhood parks. It was observed that Taman Alam Damai's comprises of many tall trees, shaded path, and secluded seating spaces than other neighbourhood parks. The lowest score of assertive elements in most of these parks suggests that the design of our neighbourhood parks is still less emphasis on social cohesion and sensory stimulation despite having many seating areas, play zones and open spaces. The findings justify Malek [19] and Ujang [21] where people hardly used the parks due to the low quality of park design, and lacking a sense of place although parks could make people relax. From the findings and observation during site assessments, it could be presumed that the design of our neighbourhood parks is sufficient to serve as a community green space. However, there is still lacking elements to bring out the emotions, and sense of place attachment to its users. Figure 3 presented a bar graph of neuro-salutogenic landscape stimuli distribution across the neighbourhood parks.

4.2 Key Elements of Neuro-Salutogenic Landscape Stimuli

It could be seen that the majority of the elements recorded a scores ranging between 40 and 50 scores from the results. The highest scores were the elements of the path with 58 scores, followed by zones (55 scores), seating area (54 scores), and social spaces (54 scores). Three elements which are landmarks (36 scores), cultural (29 scores), and historical elements (24 scores), recorded a significantly lower score than others. These results indicate that adaptive elements such as path, zones, and wayfinding were being emphasized where it is majorly found in almost every neighbourhood park in this study. Meanwhile, historical, cultural and landmarks that belong to assertive elements were rarely found in the asssesments. These results indicate a lack of cultural and heritage traits or distinctive features like landmarks being considered in the design of our neighbourhood parks. On the contrary, Deng's [16] study found out that elements like the wooden walkway, sculptures, poetry walls, poems-engraved stele, and decorative openwork windows received higher scores than roads and pavement elements in landscape preference analysis by park users. The cultural traits were also perceived as restorative attributes in their study, where people rated that rural farm experience as significantly restorative than urban scenery.

These findings are interesting where it implies that the design of our neighbourhood parks is merely designed to comply with the needs for urban green spaces as allocated by the local authorities. This justifies why most of the landscape elements and design components in our neighbourhood parks are uniformly similar. This is due to the lack of unique features or cultural elements representing the community's local identity. As the cultural background favours the relaxation score, and affecting the individual's restorative preferences [16], this is indeed time for our design professionals to consider the significance of socio-cultural components in designing neighbourhood parks. Hence, it serves as green spaces and places where people might find emotional comfort during their visit to the parks. Figure 4 shows the variation of key elements that represent the neuro-salutogenic stimuli.

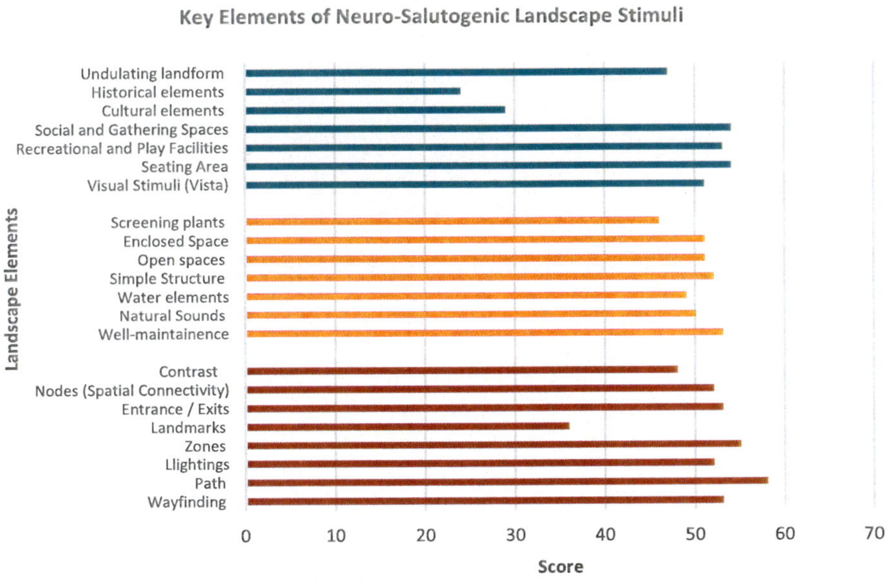

Fig. 4 The bar graph shows the variation of key elements that represent the neuro-salutogenic landscape stimuli at neighbourhood parks

5 Conclusion

Based on the theory-based model, it could be concluded that most of the elements observed at the neighbourhood parks reasonably comply with the characteristics of neuro-salutogenic landscape stimuli. Nevertheless, as a whole design, most neighbourhood parks are still inadequately portraying the excellent model of neuro-salutogenic landscape design for mitigating stress. Although the findings are preliminary, however, it revealed that our neighbourhood parks' design strongly focuses on the physical and aesthetical aspects than the behavioural aspects such as the socio-cultural aspects and identity of the local community. In the future, design professionals might find that it is essential to incorporate sensory, cultural or heritage elements, and distinctive features that bring pleasure to connect a person's emotions with the surroundings.

References

1. Song, J., et al.: Association between blue and green space availability with mental health and wellbeing. Int. J. Popul. Data Sci. (2018)
2. Banaei, M., Hatami, J., Yazdanfar, A., Gramann, K.: Walking through architectural spaces: the impact of interior forms on human brain dynamics. Front. Hum. Neurosci. (2017)
3. Silvers, J., Buhle, J.T., Ochsner, K.N.: The Neuroscience of Emotion Regulation. Curr. Opin. Behav. Sci. (Sept 2015) (2013)
4. Subhani, A., Xia, L., Malik, A.: EEG signals to measure mental stress. In: 2nd International Conference on Behavioral, Cognitive and Psychological Sciences (BCPS 2011) (2011)
5. Piefke, M., Glienke, K.: The effects of stress on prospective memory: a systematic review. Psychol. Neurosci. **10**(3), 345–362 (2017)
6. Kiroy, V.N., Warsawskaya, L.V., Voynov, V.B.: EEG after prolonged mental activity. Int. J. Neurosci. **85**(1–2), 31–43 (1996)
7. Bauer, G.F., et al.: Future directions for the concept of salutogenesis: a position article. Health Promot. Int. (2020)
8. Vinje, H.F., Langeland, E., Bull, T.: Aaron Antonovsky's development of salutogenesis, 1979 to 1994. In: The Handbook of Salutogenesis (2016)
9. Mittelmark, M.B., et al.: The Handbook of Salutogenesis (2016)
10. Dilani, A.: Architecture: the beneficial health outcomes of salutogenic design. In: Design for Health (2017)
11. Ziegler, E.: Application of a salutogenic design model to the architecture of low-income housing. Appl. Salut. Des. Model Archit. Low Income Hous. (2014)
12. Maikov, K.: Exploring the salutogenic properties of the landscape: from garden to forest (2016)
13. Maikov, K., Bell, S., Sepp, K.: An evaluation of the design of room characteristics of a sample of healing gardens. WIT Trans. Ecol. Environ. **114**, 223–232 (2008)
14. Olszewska-Guizzo, A.A., Paiva, T.O., Barbosa, F.: Effects of 3D contemplative landscape videos on brain activity in a passive exposure EEG experiment. Front. Psychiatry (2018)
15. Olszewska-Guizzo, A., Sia, A., Fogel, A., Ho, R.: Can exposure to certain urban green spaces trigger frontal alpha asymmetry in the brain?—preliminary findings from a passive task EEG study. Int. J. Environ. Res. Public Health **17**(2), 1–10 (2020)
16. Deng, L., et al.: Urban forestry & urban greening empirical study of landscape types, landscape elements and landscape components of the urban park promoting physiological and psychological restoration. Urban For Urban Green. **48**(211) (2020)

17. Deng, L., et al.: Effects of integration between visual stimuli and auditory stimuli on restorative potential and aesthetic preference in urban green spaces. Urban For Urban Green (2020)
18. Golembiewski, J.: Salutogenic design: the neural basis for health promoting environments. Des. Heal. Sci. Rev., 62–69 (2012)
19. Malek, N.A., Mohammad, S.Z., Nashar, A., Alam, B.P.: Determinant factor for quality green open space assessment in Malaysia. J. Des. Built Environ. **18**(Dec 2018), 26–36 (2020)
20. Golembiewski, J.A.: The designed environment and how it affects brain morphology and mental health. Health Environ. Res. Des. J. (2016)
21. Ujang, N., Moulay, A., Zakariya, K.: Sense of well-being indicators: attachment to public parks in Putrajaya, Malaysia. Proc. Soc. Behav. Sci. (2015)

Development of a Mobile Augmented Reality System for Radiotherapy Practitioner Training

Kinersh Gopalakrishnan, Nor Aniza Azmi, Rozilawati Ahmad, Wan Nordiana Wan Abdul Rahman, and Ashrani Aizzuddin Abd Rahni

Abstract Radiotherapy (RT) is the use of radiation to treat diseases in particular cancer. Recent advancements of imaging in RT and improved precision in treatment delivery require extensive training among the team. A good training approach need to be applied which aims to equip healthcare practitioners with a combination of essential understanding, clinical professional skills and technical competencies. This will provide accurate, precise and effective RT delivery. However, the expensive nature of high energy RT delivery systems and rapid introduction of new technology has until recently made their use in an academic training environment unfeasible. Augmented reality (AR) platforms, which can be run on mobile devices today constitute a possibility for academic training at lower cost. This paper describes the development of a proof of concept for an Android based device. We showed that the developed app can track small objects as well as a large object with a superimposed LINAC (Linear Accelerator) model. This proof of concept can thus be developed further for actual RT practitioner training.

Keywords Radiotherapy · Practitioner · Training · Augmented reality · Mobile device · Android · Unity · VisionLib · Varian Clinac iX

K. Gopalakrishnan · A. A. A. Rahni (✉)
Faculty of Engineering and Built Environment, Universiti Kebangsaan Malaysia, 43600 Bangi, Malaysia
e-mail: ashrani@ukm.edu.my

N. A. Azmi · R. Ahmad
Faculty of Health Science, Universiti Kebangsaan Malaysia, 50300 Kuala Lumpur, Malaysia

W. N. W. A. Rahman
School of Health Science, Universiti Sains Malaysia, 16150 Kubang Kerian, Malaysia

J. Usman et al. (eds.), *6th Kuala Lumpur International Conference on Biomedical Engineering 2021*, IFMBE Proceedings 86,
https://doi.org/10.1007/978-3-030-90724-2_51

1 Introduction

Radiotherapy (RT) is the use of radiation to treat diseases in particular cancer. Recent advancements of imaging in RT and improved precision in treatment delivery require extensive training among the team. A good training approach need to be applied which aims to equip healthcare practitioners with a combination of essential understanding, clinical professional skills and technical competencies. This will provide accurate, precise and effective RT delivery. However, the expensive nature of high energy RT delivery systems and rapid introduction of new technology has until recently made their use in an academic training environment unfeasible. Augmented reality (AR) platforms [1, 2], which can be run on mobile devices today constitute a possibility for academic training at lower cost.

We are aware of prior recent work, the most notable of which is the RAD-AR system [3]. However, our work differs from RAD-AR in a number of ways. RAD-AR assumes access to an actual radiotherapy treatment facility equipped with a LINAC (Linear Accelerator). As stated above, the main motivation of our work is limited access to an actual LINAC. As such, the aim of the system we wish to develop is not just to augment the environment of an actual LINAC, rather it is to recreate the LINAC itself virtually and augment this view into another environment. In this sense, the finished system will be closer to the VERT (Virtual Environment for Radiotherapy Training) [4] but achieves it using an augmented reality display. Secondly, as opposed to RAD-AR which focuses on less accessible platforms namely iOS and HoloLens, our system is developed on Android, which has a much greater user base.

The rest of the paper is structured as follows: Sect. 2 describes the main rationale of this work and the development process. Section 3 show some preliminary results of our proof of concept. Finally, Sect. 4 summarises the results and presents some avenues for future work.

2 Methodology

2.1 Overall Concept

In this work, an AR system is developed to augment a scene consisting of an actual patient treatment couch top with a virtual model of the radiotherapy machine also known as a LINAC. The overall concept is shown in Fig. 1.

For this project the LINAC modelled is the Varian Clinac iX as that is the machine used at UKM Medical Centre. The AR display on the other hand is developed to run on the Android operating system.

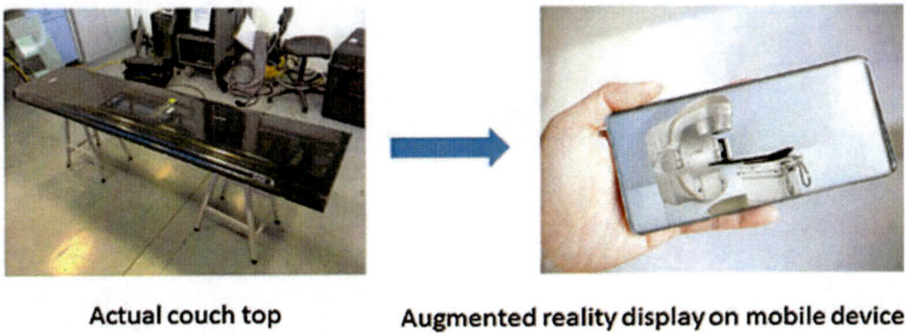

Fig. 1 Augmented reality display of a LINAC around a physical couch top on a mobile device

2.2 *Software Development*

The AR system itself is developed in Unity[1] using the visionLib[2] SDK as the tracking library. Unity is a well-known cross-platform engine for developing software interfaces consisting of 2D, 3D, virtual reality (VR) and AR interfaces. While Unity was originally developed as a game engine, it has also wide use outside of gaming.

VisionLib on the other hand is a cross-platform library for developing AR applications. It enables object tracking purely based on a shape model representing a real world object.

2.3 *LINAC Model*

As mentioned, the LINAC modelled for this project is the Varian Clinac iX. The model is constructed by referring to its dimensions as stated in technical documents. Figure 2 shows a comparison between the actual LINAC and the virtual model. The virtual model was designed using AutoCAD Fusion 360.

Before the actual model is used in the AR application, a number of small test models are used. This is shown in more details in the results section below.

[1] www.unity.com.

[2] www.visionlib.com.

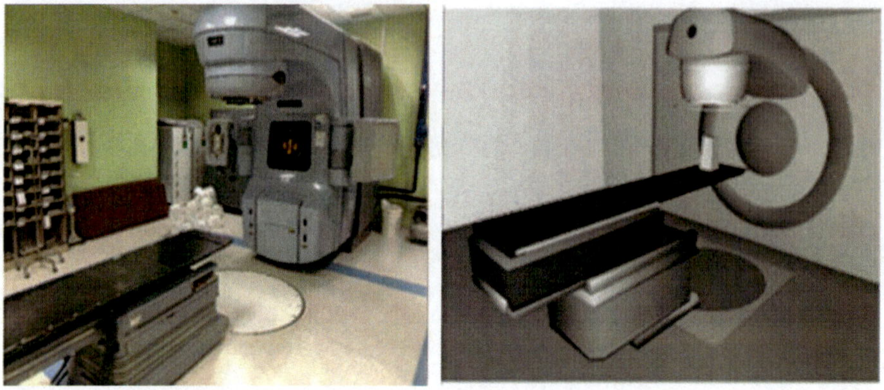

Fig. 2 Actual Varian Clinac iX LINAC (right) and the virtual model (left)

3 Results and Discussion

Testing was performed in 2 phases, with small test models and with a model of the actual Varian Clinac iX LINAC. The results are as shown in the subsections below.

3.1 *Test Models*

As a set of preliminary tests, the AR system is tested with 2 small models of increasing size: a model car and a drink can.

The model car is provided with the visionLib test app and measures around 5 cm × 5 cm × 10 cm (width, height, length). The result of the app tracking this toy car is shown in Fig. 3 below.

The app was able to track the test car when the device was moved around slowly.

The second test model used is an average (325 ml) drink can. The virtual model is constructed based on the well-known dimensions of carbonated drink cans. Figure 4 shows the test app tracking a drink can with this virtual model.

The drink can constitute a more challenging due to its shiny surface. However the test app was still able to track the can successfully.

3.2 *LINAC Model*

Tracking with an augmented LINAC model was performed in 2 stages: tracking a large object to represent the couch and tracking with the LINAC model.

Before the LINAC model is included in the app, we performed tracking with a large object. Due to limitations at the time of development, we tracked a single size

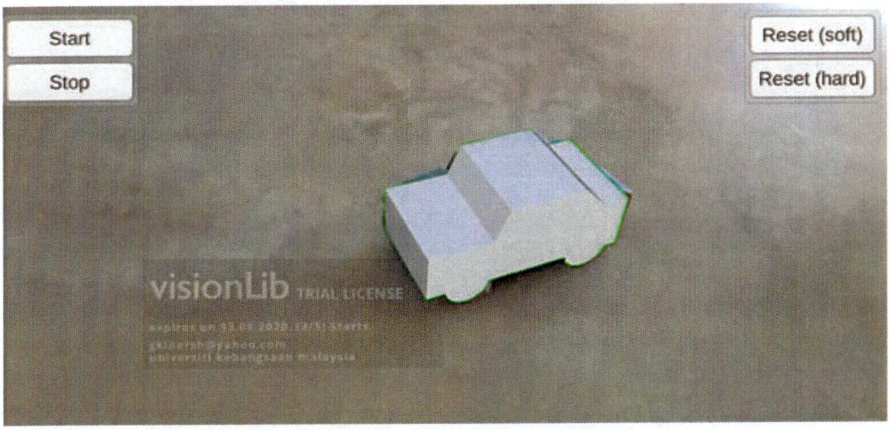

Fig. 3 Test app tracking the small model car provided in visionLib

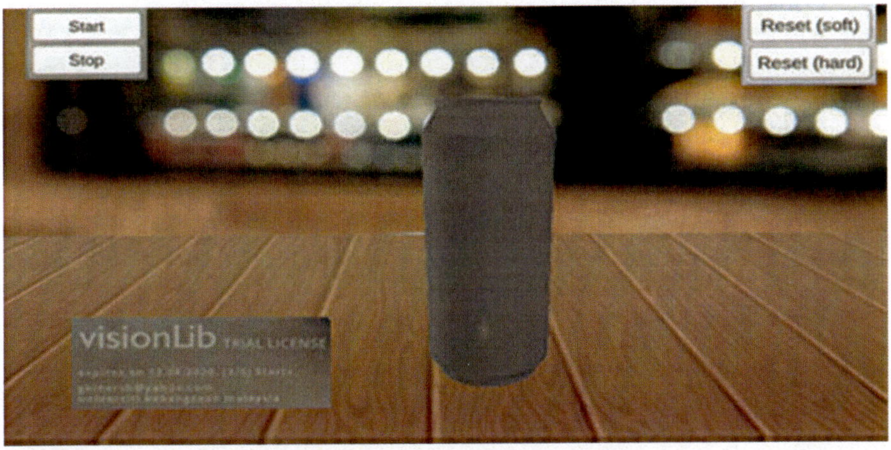

Fig. 4 Test app tracking an average carbonated drink can

mattress to represent the treatment couch. It was acceptable for this proof of concept as the length of a mattress is roughly the same length as the treatment couch (2 m) although it is slightly wider (90 cm). Figure 5 shows the app tracking an actual single size mattress.

As before, the app was able to track this much larger object.

The final development phase of this proof of concept is to superimpose the LINAC model onto the tracked mattress. Due to limitations at the time of development, the LINAC model was scaled down to roughly 50% of its actual size. Figure 6 shows the result of tracking while displaying the LINAC model.

Even with this added augmented model, the app was able to successfully track the mattress.

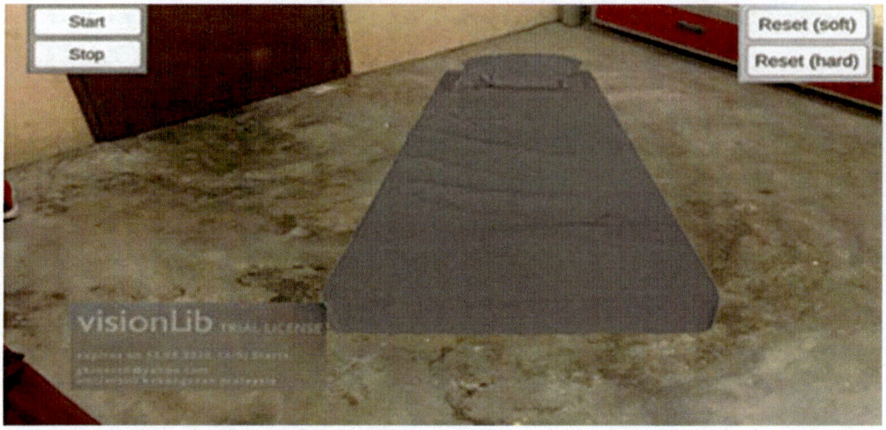

Fig. 5 Result of tracking an actual single size mattress

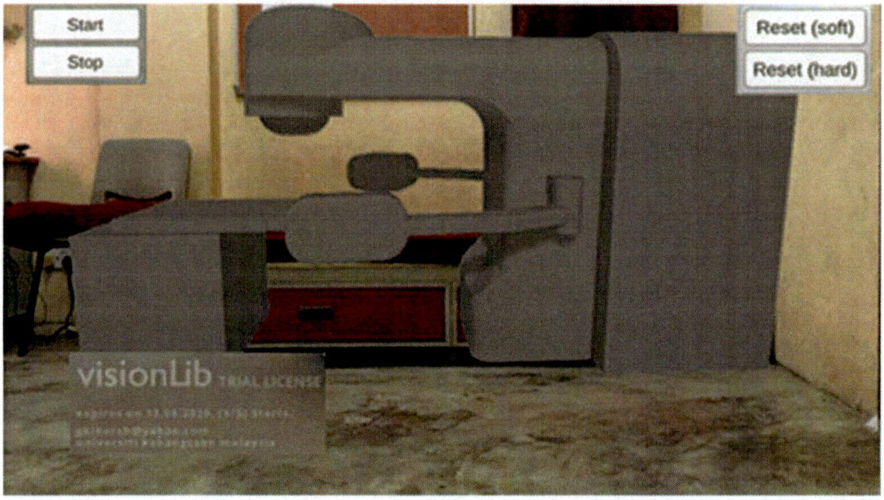

Fig. 6 Result of tracking an actual single size mattress with the LINAC model superimposed

4 Conclusion

A test app in the Android operating system was successfully developed using the Unity engine and VisionLib SDK. It successfully tracked various objects including a mattress which is comparable in size (around 2 m long) to an actual treatment couch. The final proof of concept was able to show a scaled down LINAC model around this tracked mattress.

Further development will consists of updating the LINAC model to actual size and tracking an actual treatment couch. Furthermore, the actual operation of the

LINAC and its software interface will be simulated for use in training radiotherapy practitioners.

References

1. Jin, W., Birckhead, B., Perez, B., Hoffe, S.: Augmented and virtual reality: exploring a future role in radiation oncology education and training. Appl. Radiat. Oncol. **6** (2017)
2. Servotte, J.C., Guillaume, M., Boga, D., Coucke, P.: Methodological approach for the implementation of a simulator in augmented reality in a radiation therapy department. Int. J. Healthcare Manage. **10**(3), 154–159 (2017)
3. Cosentino, F., John, N.W., Vaarkamp, J.: RAD-AR: RADiotherapy—augmented reality. In: 2017 International Conference on Cyberworlds, pp. 226–228. IEEE Computer Society, Chester, United Kingdom (2017)
4. Beavis, A.W., Page, L., Phillips, R., Ward, J.: VERT: virtual environment for radiotherapy training. World Cong. Med. Phys. Biomed. Eng. **25**(12), 236–238 (2009)

Visual Directed Deep Breathing with Heart Rate Variability Measurement in Mobile Application

Poh Foong Lee, Ming Chien Ong, Wei Liang Soon, Chean Swee Ling, and Paul E. Croarkin

Abstract Deep breathing produces positive physiological effects. There is numerous, existing mobile application that measures heart rate variability. However, the study on reporting the unknown changes of the total time interval at the resting stage before and after the deep breathing at 6 cycles per min for 3 min and data mining with the mobile application is novel. In this work, the measurement of the blood flow changes on the fingertip was employing the mobile camera and developed into an android-based mobile application for measuring the heart rate variability for pre-and post-effect of a directed 6 cycles in a min deep breathing video for 3 min. To date, a total of 204 respondents shows a total of increment of Standard Deviation of normal to normal (SDNN) 43.1 with video-directed deep breathing for 6 cycles per min for 3 min in breathing length for 3 years after the android App has launched in the Google App Store. Data mining concept with the mobile application which integrated with physical measurement enables the huge sample size recruitment globally.

Keywords Mobile application · Data mining · Deep breathing · Heart rate variability

1 Introduction

Deep breathing is a common element in mindfulness practices, such as yoga, tai chi, Reiki, and meditation [1]. Recent interest has surged in this investigation of the effects of deep breathing on human cognition [2], newly learned motor skills, [3] and age-related cognitive decline. Yadav and Mutha [3] provided the first evidence to link deep breathing to motor memory by showing that a 30-min deep breathing intervention led to a better performance in a motor skill. This improved retention in motor

P. F. Lee (✉) · M. C. Ong · W. L. Soon · C. S. Ling
Lee Kong Chian Faculty of Engineering and Science, Universiti Tunku Abdul Rahman, Kuala Lumpur, Malaysia
e-mail: leepf@utar.edu.my

P. E. Croarkin
Department of Psychiatry and Psychology, Mayo Clinic, Rochester, MN, USA

J. Usman et al. (eds.), *6th Kuala Lumpur International Conference on Biomedical Engineering 2021*, IFMBE Proceedings 86,
https://doi.org/10.1007/978-3-030-90724-2_52

skills was evident both immediately after the breathing session and maintained at a one-day break. Ferreira et al. [4] investigated the cognitive decline due to aging where the respiratory training groups had undergone seven forms of respiratory training, and deep breathing was one of the parameter. However, at the end of the experiment, the attention level of the respiratory training group was stable without a significant difference between the pre-and post-measurements. Notably, the control and aerobic exercise groups showed a significant decline in attention levels. In consideration of prior research and the fact that deep breathing is a common element in many mindfulness practices, deep breathing may be related to changes in brainwaves [5]. Conflict monitoring with video-aided mindful deep breathing [2], may also lead to improved sustained attention. A plausible mechanism underlying how deep breathing improved our cognitive control is related to the alteration of the activation of the anterior cingulate cortex (ACC), which has a role in cognitive control [2]. Greater activation of the ACC would be required to resolve conflicts such as distracting thoughts to maintain the attention placed on the deep breathing process [2]. Prior literature suggests that frontal cortex blood flow changes are affected by deep breathing [6].

This project developed a prototype to measure heart rate variability with the camera-based mobile application. Quantitative research methodology by using a questionnaire to collect data and opinions from the users was carried out. Development tools with the official Integrated Development Environment (IDE), Android Studio, that is published by Google in developing mobile application was chosen. Lastly, the SQLite database for the mobile application due to its compact and small memory usage for mobile applications was selected. The mobile application was developed based on a few research questions such as, the average successful extended time interval between heartbeat after the 3 min of video aided deep breathing video, preliminary survey outcome on understanding the preference of the user that who would choose to use this type of heart rate measurement types of deep breathing exercise, gender preference in using scientifically measurement for tracking the deep breathing progress.

In this project, the study on a total of heart rate variability changes after deep breathing was begun with the developed mobile application which was supported by the Android Kit-Kat 4.4.2, integrated with the visual deep breathing video which was improvised from the work of Cheng et al. [2, 5, 7, 8].

2 Methods

For the mobile application development to integrate the visual deep breathing and heart rate variability measurement with the camera based on the phone itself. Methods started from system development as below. The stages of prototyping for this work are shown in Fig. 1.

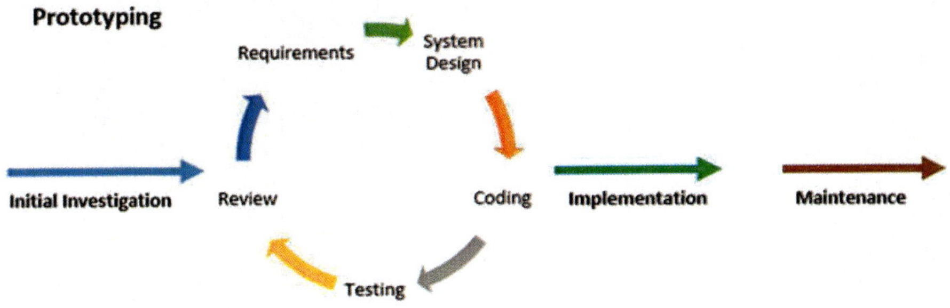

Fig.1 Architecture of the mobile application prototyping

2.1 The Description of the Mobile Application Prototype

Previous research and studies about stress, heart rate variability were being reviewed and gathered. The data collected was being analyzed to produce the requirements needed for developing the mobile application. The storyboard shows the workflow and the user interfaces of the mobile application. After the storyboard of the mobile application is signed off, the development of the prototype would then commence. The prototype is developed based on the user interface interaction at the beginning. This is followed by the users who test the prototype and give their suggestions about the prototype. Once the prototype is signed off by the users, the prototype would add in more functionalities and ready to evolve into the second version of the prototype.

Users' behavior is observed and monitored for using the prototype to enable the developers to understand further the users' requirements. The prototype is improved into the next version or the final version of the prototype. From the feedback and evaluation of the users on the prototype, the prototype is refined to improve the functionalities of the prototype to make sure it meets the requirements of the users. The final phase of the system development is achieved when the prototype finally meets the requirements of the users and the prototype is being approved and signed off by the users and stakeholders. The final prototype is evaluated with User Acceptance Testing (UAT) before the final release of the product. When the final prototype passed the UAT, it is released as a product to the customers.

2.2 Heart Rate with Mobile Camera

Pulse is generated once a sudden burst of blood to the circulatory system when the wall of heart contracted. There are currently multiple devices in the market for the use of detecting the heart rate pulse. A concept of photo plethysmography (PPG) is used to estimate the heart rate, and this concept can be achieved by using most of the smartphones that are currently in the market, but it needs to have camera and flashlight around the camera. Whenever there is a heartbeat occurs, there will be a rush of blood into the vessels as well as the blood capillaries on the fingertips as shown in Fig. 2. When the amount of blood is rich in the blood capillaries of the fingertips, lighter will be absorbed by the blood when the flashlight on the smartphone applied on the fingertips. When the light was absorbed, then there will be lower reflective index and have darker frame intensities [9]. If there is lesser blood amount in the blood capillaries, then there will be lesser light absorbed, and lighter will be getting reflected which leading to the brighter frames. With these changes in the intensity of the light that are passing through the finger can generate a pattern of waves which are like a pulse and these can be referred as the heart rate of a person. Heart Rate Variability (HRV) can be used to measure stress level of a user since HRV is the change in time intervals between adjacent heartbeats of the user, which is related to the health condition and regulatory system of the user. For a person who experiences high stress level, the HRV of the user will be lower while the HRV of user will be lower if user's autonomic nervous system is in good condition. There are several ways to measure HRV, for example: Interbeat Interval (IBI), Standard deviation of normal-to-normal intervals (SDNN) and some other methods. IBI is the time of interval between two heart beats, and SDNN will use IBI collected and calculate the standard deviation of time interval between two peak beats. Below is the formula to calculate SDNN value.

$$\mathrm{SDNN} = \sqrt{\frac{1}{\mathrm{N}-1}\sum_{j=1}^{N}\left(RR_j - \overline{RR}\right)^2}$$

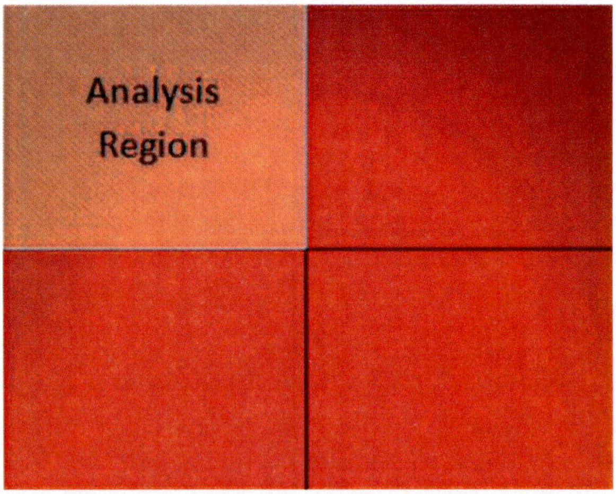

Fig. 2 Analysis region on the light intensity gathered [9]

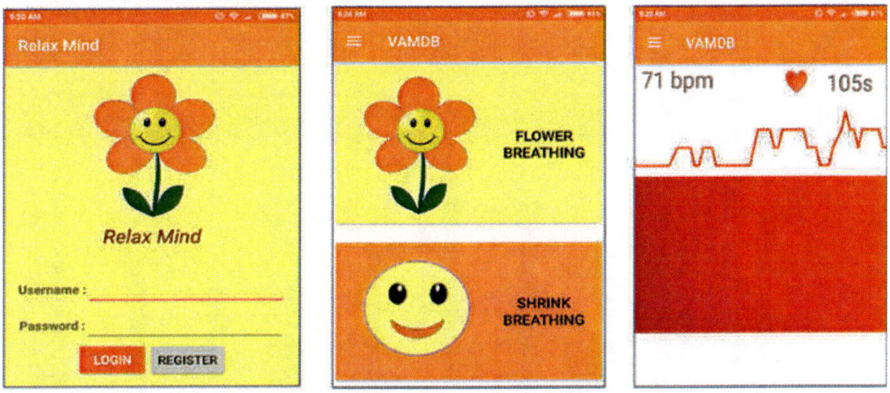

Fig. 3 **a** The registration page, **b** selecting the deep breathing training page and **c** measurement of the heart rate variability

2.3 The Prototype

Figure 3 is one of the frames that was captured during the video recording with the flashlight on. In the frame, an analysis region needs to be selected for the change of intensity of light on the frame to be determined. From this frame, we can determine that there is only red color in the frame, and hence it is only going to determine the difference in the red channel intensity of the pixel information. To get a better accuracy result, users should be holding their finger on the camera lens for longer time, and with a gentle strength applied on the camera lens as well. The display of figures in the App launched in Google App Store, https://play.google.com/store/apps/details?id=com.vamdb.asus.happyproject. Data mining was started and waiting for enough sufficient sample size to validate the average extended heart rate variability with the aided mindful deep breathing. The figure of the App as shown in Fig. 3.

3 Result

Figure 4 shows the first 10 users gave an increase in SDNN, the time interval of the total 2 min of the measurement. Video aided deep breathing for a duration of 5 min was reported to be able to improve on cognitive function and brainwaves shifting [6], in this deep breathing exercise, 3 min of 6 cycles per minute was recommended as user in general are more patience with a shorter duration. On the other hand, the heart rate variability measurement with standard of 5 min for analysis was recommended as well, but in this study, 2 min before and after of the measurement was 2 min apart.

The App has been launched in the Google App Store for data mining purposes on its own without any promotion for 3 years. It happens that the 95 of female users and 105 male users from this total of 204 respondents worldwide, as in Fig. 5. The

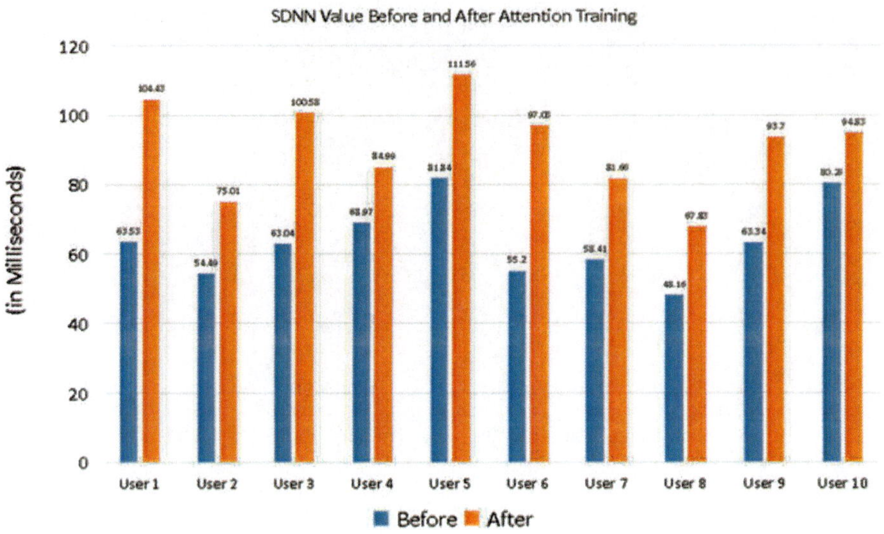

Fig. 4 Outcome data from 10 initial users

Fig. 5 Gender distribution of respondents 3 years after launching the mobile application

Gender	Number
Male	95
Female	109

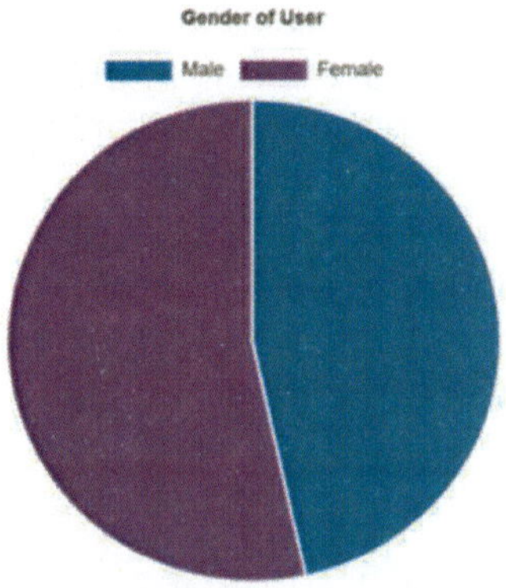

outcome from administrative Website, has drawn the average SDNN of 43.1 from total of 204 respondents, consists of 43.1% of increment as shown in Fig. 6.

SDNN	Millseconds
Before	92.794
After	132.785

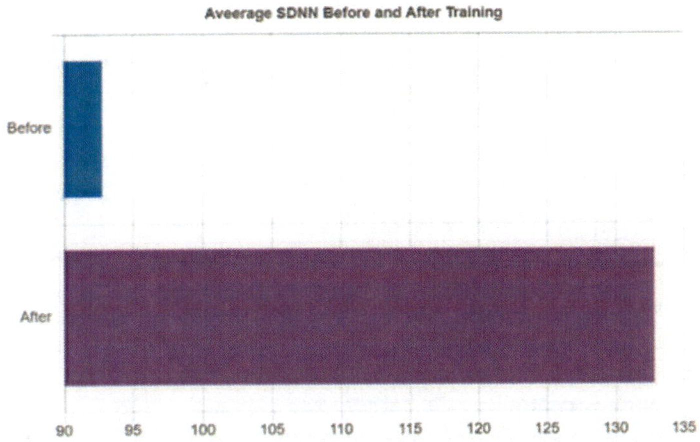

Fig. 6 Total of 204 respondents after 3 years of App launching from data mining, the average SDNN was found to be 40 ms, 43.1% of increment

4 Discussion

Total of 204 with almost equal of users consists of male and female. The 3 min video directed deep breathing has successfully obtained an average of the inter-beat interval (IBI) increase in its SDNN of total of 40 ms from the total sample size of 204 respondents through mobile application. The increase in IBI after deep breathing is promising since numerous reports has been showing the carry-over effects of deep breathing on the HRV measurement. Prinsloo et al. [10], by using an HRV biofeedback-induced deep breathing intervention, had evaluated the changes in the HRV indices during baseline, intervention, and a post-intervention period and reported that during the intervention (lasting for 10 min), both the SDNN, total power and LF power were significantly larger than the control group whereas during the post-intervention period, the intergroup differences disappeared. Meanwhile, Tharion et al. [11] had investigated the changes in the HRV measurement after one month of practicing deep breathing at 6 breaths per minute, once every day for 30 min.

Another study with heart rate variability with video aided mindful deep breathing for short duration had shown a positive impact on reducing depressive feeling after 7 days of consecutively practice for 5 min for each min with 6 deep breath per day [8]. In this study, the outcome of average extended time internal between each pulse was aimed by integrated 6 deep breathing per minute with video aided for 3 min in duration into the smartphone application. Meanwhile, the similar team had applied the 3 min video aided deep breathing in pain management among athletes [7].

When users use their smartphone camera to measure HRV, there might be some noises occurred which may cause the inaccurate of the result. These noises might be caused by the movement of fingers during measurement and the insensitive of smartphone camera. Besides that, another limitation of this application is that we can keep track of the users' finger during the measurement, thus the measuring process will continue although users leave their fingers from the camera. For future work, the development of the IOS version for the mobile application should be included.

5 Conclusions

The aim of the study to promote and maintain wellness of body and mind through scientific measurement with heart rate variability for the users had successfully developed for the community. The measurement based on the PPG concept can detect the heart rate through accessing to the camera and lighting features from the phone, enabling anyone access to the mobile application to enjoy the tool without needed to purchase any instrument. In addition, the users had contributed to the strength of information on total of average extended time interval in milliseconds counts after the 3 min of video aided deep breathing exercise. Total per time of usage for before and after, with the deep breathing practice, are 7 min, therefore, the user can enjoy a total of 7 min of interaction time with the mobile application for the wellness exercise.

References

1. Brown, R.P., Gerbarg, P.L.: Yoga breathing, meditation, and longevity. Ann. N. Y. Acad. Sci. **1172**, 54–62 (2009). https://doi.org/10.1111/j.1749-6632.2009.04394.x
2. Cheng, K.S., Chang, Y.F., Han, R.P.S., Lee, P.F.: Enhanced conflict monitoring via a short-duration, video-assisted deep breathing in healthy young adults: an event-related potential approach through the Go/NoGo paradigm. PeerJ **2017**(10). https://doi.org/10.7717/peerj.3857
3. Yadav, G., Mutha, P.K.: Deep breathing practice facilitates retention of newly learned motor skills. Sci. Rep. **6**(1), 1–8 (2016). https://doi.org/10.1038/srep37069
4. Ferreira, L., Tanaka, K., Santosgalduróz, R.F., Galduróz, J.C.F.: Respiratory training as strategy to prevent cognitive decline in aging: a randomized controlled trial. Clin. Interv. Aging **10**, 593–603 (2015). https://doi.org/10.2147/CIA.S79560
5. Cheng, K.S., Han, R.P.S., Lee, P.F.: Neurophysiological study on the effect of various short durations of deep breathing: a randomized controlled trial. Respir. Physiol. Neurobiol. **249**, 23–31 (2018). https://doi.org/10.1016/j.resp.2017.12.008
6. Cheng, K.S., Lee, P.F.: A physiological/model study on the effects of deep breathing on the respiration rate, oxygen saturation, and cerebral oxygen delivery in humans. Neurophysiology **50**(5), 351–356 (2018). https://doi.org/10.1007/s11062-019-09761-4
7. Ramalingam, V., Cheng, K.S., Singh Sidhu, M., Foong, L.P.: A pilot study: neurophysiological study on the effect of chronic ankle pain intervene with video assisted mindful deep breathing,

pp. 388–393. Institute of Electrical and Electronics Engineers (IEEE) (2019). https://doi.org/10.1109/iecbes.2018.8626731

8. Cheng, K.S., Croarkin, P.E., Lee, P.F.: Heart rate variability of various video-aided mindful deep breathing durations and its impact on depression, anxiety, and stress symptom severity. Mindfulness **10**(10), 2082–2094 (2019).https://doi.org/10.1007/s12671-019-01178-8
9. Visvanathan, A., Banerjee, R., Misra, A., Choudhury, A.D., Pal, A.: Effects of fingertip orientation and flash location in smartphone photoplethysmography. In: Proceedings of the 2014 International Conference on Advances in Computing, Communications and Informatics, ICACCI 2014, pp. 468–471. Institute of Electrical and Electronics Engineers Inc. (2014). https://doi.org/10.1109/ICACCI.2014.6968536
10. Prinsloo, G.E., Derman, W.E., Lambert, M.I., Laurie Rauch, H.G.: The effect of a single session of short duration biofeedback-induced deep breathing on measures of heart rate variability during laboratory-induced cognitive stress: a pilot study. Appl. Psychophysiol. Biofeedback **38**(2), 81–90 (2013). https://doi.org/10.1007/s10484-013-9210-0
11. Tharion, E., Samuel, P., Rajalakshmi, R., Gnanasenthil, G., Subramanian, R.K.: Influence of deep breathing exercise on spontaneous respiratory rate and heart rate variability: a randomised controlled trial in healthy subjects. Indian J. Physiol. Pharmacol. **56**(1), 80–87 (2012)

Feature Selection for Identification of Fake Profiles on Facebook

John Benyen Munga and Prabu Mohandas

Abstract Technology is advancing at a breakneck speed these days. Online Social Network (OSN), which has become a part of everyone's life in terms of making new friends and keeping track of friends and their interests. Social networking sites make social life better, but there are many problems when using these Social Media sites, especially Facebook. Problems i.e., privacy, offline, hacking are mainly done through fake profiles. Researchers found that 20–40% of profiles on social networking sites such as Facebook are fake profiles. So, the problem is to build an accurate model to detect if a Facebook profile is a fake profile based on the user's social activity using machine learning techniques. As it is an automatic detection technique, machine can make it easier for the sites to manage the huge number of profiles, which cannot be done manually. There are many previous works on the identification of fake profiles. So this paper proposes the minimal set of generic features to identify the fake profiles on Facebook and the study determines that minimized set of main features are significant in the detection of the fake accounts on Facebook.

Keywords Online social networks · Fake profiles · Machine learning · Classification · Features based techniques

1 Introduction

Social Media is an application or website that allows users to create and share content or participate in social networking. Marketers use Social Media to have a voice and engage with their peers, consumers, and potential customers. It aids in the delivery of the message in a conversational and relaxed manner. Facebook is one of the huge Social Media platforms for businesses to reach out to potential clients. Using Social Media platforms has a range of benefits, but with that has come inevitable issues like cyberbully, fake profile etc. [1, 2].

J. B. Munga (✉) · P. Mohandas
National Institute of Technology Calicut, Calicut, Kerala 673601, India

J. Usman et al. (eds.), *6th Kuala Lumpur International Conference on Biomedical Engineering 2021*, IFMBE Proceedings 86,
https://doi.org/10.1007/978-3-030-90724-2_53

A fake profile is a Social Media depiction of a person, organization, or enterprise that does not exist in real life. These accounts genuine people's names and identities to access specific people and their target audience. Fake profiles are not authentic, i.e., those created by people who pretend to be someone they are not and engage in destructive and unwanted behaviour. People use online imitation and social engineering to construct fake profiles to malign a person or group.

Various Machine Learning algorithms like Neural Network, Random Forest, and Support Vector Machines can be used for detecting the fake profiles on Social Media.

Machine learning is a branch of computer science that deals with the study of algorithms with the ability to learn [3–5]. According to the importance of Social Media's effect on society, this research aims to detect the fake profile accounts from Facebook online social network. In Sect. 2 of this paper, literature review is analyzed, and the observations are mentioned. In Sect. 3, problem statement is defined. In Sect. 4, proposed method are described. In the Sect. 5, result analysis is done. In Sect. 6, the conclusion of this thesis work along with future scope is mentioned.

2 Literature Review

Various studies have been presented to detect fake accounts using various methods. A feature based detection technique is used in this study. This approach is based on monitoring the behaviour of the user, such as his number of posts, status, friends, etc. this concept is based on the assumption that genuine accounts usually behave differently than the fakes, so detecting this behavior will lead to the revealing of the fake accounts.

Table 1 shows different approaches studied by the researchers briefly. Different datasets used and the initial estimations are shown.

According to Ramalingam and Chinnaiah [7] network bot detection can be classified into three categories: feature or content-based defense, network structure or

Table 1 Comparing approaches

S. No.	Author details and year	Data-set	Approach	Estimation
1	Ramalingam and Chinnaiah (2017)	None	Exploring various detection techniques	Identifies possible future developments
2	Manuel Eagle	Fb, Twitter	COMPA [6]	The behavior of normal users are stable compared to compromised users
3	Shama (2019)	Fb	Neural Networks	Increase accuracy by training with larger datasets
4	Faraz Ahmed	Fb, Twitter	Features based	False positive rates, detection rates

graph-based defense and a combination of both. The vast amount of data available on online social networking sites has enticed researchers to mine the data and investigate issues that concern the social networking community. The authors presented significant work on spam detection on OSN's [8]. The authors compared three different classification models. Individual datasets scraped from Facebook and Twitter networks were used in the study. The authors analysed the efficiency of all three methods and concluded that four basic components make up social networks—interactions, posts/tweets, URLs, and tags/mentions. Collected 11 matching features from both Facebook and Twitter. Evaluated the 11 features using three different classification algorithms. In the next stage, authors shared their observations about the importance of each feature as they deleted one at a time [9].

Based on all the papers studied below are the observations made.

2.1 *Analysis and Validation*

In [10] authors started with 21 attributes, chosen to use only features that have a direct impact on the outcomes. Later removed all the unnecessary attributes/features making it down to just 4 attributes. This method can be used on the datasets which have very less features but it ignores lot of features which can contribute in detecting the fake profiles and Facebook has a lot features. Authors concluded that Random Forest method outperforms the Decision Tree approach with an accuracy 99.64 compared to 99.28.

In [11] authors chose the most used features and processed to preprocess the features. Features are chosen generically with the main focus on Neural Network and Random Forest. Authors concluded that both Neural Network and Random Forest generate similar accuracy of 91.

In [9] authors analyzed the similar features in both Facebook and Twitter utilized the publicly available Java API "HTML Parser", for gathering the required information for datasets of FB and Twitter. Features are limited to 11 because the features should be in match with the features in Twitter. Authors concluded that the best approach/algorithm for Facebook is decision tree for the features used.

In [12] authors started with a 22 features data set and after applying the 5-cross validation in 3 rounds authors concluded it to 6 useful features (Table 2).

Table 2 Comparing performances

S. No.	Author details	Accuracy	Precision	Detection rate
1	Elyusufi	99.64%	N/A	N/A
2	Shama	91%	N/A	N/A
3	Ahmed	N/A	N/A	95.7%
4	El Azab	N/A	99%	N/A

2.2 Findings

Feature based and hybrid technique approaches give better accuracy to find fake profiles. Because initially researchers aren't convinced that machine can learn according to the fake profile. Now researchers are using many machine learning classification algorithms to detect fake profiles and also fake news/posts. Method [11] can be used on the datasets which have very less features but it ignores lot of features which can contribute in detecting the fake profiles and Facebook has a lot features. Authors concluded that Random Forest method outperforms the Decision Tree approach. It is also noted that both Neural Network and Random Forest generate similar accuracy. In [11] method used 5 algorithms and concluded that the each algorithms show the best results when the features with the at-least 0.5 information gain are used and authors trimmed down the features to 7. It is also further mentioned that it can be applied on the Facebook with minor changes, however it needed a proper dataset.

To overcome all the limitations mentioned in the analysis and findings, the model should be built on feature based and features should be minimal set with the most contribution on finding in the fake profile. As minimal as possible model should not overlook the features that can contribute. Model needs a dataset with more features and should apply ML algorithms according to the attributes that are in the dataset, based on information gain.

3 Problem Definition

Build an accurate model to detect if a Facebook profile is fake or genuine with limited profile information by finding the most significant features of all the features in the Facebook.

4 Proposed Method

A dataset of 1337 fake and 1481 genuine profiles is gathered with many attributes such as friends count, followers count, status count etc. are included. From the dataset used, more than 80% of the accounts are used for data training and the other 20% of accounts are used for data analysis. Dataset collected consists of 25 features. The proposed model consists of 2 rounds round 1 (Fig. 1) and round 2 (Fig. 2), all the 25 features 'Table 3' consisted are used for round 1. Based on the information gain calculated and number of N/A values, features are trimmed down to 5 features 'Table 4' for round 2. Of these 2 rounds accuracy should be greater in round 2 compared to round 1 as the features used for the round 2 have better information gain [12].

The following are the steps involved before the data preprocessing:

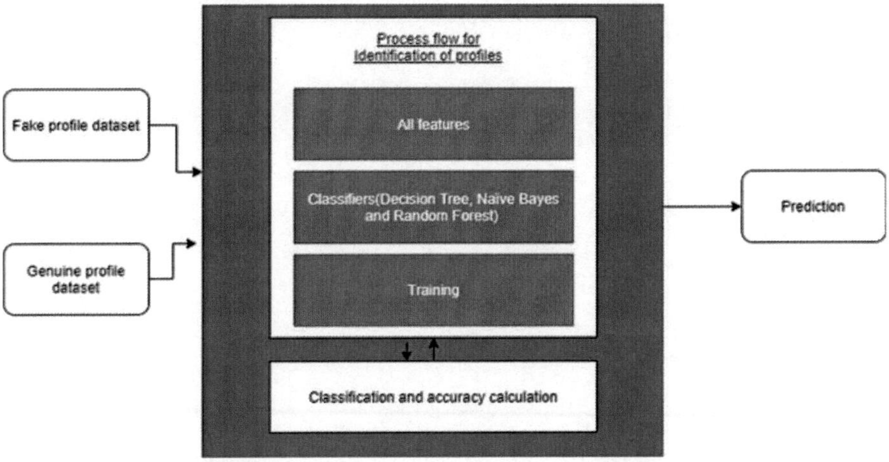

Fig. 1 Model design for round 1

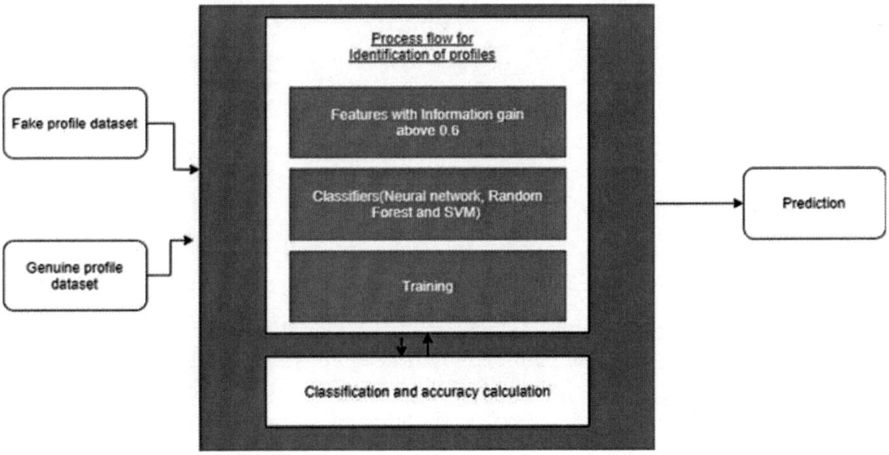

Fig. 2 Model design for round 2

- Calculation of Entropy.
- Calculation of Information Gain.
- Selection of attributes for round 1 and round 2.

The following are the steps involved in data preprocessing:

- Elimination of Noisy data.
- Handling missing data.
- Data augmentation.

Table 3 Attributes for round 1

Attribute	Information gain	N/A count
Name	1.002416621	0
statusescount	0.84053497	0
Followerscount	0.658579642	0
friendscount	0.525472722	0
Favouritescount	0.723996884	0
listedcount	0.319974575	0
url	0.178517293	2355
Lang	0.735168964	0
timezone	0.505383205	1749
defaultprofile	0.506225096	1090
defaultprofileimage	0.000006620	2810
geoenabled	0.287918625	2097
profilebannerurl	0.454456611	1831
profileusebackgroundimage	0.023668668	58
profilebackgroundimageurlht	tps0.512665804	0
profiletextcolor	0.188836515	0
profilesidebarbordercolor	0.443867996	0
profilebackgroundtile	0.179122855	2329
profilesidebarfillcolor	0.349709713	0
profilebackgroundimageurl	0.499174359	0
profilebackgroundcolor	0.414091645	0
profilelinkcolor	0.364044981	0
utcoffset	0.505383205	1749
protected	0.00458163	2818
verified	0	2818

Table 4 Attributes for round 2

Attribute	Information gain	N/A count
statusescount	0.84053497	0
Lang	0.733219899	0
favouritescount	0.723996884	0
Followerscount	0.658579642	0
Friendscount	0.525472722	0

One of the main limitation from the previous works, to minimize the set of features many features which can contribute to identifying fake profiles are ignored in order to overcome this limitation data argumentation is used in the model preprocessing. Apart from the five features proposed in Table 4 three more attributes are added using data argumentation. The columns added are

- Gender: Gender of the profile was predicted using Sex machine package by giving username as input.
- Account age: Account age is calculated using the created at column.
- Location: Location is in string format converted to integer using the label encoding.

Dataset is generated for each round respectively. 1st round consists of dataset with all features. Features with the null values are filled randomly using label encoding. 2nd round consists of dataset with limited features which doesn't consists of any null values. The processed data is now ready to be trained for the model after the data augmentation has been completed. Three different classification algorithms, namely Random Forest, SVM, and Neural Networks, are applied to the available dataset to obtain three different models. Values for accuracy, precision, recall, and other metrics after testing the three models with the test dataset are estimated.

5 Results

The Classification report with the precision, recall and f1-score for the Random Forest classifier, SVM and Feed forward Neural Network respectively is (Figs. 3, 4, and 5),

Confusion matrix for the Random Forest classifier, SVM and Feed forward Neural Network respectively is (Table 5),

All three algorithms are run separately with both round 1 and round 2. Increase in the accuracy can be observed from round 1 to round 2 because features chosen in the round 2 are best possible feature set (Table 6).

	precision	recall	f1-score	support
Fake	0.99	1.00	1.00	287
Genuine	1.00	0.99	1.00	277
micro avg	1.00	1.00	1.00	564
macro avg	1.00	1.00	1.00	564
weighted avg	1.00	1.00	1.00	564

Fig. 3 Random Forest

	precision	recall	f1-score	support
Fake	1.00	1.00	1.00	296
Genuine	1.00	1.00	1.00	268
micro avg	1.00	1.00	1.00	564
macro avg	1.00	1.00	1.00	564
weighted avg	1.00	1.00	1.00	564

Fig. 4 Support vector machine

	precision	recall	f1-score	support
Fake	0.93	0.97	0.95	274
Genuine	0.97	0.93	0.95	289
micro avg	0.95	0.95	0.95	563
macro avg	0.95	0.95	0.95	563
weighted avg	0.95	0.95	0.95	563

Fig. 5 Neural network

Table 5 Confusion matrix

Random Forest		SVM		Neural network	
287	0	295	1	252	3
2	275	1	267	30	278

Table 6 Accuracy table

S. No.	ML algorithm	Round 1 (%)	Round 2 (%)
1	Random Forest classification	96.45	99.46
2	Support vector machine classification	94.85	99.64
3	Feed forward neural network classification	48.49	94.13

6 Conclusion and Future Work

In this research, Machine Learning model is built which work efficiently and is able to detect the fake accounts with limited profile information, the proposed approach was based on determining the effective features for the detection process. The features collected have been filtered using the entropy and information gain. From 25 attributes, the proposed approach has reached only eight effective attributes for fake accounts detection with five determined based on information gain. Using 2 rounds it's further illustrated with different algorithms, how the minimal set of features with higher information gain gives a better accuracy. As the part of future work, properties of each feature can be studied by removing each feature individually and combining with other features. Model can also be implemented on other social websites like Instagram with some minor changes.

References

1. Cao, Q., Sirivianos, M., Yang, X., Munagala, K.: Combating friend spam using social rejections. In: 2015 IEEE 35th International Conference on Distributed Computing Systems, pp. 235–244 (2015). https://doi.org/10.1109/ICDCS.2015.32
2. Wani, S.Y., Kirmani, M.M., Ansarulla, S.I.: Prediction of fake profiles on Facebook using supervised machine learning techniques-a theoretical model. Int. J. Comput. Sci. Inf. Technol. (IJCSIT) **7**(4), 1735–1738 (2016)
3. Bishop, C.: Pattern Recognition and Machine Learning, pp. 295–300. IEEE (2011)
4. Mitchell, T.: The discipline of machine learning: Carnegie Mellon University. Carnegie Mellon University, School of Computer Science, Machine Learning Department (2006)
5. Witten, I.H., Frank, E.: Data Mining: Practical Machine Learning Tools and Techniques, 3rd ed. Morgan Kaufmann (2011)
6. Egele, M., Stringhini, G., Kruegel, C., Vigna, G.: Towards detecting compromised accounts on social networks. IEEE Trans. Dependable Secure Comput. **14**(4), 447–460 (2017). https://doi.org/10.1109/TDSC.2015.2479616,1July-Aug
7. Ramalingam, D., Chinnaiah, V.: Fake profile detection techniques in large-scale online social networks: a comprehensive review. Comput. Electr. Eng. **65**, 165–177 (2018)
8. Stringhini, G., Kruegel, C., Vigna, G.: Detecting spammers on social networks. In: Proceedings of the 26th Annual Computer Security Applications Conference, pp. 1–9. ACM, (2010)
9. Ahmed, F., Abulaish, M.: A generic statistical approach for spam detection in online social networks. IJRTE (2013)
10. Elyusufi, Y., Elyusufi, Z., Kbir, M.A.: Social networks fake profiles detection using machine learning algorithms. In: Innovations in Smart Cities Applications, 3 edn., pp. 30–40 (2020)
11. Shama, S.K., Siva Nandini, K., Bhavya Anjali, P., Devi Manaswi, K.: Fake profile identification in online social networks. IJRTE **9**(4), 11190–11194 (2019)
12. El Azab, A., Idrees, A.M., Mahmoud, M.A., Hefny, H.: Fake account detection in Twitter based on minimum weighted feature set. IEEE **10**(1), 13–18 (2016)

Tissue Engineering and Clinical Management

Feasibility of Using Saliva Samples and Laser-Induced Breakdown Spectroscopy for Dental Screening During Pandemic

Syafriandi, Siti Norhayati Md Yassin, Siti Norbaieah Mohd Hashim, Maheza Irna Mohamad Salim, Rania Hussein AlAshwal, Asnida Abdul Wahab, Mariaulpa Sahalan, Hum Yan Chai, and Lai Khin Wee

Abstract Recent studies show that dental caries affect more than half of the adult population globally, with the socially disadvantaged groups being majorly affected. The purpose of this study is to investigate the feasibility of using Laser-Induced Breakdown Spectroscopy (LiBS) as a method of early caries screening in adults through the detection of caries elements dissolved in saliva. This experiment involved 25 students of School of Biomedical Engineering and Health Sciences, Universiti Teknologi Malaysia. Parameters that are considered in this study are pH of the saliva and spectroscopic analysis of other elements such as Na and Ca. The data were statistically analysed to evaluate the significance differences of these elements in all group levels by using One-Way ANOVA. Results show that there is a significant difference in Calcium and Sodium intensity values between the mild, moderate, and severe caries groups. Additionally, pH level also shows a significant difference between the groups. This research concluded that LIBS allows for absolute and quantitative analysis of elements contained in saliva without examining patients' teeths and is useful as a fast and accurate oral health screening method for the community as LiBS could provide not only caries detection but also determining the caries severity level. Thus, this investigation proves that analysis of saliva samples using LiBS can be an alternative or future method in screening dental caries and applicable especially during pandemic situations.

Syafriandi · S. N. M. Yassin · S. N. M. Hashim · M. I. M. Salim (✉) · R. H. AlAshwal · A. A. Wahab · M. Sahalan
Diagnostic Research Group, School of Biomedical Engineering and Health Sciences, Faculty of Engineering, Universiti Teknologi Malaysia, 81310 Johor, Malaysia
e-mail: maheza@biomedical.utm.my

L. K. Wee
Department of Biomedical Engineering, Faculty of Engineering, Universiti Malaya, Kuala Lumpur, Malaysia

H. Y. Chai
Lee Kong Chian Faculty of Engineering and Science, Universiti Tun Abdul Razak Malaysia, Kuala Lumpur, Malaysia

J. Usman et al. (eds.), *6th Kuala Lumpur International Conference on Biomedical Engineering 2021*, IFMBE Proceedings 86,
https://doi.org/10.1007/978-3-030-90724-2_54

Keywords Dental caries · LiBS · Background analysis · pH of saliva

1 Introduction

According to the World Health Organization WHO [19], dental caries is the most common disease of all health conditions and affects almost half of the world's population. Data from the Ministry of Health, Malaysia on trend of decayed teeth among Malaysian population aged 16 years old and below shows that more than 60% of them have caries [10] and the statistic is reducing to 43.1% of 16 years old Malaysian in 2018 report [8]. Dental caries are characterized by a slow evolution that leads to the destruction of hard tissues of teeth. The destruction is led by a progressive demineralization process. There are three main factors that can be taken as the main factors of dental caries or tooth decay [13] including a susceptible tooth, bacteria, and diet such as sugar and carbohydrate intakes which simultaneously present over the times to accumulate caries. It develops through gradual complex biological interactions of acid-forming bacteria, fermentable carbohydrates and host factors such as the teeth and saliva. A correct and precise screening assessment of caries status is necessary for tooth decay prevention and management [2, 18]. At this moment, oral hygiene evaluation is conducted based on the standard criteria given by WHO using the visual-tactile method. Clinical examination is basically a visual evaluation which is often inadequate when used solely for caries assessment [1]. Additionally, Mohanraj et al. [9] stated that this method shows inadequate validity with poor sensitivity and moderate specificity. This indicates that this approach is an inexact method which results in over-diagnosis and under-diagnosis, which leads to studies of finding quantitative detection tools [9].

Saliva provides several mechanisms to protect the teeth such as elimination of microorganisms, buffering actions to neutralize acid, and clearance of food debris and sugar [4]. Evaluating the causative factors in the saliva of individuals at risk to dental caries can pave the way to make recommendations that will cater specifically to the individual's needs. Many benefits exist for both patients and dentists by introducing saliva testing as part of practice philosophy [12]. Zhang et al. [22] stated that human saliva appears to possess a notable role in the health of the oral cavity and of the body as a whole. Salivary factors such as low rate, urea, buffering capacity and neutralization capability play an important role in preventing dental erosion [11, 22].

Laser-induced breakdown spectroscopy (LiBS) is a rapid multi-elemental analytical technology which uses spectroscopic analysis of the radiation emitted by laser-induced plasma [6]. Sasazawa et al. [14] claim that by using laser-induced breakdown spectroscopy (LiBS) to detect caries, this method enables absolute and quantitative analysis of elements contained in teeth. In this study, saliva samples collected from adult subjects were analyzed using the LiBS system to investigate the level of caries element intensity for caries severity identifications via the determination of different peaks of the analyzed samples along with other parameters such as pH.

2 Materials and Method

All subjects were asked to fill up informed consent at the beginning of the experiment. A series of questions extracted from the WHO oral health questionnaire to probe the subject's oral health were also given [17, 20]. Sample of saliva was then collected for analysis. Subjects were asked to do self-examination of their own oral health for them to answer the questions properly. 25 adults aged 19–25 years old were involved in this study. Passive drool technique is applied as the methods for saliva collection in order to maintain consistency in the type of sample collected. The saliva samples were collected at least 30 min before meals and at least 10 min after brushing or rinsing to reduce diurnal variability effects on saliva composition. 5 ml droplets of saliva from the adult was collected passively to maintain the consistency of the saliva. The saliva was kept in a collection cup labelled with the subject's name and ID. The collected saliva was preserved using a cooling box before further processing at the laboratory and categorized into mild, moderate and severe caries according to mouth score.

Saliva samples from every caries category were analyzed within 2 h after collection to control the quality of the saliva and to avoid any effect of saliva decomposition. pH of the saliva was analyzed using a digital meter, PB-10, Sartorius and it was first tested using a standard solution (pH 10) as control before carrying out sample measurement. All pH values were recorded in Microsoft Excel for statistical analysis.

The collected saliva (5 ml) was then put on a laser-induced breakdown spectroscopy's sample holder. Background test involving different types of sample holders was conducted in order to determine chemical elements that may present in sample holders to be omitted during saliva analysis. Laser-induced breakdown spectroscopy (LiBS) is a rapid multi-elemental analytical technology which uses spectroscopic analysis of the radiation emitted by laser-induced plasma. LiBS enables fast identification of the chemical composition by determining the different peaks of the analyzed samples. The surface of the saliva was radiated by using the Nd:YAG laser as the source of excitation. Emission spectrums captured by spectrometers were stored and displayed by using SpectraSuite software. The analysis was made in SpectraGryph software to identify the position of the peaks following the National Institute of Standards and Technology (NIST) Atomic Spectra Database Lines Data. The results obtained were then statistically analyzed using One-Way ANOVA with $P < 0.05$ will be counted as statistically significant, whilst highly significant is when the value of $P < 0.001$.

3 Result

From the self-examination mouth scores, the respondents involved for this project were categorized as mild caries (7), moderate caries (9) and severe caries (8) following the American Dental Association 2015 classifications. The mild caries scores are based on the number of tooth lesions indicated by the existence of white or brown spots on the hard surface of the teeth and enamel has lost its gloss. Additionally, 9 respondents with obvious or visible damage of the enamel and demineralization were classified as moderate caries. Lastly, Holes or obvious cavitated teeth were found on 8 respondents and classified as severe caries.

3.1 Determination of pH Level

Figure 1 shows the result for pH level. From the result the mean pH level of mild caries is higher than moderate and severe caries. This shows that subjects with severe dental caries have a more acidic saliva. This result is in agreement with the previous study reported by Shetty et al. [16]. Result for mild caries shows an outlier value of pH 7.69. This may be contributed by the high concentration of fluoride after brushing teeth that increase the pH level of the saliva as reported [15].

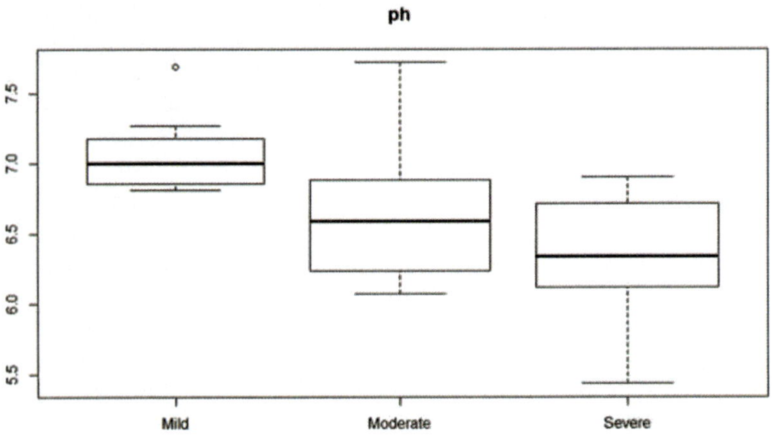

Fig. 1 pH level of saliva with mild, moderate and severe caries

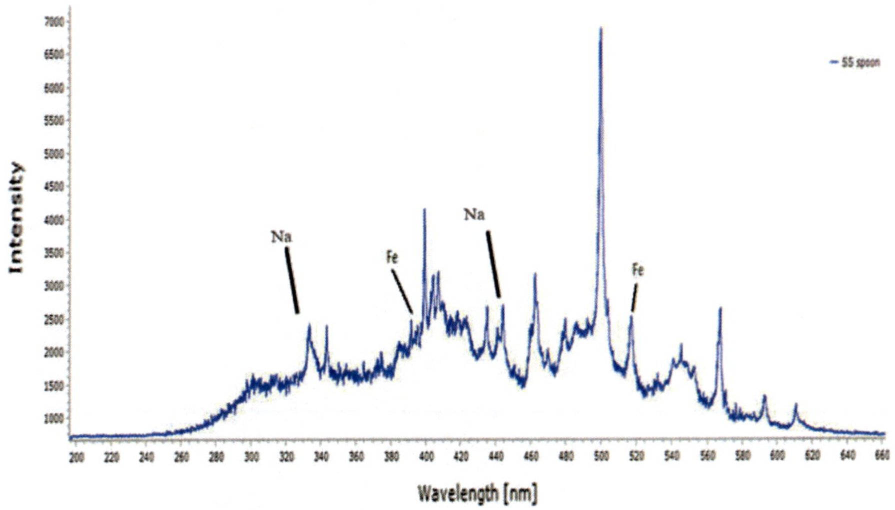

Fig. 2 Spectrum of a stainless steel spoon

3.2 *Results of LiBS Analysis*

3.2.1 Background Analysis

Before saliva sample analysis was conducted, background analysis was done to ensure that the LiBS spectrum from saliva is not influenced by the background or sample holder spectrum. In this study, a wooden spoon, a plastic bowl, and a stainless-steel spoon were used to identify a suitable background for the sample. Result shows that the stainless-steel background contains Fe elements as shown in Fig. 2.

3.2.2 Background and Saliva Sample Comparison

The saliva samples were analyzed using LiBS for 4 times per sample to ensure accuracy and consistency of the result. Figure 3 shows the LiBS spectrum from a saliva sample and a stainless-steel background with elements of calcium (Ca) and sodium (Na) found in the sample. The background spectrum is indicated by the yellow line and the saliva sample is indicated by a blue line.

The first peak of Ca is found at 393.37 nm, and the second peak is located at 396.85 nm. The same results were reported by Choi et al. (2014) in their research for calcium ions investigation using LiBS.

As for sodium, three peaks were found in the result. However, only the peak at 318 nm was considered as the other 2 peaks were found in the background spectrum.

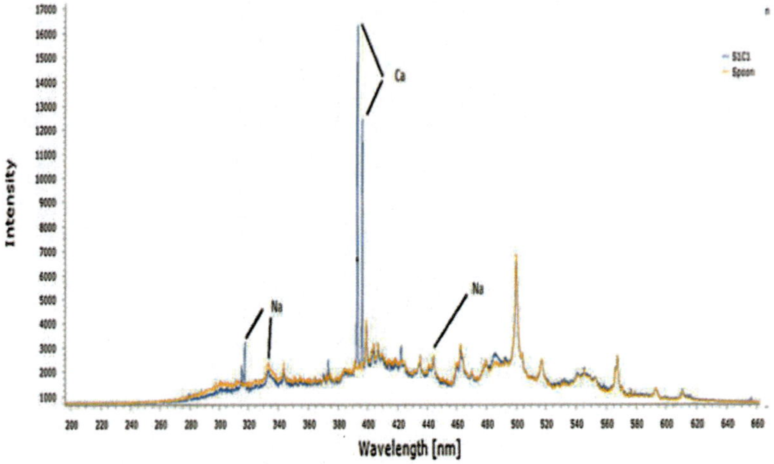

Fig. 3 Background and saliva sample spectrum

Levels of calcium elements at wavelength 396.85 nm and 393.37 in mild, medium and severe caries samples are shown in Fig. 4a, b. Severe caries is shown to have a lower level of calcium content in saliva compared to moderate and mild caries levels at both wavelengths.

On the other hand, levels of sodium at wavelength 318 nm in mild, moderate and severe groups also showed a similar trend as calcium. Sodium level is lowest in the severe group followed by moderate and lastly the level is highest for mild groups. Figure 5 shows the result for sodium.

All the parameters were then analyzed by using One-Way ANOVA to see the significance difference and the result is shown in Table 1.

From Table 1, all parameters are significantly different for every group. A significant result is found when the *P*-value or critical value of our finding is less than 0.05, whilst a highly significant difference is when $P < 0.01$ [7]. For pH level, the difference in results for each group is highly significant. Similar findings were found by Shetty et al. [16] on their measurement on pH of dental caries. Fiyaz et al. [3] also find there is a significant difference in the amount of calcium in the caries group. Sasazawa et al. [14] and Gazmeh et al. [5] found there is an increase of calcium intensity in the healthier dental patients As for Na, there is a statistically high significant difference among the groups. The similar result discussed by Zahir and Sarkar [21] whereas there is a highly significant difference between caries groups patients.

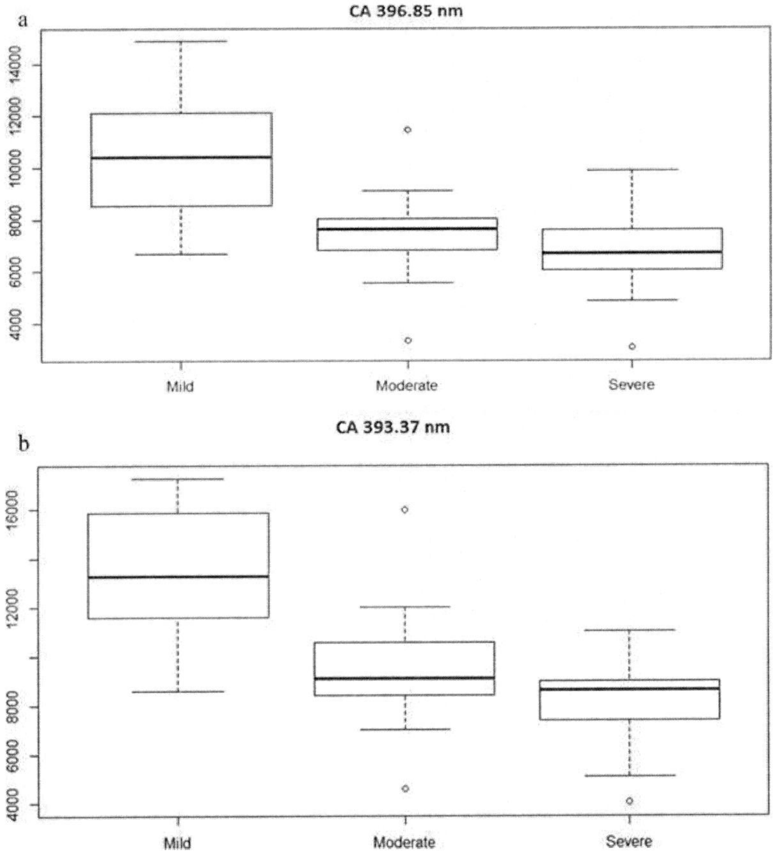

Fig. 4 **a**, **b** Calcium elements present in saliva with mild, moderate and severe caries at wavelength 396.85 nm and 393.37 nm respectively

4 Conclusion

Saliva analysis by using LiBS can determine the elements in the sample such Na and Ca. The statistical analysis managed to show that all parameters observed in this study have significant differences between the three groups which are mild, moderate, and severe caries especially for intensity levels of Ca, Na and pH levels. Thus, this investigation proves that analysis of saliva samples using LiBS can be an alternative or future method in screening dental caries and applicable especially during pandemic situations.

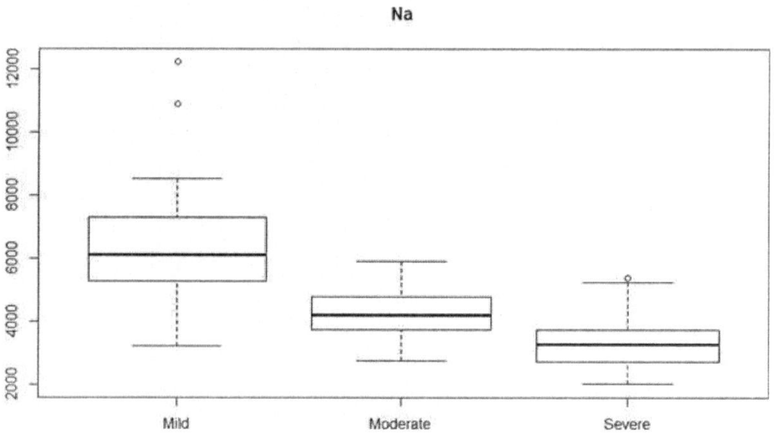

Fig. 5 Sodium level in mild, moderate and severe group

Table 1 Results of one-way Anova

	Caries groups			*P*-value
	Mild	Moderate	Severe	
	Mean	Mean	Mean	
Salivary pH	7.07	6.68	6.33	0.017
Ca (392.98 nm)	13,373.98	9467.91	8203.14	2.89E−17
Ca (396.47 nm)	10,466.60	7402.50	6745.79	1.86E−15
Na (317.59 nm)	6415.51	4247.83	3346.20	1.46E−15

Acknowledgements The Authors would like to thanks Universiti Teknologi Malaysia for the research funding under the RUG Scheme Vot number 15J83.

References

1. Chu, C.H., Chung, B.T.O., Lo, E.C.M.: Caries assessment by clinical examination with or without radiographs of young Chinese adults, 265–268 (2008)
2. Engelmann, J.L., Tomazoni, F., Machado, M.D., Ardenghi, T.M.: Association between dental caries and socioeconomic factors in school children—a multilevel analysis. **27**, 72–78 (2016)
3. Fiyaz, M., Ramesh, A., Ramalingam, K., Thomas, B., Shetty, S., Prakash, P.: Association of salivary calcium, phosphate, pH and flow rate on oral health: a study on 90 subjects. J. Indian Soc. Periodontol. **17**(4), 454 (2013)
4. Gao, X., Koh, D., Hsu, C.-Y.S.: Salivary biomarkers for dental caries. **70**(93), 128–141 (2016)
5. Gazmeh, M., Bahreini, M., Tavassoli, S.H.: Discrimination of healthy and carious teeth using laser-induced breakdown spectroscopy and partial least square discriminant analysis. Appl. Opt. **54**(1), 123 (2014)

6. Gazmeh, M., Bahreini, M., Tavassoli, S.H., Asnaashari, M.: Qualitative analysis of teeth and evaluation of amalgam elements penetration into dental matrix using laser induced breakdown. Spectroscopy **6**(2), 67–73 (2015)
7. Laerd Statistics.: One-way ANOVA—an introduction to when you should run this test and the test hypothesis. Laerd Statistics (2019)
8. Ministry of Health Malaysia.: Annual report 2016 (2018)
9. Mohanraj, M., Prabhu, V.R., Senthil, R.: Diagnostic methods for early detection of dental caries—a review. Int. J. Pedodontic Rehabil. **1**(1), 29–36 (2016)
10. 2019 Oral Health Report, Oral Health program, Ministry of Health Malaysia, https://ohd.moh.gov.my/images/pdf/annual_rpt/annual_rpt19.pdf
11. Piangprach, T., Hengtrakool, C., Kukiattrakoon, B., Kedjarune-Leggat, U.: The effect of salivary factors on dental erosion in various age groups and tooth surfaces. J. Am. Dent. Assoc. **140**(9), 1137–1143 (2009)
12. Prabhakar, A., Akanksha, G., Deepak, M., Sugandhan, S.: Diagnostic applications of saliva in dentistry. **2**(Dec), 7–13 (2009)
13. Quock, R.L.: Dental Caries: A current understanding and implications. **1**(1), 1–4 (2015)
14. Sasazawa, S., Kakino, S., Matsuura, Y.: Optical-fiber-based laser-induced breakdown spectroscopy for detection of early caries. J. Biomed. Optics **20**(6), 065002 (2015)
15. Setiawan, S., Haroen, E.R., Hadidjah, D.: The difference in saliva pH before and after brushing with fluoride containing toothpaste and without toothpaste. Padjajaran J. Dentist. **1**, 139–142 (2008)
16. Shetty, C., Hegde, M.N., Devadiga, D.: Correlation between dental caries with salivary flow, pH, and buffering capacity in adult south Indian population: an in-vivo study. Int. J. Res. Ayur. Pharm. **4**(2), 219–223 (2013)
17. World Health Organization.: Oral Health Survey Basic Methods, 89 (2013)
18. World Health Organization.: WHO Expert Consultation on Public Health Intervention against Early Childhood Caries Report of a Meeting, (January), 26–28 (2016). Retrieved from http://apps.who.int/iris/bitstream/handle/10665/255627/WHO-NMH-PND-17.1-eng.pdf;jsessionid=C1CD11587248693F9411C17918FB4C3C?sequence=1
19. World Health Organization.: Sugars and dental caries. WHO Technical Information Note, (October), 1–4 (2017)
20. Young, D.A., Nový, B.B., Zeller, G.G., Hale, R., Hart, T.C., Truelove, E.L.: The American dental association caries classification system for clinical practice. Am. Dental Asso. **146**(February), 79–86 (2015)
21. Zahir, S., Sarkar, S.: Study of trace elements in mixed saliva of caries free and caries active children. J. Indian Soc. Pedod. Prev. Dent. **24**(1), 27–29 (2006)
22. Zhang, C.Z., Cheng, X.Q., Li, J.Y., Zhang, P., Yi, P., Xu, X., Zhou, X.D.: Saliva in the diagnosis of diseases. Int. J. Oral Sci. **8**(3), 133–137 (2016)

Determination of Suitable Bioactive Glass-Polymer Film Conditioned Medium Extracts for Potential Applications in Tissue Regeneration: A Preliminary Study

Siti Fatimah Samsurrijal, Siti Noor Fazliah Mohd Noor, Mamun Khan Sujon, and Khirun Musa

Abstract Composite film combining bioactive particles with natural and synthetic polymer has received greater attention for enhanced cytocompatibility properties. The current study aimed to determine human mesenchymal stem cells (HMSC) responses towards different concentration of bioactive glass/poly-Ɛ-caprolactone/chitosan (BG/PCL/CS) films conditioned medium extract using Alamar Blue assay. The samples were incubated in simulated body fluid (SBF) and the pH was assessed during the 21 days of incubation. Briefly, BG/PCL/CS at optimize weight percentages in acetic acid solution were prepared using solvent casting method and left to dry under fume hood for 48 h. The BG/PCL/CS films were incubated in culture medium at 200 mg/ml for 24 h at 37 °C and was serially diluted until 0.78 mg/ml with culture medium and supplemented before exposure to HMSC. The effects of the conditioned mediums are not consistent and not in dose dependent order towards HMSC cell's viability and proliferation. Higher conditioned medium extracts concentration tends to reduce cell proliferation. The pH of the samples tends to approach equilibrium at pH 7 for 21 days duration when incubated in SBF that may be contributed by the sample's compositions. Thus, suitable concentration or dose ratio of the samples is important to reduce cytotoxicity before further biocompatibility assessment is conducted.

Keywords Bioactive glass · Poly-Ɛ-caprolactone · Chitosan

S. F. Samsurrijal · S. N. F. M. Noor (✉) · M. K. Sujon · K. Musa
Craniofacial and Biomaterial Sciences Cluster, Advanced Medical and Dental Institute, Universiti Sains Malaysia, 13200 Kepala Batas, Pulau Pinang, Malaysia
e-mail: fazliah@usm.my

S. N. F. M. Noor
Dental Stimulation and Virtual Learning, Research Excellence Consortium, Advanced Medical and Dental Institute, Universiti Sains Malaysia, 13200 Kepala Batas, Pulau Pinang, Malaysia

J. Usman et al. (eds.), *6th Kuala Lumpur International Conference on Biomedical Engineering 2021*, IFMBE Proceedings 86,
https://doi.org/10.1007/978-3-030-90724-2_55

1 Introduction

Development of three-dimensional (3D) scaffold for tissue engineering nowadays are geared towards combination of bioactive materials, natural such as chitosan (CS) and synthetic polymers such as poly-Ɛ-caprolactone (PCL) since these combinations results in superior scaffold intended for designated applications [1].

Bioactive glasses (BG) combined with polymers such as polycaprolactone and poly-lactic acid has potential in replacing common paste for skin or mucosal ulcers where BG-polymer film may provide easy applications, able to be retained and covering ulcers during healing period in acute and chronic wounds [2, 3]. Furthermore, these bioactive glasses can be tuned in its composition for soft tissue healing with addition ions such as magnesium or cobalt which promoted antibacterial properties and angiogenesis [4].

Bioactive glasses have the capability to develop a surface bonding with living tissues and stimulate a cellular response for healing and remodelling which can be used for both hard and soft tissue engineering purposes. These are biodegradable materials applicable in many clinical fields including dentistry, oral and maxillofacial and orthopaedics, osteogenesis and as means of ion delivery for antimicrobial effects [4]. These bioactive materials can degrade or being soluble in an aqueous media by ionic dissolutions of respective ions. The degradation rate can be regulated by chemical modifications into glass chemistry depending upon functional needs [5].

Ulceration is a widespread problem for certain medical conditions [6] and wound on skin following major surgery requires the need for use of patch for covering defective area. The use of synthetic and non-degradable plaster posed the need for patient to remove it and changed of plaster dressing not only creates pain but also clinical waste that sometimes are not disposed properly. Hence, there is a need to produce a suitable patch that can be used clinically, degrades over certain period and non-toxic. The incorporation of BG into the BG/PCL/CS patch will aid in bioactivity since BG is able to release bio-actives for stimulating new cell layer and promote tissue regeneration.

A wound healing material for external use must be able to maintain moisture and allowing skin to breathe while providing protection from inflammation and enhance skin fibroblast proliferation, which can be provided by CS. The addition of CS will help to enhance its process due to its antimicrobial and structural properties. For structural integrity, CS has been observed to produce crosslinking of nanofibers which are treated with heat to form water stable membranes and water absorption capabilities [7]. Addition of PCL of into the composite film patch will add strength and provide structural support for the film. PCL is FDA approved and commonly used in many biomedical field [8].

2 Materials and Methods

2.1 *Chemicals and Media*

Tetraethyl Orthosilicate (TEOS), Triethyl Phosphate (TEP), sodium nitrate and calcium nitrate tetrahydrate, low molecular weight chitosan (MWavg = 120 KDa) and poly-Ɛ-caprolactone (MWavg = 80,000) were purchased from Sigma-Aldrich (UK). Human mesenchymal stem cell from Lonza (Basel, Switzerland) and cell culture materials Dulbecco´s Modified Eagle's Medium (DMEM), fetal bovine serum (FBS), antibiotic–antimycotic were purchased Gibco Invitrogen Technologies (UK). All other reagents used were of analytical or microbiological grade purchased from Merck (Darmstadt, Germany).

2.2 *Bioactive Glass Synthesis*

Sol–gel BG were synthesized according to previous published study [9] where the glass fabrication involves mixing of vital compounds such as deionized water, 2 N nitric acid, TEOS, TEP, sodium nitrate and calcium nitrate tetrahydrate. The mixture will be left stirred overnight to achieve gelling state. The semi-gelation mixture will then be further gelled at 35 °C in the oven for 3 days before the sealed container containing the gelled mixture is then aged at 60 °C for 2 days. The mixture is then subjected to 110 °C for 2 days to ensure it is fully dried before the samples will then be sintered at 700 °C for 1 h. The sol gel BG powder is then will be grounded and sieved to achieve powder with particle size less than 50 μm.

2.3 *BG/PCL/CS Patch Synthesis*

The patch was synthesized using solvent casting method. Briefly, BG (10 weight percent, wt%), CS (10 wt%) and PCL (80 wt%) were dissolved in 100.0% (w/v) acetic acid, stir overnight for 16 h at 500 rpm and then poured inside a PTFE mold and left to dry for 48 h under fume hood. Once dried, the patch was removed from the mold and kept inside a desiccator until further tests.

2.4 *PH Analysis in Simulated Body Fluids*

The simulated body fluid (SBF) was prepared based on procedures described by Kokubo and Takadama [10]. The patch was incubated in SBF at a liquid/solid ratio of 50 mg/ml and placed inside an incubator shaker at 37 °C and the solution pH was recorded at designated time points (Days 1, 4, 7, 14 and 21).

2.5 Determination of Suitable Dosage for BG/PCL/CS Extracts Using Alamar Blue Assay

The patch was sterilized by UV exposure for 40 min on each side and then incubated with DMEM (200 mg/ml) inside an incubator shaker for 24 h at 37 °C [11] followed by sterile filtration using 0.22 μm syringe filter and kept at −20 °C. Prior to exposure to HMSC, the BG/PCL/CS conditioned medium extracts were serially diluted until 0.78 mg/ml and supplemented with 10% FBS and 1% A/A inside a vented T25 cm^2 flask and placed inside a CO_2 incubator at 37 °C overnight for pH stabilization prior to use on cells.

The HMSC was seeded with a seeding density of 5×10^3 cells/cm^2 inside a 96-well plate for 24 h and the next day was exposed to varying concentration of BG/PCL/CS extracts for another 24 h and the cells responses were assessed using Alamar Blue (Life Technologies) assays. Briefly, old medium was removed, and cells were wash using 100 μl of DPBS and then 150 μl of 10% (v/v) AB in DMEM with no phenol red (Gibco) was added per well (including one with no cells to be used as blank) and the well plates were further incubated for 2 h at 37 °C and then, 100 μl of the reaction product was transferred to a black Costar 96-well plate. The fluorescence of AB was read at an excitation wavelength of 544 nm and emission of 590 nm using a microplate reader (FLUOstar Omega, BMG Labtech).

2.6 Statistical Analysis

The experiment was conducted at least twice with four ($N = 4$) replicates and data was reported as mean ± standard error of mean (Mean ± SE). The data were analyzed using SPSS version 26.0 (IBM, Armonk, USA) using one-way analysis of variance (ANOVA) with subsequent *Bonferroni* post-hoc test with P value less than 0.05 as statistically significant.

3 Results and Discussion

3.1 pH Changes of BG/PCL/CS Patch in SBF

The pH profiles of PCL samples inside the SBF show almost comparable trend with the control SBF showing a steady profile from initial samples incubation until day

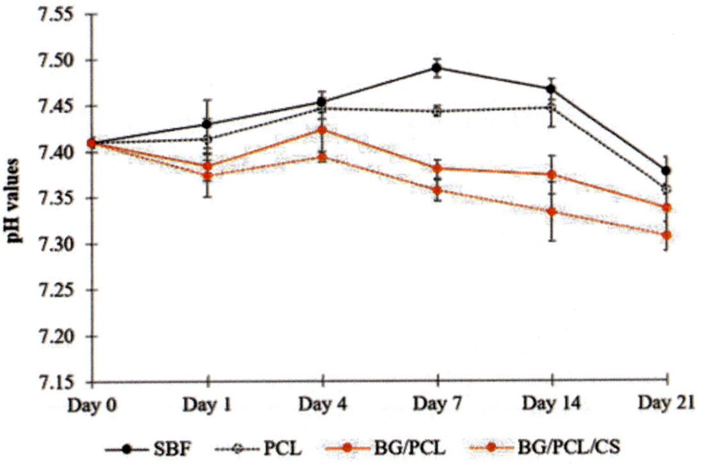

Fig. 1 The pH profiles of samples incubated in SBF throughout the 21 days of incubation

14 which tend to decrease to below pH 7.4 at day 21 (Fig. 1). Nonetheless, the pH of the samples containing BG (BG/PCL and BG/PCL/CS) show a decreasing trend from pH 7.4 towards pH 7.3 in which the pH values for BG/PCL/CS were lower compared to BG/PCL only. The addition of BG within the samples may provide buffering effect leading to lower pH towards stabilization at pH 7. A study reported that scaffolds containing 45S5 BG (PCL/50-45S5) and strontium (PCL/50-SrBG) showed higher pH at 7.75 and 7.82 after initial incubation which then reduced and fluctuated between pH 7.65 and 7.35 throughout 10 weeks immersion in α-MEM and this is contributed by the BG dissolutions into the immersion media, and the initial pH increase aided the apatite formation while the subsequent reduction in pH over time is likely caused by the gradual apatite formation [12]. The authors believed that the use of medium from a controlled source is more reliable and reflective towards cell culture studies using the same culture media [13].

Furthermore, the presence of CS also reduces the sample's pH towards pH 7.0 compared to BG/PCL only since time is needed for balancing the pH values which tend to be lower at the final when equilibrium is achieved [1]. The solubility, biological activity and ion exchange ability of samples containing CS is influenced by CS degree of deacetylation [14]. BG scaffolds impregnated with CS and PCL were incubated in SBF for up to 8 weeks where the results showed that CS influenced the bioactivity of the BG by enhancing mineralization [1].

In the current study, the SBF solution was not replaced during the 21 days incubation which may have resulted in lower pH for BG/PCL and BG/PCL/CS. A study replenished the SBF once every four weeks since the pH of the incubation media is influenced by the polymer coating degradation and BG dissolution [1] since the CS and PCL may release different organic degradation product that affects the pH of the SBF.

3.2 *HMSC Responses Towards BG/PCL/CS Extracts Conditioned Medium*

This preliminary study is to determine the toxic dose that reduces HMSC viability. Based on suggestion by ISO 10993-part 5, the material is incubated for 24 h at 37 °C with dose of 200 mg/ml [11] to prepare the material extracts usually known as the conditioned medium. Since no previous data is available for the current sample, serial dilution of the dose was carried out to ensure that future preparation of the film for direct cell seeding will not create toxic effects to the cells using AB assay. Serial dilution of 200 mg/ml extracts until 0.78 mg/ml were performed and the results showed the 200 mg/ml for BG/PCL and BG/PCL/Cs conditioned medium extracts were toxic to the cells (Fig. 2). At high dose (200 mg/ml), the BG concentration inside the medium is higher contributed by the increased in the weight percentages of the BG components; the sol–gel BG was fabricated based on a 45S5 system containing SiO_2–CaO–NaO–P_2O_5 and earlier study showed that higher NaO content is toxic to cells [15]. The gold standard 45S5 system modifications are performed through substitution of CaO and NaO with other components such as cobalt oxide [16], strontium oxide [17], and lithium oxide [18] are geared towards developing BG with enhanced angiogenesis, hard tissue repair and regeneration. BG conditioned medium in α-MEM (45S5/LiO, Li25, Li50 and Li100) at 6, 60 and 300 mg/ml incubated at specific time frame were exposed to mouse fibroblast MC3TC-E1 for 24 h and the results showed that cells exposed to the BG conditioned media at 300 mg/ml had significantly lower metabolic activity suggesting that the higher dose were toxic to cells [18].

Overall, HMSC seeded on BG/PCL/CS patch showed acceptable cell viability despite the fluctuation of the dose with cells exposed to 3.12 mg/ml had the highest

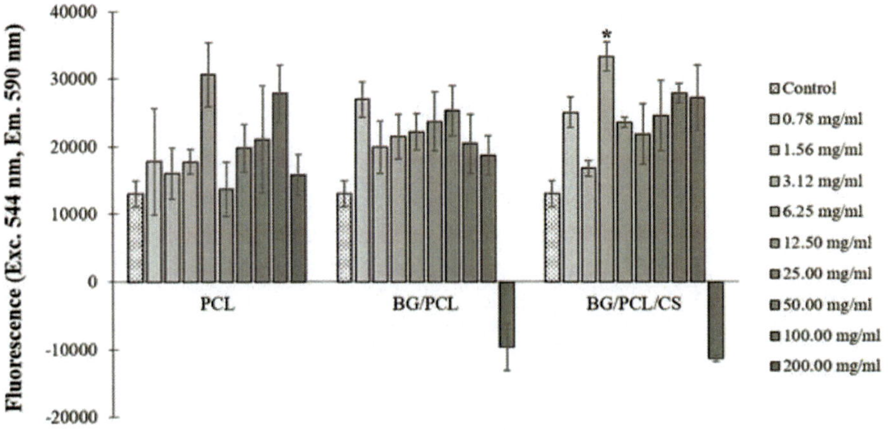

Fig. 2 The BG/PCL and BG/PCL/CS extracts at 200 mg/ml are toxic to the cells. ($P < 0.05$ when compared to PCL and BG/PCL)

viability compared to the other doses. This may highlight that a certain BG dose maybe suitable for cells [14, 15]. HMSC exposed to BG/PCL extract is not dose dependent and beginning to show reduced cell viability at 50 mg/ml. The cell viability differences when exposed to BG/PCL and BG/PCL/CS extracts at higher dose is contributed by the CS presence in which cells showed higher viability in BG/PCL/CS at 50 and 100 mg/ml. CS addition in the BG/PCL/CS samples may have slowed down the release of BG into the surrounding and reduces mechanical degradation of the film while enhancing its bioactivity [1], hence the better cell viability observed at doses lower than 100 mg/ml. However, this needs further exploration towards several types of cells and future works should address this issue since the material is targeted for wound healing use, human skin fibroblasts should be the next evaluation target. Besides, different cells will provide different responses and the cells chosen must reflect the intended application of the film. Furthermore, other parameters should be included in biocompatibility assessments such as scratch assay, functional assay for skin fibroblast and gene expression study.

4 Conclusion

The study implies the effects of different BG/PCL/CS conditioned medium extracts on HMSC where concentration at 200 mg/ml is toxic to the cells. Despite fluctuation of certain dose from 0.78 mg/ml to 100 mg/ml, the 3.12 mg/ml of BG/PCL/CS conditioned medium extract showed highest HMSC cell viability when compared to other concentration which may highlights certain dose may be suitable for certain types of cells.

The pH of the samples overall showed a decreasing trend towards pH 7.0 at final equilibrium and longer duration is needed with medium replenishment at certain time points to avoid saturation of samples dissolution into the SBF which may contribute to plateau pH value.

Acknowledgements The authors would like to thank the Ministry of Education (MOE) through Prototype Research Grant Scheme (PRGS) Project No. PRGS/2/2020/SKK07/USM/02/2 (203.CIPPT.6740075).

References

1. Motealleh, A., Eqtesadi, S., Pajares, A., Miranda, P.: Enhancing the mechanical and in vitro performance of robocast bioglass scaffolds by polymeric coatings: effect of polymer composition. J. Mech. Behav. Biomed. Mater. **84**, 35–45 (2018)
2. Naseri, S., Lepry, W.C., Nazhat, S.N.: Bioactive glasses in wound healing: hope or hype? J. Mater. Chem. B **5**(31), 6167–6174 (2017)

3. Kargozar, S., Montazerian, M., Fiume, E., Baino, F.: Multiple and promising applications of Strontium (Sr)-containing bioactive glasses in bone tissue engineering. Front. Bioeng. Biotechnol. **7**, 161 (2019)
4. Jones, J.R.: Reprint of: review of bioactive glass: from Hench to hybrids. Acta Biomater. **23**, S53-82 (2015)
5. Maçon, A.L.B., Page, S.J., Chung, J.J., Amdursky, N., Stevens, M.M., Weaver, J.V.M., et al.: A structural and physical study of sol-gel methacrylate-silica hybrids: intermolecular spacing dictates the mechanical properties. Phys. Chem. Chem. Phys. **17**(43), 29124–29133 (2015)
6. Janowska, A., Dini, V., Oranges, T., Iannone, M., Loggini, B., Romanelli, M.: Atypical ulcers: diagnosis and management. Clin. Interv. Aging **14**, 2137–2143 (2019)
7. Yao, Q., Li, W., Yu, S., Ma, L., Jin, D., Boccaccini, A.R., et al.: Multifunctional chitosan/polyvinyl pyrrolidone/45S5 Bioglass® scaffolds for MC3T3-E1 cell stimulation and drug release. Mater. Sci. Eng. C **56**, 473–480 (2015)
8. Woodruff, M.A., Hutmacher, D.W.: The return of a forgotten polymer—Polycaprolactone in the 21st century. In: Progress in Polymer Science (Oxford), vol. 35. Elsevier Ltd, pp. 1217–1256 (2010)
9. Aliaa, N.S.N.S., Fazliah, M.N.S.N., Fatimah, S.S., Syazana, A.N.: Synthesis and characterization of PLA-PEG biocomposite incorporated with sol-gel derived 45S5 bioactive glass. Materials Today: Proc., 982–988 (2019)
10. Kokubo, T., Takadama, H.: How useful is SBF in predicting in vivo bone bioactivity? Biomaterials **27**(15), 2907–2915 (2006)
11. Salgado, A.J., Figueiredo, J.E., Coutinho, O.P., Reis, R.L.: Biological response to premineralized starch based scaffolds for bone tissue engineering. J. Mater. Sci. Mater. Med. **16**(3), 267–275 (2005)
12. Poh, P.S.P., Hutmacher, D.W., Holzapfel, B.M., Solanki, A.K., Stevens, M.M., Woodruff, M.A.: In vitro and in vivo bone formation potential of surface calcium phosphate-coated polycaprolactone and polycaprolactone/bioactive glass composite scaffolds. Acta Biomater. **30**, 319–333 (2016)
13. Poh, P.S.P., Hutmacher, D.W., Stevens, M.M., Woodruff, M.A.: Fabrication and in vitro characterization of bioactive glass composite scaffolds for bone regeneration. Biofabrication **5**(4), 45005 (2013)
14. Yin, J., Xu, L.: Batch preparation of electrospun polycaprolactone/chitosan/aloe vera blended nanofiber membranes for novel wound dressing. Int. J. Biol. Macromol. **160**, 352–363 (2010)
15. Wallace, K.E., Hill, R.G., Pembroke, J.T., Brown, C.J., Hatton, P.V.: Influence of sodium oxide content on bioactive glass properties. J. Mater. Sci. Mater. Med. **10**(12), 697–701 (1999)
16. Azevedo, M.M., Tsigkou, O., Nair, R., Jones, J.R., Jell, G., Stevens, M.M.: Hypoxia inducible factor-stabilizing bioactive glasses for directing mesenchymal stem cell behavior. Tissue Eng—Part A **21**(1–2), 382–389 (2015)
17. Gentleman, E., Fredholm, Y.C., Jell, G., Lotfibakhshaiesh, N., O'Donnell, M.D., Hill, R.G., et al.: The effects of strontium-substituted bioactive glasses on osteoblasts and osteoclasts in vitro. Biomaterials **31**(14), 3949–3956 (2010)
18. da Silva, J.G., Babb, R., Salzlechner, C., Sharpe, P.T., Brauer, D.S., Gentleman, E.: Optimisation of lithium-substituted bioactive glasses to tailor cell response for hard tissue repair. J. Mater. Sci. **52**(15), 8832–8844 (2017)
19. Ciraldo, F.E., Boccardi, E., Melli, V., Westhauser, F., Boccaccini, A.R.: Tackling bioactive glass excessive in vitro bioreactivity: Preconditioning approaches for cell culture tests. Acta Biomater. **75**, 3–10 (2018)
20. Nommeots-Nomm, A., Labbaf, S., Devlin, A., Todd, N., Geng, H., Solanki, A.K., et al.: Highly degradable porous melt-derived bioactive glass foam scaffolds for bone regeneration. Acta Biomater. **57**, 449–461 (2017)

Cellulose Isolation from Oil Palm Empty Fruit Bunch (OPEFB) via Alkaline Hydrogen Peroxide Treatment

Nurul Athirah Syafiqah Mohamad Zulkifli, Farina Muhamad, and Bee Chin Ang

Abstract Waste-derived biomaterial is one of the approaches to support environmental sustainability by practising waste recycling and reducing the use of natural, raw materials. In Malaysia, oil palm empty fruit bunch (OPEFB) is one of the underutilized lignocellulosic waste which is commonly disposed due to its large production from palm oil extraction milling. Its high cellulose content makes it suitable for waste-derived cellulose synthesis whereby it can be extracted via alkaline hydrogen peroxide mechanism. The OPEFB waste was treated with 5% (v/v) hydrogen peroxide at pH 11.5, 70 °C for 90 min. The colour change of the sample was observed and its chemical structure was analyzed using FTIR. The result revealed that the colour of the sample changed from brown to white after the chemical treatment. The FTIR analysis showed that there was bound lignin and hemicellulose on the sample based on the weak intensity of the compounds indicative peak, suggesting that the cellulose obtained via this method was not 100% pure. This research work suggests more study on the percentage of the residual lignin and hemicellulose and its effect on the cytotoxicity of the cellulose as a biomaterial for biomedical application.

Keywords Cellulose isolation · Oil palm empty fruit bunch (OPEFB) · Hydrogen peroxide

N. A. S. Mohamad Zulkifli · F. Muhamad (✉)
Department of Biomedical Engineering, Faculty of Engineering, Universiti Malaya, Kuala Lumpur, Malaysia
e-mail: farinamuhamad@um.edu.my

B. C. Ang
Department of Chemical Engineering, Faculty of Engineering, Universiti Malaya, Kuala Lumpur, Malaysia

F. Muhamad · B. C. Ang
Center of Advanced Materials, Faculty of Engineering, Universiti Malaya, Kuala Lumpur, Malaysia

J. Usman et al. (eds.), *6th Kuala Lumpur International Conference on Biomedical Engineering 2021*, IFMBE Proceedings 86,
https://doi.org/10.1007/978-3-030-90724-2_56

1 Introduction

Environmental sustainability is one of the important pillars of sustainable development goals (SDG) aligned by the United Nations (UN). It was highlighted in the 12th SDG goal which is "Responsible Consumption and Production" whereby one of the targets is to cut down the production of waste through prevention, reduction, recycling and reuse by 2030 [1]. In promoting environmental sustainability for biomaterials application, valorization of biomass has opened a new avenue in biomaterials fabrication which includes deriving functional biopolymer from the underutilized biomass such as lignin, cellulose, chitosan and silk.

Cellulose is one of the biopolymers that can be found in abundance in nature. However, cellulose extraction from biomass and waste such as rye straw, wheat straw, oil palm empty fruit bunch (OPEFB) and paper waste should become the new direction to produce a functional biomaterial for biomedical application. Apart from solving the waste generation arise from improper waste management, the recycling of the underutilized lignocellulosic waste can provide a cheaper alternative for biomaterial fabrication as compared to resorting the cellulose from the market industry which is not cost-effective.

Chemical treatment using hydrogen peroxide, sodium chlorite and sodium hypochlorite are among the common treatment used to isolate the cellulose from the waste which is also known as bleaching treatment. In this process, the bleaching agents are responsible for the delignification and hemicellulose dissolution from the fibres, leaving only the cellulosic structure after the treatment. The degree of delignification and hemicellulose dissolution varies depending on the type of bleaching agent used. According to Sun et al. [2], cellulose isolation by using sodium chlorite is more effective as compared to hydrogen peroxide. Nevertheless, there is some issue with regards to the toxicity of the byproduct of cellulose isolation by using sodium chlorite. Nazir et al. [3] reported that the chlorite from the acidified sodium chlorite; a common reagent for cellulose isolation may generate a chlorine radical which reacts and disintegrates the lignocellulosic material to become a very toxic organochlorine. This was supported by Lamaming et al. [4] who have mentioned that the use of the conventional chlorine-based reagents may impose a negative impact on human health and also on the environment. Thus, a non-chlorine based bleaching agent such as hydrogen peroxide is found to be a better alternative to extract the cellulose from the waste.

Several research works have been carried out to isolate the cellulose from waste such as office paper waste [5], oil palm biomass [6, 7], banana peels [8] and bagasse [9]. In Malaysia, the oil palm industry is one of the most significant sectors that drive the economy of the country. The palm oil extracted is only accounted for ~10% and another ~90% is left as biomass, which becomes a challenge in terms of its disposal [10, 11]. The oil palm by-product is produced from pruning, harvesting, milling and replanting activities [12]. There are six main types of biomasses produced which are oil palm fronds (OPF), oil palm trunks (OPT), empty fruit bunches (EFB), palm kernel shells (PKS), mesocarp fibres (MF) and palm oil mill effluent (POME). To address this issue, these oil palm wastes were utilized in various applications in an effort to reduce the waste disposal. Such examples are OPF and OPT were used as animal feedstock [13], MF was exploited for boiler fuel, PKS was recycled as road paving material [14] whereas EFB was converted into soil conditioner [15, 16], bio-oil [17] and fibreboard [18]. However, in the case of bio-oil from EFB, the pyrolysis process will produce a very complex bio-oil due to its high water content and viscosity, which makes it difficult for commercialization [19]. Furthermore, despite these various efforts, there are still a large amount of biomass to be handled which makes the only option left is to either burn them or left at the plantations, which lead to environmental problems and underutilization of lignocellulosic feedstock [20].

In this research work, the objective is to isolate the cellulose from the OPEFB waste by using hydrogen peroxide as the bleaching agent with the aim of further use this biomaterial for biomedical application. The colour change and chemical structure of the end product will be compared with the raw sample for any differences.

2 Materials and Method

2.1 Materials

Oil palm empty fruit bunch (OPEFB) waste collected from Kilang Panji Alam Sawit Sdn Bhd (Kemaman, Terengganu). Sodium hydroxide (NaOH) (Fisher Scientific), Hydrogen peroxide (H_2O_2) (35%) (R&M Chemicals), Denatured ethanol (Chemical Industries (Malaya) Sdn. Bhd.). All chemicals were used as received.

2.2 OPEFB Pretreatment

OPEFB fibres were physically separated, washed with tap water and detergent and rinsed several times to remove soils and dirt from the fibres [3]. Rinsing with tap water was done thoroughly until the used water changed from dark brown to colourless. The cleaned fibres were dried in the oven at 70 °C and proceeded with grinding by using a coffee grinder. The ground OPEFB was then sieved to pass through 150 μm mesh. The ground fibres were labelled as raw OPEFB and dewaxed with 150 mL 70% (v/v) ethanol by using Soxhlet apparatus for six hours to remove wax and oils. The fibres were filtered and washed with distilled water two to three times to remove traces of alcohol. After washing, the dewaxed fibres were dried at 70 °C and kept in a desiccator before further use.

2.3 Cellulose Isolation

The cellulose isolation from OPEFB was based on the methodology by Rayung et al. [21] with some modifications on the ratio of sample to the hydrogen peroxide. Briefly, alkaline bleaching was used as a treatment to isolate the cellulose from OPEFB fibres. The treatment was started by subjecting the dewaxed raw OPEFB in 5% (v/v) hydrogen peroxide at pH 11.5 (adjusted with 6% (wt/v) sodium hydroxide) for 90 min at 70 °C with sample to hydrogen peroxide ratio of 4: 100 (g mL^{-1}). This ratio was chosen because according to Gould [22], the alkaline bleaching using hydrogen peroxide was most effective at this ratio. Following the alkaline bleaching, the sample obtained was filtered and washed with distilled water until neutral pH was achieved. Finally, the sample was dried in an oven at 50 °C for 24 h. This bleached sample was labelled as cellulose-OPEFB.

2.4 Macroscopic Observation

The macroscopic differences of the sample before and after alkaline bleaching treatment was done in terms of its appearance. The images were taken by using a phone camera and processed in the Adobe Photoshop Version 2018 software to remove the appearance of shadows.

2.5 Fourier Transform Infrared Spectroscopy (FTIR) Analysis

FTIR analysis was carried out to confirm the removal of non-cellulosic structure such as lignin and hemicellulose from the fibres. The characterization was done by using Perkin Elmer Spectrum 400 FTIR Spectrometer with scan range in between 400 and 4000 cm^{-1}.

3 Results

3.1 Macroscopic Observation

Figures 1 and 2 show the difference in the appearance of the OPEFB fibres before and after the alkaline bleaching treatment respectively. It can be observed that the colour of the fibres changed significantly after the bleaching process whereby it turned into white as compared to the original sample which was brown.

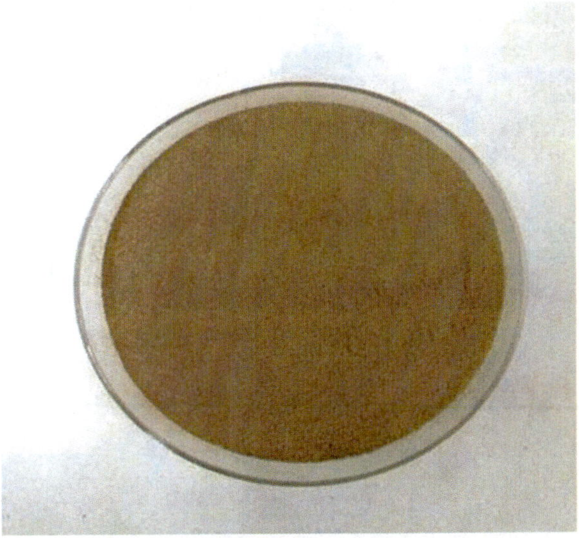

Fig. 1 Raw OPEFB

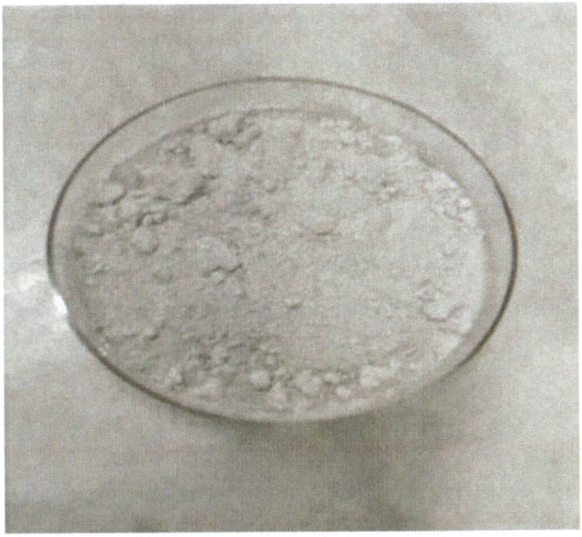

Fig. 2 Cellulose OPEFB

3.2 FTIR Analysis

Figure 3 shows the FTIR spectra of the raw OPEFB and cellulose OPEFB. The peaks around 3300 cm^{-1} and 2900 cm^{-1} represented the stretching of –OH and C–H functional groups respectively [23, 24]. A peak around 1500 cm^{-1} was presented in both spectra, which represent the C=C functional group, indicating the aromatic ring of lignin [21, 25]. However, the intensity of this peak decreased after the alkaline

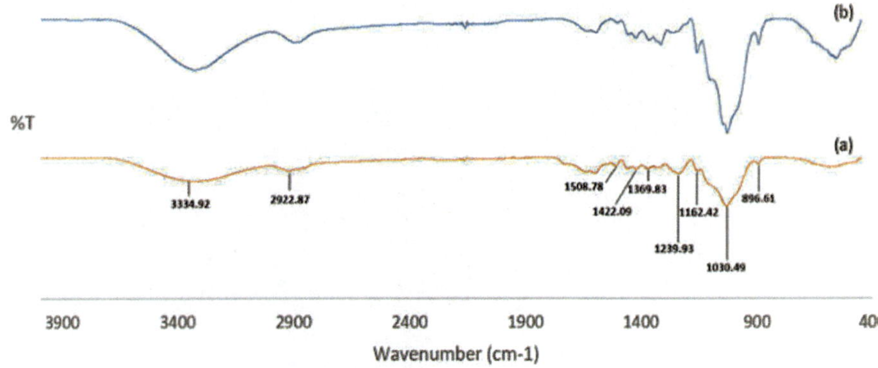

Fig. 3 FTIR spectra of **a** raw OPEFB and **b** cellulose OPEFB

bleaching treatment which implies partial removal of lignin from the fibres. The bending of $-CH_2$ and aromatic ring of polysaccharide were presented in all spectra at peaks around 1420 cm^{-1} and 1369 cm^{-1} respectively [24]. A significant difference in the spectrum was noted at peak 1239.93 cm^{-1} which can be associated with aryl alkyl ether of lignin or C=C and C=O of hemicellulose [25–27]. This peak was shown to be sharply decreased and broader in the cellulose OPEFB sample as compared to the raw OPEFB sample, suggesting that these compounds were mostly removed from the sample. Asymmetrical deformation of C–O–C band was shown at peak 1162 cm^{-1} in both spectra [25]. Peaks at 1030 and 896 cm^{-1} showed the stretching of C–O and C–H of pyranose ring skeleton and β-glycosidic linkage of cellulose, indicating that the structure of the cellulose was not affected throughout the chemical treatment [3, 24, 26]. It was observed that peak 1162, 1030 and 896 cm^{-1} were more prominent after the alkaline bleaching treatment. These changes in spectrum demonstrate the partial hemicellulose dissolution and removal of lignin from the sample.

4 Discussion

In this work, cellulose isolation was done via alkaline bleaching which is based on the alkaline peroxide mechanism. In this treatment, sodium hydroxide was added drop-wise into the hydrogen peroxide producing a solution with pH of more than 11.5 which caused the hydrogen peroxide to dissociate, forming hydroperoxide anion (HOO^-) [22, 28].

$$H_2O_2 + OH^- \rightarrow HOO^- + H_2O \tag{1}$$

This anion is an active bleaching species that attacked the ethylenic and carbonyl groups of the lignin, leading to the conversion of chromophore groups of lignin such as quinones, cinnamaldehyde and ring-conjugated ketoses to nonchromophoric species [29]. This consequently bleached the fibres as shown in Fig. 2, whereby the colour of the fibres turned into white after the chemical treatment. The hydroperoxide anion also reacted with the undissociated hydrogen peroxide to produce highly reactive hydroxyl radicals ($HO^{\cdot}$) and superoxide anion radicals ($O_2^{-\cdot}$) [22].

$$H_2O_2 + HOO^- \rightarrow HO^{\cdot} + O_2^{-\cdot} + H_2O \quad (2)$$

These radicals caused the delignification and hemicellulose breakdown from the fibres. This is shown in the cellulose OPEFB sample whereby there was a decrease in intensity of FTIR peaks at 1500 and 1239.93 cm^{-1}. The weak intensity at peak 1500 cm^{-1} indicates that there was some bound lignin in the sample, implying that lignin was partially removed during the treatment. This agrees with other research works which used the same mechanism with different parameters whereby lignin indicative peak with weak intensity was detected after the bleaching treatment by using the hydrogen peroxide [21, 29, 30].

The broad, low intensity peak 1239.93 cm^{-1} of hemicellulose is consistent with the result obtained by Lamaming et al. [26] whereby in their study, the hemicellulose indicative peak was sharply decreased after bleaching treatment with acidified sodium chlorite and potassium hydroxide. However, in another study that carried out the cellulose extraction via alkaline peroxide mechanism, this hemicellulose peak was absent after the extraction process with 35% hydrogen peroxide concentration. Nevertheless, it was reported that bound hemicellulose was still presented in the bleached sample based on the chemical composition analysis [27].

This study supports the previous literature that the use of alkaline hydrogen peroxide can only partially remove the lignin from the raw fibres. Furthermore, the presence of hemicellulose residue was parallel with other research work that used sodium chlorite as the bleaching agent. However, FTIR analysis should be further supported with the quantitative analysis whereby the percentage of the bound lignin and hemicellulose should be calculated to evaluate the weight ratio of these bound compounds and the purity of the sample. According to Nakasone and Kobayashi [31], the impurity of the cellulose involving lignin can be reduced by pre-treating the sample with sodium hydroxide for prolong time. In this study, the authors pre-treated the sugarcane bagasse with 10% sodium hydroxide for different periods which were 1, 6 and 12 h prior to bleaching with sodium hypochlorite. The result showed that the sample that was treated with sodium hydroxide for 12 h had the lowest lignin bound percentage which was 0.68%. This suggests more improvement to this current study in order to obtain high purity cellulose. Furthermore, the cytotoxicity study of the sample should also be carried out in order to evaluate the effect of residual lignin and hemicellulose in cellulose for biomedical application.

The obtained cellulose from waste is beneficial as a biomaterial due to its resemblance with the hard tissue in terms of its mechanical properties, which suggests its further application as a bone graft in bone substitution [32]. Moreover, cellulose has been explored as a promising candidate in hybrid material fabrication whereby cellulose hybrid materials can be suited for bone tissue engineering application [32] and drug delivery [33].

5 Conclusion

Cellulose has been successfully isolated from the OPEFB waste with some bound lignin and hemicellulose residue in the sample. This was confirmed by the colour of the sample after the alkaline hydrogen peroxide treatment and FTIR spectra which showed the peak representing the presence of lignin and hemicellulose but with low intensity. This work suggests further research on the evaluation of the purity percentage of the cellulose and the impact of these residues on the cytotoxicity of the material for biomedical application.

References

1. United Nations. https://www.un.org/development/desa/disabilities/envision2030-goal12.html. Last accessed 15 May 2021
2. Sun, J.X., Sun, X.F., Zhao, H., Sun, R.C.: Isolation and characterization of cellulose from sugarcane bagasse. Polym. Degrad. Stab. **84**(2), 331–339 (2004)
3. Nazir, M.S., Wahjoedi, B.A., Yussof, A.W., Abdullah, M.A.: Eco-friendly extraction and characterization of cellulose from oil palm empty fruit bunches. BioResources **8**(2), 2161–2172 (2013)
4. Lamaming, J., Hashim, R., Leh, C.P., Sulaiman, O.: Properties of cellulose nanocrystals from oil palm trunk isolated by total chlorine free method. Carbohyd. Polym. **156**, 409–416 (2017)
5. Orue, A., Santamaria-Echart, A., Eceiza, A., Peña-Rodriguez, C., Arbelaiz, A.: Office waste paper as cellulose nanocrystal source. J. Appl. Polym. Sci. **134**, 45257 (2017)
6. Daud, W.R.W., Kassim, M.H.M., Mohamded, M.A.S.: Cellulose phosphate from oil palm biomass as potential biomaterials. BioResources **6**(2), 1719–1740 (2011)
7. Mohamad Haafiz, M.K., Eichhorn, S.J., Hassan, A. Jawaid, M.: Isolation and characterization of microcrystalline cellulose from oil palm biomass residue. Carbohyd. Polym. **93**(2), 628–634 (2013)
8. Tibolla, H., Pelissari, F.M., Martins, J.T., Vicente, A.A., Menegalli, F.C.: Cellulose nanofibers produced from banana peel by chemical and mechanical treatments: characterization and cytotoxicity assessment. Food Hydrocoll. **75**, 192–201 (2018)
9. de Oliveira, F.B., Bras, J., Pimenta, M.T.B., da Silva Curvelo, A.A., Belgacem, M.N.: Production of cellulose nanocrystals from sugarcane bagasse fibers and pith. Indus. Crops Prod. **93**, 48–57 (2016)
10. Kurnia, J.C., Jangam, S.V., Akhtar, S., Sasmito, A.P., Mujumdar. A.S.: Advances in biofuel production from oil palm and palm oil processing wastes: a review. Biofuel Res. J. **3**(1), 332–346 (2016)
11. Abdullah, N., Sulaiman, F., Aliasak, Z.: A case study of pyrolysis of oil palm wastes in Malaysia. In: AIP Conference Proceedings, pp. 331–336. American Institute of Physics (2013)
12. Loh, S.K.: The potential of the Malaysian oil palm biomass as a renewable energy source. Energy Convers. Manage. **141**, 285–298 (2017)
13. Awalludin, M.F., Sulaiman, O., Hashim, R., Nadhari, W.N.A.W.: An overview of the oil palm industry in Malaysia and its waste utilization through thermochemical conversion, specifically via liquefaction. Renew. Sustain. Energy Rev. **50**, 1469–1484 (2015)
14. Sulaiman, F., Abdullah, N., Gerhauser, H., Shariff, A.: An outlook of Malaysian energy, oil palm industry and its utilization of wastes as useful resources. Biomass Bioenerg. **35**(9), 3775–3786 (2011)
15. Yusoff, S.: Renewable energy from palm oil–innovation on effective utilization of waste. J. Clean. Prod. **14**(1), 87–93 (2006)

16. Shuit, S.H., Tan, K.T., Lee, K.T., Kamaruddin, A.H.: Oil palm biomass as a sustainable energy source: a Malaysian case study. Energy **34**(9), 1225–1235 (2009)
17. Abdullah, N., Sulaiman, F., Gerhauser, H.: Characterisation of oil palm empty fruit bunches for fuel application. J. Phys. Sci. **22**(1), 1–24 (2011)
18. Prasertsan, S., Prasertsan, P.: Biomass residues from palm oil mills in Thailand: an overview on quantity and potential usage. Biomass Bioenerg. **11**(5), 387–395 (1996)
19. Geng, A.: Conversion of oil palm fruit bunch to biofuels. In: Liquid, Gaseous and Solid Biofuels: Conversion Techniques, pp. 479-490. InTech Open Access Publisher, London (2013)
20. Onoja, E., Chandren, S., Razak, F.I.A., Mahat, N.A., Wahab, R.A.: Oil palm (Elaeis guineensis) biomass in Malaysia: the present and future prospects. Waste and Biomass Valorization **10**(8), 2099–2117 (2019)
21. Rayung, M., Ibrahim, N.A., Zainuddin, N., Saad, W.Z., Razak, N.I.A., Chieng, B.W.: The effect of fiber bleaching treatment on the properties of poly (lactic acid)/oil palm empty fruit bunch fiber composites. Int. J. Mol. Sci. **15**(8), 14728–14742 (2014)
22. Gould, J.M.: Studies on the mechanism of alkaline peroxide delignification of agricultural residues. Biotechnol. Bioeng. **27**(3), 225–231 (1985)
23. Khalil, H.P.S.A., Ismail, H., Rozman, H.D., Ahmad, M.N.: The effect of acetylation on interfacial shear strength between plant fibres and various matrices. Eur. Polym. J. **37**(5), 1037–1045 (2001)
24. Kargarzadeh, H., Ahmad, I., Abdullah, I., Dufresne, A., Zainudin, S.Y., Sheltami, R.M.: Effects of hydrolysis conditions on the morphology, crystallinity, and thermal stability of cellulose nanocrystals extracted from kenaf bast fibers. Cellulose **19**(3), 855–866 (2012)
25. Ching, Y.C., Ng, T.S.: Effect of preparation conditions on cellulose from oil palm empty fruit bunch fiber. BioResources **9**(4), 6373–6385 (2014)
26. Lamaming, J., Hashim, R., Sulaiman, O., Leh, C.P., Sugimoto, T., Nordin, N.A.: Cellulose nanocrystals isolated from oil palm trunk. Carbohyd. Polym. **127**, 202–208 (2015)
27. Tuerxun, D., Pulingam, T., Nordin, N.I., Chen, Y.W., Kamaldin, J.B., Julkapli, N.B.M., Lee, H.V., Leo, B.F., Johan, M.R.B.: Synthesis, characterization and cytotoxicity studies of nanocrystalline cellulose from the production waste of rubber-wood and kenaf-bast fibers. Eur. Polym. J. **116**, 352–360 (2019)
28. Sun, R.C., Tomkinson, J., Ma, P.L., Liang, S.F.: Comparative study of hemicelluloses from rice straw by alkali and hydrogen peroxide treatments. Carbohyd. Polym. **42**(2), 111–122 (2000)
29. Fang, J.M., Sun, R.C., Tomkinson, J.: Isolation and characterization of hemicelluloses and cellulose from rye straw by alkaline peroxide extraction. Cellulose **7**(1), 87–107 (2000)
30. Tezcan, E., Atıcı, O.: Isolation of cellulose and hemicellulose by using alkaline peroxide treatment at room temperature from wasted fall leaves. Nat. Eng. Sci. **2**(2), 100–110 (2017)
31. Nakasone, K., Kobayashi, T.: Cytocompatible cellulose hydrogels containing trace lignin. Mater. Sci. Eng., C **64**, 269–277 (2016)
32. Salama, A., El-Sakhawy, M.: Regenerated cellulose/wool blend enhanced biomimetic hydroxyapatite mineralization. Int. J. Biol. Macromol. **92**, 920–925 (2016)
33. Salama, A., El-Sakhawy, M., Kamel, S.: Carboxymethyl cellulose based hybrid material for sustained release of protein drugs. Int. J. Biol. Macromol. **93**, 1647–1652 (2016)

Identifying Bioglass and Liquid Exfoliation of Graphite/MWCNT Mixtures Through UV–Vis Spectroscopy

Siti Fatimah Samsurrijal, Nik Syahirah Aliaa Nik Sharifulden, Nur Syazana Azizan, David Yi San Chau, and Siti Noor Fazliah Mohd Noor

Abstract Carbon allotropes such as graphene and multiwalled carbon nanotube (MWCNT) are studied for an extensive range of applications. Various exfoliation techniques were employed to yield the best form of generated allotropes. Liquid phase exfoliation utilizes the technique of sonication of these allotropes in the solvent, results in the best desired form of the high quality, safe, simple and economically viable final product. This study discusses liquid-phase exfoliation of graphene and MWCNT in chloroform. Their absorbance intensity has shown a contrast solubility profile with respect to different weight percentages of each allotrope. The comparative study was further analyzed with modification of bioglass (BG) within the suspensions, of which hazards in agglomerations of allotropes' particles as concentration increases could potentially give a prevention insight for better preparation and processing materials formulation. Hence the study aims in reporting UV absorbance intensity of various weight percentages of liquid exfoliated graphene and MWCNT particles, with the addition of BG in chloroform due to their unique structures and remarkable properties and their exploitation in diverse potential applications, including the biomedical engineering field especially in the field of bone tissue engineering.

Keywords Graphene · MWCNT · Bioglass

S. F. Samsurrijal · N. S. Azizan · S. N. F. M. Noor (✉)
Craniofacial and Biomaterial Sciences Cluster, Advanced Medical and Dental Institute, Universiti Sains Malaysia, Bertam Campus, 13200 Kepala Batas, Pulau Pinang, Malaysia
e-mail: fazliah@usm.my

N. S. A. N. Sharifulden · D. Y. S. Chau
Division of Biomaterials and Tissue Engineering, UCL Eastman Dental Institute, University College London, Royal Free Hospital, Rowland Hill Street, London NW3 2PF, UK

S. N. F. M. Noor
Dental Stimulation and Visual Learning, Research Excellence Consortium, Advanced Medical and Dental Institute, Universiti Sains Malaysia, Bertam Campus, 13200 Kepala Batas, Pulau Pinang, Malaysia

J. Usman et al. (eds.), *6th Kuala Lumpur International Conference on Biomedical Engineering 2021*, IFMBE Proceedings 86,
https://doi.org/10.1007/978-3-030-90724-2_57

1 Introduction

Graphene, known to be a wonder material, made its experimental breakthrough in 2004 via micromechanical exfoliation from graphite. It comprises sp^2 bonded carbon atoms arranged in a honeycomb lattice two-dimensional (2D) single layer. Knowing to exhibit various and distinct mechanical, physical, electrical and thermal properties, graphene has been extensively studied in several applications in its early research stage, including supercapacitors, energy storage, sensors and nanocomposites [1, 2]. Graphene compiles and demonstrates unique properties by having high surface area, high Young's modulus, excellent thermal and electrical characteristics and distinct optical properties making the material attractive for exploitation in the biomedical field. Current and ongoing research on utilizing graphene and its derivatives range from drug delivery, biosensing to the development of biomedical devices for healthcare engineering applications [3–5].

To date, various techniques have been employed to generate graphene. Importantly, considering the dynamic and detailed development of the various industries, significant efforts were devoted to ensuring that a reproducible, non-structural defective, and high-quality material could be obtained. In brief, the preparation of graphene can be categorized as either a "bottom-up" or a "top-down" approach. The former category can be further divided into examples such as epitaxial growth and chemical vapour deposition (CVD), which enable the production of large-sized graphene. However, these approaches display some drawbacks in producing limited dimensions and utilize very high working temperatures, hence hindering the production of high-quality graphene that is usually economically viable [6]. Meanwhile, examples of top-down approaches such as pioneers mechanical cleavage and the Hummers' method are much more desirable as they are able to yield graphene at reasonably low cost: however, both methods suffer from low-scale production and generate graphene with structural defects [6, 7]. As such, a more reliable top-down method to produce graphene via liquid-phase exfoliation has gained significant interest as it is not only able to produce high-quality graphene but is also simple, safe, and economically viable [1, 8].

Liquid phase exfoliation of graphene is the action of utilizing sonication in exfoliating a monolayer or few-layer defect-free graphene from graphite in the solvent. The mechanism purposely detaches the Van der Waals forces between graphene layers, within graphite, via propagation of cavitation bubbles from ultrasonic waves through the medium, which induces physical or chemical surface tension within the molecules between the solvent and the forces [1, 6]. There are various solvents studied in exfoliating graphene via liquid-phase exfoliation, with the majority having a surface tension value around 40–50 mJ/m^2 [9]. Some of the most commonly used solvents include DMF (N, N-Dimethylformamide), ODCB (ortho-dichlorobenzene), and chloroform. Each solvent requires a different sonication period which consequently generates graphene at different concentrations [9].

Meanwhile, another form of carbon allotrope, multiwalled carbon nanotubes (MWCNTs), has also gained much interest within the research environment due to its optical, mechanical and electrical properties. MWCNTs are essentially rolled graphene sheets that allures to it having similar characteristics to graphene. However, due to the high aspect ratio and stronger π–π interactions between the tubes, MWCNTs are hindered by their solubility in organic and aqueous solvents, leading to the consequent aggregation in these media and also difficulties in large-scale processing and manufacture [10, 11]. As such, the functionalization of these carbon allotropes is one of the most studied areas to improve their native solubility and contribute to the overall characteristics of composites especially for novel applications such as biomedical and healthcare engineering.

On the other hand, bioactive glass (BG) is a type of bio-ceramics that exhibits biocompatibility, biodegradability and excellent bioactivity, antibacterial and anti-inflammatory properties [12]. This material can also form an apatite layer on its surface upon contact with physiological fluid, which subsequently induces angiogenesis [13]. The exploitation and modification of BG have always been the subject of interest due to the natural brittleness of BG's structure where its distinct features support and improve cells adhesion either by itself or when being incorporated into biomaterials, offers a great deal of potential to many applications.

Therefore, this study reports in detail the generation of graphene via liquid-phase exfoliation in chloroform with respect to the different weight percentage of graphite powder, alongside an additional comparative study against MWCNT. Subsequently, this present study will provide a comparative insight into the absorbance intensity, via UV–Vis analyses, between graphene and MWCNT. In addition, functionalization of the material with BG suspension in chloroform will be assessed and may allow its exploitation in a wide range of diverse applications that include materials science, drug delivery and tissue engineering.

2 Materials and Methods

2.1 Materials

Graphite powder (Cat. No: 104206, Supelco, Merck KGaA, Darmstadt, Germany), multiwalled carbon nanotubes (MWCNTs) (UN19FMW011, Nano Malaysia, USM), 45S5 bioactive glass powder (BG) was synthesized as previously reported [14], chloroform (Sigma Aldrich, Malaysia).

2.2 Exfoliation of Graphene

Liquid exfoliation of graphene was performed in chloroform containing graphite powder in different weight percentages (wt%) from 1.56, 3.125, 6.25 and 12.5 wt%. The solutions were then subjected to sonication using a tabletop sonicator at room temperature (Bandelin, Sonorex) for 120 min, subsequently followed by centrifuge (Eppendorf 5810R, Germany) at 4000 rpm for 30 min [6]. Chloroform without graphite powder was used as a control.

2.3 *Exfoliation of Multiwalled Carbon Nanotubes (MWCNTs)*

Similarly to graphene, MWCNTs were prepared via liquid exfoliation in chloroform with different wt% of 1.56, 3.125, 6.25 and 12.5 wt%. Based on a previous study, MWCNTs require a shorter sonication time of around 10 min [15] before centrifuged at 4000 rpm for 30 min.

2.4 *Preparation of BG Suspension*

BG powder (BG) was prepared according to a previously published paper [14]. The powder was dissolved in chloroform at different wt% of 1, 5, 10, 20 and 30 wt%. In order to obtain a homogenous solution, the mixtures were dispersed via sonication for 120 min before being centrifuged at 4000 rpm for 30 min.

2.5 *Preparation of Graphene/BG and MWCNT/BG Suspension*

Both graphite (G) and MWCNT powder (3 and 6 wt%) was combined with BG powder (1 and 2.5 wt%), with chloroform as the control. Graphite-BG (G-BG) and MWCNT-BG solutions were then subjected to liquid exfoliation by sonicating for 120 min and 10 min respectively, before both were centrifuged at 4000 rpm for 30 min.

2.6 *Absorbance Intensity Study of Exfoliated Suspension*

The absorbance intensity of exfoliated suspensions was studied and analyzed via a UV–Vis spectrometer (Fluostar Omega, BMG Labtech, Germany). The intensity of the suspensions was read at a wavelength between 220 to 800 nm, with chloroform used as the background inside a 96-well plate (Nunclon, Delta Surface, ThermoScientific) with three replicates for each sample.

2.7 *Statistical Analysis*

The samples were prepared in triplicates in the 96-well plate, and the results are presented as mean values and standard deviation (Mean ± SD). All the data were statistically analyzed via OriginLab software (Origin Lab, Northampton, USA) and SPSS Version 26 (IBM Inc, Armonk, NY, USA).

3 Results and Discussions

3.1 *Exfoliation of Graphene in Chloroform*

Figure 1 shows broad peaks of graphene intensity for different weight percentages recorded at around 255 and 290 nm. Although more significant peaks are expected similar to other previous studies [16–18], however, the broad peaks obtained in this work might most likely due to batch-to-batch variation of the starting material and the limited maximum absorbance range detected by the machine. Nonetheless, the appearance of anticipated characteristic absorption peak approximately at ~270 nm

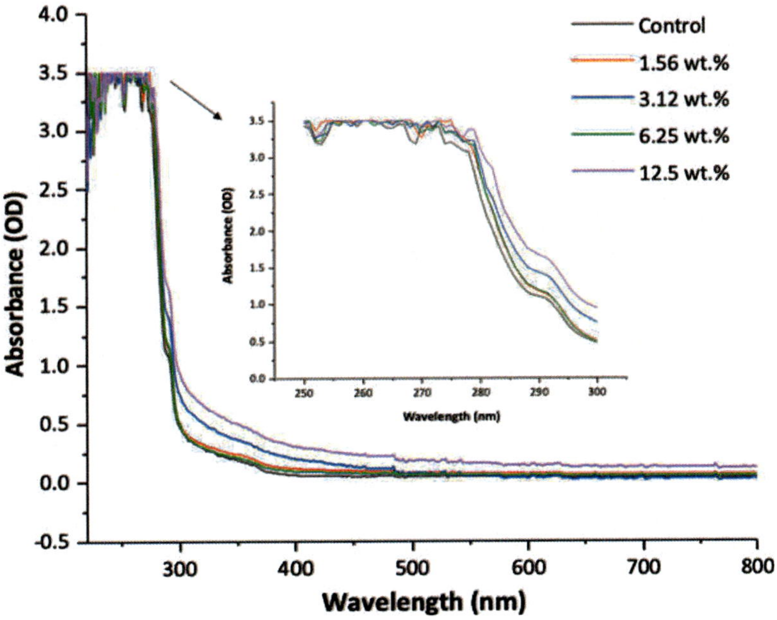

Fig. 1 UV absorbance intensity of different weight percentage of liquid exfoliated graphene in chloroform. Insert figure shows an apparent plateau absorption region ranging from 250 to 300 nm

wavelength was seen, indicating graphene dispersion for all different weight percentages of graphite powder that corresponds to the restored (–conjugation network transition of C–O bonds of graphene [5, 6]. The UV absorbance peaks show an increasing trend, clearly shown in the wavelengths range from 280 nm towards 500 nm, as the weight percentage of graphite increases from 1.56 to 12.5 wt%. However, the graphite powder at 6.25 wt%, shows low absorbance intensity in the range almost similar to that of the control sample, between the wavelengths range from 300 to 800 nm. This decrease is likely due to the potential starting of agglomeration of graphite powder or sample error where the graphite powder was accidentally included in the well plate during reading inside the microplate reader. The general profile trend displays in Fig. 1 shown an increment in radiation being absorbed as the concentration increases, as absorbance is directly proportional to concentration.

3.2 *Exfoliation of Multiwalled Carbon Nanotubes (MWCNTs) in Chloroform*

For MWCNT in chloroform, Fig. 2 shows a similar broad peaks appearance to UV absorbance intensity of different weight percentage of liquid exfoliated graphene in chloroform. The absorbance bands can be seen at approximately ~262 nm, attributed

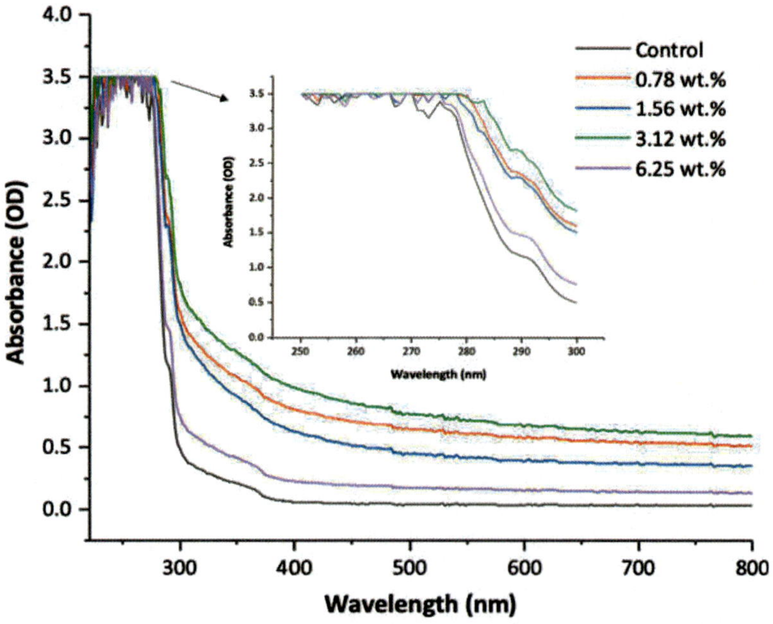

Fig. 2 UV absorbance intensity of different weight percentage of liquid exfoliated MWCNT in chloroform. Insert figure shows an apparent plateau absorption region ranging from 250 to 300 nm

to C=C bonds and also the dispersion into individual nanotubes of MWCNTs [10]. However, the results show opposite trend to graphene, whereby decreasing the MWCNT weight percentages increases absorbance intensity. An exception is observed for the 3.12 wt% MWCNT sample that demonstrated the highest absorbance intensity profile, which corresponds to wavelength range between 300 and 800 nm, for liquid exfoliation of MWCNT in chloroform. This shows that MWCNT is the most stable at 3.12 wt% with minimal agglomeration sign, possibly due to the lowest Van der Waals forces between the particle and solvent, which prevents the dynamic entanglement process. This weight percentage can potentially be addressed as the optimized concentration of MWCNT sonicated in chloroform. However, further exploration is needed since the sonication time was chosen to be within 10 min only in this work. The trend exhibited by MWCNTs shows that as concentration increases, absorbance intensity decreases, which indicates the presence of sedimentation of large particles due to agglomeration within MWCNTs [19]. This may be attributed to the air bubbles formed naturally through bridging during sonication of MWCNT that undoubtedly promotes agglomeration.

3.3 Exfoliation of BG Suspension in Chloroform

A comparative study for BG suspension in chloroform before adding graphene and MWCNT is shown in Fig. 3. An extensive absorption band of BG at approximately 200–300 nm similar to other published paper [20] was observed, indicating the presence of Fe^{3+} and Fe^{2+} iron impurities in the reactant. The presence of these ions resulted in intense broad band of UV absorbance intensity in a range from 200 to 300 nm which might be possible due to the presence of more than one site of both iron species of Fe^{3+} and Fe^{2+} that can be detected in glasses [20]. As the concentration of the BG increases from 1 to 20 wt%, the absorbance spectroscopy shows increased intensity in the visible range of wavelength from 300 to 500 nm. A drop in the absorbance intensity at the higher weight percentage of BG (i.e. 30 wt%) is observed, which may occur due to the commencement of particle agglomeration.

3.4 Exfoliation of Graphene/BG Suspension in Chloroform

As for graphene-BG suspensions, Fig. 4 demonstrates that absorbance intensity increases proportionally to the concentration of the material; the highest intensity being graphite (6 wt%) and BG powder (2.5 wt%), as shown in Fig. 4b. This shows the complementary relationship between both materials with the enhancement of absorbance intensity after the addition of BG. The selection for graphite and BG concentrations were based on previous sections, where average range of graphite was selected, and subsequently improvising the formulation with low concentration of BG to observe any possible effects induced by BG within the suspensions.

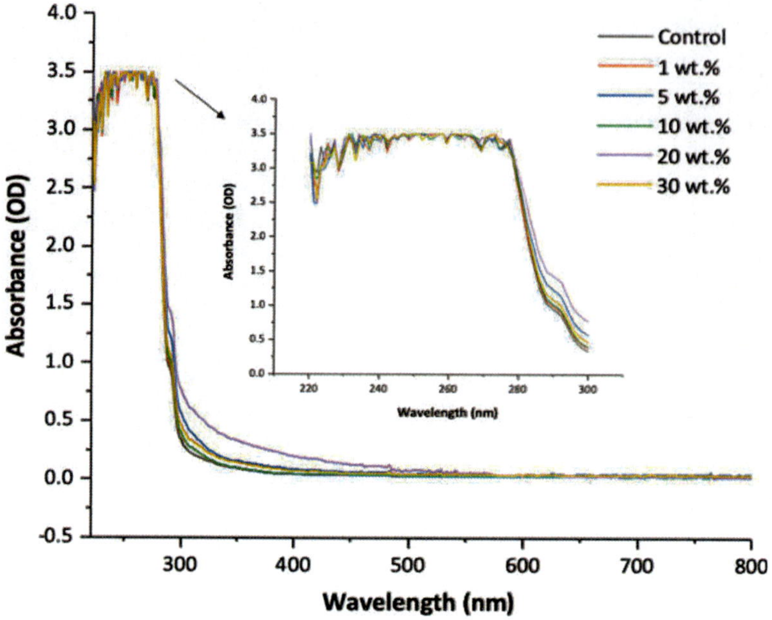

Fig. 3 UV absorbance intensity of different weight percentage of BG suspension in chloroform. Insert figure shows an apparent plateau absorption region ranging from 250 to 300 nm

The BG concentration was chosen to be less than 10 wt% since higher BG resulted in agglomeration within the suspension (data not shown). Furthermore, the results illustrate a stable exfoliation of graphene with similar trend shown in Fig. 1. Interestingly, at even higher concentration of graphite 6 wt%, which previously shown low absorbance intensity as compared to other concentrations as discussed in Sect. 3.1, displays no signs of agglomeration after addition of BG. It is assumed that addition of BG plays an important role in enhancing the solubility feature of graphene in chloroform. This being a vital characteristic in any physiological application.

3.5 Exfoliation of MWCNT/BG Suspension in Chloroform

On the other hand, Fig. 5 shows a trend which displays further agglomeration drawbacks of MWCNTs at higher concentration (6 wt%). MWCNTs has shown the most stable state and higher intensity at a weight percentage of 3 wt% with the addition of 2.5 wt% BG, in contrast to a higher concentration of MWCNTs as depicted in Fig. 5a, b. In comparison to Fig. 2, a drop in absorbance intensity values can be seen for all concentrations of MWCNTs, even after incorporation of BG, which might be due to either further agglomerations of both particles or dominant of lower absorbance

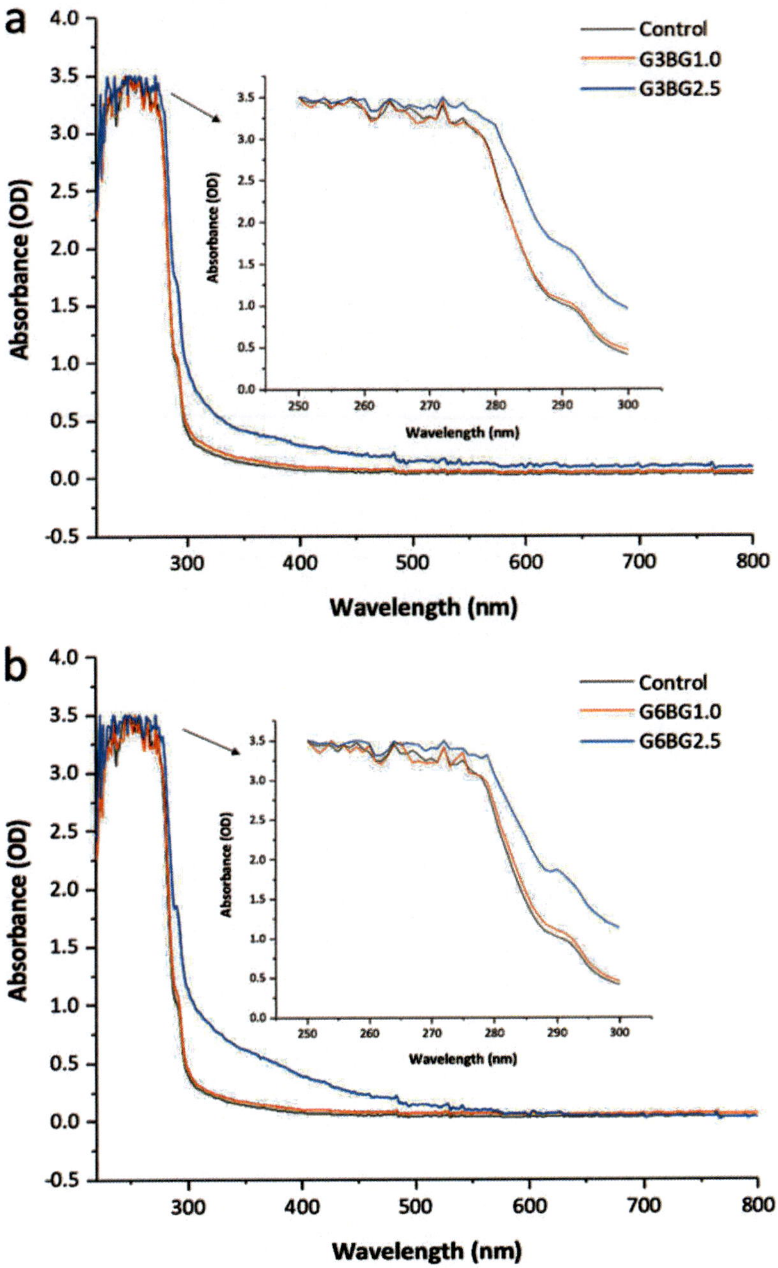

Fig. 4 UV absorbance intensity of liquid exfoliated graphene-BG suspension in chloroform. Different weight percentages of graphite (G) and BG used for comparisons as shown in **a** 3 wt% of G exfoliated with 1 and 2.5 wt% of BG, respectively and **b** 6 wt% of G exfoliated with 1 and 2.5 wt% of BG, respectively. Insert figures show respective clearer plateau absorption region ranging from 250 to 300 nm

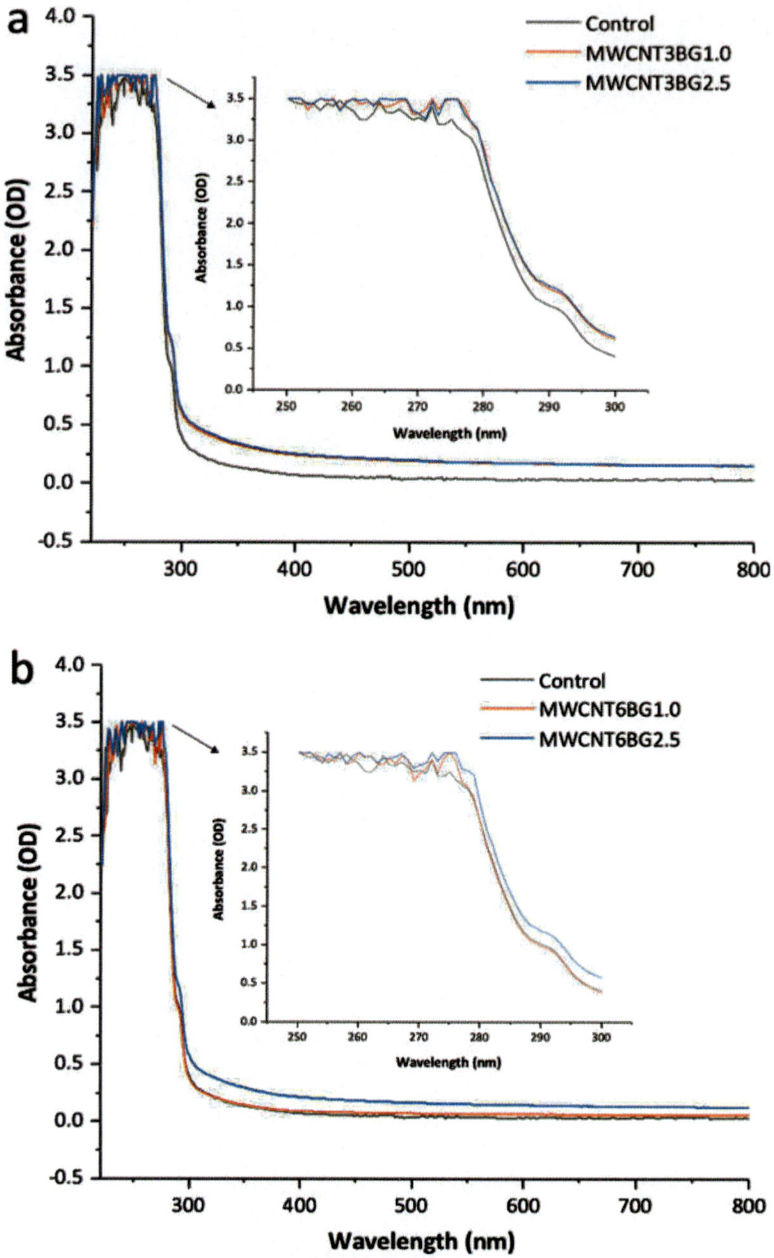

Fig. 5 UV absorbance intensity of different weight percentage of MWCNT-BG suspension in chloroform (shown in **a**) 3 wt% of MWCNT exfoliated with 1 and 2.5 wt% of BG respectively and **b** 6 wt% of MWCNT exfoliated with 1 and 2.5 wt% of BG respectively. Insert figures show respective clearer plateau absorption region ranging from 250 to 300 nm

intensity values BG upon addition to MWCNTs. The drawback is seen somehow to hinder the processing ability of these two superior materials.

Such selections for MWCNT concentrations were based on most affected and average values as discussed in Sect. 3.2, whereby low concentrations of BG were chosen to study any possible effects within the suspensions in reducing the agglomerations of the particles.

4 Conclusions

A comparative study on absorbance intensity between exfoliation of graphene and MWCNT, respectively, with the addition of BG in chloroform has been discussed. Graphene demonstrates greater composition stability upon the liquid exfoliation in chloroform, which is further improved by the addition of BG compared to BG on MWCNTs. This characteristic is crucial to illustrate the complementary relationship between both types of materials-corresponding to their solubility profile, which affects cell adhesion in contact with a physiological fluid. In contrast, MWCNTs demonstrate an inverse relationship before and after the addition of BG due to agglomeration effects, which may cause limitations in the preparation and processing of materials, especially in key, surface-dependent applications such as biomedical engineering therapies.

Future studies following on from the current findings where further characterizations, for example, analyzing morphology and composition of the composite materials, are highly anticipated. These observations are vital in confirming the synthesized materials and extending into a biological study which will further evaluate the functionality of BG in facilitating and enhancing the overall composite, especially with graphene. The findings of this research may potentially contribute to study the enhancement of BG towards exfoliation of nanoparticles (graphite and MWCNT) in solvent (chloroform), by reducing the usual agglomeration effects encountered by nanoparticles in suspensions.

Acknowledgements The authors acknowledged the support from the Ministry of Higher Education under the Fundamental Research Grant Scheme No. FRGS/1/2018/STG07/USM/02/13 (203.CIPPT.6711664).

Conflict of Interest The authors declare no conflict of interests.

References

1. Xu, Y., Cao, H., Xue, Y., Li, B., Cai, W.: Liquid-phase exfoliation of graphene: an overview on exfoliation media, techniques, and challenges. Nanomaterials **8**(11) (2018)
2. Singh, R., Charu Tripathi, C.: Electrochemical exfoliation of graphite into graphene for flexible supercapacitor application. Mater. Today Proc. **5**(1), 1125–1130 (2018)

3. Shang, L., et al.: Graphene and graphene oxide for tissue engineering and regeneration. No. January. Elsevier Inc. (2019)
4. Wu, M.C., Deokar, A.R., Liao, J.H., Shih, P.Y., Ling, Y.C.: Graphene-based photothermal agent for rapid and effective killing of bacteria. ACS Nano **7**(2), 1281–1290 (2013)
5. Hu, Y., Wang, K., Zhang, Q., Li, F., Wu, T., Niu, L.: Decorated graphene sheets for label-free DNA impedance biosensing. Biomaterials **33**(4), 1097–1106 (2012)
6. Uran, S., Alhani, A., Silva, C.: Study of ultraviolet-visible light absorbance of exfoliated graphite forms. AIP Adv. **7**(3) (2017)
7. Salaheldin, T.A., Loutfy, S.A., Ramadan, M.A., Youssef, T., Mousa, S.A.: Ir-enhanced photothermal therapeutic effect of graphene magnetite nanocomposite on human liver cancer HepG2 cell model. Int. J. Nanomed. **14**, 4397–4412 (2019)
8. Kerkeni, L., et al.: We are IntechOpen, the world's leading publisher of Open Access books built by scientists, for scientists TOP 1%. Intech, no. tourism, p. 13 (2016)
9. Liscio, A., et al.: Exfoliation of few-layer graphene in volatile solvents using aromatic perylene diimide derivatives as surfactants. ChemPlusChem **82**(3), 358–367 (2017)
10. Xu, L., Ye, Z., Cui, Q., Gu, Z.: Noncovalent nonspecific functionalization and solubilization of multi-walled carbon nanotubes at high concentrations with a hyperbranched polyethylene. Macromol. Chem. Phys. **210**(24), 2194–2202 (2010)
11. Hanumansetty, S., O'Rear, E., Resasco, D.E.: Encapsulation of multi-walled carbon nanotubes with copolymer to disperse in aqueous media. J. Polym. Res. **24**(12), 1–10 (2017)
12. Ilyas, et al., K.: In-vitro investigation of graphene oxide reinforced bioactive glass ceramics composites. J. Non. Cryst. Solids **505**(July 2018), 122–130 (2019)
13. Eqtesadi, S., Motealleh, A., Wendelbo, R., Ortiz, A.L., Miranda, P.: Reinforcement with reduced graphene oxide of bioactive glass scaffolds fabricated by robocasting. J. Eur. Ceram. Soc. **37**(12), 3695–3704 (2017)
14. Aliaa, N.S.N.S., Fazliah, M.N.S.N., Fatimah, S.S., Syazana, A.N.: Synthesis and characterization of PLA-PEG biocomposite incorporated with sol-gel derived 45S5 bioactive glass. Mater. Today Proc. **17**, 982–988 (2019)
15. Staudinger, U., Krause, B., Steinbach, C., Pötschke, P., Voit, B.: Dispersability of multiwalled carbon nanotubes in polycarbonate-chloroform solutions. Polymer (Guildf) **55**(24), 6335–6344 (2014)
16. Vacacela Gomez, et al., C.: The liquid exfoliation of graphene in polar solvents. Appl. Surf. Sci. **546**(Sept 2020), 149046 (2021)
17. Duan, D., et al.: Efficient exfoliation of graphite in chloroform with a pyrene-containing hyperbranched polyethylene as stabilizer to render pyrene-functionalized high-quality graphene. Carbon N. Y. **136**, 417–429 (2018)
18. Noroozi, M., Zakaria, A., Radiman, S., Wahab, Z.A.: Environmental synthesis of few layers graphene sheets using ultrasonic exfoliation with enhanced electrical and thermal properties. PLoS ONE **11**(4), 1–17 (2016)
19. Eremin, Y.S., Kolesnikova, A.A., Grekhov, A.M.: Agglomeration and sedimentation of MWCNTS in chloroform. Phys. Procedia **72**, 56–61 (2015)
20. El-Tablawy, S.Y., Abd-Allah, W.M., Araby, E.: Efficacy of irradiated bioactive glass 45S5 on attenuation of microbial growth and eradication of biofilm from AISI 316 L discs: in-vitro study. SILICON **10**(3), 931–942 (2018)

Increasing the Bacterial Cellulose Yield by Supplementation of Static Culture Medium

Farhana Islam and M. Tarik Arafat

Abstract High production costs and low production rates often restrict the use of bacterial cellulose (BC) at the industrial scale despite having excellent unique properties and potential. In this study, BC was produced by *Enterobacter amnigenus* GH-1, which was isolated from rotten apples and identified by gram staining reaction. Attempts were taken to enhance yield by supplementing the culture medium with two water-soluble polysaccharides: gelatin and acacia and oil. Here, the polysaccharides acted as a growth factor for bacteria and the oil facilitated the supply of sufficient oxygen and nutrients to the microorganisms. Results showed that the yield of cellulose increased significantly by 900% over the standard medium when the medium contained gelatin in the presence of oil by the dual effect of polysaccharide and oil. Moreover, enhancement of yield using medium thickening polysaccharides in the static culture medium could be possible due to the presence of oil as oil could continue to supply oxygen and nutrients to bacteria. On the other hand, gelatin and acacia, when used alone made the medium viscous resulting in a shortage of oxygen and nutrients in the medium. ATR-FTIR result confirmed the presence of functional groups of cellulose at the obtained white pellicle.

Keywords Bacterial cellulose · Yield · Oil

1 Introduction

Polysaccharides are the most common natural polymers on earth. They are long chains of carbohydrate molecules composed of monosaccharide units with the general formula $C_6H_{10}O_5$ bound together by glycosidic linkages. Their structure can range from linear e.g. cellulose to highly branched e.g. glycogen [1]. Cellulose is the most plentiful naturally occurring polysaccharide in nature obtained from

F. Islam · M. T. Arafat (✉)
Department of Biomedical Engineering, Bangladesh University of Engineering and Technology (BUET), Dhaka 1205, Bangladesh
e-mail: tarikarafat@bme.buet.ac.bd

J. Usman et al. (eds.), *6th Kuala Lumpur International Conference on Biomedical Engineering 2021*, IFMBE Proceedings 86,
https://doi.org/10.1007/978-3-030-90724-2_58

sustainable sources. Up to 15,000 D-glucose residues (a glucan) link by $\beta(1 \rightarrow 4)$ glycosidic bonds to form this linear polymer [2].

The main dominant pathway to obtain cellulose is from plants. It is renewable, cheap, and biodegradable. However, plant cellulose coexists with lignin and other polysaccharides, e.g., hemicellulose [3]. In order to get pure cellulose from plants, physical and chemical treatment and other purification processes are needed. Meanwhile, the purity of cellulose has become increasingly important in biomedical applications. Cellulose can also be synthesized by bacteria, fungi, and algae [4]. The discovery of bacterial cellulose was first reported by A. J. Brown in 1886 [5]. During the synthesis process, inside the bacterial body, glucose chains are produced. They extrude out through tiny pores present on the cell and combine to form nano-sized fibers, generating a web-shaped network structure with many empty spaces between the fibers. Bacterial cells get entrapped in the complex cellulose network, frequently enhancing the population at the air–liquid medium. The polymer matrix facilitates nutrient supply and helps in the adhesion of cells onto any attainable surface. The synthesis of BC production involves two consecutive mechanisms: synthesis of uridine-5′-diphosphate-α-D-glucose (UDP-glucose), finally polymerization of glucose into long un-branched chains [6]. Thus, cellulose formation by laboratory bacterial culture is an fascinating access to pure cellulose.

Bacterial cellulose (BC) is an advantageous biomaterial having highly potential applicability in different biomedical sectors [7]. BC is characterized by high levels of biocompatibility, moisture-holding capacity, mechanical stability, and purity. It provides a supportive environment for wound healing and is suitable for controlled drug delivery, tissue engineering, and bio-sensing fields [8]. BC can be synthesized from both specific gram-negative bacteria species: *Acetobacter*, *Agrobacterium, Azobacter, Salmonella, Rhizobium,* and gram-positive bacteria species: *Sarcina ventriculi. Enterobacter* sp. producing bacterial cellulose was turned up for the first time in 2001 [9]. Several methods are being used to produce BC. Among them, static culture is a comparatively simple, low-tech, and widely used method than the other methods [10]. Different culture medium and medium composition and culture conditions have been studied to observe the effect on BC production over the last many years [11]. However, the number of pellicles formed in the static medium is relatively lower because the pellicles act as an effective barrier at the air/liquid interface in the static medium. This barrier is formed between oxygen on one side and nutrients on the other side as a result which sufficient oxygen cannot reach the cellulose-producing bacteria. Hence, the growth of cells slows down.

Low yield rate and comparatively high production cost have limited use of BC as an alternative to plant cellulose. Effective BC-producing strain and optimized culture conditions are the primary requirements for using BC in industrial applications. Several approaches have been studied for decades to find a process that can significantly increase the yield of BC [12]. These efforts have been escalated in recent years owing to the outstanding application of BC in the aforementioned biomedical fields. In addition, there have been attempts to increase yield and lower cost by synthesizing using industrial and foodstuff wastes like vegetable and food waste, molasses, glycerol, etc. [13]. Besides, different additives such as polysaccharides: agar, sodium alginate [14], xanthan, organic acids, ethanol, fruit juices [12], oil [15] have been used to increase yield. It has been shown that the addition of water-soluble polysaccharides reduces the shear stress of BC by enhancing the relative viscosity of the medium to form uniform pellets, and it delays BC coagulation and stimulates cell growth and BC production [16, 17]. On the contrary, these medium thickening polysaccharides decrease BC yield in static culture since there is no shear stress acting on there, hindering nutrient supply by making the medium viscous. In this study, an approach has been taken to explore more effective alternatives to the existing processes, and efforts have been made to increase yield more than the existing best processes give. Two water-soluble polysaccharides: Gelatin and acacia, have been employed in the static culture of BC to observe the effect on BC production in the presence of oil, which has been earlier proven to supply sufficient oxygen and nutrient supply to the microorganisms in the medium. Bacteria were extracted from rotten apples and identified by the gram staining method. The obtained BC pellicles have been characterized by attenuated total reflection Fourier transform infrared spectroscopy (ATR-FTIR). Statistical optimization has also been performed.

2 Experimental Set-Up and Methodology

2.1 Materials

Glucose, Peptone, Yeast Extract, Disodium phosphate, Bacteriological agar, and Citric acid were purchased from Sigma Aldrich. Gelatin and acacia were purchased from Research Lab. Bacterial strain *Enterobacter amnigenus* GH-1 was extracted from rotten apples.

2.2 Isolation and Screening of Microorganisms

Standard Hestrin-Schramm (HS) medium composed of 2% glucose (w/v), 0.5% peptone (w/v), 0.5% yeast extract (w/v), 0.115% citric acid (w/v), and 0.27% disodium phosphate (w/v) was employed to extract microorganism from rotten apple as well as to culture those extracted bacteria for producing cellulose. Medium pH was adjusted to 6. Rotten apples were cut into small pieces and put into 100 ml sterile saline containing conical flasks. In order to detach the surface microbiota, the flask was kept in a shaker for 30 min at room temperature. 0.5 ml extract from the flask was added to 10 ml of HS medium with 0.5% (v/v) ethanol, 0.2% (v/v) acetic acid and 0.02% (w/v) cycloheximide into a test tube. It was then kept at room temperature for 24 h of incubation. After that, 1 ml of enriched sample from the test tube was inoculated into 100 ml of HS medium and incubated at room temperature for 14 days. Flasks were kept for growth and observed for pellicle formation.

2.3 Microorganism Culture

Sterile phosphate buffer solution was used to serially dilute white pellicle culture grown on the air/liquid surface of the medium. 0.1 ml of appropriate dilutions were then spread onto the HS agar medium plate containing 1.5% (w/v) bacteriological agar and incubated at 37 °C to get an isolated bacterial colony.

2.4 BC Production and Purification

100 ml of standard HS medium (pH 6.0) was inoculated with a single bacterial colony and incubated at 28 °C for 7 days for cellulose pellicle formation. Formation of pellicle started at the air/liquid interface on the 3rd or 4th day of incubation. The pellicle was carefully removed after 7 days of incubation and immersed in 2% NaOH solution. Then transferred to DI water and boiled for 30 min and then washed again thoroughly with DI water. Drying was carried out in an oven at 65 °C overnight before further characterization. In the next step, to increase the yield of BC, Oil, gelatin, and acacia were used as additives, and several combinations of three of these variables have been made to examine the effect. Firstly, two types of oil were used to differentiate the effect. Next, the medium was complemented with medium thickening agent gelatin and acacia alone. Finally, how gelatin and acacia work in the presence of oil is examined. 1% (v/v) oil was used. Two different percentages of gelatin and acacia were used: in one experiment, gelatin and acacia were used 0.04% (w/v) and 0.06% (w/v), respectively, and in another experiment, both percentages were increased to 0.5% (w/v). Samples were labeled as control, HS + RO, HS + PO, HS + G, HS + A, HS + PO + G, HS + PO + A, HS + PO + G + A where control represents a medium with only standard HS medium without any additives and HS, RO, PO, G, A represent standard HS medium, rice oil, palm oil, gelatin, and acacia, respectively. For example, HS + PO + G + A represents standard HS culture medium is supplemented with palm oil, gelatin, and acacia.

3 Characterization

Attenuated total reflection Fourier transform infrared spectroscopy (ATR-FTIR) spectrum was recorded by Nicolet iS5 ((Nicolet Instrument Corporation, WI, USA) FTIR Spectrometer with an accumulation of 40 scans at room temperature in the range of 500–4000 with spectral resolution 2.

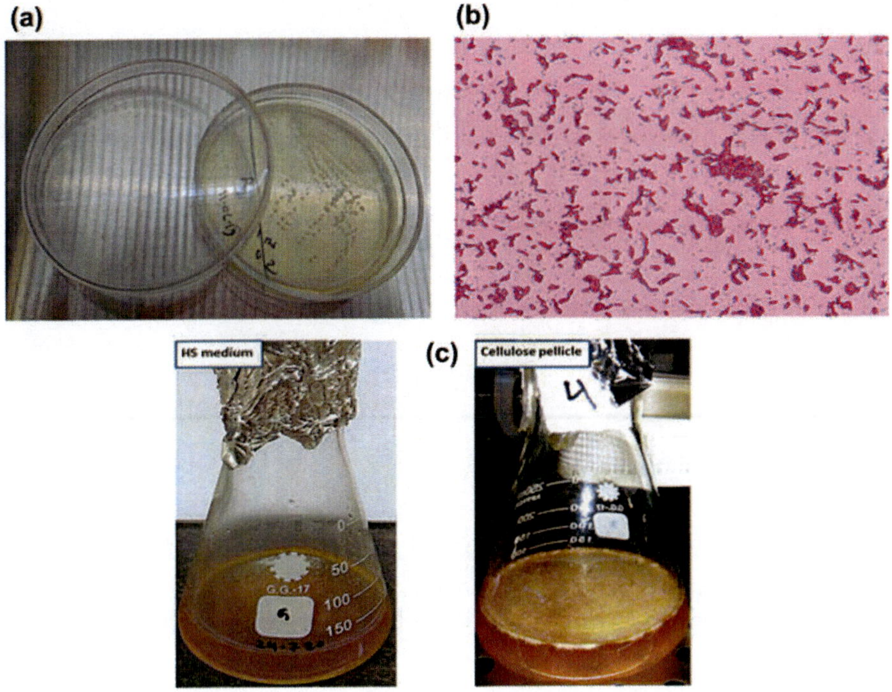

Fig. 1 **a** bacterial colony on the agar plate **b** gram staining reaction proved gram-negative bacteria obtained and **c** formation of cellulose pellicle at the air/liquid interface

4 Results and Discussion

4.1 Identification and Gram Staining of BC-Producing Microorganism

Isolated single colonies were observed on the agar plate shown in Fig. 1a. The pure colony was slimy, smooth, and cream in color. *Enterobacter amnigenus* GH-1 are gram-negative bacteria, and in gram staining reaction test, they show pink/red color like found in the test shown in Fig. 1b.

4.2 Statistical Optimization of BC Yield

A white pellicle was observed at the air/liquid interface of the conical flask, as shown in Fig. 1c. Comparative results are shown in Fig. 2. The yield of BC increased about 200% in HS + PO than the control concluding that palm oil works better than rice oil in BC production. When gelatin and acacia were added alone, HS + G and HS

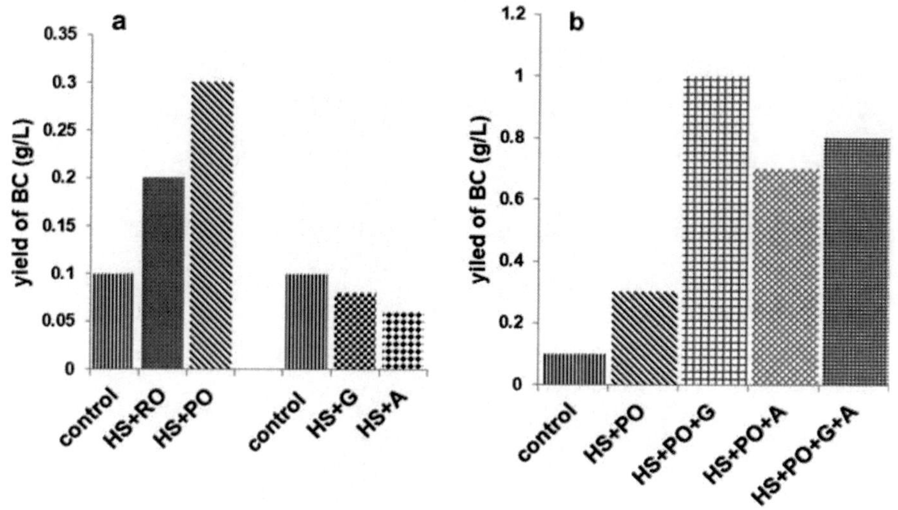

Fig. 2 The yield of BC synthesized by *Enterobacter* in control HS medium and **a** HS medium supplemented with two oils: rice oil (RO) and palm oil (PO) and medium thickening water-soluble polysaccharide gelatin (G) and acacia (A) and **b** HS medium supplemented with gelatin (G) and Acacia (A) in the presence of palm oil (PO). The yield of cellulose was highest for HS + PO + G around 900%

+ A samples showed a decreased yield of BC than control as these polysaccharides cause a shortage in supply of nutrients by increasing viscosity of the medium, but the addition of oil compensated this shortcoming. Figure 2 shows that when the medium is complemented with oil and medium thickening agent, yield increased up to 900% than the control; HS + PO + G showed the highest amount of yield. The selection of a suitable polysaccharide with a proper percentage is critical [18]. For example, when gelatin percent was increased to 0.5%, the yield decreased as BC production impeded when the medium became more viscous. On the other hand, when acacia concentration 0.06% is used, no cellulose was produced, whereas at 0.5% concentration, cellulose formed, suggesting a lower concentration was used earlier.

Normally in the production of BC, a glucose medium is used. There is a tendency of sinking movement of cellulose pellicle as there works a downward force due to the density of BC pellicle being slightly higher than the glucose medium because cellulose is a polymer of glucose [19]. The sinking process helps in increasing the availability of nutrients and oxygen, which are critical to BC formation and the formation of new sticking cellulose layers on top of the primary layer. But normally, opposite to sinking downward force, the rough surface of the vessel applies upward frictional force trying to hinder the sinking process, thus decreasing BC production. Oil has a tremendous effect on increasing bacterial cellulose yield. It was observed that the addition of oil reduces these frictional forces enabling the sinking process and allowing sufficient nutrients and oxygen to the top layer. It works in the following process; it forms a cone shape in the flask, BC mass deposited at the lower part of the structure leaving free fresh medium at the top to allow bacteria cells to produce BC. This process is self-fueling and escalating as a new layer of cellulose forms after the previous layer sinks. This can be continued up to four coherent.

Oil droplets tend to adapt a funnel form within cellulose according to the law of physics, where the base of the funnel directs at the surface of the medium. At the same time, oil being hydrophobic pushes back the cellulose matrix, which consists of >98% of water. These two opposing processes create spaces in between, which are accessible to oxygen in the air and possibly facilitate oxygen exchange within deeper layers of cellulose membranes [15]. On the other hand, added polysaccharides: gelatin and acacia enhance the growth of bacteria significantly [20]. This dual effect together enhanced the yield of cellulose more than oil alone does.

4.3 ATR-FTIR

The presence of cellulose was confirmed by ATR-FTIR, shown in Fig. 3. A broad absorption band of the hydroxyl group appears 3400 cm^{-1} [21]. The C–H stretching bands of $-CH_3$ and $-CH_2$ groups are observed at 2900 cm^{-1}. The peak at 1640 cm^{-1} corresponds to H–OH vibration of absorbed water molecules in BC. Glycosidic C–O–C stretching vibration is observed at 1000 cm^{-1} [22].

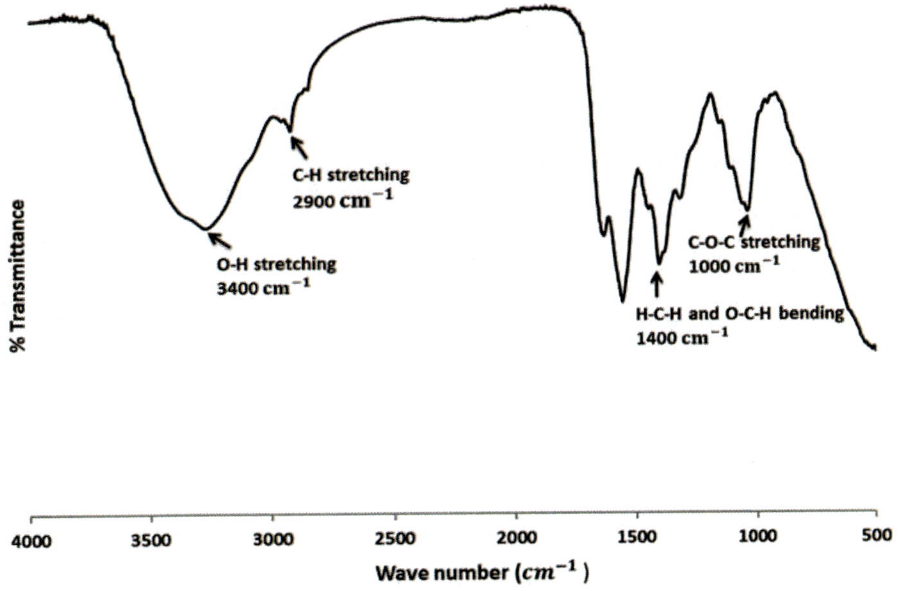

Fig. 3 ATR-FTIR spectrum shows functional groups of cellulose produced by *Enterobacter amnigenus* GH-1 isolated from rotten apple

5 Conclusion

In this present study, *Enterobacter amnigenus* GH-1 was successfully isolated from rotten apple and could produce cellulose pellicle in a static culture medium. A significant increase of BC could be achieved by a simple method using polysaccharide additives and oil into the culture medium. The limitation of using water-soluble medium thickening polysaccharides in static culture in the production of BC was successfully eliminated by using oil. Oil supplies oxygen and nutrient to the microorganism, which was earlier hindered in the absence of oil due to the viscous nature of the medium. These polysaccharides are also a source of growth factors for bacteria. As a result, polysaccharides in combination with oil enhanced yield by a significant amount. ATR-FTIR confirmed the presence of cellulose in the obtained pellicle. Our further study aims at evaluating useful properties, e.g., swelling, mechanical strength, cytotoxicity of BC, to investigate that the new technique used to increases yield would not cause depression of any of these properties. Therefore, this simple technique indicates a new strategy in the study of enhancing bacterial cellulose yield and demands further investigation of its functional properties for application in various biomedical fields.

Acknowledgements The research project was conducted under grant no: DAERS/CASR/R-1/2020/DR-330(53) supported by Bangladesh University of Engineering and Technology (BUET).

References

1. Atkins, E.: Conformations in polysaccharides and complex carbohydrates. **8**, 375–387 (1985)
2. Yan, H., Chen, X., Song, H., Li, J., Feng, Y., Shi, Z., Wang, X., Lin, Q.: Food Hydrocolloids Synthesis of bacterial cellulose and bacterial cellulose nanocrystals for their applications in the stabilization of olive oil pickering emulsion. Food Hydrocoll. **72**, 127–135 (2017). https://doi.org/10.1016/j.foodhyd.2017.05.044
3. Portela, R., Leal, C.R., Pedro, L.: Minireview Bacterial cellulose : a versatile biopolymer for wound dressing applications 2019 (2020). https://doi.org/10.1111/1751-7915.13392
4. Lin, W., Lien, C., Yeh, H., Yu, C., Hsu, S.: Bacterial cellulose and bacterial cellulose—chitosan membranes for wound dressing applications. Carbohydr. Polym. **94**, 603–611 (2013). https://doi.org/10.1016/j.carbpol.2013.01.076
5. Chen, X., Yuan, F., Zhang, H., Huang, Y., Yang, J., Sun, D.: Recent approaches and future prospects of bacterial cellulose-based electroconductive materials. J. Mater. Sci. (2016). https://doi.org/10.1007/s10853-016-9899-2
6. Römling, U., Galperin, M.Y.: Bacterial cellulose biosynthesis: diversity of operons, subunits, products, and functions. 1–13 (2015). https://doi.org/10.1016/j.tim.2015.05.005
7. Sharma, C., Bhardwaj, N.K.: Bacterial nanocellulose: present status, biomedical applications and future perspectives. Mater. Sci. Eng. C. **104**, 109963 (2019). https://doi.org/10.1016/j.msec.2019.109963
8. Eslahi, N., Mahmoodi, A., Mahmoudi, N., Zandi, N.: Processing and properties of nanofibrous bacterial cellulose-containing polymer composites: a review of recent advances for biomedical applications. Polym. Rev. **0**, 1–27 (2019).https://doi.org/10.1080/15583724.2019.1663210

9. Gupta, B.S.H.S.G.: Production of bacterial cellulose from Enterobacter amnigenus GH-1 isolated from rotten apple. 1823–1828 (2010). https://doi.org/10.1007/s11274-010-0363-1
10. Hong, F., Qiu, K.: An alternative carbon source from konjac powder for enhancing production of bacterial cellulose in static cultures by a model strain Acetobacter aceti subsp. xylinus ATCC 23770. Carbohydr. Polym. **72**(3), 545–549 (2008)
11. Reiniati, I., Hrymak, A.N., Margaritis, A.: Critical reviews in biotechnology recent developments in the production and applications of bacterial cellulose fibers and nanocrystals. **8551** (2017). https://doi.org/10.1080/07388551.2016.1189871
12. Islam, M.U., Ullah, M.W., Khan, S., Shah, N., Park, J.K.: Strategies for cost-effective and enhanced production of bacterial cellulose. Int. J. Biol. Macromol. **102**, 1166–1173 (2017). https://doi.org/10.1016/j.ijbiomac.2017.04.110
13. Tsouko, E., Kourmentza, C., Ladakis, D., Kopsahelis, N., Mandala, I., Papanikolaou, S., Paloukis, F., Alves, V., Koutinas, A.: Bacterial cellulose production from industrial waste and by-product streams. Int. J. Mol. Sci. **16**, 14832–14849 (2015). https://doi.org/10.3390/ijms160714832
14. Cheng, K.C., Catchmark, J.M., Demirci, A.: Effect of different additives on bacterial cellulose production by Acetobacter xylinum and analysis of material property. Cellulose **16**, 1033–1045 (2009). https://doi.org/10.1007/s10570-009-9346-5
15. Żywicka, A., Junka, A.F., Szymczyk, P., Chodaczek, G., Grzesiak, J., Sedghizadeh, P.P., Fijałkowski, K.: Bacterial cellulose yield increased over 500% by supplementation of medium with vegetable oil. Carbohydr. Polym. **199**, 294–303 (2018). https://doi.org/10.1016/j.carbpol.2018.06.126
16. Chao, Y., Mitarai, M., Sugano, Y., Shoda, M.: Effect of addition of water-soluble polysaccharides on bacterial cellulose production in a 50-L airlift reactor. Biotechnol. Prog. **17**, 781–785 (2001). https://doi.org/10.1021/bp010046b
17. Research Commons at the University of Waikato Copyright Statement: Production of Bacterial Cellulose Using Low-cost Media A thesis of Doctor of Philosophy in Engineering at The University of Waikato by Azila Binti Adnan, 1994 (1994)
18. Mohamad, N., Mohd Amin, M.C.I., Pandey, M., Ahmad, N., Rajab, N.F.: Bacterial cellulose/acrylic acid hydrogel synthesized via electron beam irradiation: accelerated burn wound healing in an animal model. Carbohydr. Polym. **114**, 312–320 (2014). https://doi.org/10.1016/j.carbpol.2014.08.025
19. Phruksaphithak, N., Kaewnun, C., O-Thong, S.: Bacterial cellulose production and applications, Sci. Eng. Heal. Stud. **13**, 1–7 (2019). https://doi.org/10.14456/sehs.2019.1
20. Ishida, T., Mitarai, M., Sugano, Y., Shoda, M.: Role of water-soluble polysaccharides in bacterial cellulose production. Biotechnol. Bioeng. **83**, 474–478 (2003). https://doi.org/10.1002/bit.10690
21. Wood, D., Salusso, C.J.: Production and characterization of bacterial cellulose fabrics. In: International Textile and Apparel Association Proceedings, pp. 11–13 (2015)
22. Oliveira, R.L., Vieira, J.G., Barud, H.S., Assunção, R.M.N., Filho, G.R., Ribeiro, S.J.L., Messadeqq, Y.: Synthesis and characterization of methylcellulose produced from bacterial cellulose under heterogeneous condition. J. Braz. Chem. Soc. **26**, 1861–1870 (2015). https://doi.org/10.5935/0103-5053.20150163

Novel Method of Producing Free-Standing SU8-Based Carbon Scaffold as Biomedical Engineering Application

Vieralynda Vitus, Fatimah Ibrahim, and Wan Safwani Wan Kamarul Zaman

Abstract For the first time, this paper highlighted the method of detaching SU8-based carbon scaffolds from substrates using the acid treatment method. This finding provides a method to detach pyrolysed scaffolds from a substrate without the need to scrap the pattern. Briefly, the scaffold patterns were fabricated using photolithography and the pyrolysis method. Then, various attempts of detaching the carbon scaffold by using acids were investigated include H_2SO_4, HNO_3, H_2O_2, and H_2SO_4/HNO_3. Under 60 min treatment of HNO_3 with stirring and non-stirring conditions has led to the detachments of pyrolysed SU8 without visible defect on the structure. This finding provides a free-standing SU8-based carbon scaffold that could be easily incorporated into hydrogel or other composites materials to form a conductive 3D in vitro model for biological application. Hence, these novel detachment methods provide new knowledge to detach SU8-based carbon scaffolds, while performing surface treatment to improve the surface properties of carbon scaffolds. The findings of this study improve the potential of SU8-based carbon scaffolds as tools in future biological applications.

Keywords Detachment method · Free standing carbon scaffold · SU8-based carbon scaffold · Acid treatment

V. Vitus · F. Ibrahim · W. S. Wan Kamarul Zaman (✉)
Department of Biomedical Engineering, Faculty of Engineering, Universiti Malaya, 50603 Kuala Lumpur, Malaysia
e-mail: wansafwani@um.edu.my

Centre for Innovation in Medical Engineering (CIME), Department of Biomedical Engineering, Faculty of Engineering, Universiti Malaya, 50603 Kuala Lumpur, Malaysia

F. Ibrahim
Centre for Printable Electronics, Universiti Malaya, 50603 Kuala Lumpur, Malaysia

J. Usman et al. (eds.), *6th Kuala Lumpur International Conference on Biomedical Engineering 2021*, IFMBE Proceedings 86,
https://doi.org/10.1007/978-3-030-90724-2_59

1 Introduction

Carbon materials have been extensively and widely studied in various fields of application. Currently, carbon from polymer precursors has made its way as a potential tool in biomedical applications due to their flexibility and customisable ability in fabrications [1]. To date, the negative photoresist SU8 polymer was widely employed in producing nano- and micro-scale scaffolds through MEMS technology to fabricate patterns similar to the extracellular matrix of cells [2]. Based on previous studies, the SU8-based carbon scaffold has shown to be biocompatible and could influence cells behaviours. Plus, the carbon-based scaffold's electroconductive properties support the growth of electro-active cells such as cardiac cells, neural cells, and skeletal cells [3–5]. However, the surface of the SU8-based carbon scaffold is insufficiently hydrophilic, which is less favour by cells. Thus, surface treatments were utilized to improve the hydrophilicity of the SU8-based scaffold.

Commonly, the surface treatments performed on carbon materials is to improve the surface wettability and adhesion properties, which affect the biocompatibility of carbon [6]. Among the current surface treatment methods employed on carbon materials are wet chemical treatments using an acid solution. Various acid solutions and mixtures include HCL, HNO_3, H_2SO_4, H_2SO_4/HNO_3, H_2SO_4/NaOH, were utilized [7–10]. Acid treatment on carbon materials is mainly done on carbon nanotubes and other carbon powder [9, 11–13]. However, there is no report yet on the ability of acid treatments to loosen the interfacial adhesion strength, which led to the detachment of carbon scaffold from substrates.

Currently, most of the studies utilising SU8 polymer in the production of SU8-based carbon scaffolds are attached to a substrate for example, fabrication of SU8 micro pattern on silicon wafer [14]. Based on previous studies, the detachment method of SU8 polymer from substrate has been widely employed to obtain free-standing devices or structures from coating materials to the sacrificial layer. For instance, Microchem Omnicoat was used as substrate's coater prior to the deployment of SU8 for easy removal of SU8 structure from the substrate [15]. Others use the PDMS layer to easily detach the SU8 structure from the substrate [16, 17]. In comparison, Jang et al. [18] utilised chrome/gold as a sacrificial layer to release the SU8 structure. Meanwhile, Chiriacò et al. [19] applied Lift-Off Resist as a sacrificial layer for easy peel off to obtain a free-standing SU8 structure. However, although various method to release SU8 polymer structure from substrate has been developed, the method to release pyrolysed SU8 carbon structure from substrates remains unexplored.

Therefore, in this manuscript, we present for the first time the methods to detach SU8-based carbon scaffold from a substrate that simultaneously undergoes surface functionalisation. Through this finding, a free-standing SU8-based carbon scaffold was obtained. The free-standing SU8-based carbon scaffold could be potentially incorporate into hydrogel or other composites materials to create a conductive 3D carbon model for in vitro biological application.

2 Methods

2.1 *Fabrication of SU8-Based Carbon Scaffold on Substrates*

Firstly, the fused silica wafer was clean with acetone, isopropanol, and distilled water. Followed by drying with nitrogen gas and further drying on the hot plate at 200°C for 1 h. Subsequently, spin coating of SU8 3035 photoresists on substrates at 3000 rpm speed to obtain 35 μm height. Next, the SU8 was soft baked at 105°C for 20 min on the hot plate and then exposed to UV light for 25 s under the photomask. After that, the SU8 was post baked at 105°C for 6 min followed by the development step using SU8 developer and final bake at 190°C for 1 h. Finally, the substrates were subjected to pyrolysis process to obtain carbonised patterns at 900°C in the furnace (Nabertherm more than heat 30–3000°, P330, Germany) under a continuous flow of nitrogen gas with a flow rate of 2 cc/min.

2.2 *Acid Treatment on SU8-Based Carbon Scaffold from Substrates*

The process of detaching the pyrolysed SU8 from substrates was performed by using H2SO4, HNO3, H2SO4/HNO3, and H2O2. The process was performed at 60°C in 30 min intervals with and without stirring conditions of 180 rpm speed on a hot plate. After that, the pyrolysed SU8 pattern was washed with running tap water, and a pH meter was used to check the pH level to ensure all acid remnants had been removed.

2.3 *Fabrication of SU8-Based Scaffold on Substrates with Kapton Tape*

Prior to spin coating, the Kapton tape was applied on the microscope glass slide, followed by spin coating of SU8 at 3000 rpm speed. Next, the SU8 was soft baked at 65°C for 20 min on a hot plate and exposed to UV light for 15 s and post baked at 95°C for 5 min on a hot plate. Then, the UV exposed SU8 patterns were immersed in SU8 developer for 1 h. After that, the SU8 structure was peeled off from the substrate. Lastly, it was subjected to a final bake at 190°C for 1 h on a hot plate. The overall process as in Fig. 1.

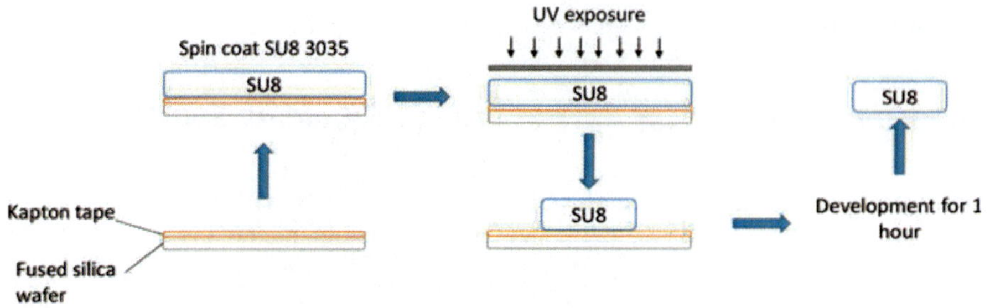

Fig. 1 Detachment method by using Kapton tape on SU8 polymer

2.4 *Pyrolysis Process of the Detached SU8-Based Scaffold*

Prior to pyrolysis, the detached SU8-based scaffold was sandwiched between two pieces of fused silica wafer and placed on a ceramic boat and then placed the ceramic boat in the centre of the furnace tube. Then, the pyrolysis process was performed at 900°C in the furnace (Nabertherm more than heat 30–3000°, P330, Germany) under a continuous flow of nitrogen gas with a flow rate of 2 cc/min.

3 Results and Discussion

Based on the investigation, H_2SO_4 treatments on both stirring and non-stirring conditions resulted in visible structural damage at 60- and 120-min treatments, and the pyrolysed SU8 pattern remains attached on the substrate. On both HNO_3 conditions at 30 min treatment, the bottom attached parts of the SU8-based carbon scaffold on the substrate visibly began to detach (see Fig. 2). At 60 min, HNO_3 treatment on both conditions has led to the detachment of pyrolysed SU8 from substrates without visible damage. The H_2O_2 treatments on pyrolysed SU8 under both treatment conditions do not lead to the detachment of carbon structure, and no visible damage was seen. Lastly, the treatments under the mixture of H_2SO_4/HNO_3 on both conditions led to the detachment of carbon structure, but severely damage patterns were obtained (see Table 1).

Therefore, visually the most suitable acid treatment to detach the pyrolysed scaffold from fused silica substrate is through 60 min treatment of HNO_3 either in stirring or non-stirring conditions.

Additionally, in this study, we also attempted to detach the SU8 polymer structure prior to the pyrolysis process by using Kapton tape as a release layer. However, through this investigation, the pyrolysis process on the detached SU8 polymer structure resulted in extreme shrinkage, breakage, and curling of SU8-based carbon structure (see in Fig. 3d). These may be due to the stress of interfacial shear strength under a high heat temperature environment [20]. Therefore, detaching the scaffold prior to

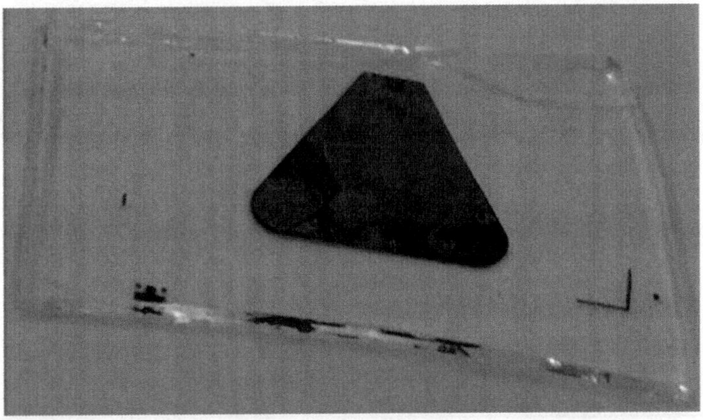

Fig. 2 The bottom attached part of SU8-based carbon scaffold on fused silica wafer. The darker colour indicates the scaffold still adhere to the substrate, whereas the greyish colour indicates the scaffold is no longer attached to the substrate

the pyrolysis process is not feasible. Thus, this is the main reason we utilised acid treatments after the pyrolysis process of the SU8-based scaffold.

4 Conclusion

This study describes a simple, time-saving, cost-effective method to detach SU8-based carbon scaffold while simultaneously performing surface functionalisation. To our knowledge, this is the first investigation to detach pyrolysed SU8-based scaffold. Further studies will be conducted in the future to understand better the effect of acid treatment towards the detachment of SU8-based carbon scaffold and the potential use of free-standing SU8-based carbon scaffold in biomedical engineering applications.

Table 1 Findings of acid treatments on SU8-based carbon scaffold

Treatment period	30 min				60 min				120 min			
Conditions	Stirred		Not stirred		Stirred		Not stirred		Stirred		Not stirred	
Findings	Da/UD	De/A	Da/UD	De/A	Da/UD	De/A	Da/UD	De/A	Da/UD	De/A	Da/UD	De/A
H_2SO_4	Da	A	Da	A	Da	A	Da	A	Da	A	Da	A
HNO_3	UD	A	UD	A	UD	De	UD	De	–	–	–	–
H_2O_2	UD	A	UD	A	UD	A	UD	A	UD	A	UD	A
H_2SO_4/HNO_3	Da	De	Da	De	Da	De	Da	De	Da	De	Da	De

*Da = Damaged pattern; UD = Undamaged pattern; De = Pattern detached; A = Pattern attached

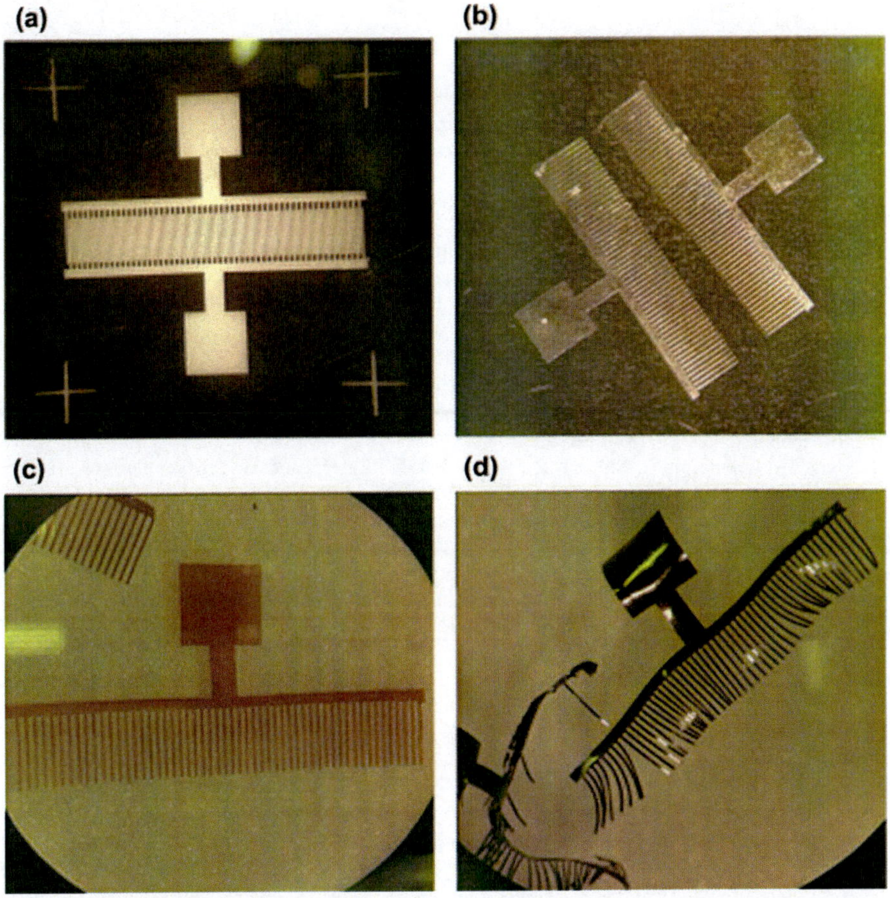

Fig. 3 Detached SU8 polymer pattern by Kapton tape method. **a** Pattern on photomask; **b** Detached SU8 patterns under the microscope; **c** SU8 pattern after final bake; **d** Pyrolysed detached SU8 pattern

Acknowledgements This study was supported by University Malaya Impact-Oriented Interdisciplinary Research Grant Program (IIRG007-19HWB).

Conflicts of Interest The authors declare that they have no conflicts of interest.

References

1. Mishra, R., Pramanick, B., Maiti, T., Bhattacharyya, T.: Glassy carbon microneedles—new transdermal drug delivery device derived from a scalable C-MEMS process. Microsyst. Nanoeng. **4** (2018). https://doi.org/10.1038/s41378-018-0039-9

2. Caviglia, C., Carletto, R.P., De Roni, S., Hassan, Y.M., Hemanth, S., Dufva, M., Keller, S.S.: In situ electrochemical analysis of alkaline phosphatase activity in 3D cell cultures. Electrochimica Acta **359**, 136951 (2020)
3. Amato, L., Heiskanen, A., Caviglia, C., Shah, F., Zór, K., Skolimowski, M., Madou, M., Gammelgaard, L., Hansen, R., Seiz, E., Ramos, M., Ramos Moreno, T., Martinez Serrano, A., Keller, S., Emnéus, J.: Pyrolysed 3D-carbon scaffolds induce spontaneous differentiation of human neural stem cells and facilitate real-time dopamine detection. Adv. Func. Mater. **24** (2014). https://doi.org/10.1002/adfm.201400812
4. Fuhrer, E., Bäcker, A., Kraft, S., Gruhl, F.J., Kirsch, M., MacKinnon, N., Korvink, J.G., Sharma, S.: 3D carbon scaffolds for neural stem cell culture and magnetic resonance imaging. Adv. Healthc. Mater. **7**(4) (2018). https://doi.org/10.1002/adhm.201700915
5. Martins, A.M., Eng, G., Caridade, S.G., Mano, J.F., Reis, R.L., Vunjak-Novakovic, G.: Electrically conductive chitosan/carbon scaffolds for cardiac tissue engineering. Biomacromol **15**(2), 635–643 (2014)
6. Imaninezhad, M., Schober, J., Griggs, D., Ruminski, P., Kuljanishvili, I., Zustiak, S.P.: Cell attachment and spreading on carbon nanotubes is facilitated by integrin binding. Front. Bioeng. Biotechnol. **6**, 129 (2018)
7. Eyni, H., Ghorbani, S., Shirazi, R., Salari Asl, L., Beiranvand, S.P., Soleimani, M.: Three-dimensional wet-electrospun poly(lactic acid)/multi-wall carbon nanotubes scaffold induces differentiation of human menstrual blood-derived stem cells into germ-like cells. J. Biomater. Appl. **32**(3), 373–383 (2017)
8. Zhao, C., Andersen, H., Ozyilmaz, B., Ramaprabhu, S., Pastorin, G., Ho, H.K.: Spontaneous and specific myogenic differentiation of human mesenchymal stem cells on polyethylene glycol-linked multi-walled carbon nanotube films for skeletal muscle engineering. Nanoscale **7**(43), 18239–18249 (2015)
9. Pak, S.-H., Jeon, M.-J., Jeon, Y.-W.: Study of sulfuric acid treatment of activated carbon used to enhance mixed VOC removal. Int. Biodeterior. Biodegradation **113**, 195–200 (2016)
10. Woodhead, A.L., de Souza, M.L., Church, J.S.: An investigation into the surface heterogeneity of nitric acid oxidized carbon fiber. Appl. Surf. Sci. **401**, 79–88 (2017)
11. Zhang, Q., Li, K., Fan, Q., Xia, X., Zhang, N., Xiao, Z., Zhou, W., Yang, F., Wang, Y., Liu, H.: Performance improvement of continuous carbon nanotube fibers by acid treatment. Chin. Phys. B. **26**(2), 028802 (2017)
12. Rocha, P.D., Franca, A.S., Oliveira, L.S.: Batch and column studies of phenol adsorption by an activated carbon based on acid treatment of corn cobs. Int. J. Eng. Technol. **7**(6), 459 (2015)
13. Li, Y., Zhang, D., Feng, X., Xiang, Q.: Enhanced photocatalytic hydrogen production activity of highly crystalline carbon nitride synthesized by hydrochloric acid treatment. Chin. J. Catal. **41**(1), 21–30 (2020). https://doi.org/10.1016/S1872-2067(19)63427-3
14. Ferraro, R.M., Ginestra, P., Giliani, S., Ceretti, E.: Carbonization of polymer precursors substrates to direct human iPSC-derived neurons differentiation and maturation. Procedia CIRP **89**, 39–44 (2020). https://doi.org/10.1016/j.procir.2020.05.116
15. Pinto, V.C., Sousa, P.J., Cardoso, V.F., Minas, G.: Optimized SU-8 processing for low-cost microstructures fabrication without cleanroom facilities. Micromachines **5**(3), 738–755 (2014)
16. Patel, J.N., Gray, B.L., Kaminska, B., Wu, N.-C., Gates, B.D.: SU-8-and PDMS-based hybrid fabrication technology for combination of permanently bonded flexible and rigid features on a single device. J. Micromech. Microeng. **23**(6), 065029 (2013)
17. Baëtens, T., Pallecchi, E., Thomy, V., Arscott, S.: Metallized SU-8 thin film patterns on stretchable PDMS. J. Micromech. Microeng. **29**(9), 095009 (2019)
18. Jang, J., Jang, J.H., Choi, H.: MEMS flexible artificial basilar membrane fabricated from piezoelectric aluminum nitride on an SU-8 substrate. J. Micromech. Microeng. **27**(7), 075006 (2017)

19. Chiriacò, M.S., Bianco, M., Amato, F., Primiceri, E., Ferrara, F., Arima, V., Maruccio, G.: Fabrication of interconnected multilevel channels in a monolithic SU-8 structure using a LOR sacrificial layer. Microelectron. Eng. **164**, 30–35 (2016). https://doi.org/10.1016/j.mee.2016.07.006
20. Natu, R., Islam, M., Gilmore, J., Martinez-Duarte, R.: Shrinkage of SU-8 microstructures during carbonization. J. Anal. Appl. Pyrol. **131**, 17–27 (2018)

The Effect of microRNA Targeting IL-17RA in the Regulation of RANKL and OPG Expressions in Stem Cells from Human Exfoliated Deciduous Teeth

Wan Khairunnisaa Wan Nor Aduni, Rashidi Dzul Keflee, See Too Wei Cun, and Asma Abdullah Nurul

Abstract microRNA is a small RNA molecule able to regulate gene expressions at post transcription level, either via mRNA degradation or translational repression. This study is designed to determine the potential microRNA targeting IL-17RA and its effects towards OPG and RANKL expressions in SHED. Complex filtration process via in silico study, using the most recent algorithmically programmes (DIANA-micro T CDS, mirWalk v2.0, and TargetScan v7.1) was done to predict potential microRNA. The concentration of 25, 50, and 100 nM microRNA targeting GAPDH were optimized to determine the most efficient downregulation activity. The result showed that 50 nM microRNA mimic transfected for 48 h resulted in the lowest level of GAPDH mRNA expression measured by quantitative real time PCR. Following microRNA optimization, SHED were grown for 7 days in complete α-mem supplemented with osteoinducing reagents and treated with 50 ng/mL IL-17A to enhance osteogenic differentiation. Treated cells were then transfected with 50 nM of predicted microRNA (hsa-miR-4524a-3p and hsa-miR-6761-5p) for 48 h. The expressions of IL-17RA, OPG and RANKL were measured by qPCR and normalized with β-actin. The microRNA mimic hsa-miR-4524a-3p downregulated IL-17RA expression more than the microRNA mimic hsa-miR-6761-5p ($p < 0.01$). Additionally, both OPG and RANKL expressions were downregulated by both mimics, although only OPG expression was significantly decreased. These findings highlight the importance of microRNA targeting IL-17RA and its effects on regulating the expressions of OPG and RANKL in SHED, implying a role in the bone metabolism process.

Keywords Bone · Interleukin-17A · microRNA · Osteogenic differentiation · Osteoprotegerin · RANKL · SHED

W. K. Wan Nor Aduni · S. T. Wei Cun · A. A. Nurul (✉)
School of Health Sciences, Universiti Sains Malaysia, 16150 Kubang Kerian, Kelantan, Malaysia
e-mail: nurulasma@usm.my

R. Dzul Keflee
Department of Molecular Medicine, Faculty of Medicine, Universiti Malaya, 50603 Kuala Lumpur, Malaysia

J. Usman et al. (eds.), *6th Kuala Lumpur International Conference on Biomedical Engineering 2021*, IFMBE Proceedings 86,
https://doi.org/10.1007/978-3-030-90724-2_60

1 Introduction

Bone metabolism is a complex mechanism of bone growth and bone resorption, which entails a vital interaction between osteoblast and osteoclast. The mechanisms are regulated by several cell types and molecular signalling pathways. The RANK/RANKL/OPG signalling pathway has received the greatest attention in the field of bone metabolism and is critical for bone remodelling. Receptor activator of NF-κB (RANK) is a TNF receptor superfamily homotrimeric transmembrane protein, whereas receptor activator of NF-κB ligand (RANKL) is membrane-bound osteoblasts or secreted by activated T cells. Meanwhile, osteoprotegerin (OPG) can act as a soluble decoy receptor for RANKL which is secreted by various cell types including osteoblasts [1]. RANK is a signalling receptor for RANKL and the binding between those two will induce osteoclast differentiation, whereas OPG will act as a negative regulator of RANK signalling, thus inhibits osteoclastogenesis [2].

Stem cells from human exfoliated deciduous teeth (SHED) possess self-renewal capacity and able to differentiate into multiple cell lineages including osteogenic lineage differentiation. Those capabilities make the cells as a promising cell source for bone tissue regeneration [3]. It has been reported that after 4 weeks supplemented with osteoinducing reagents, SHED developed Alizarin red-positive nodules, indicating calcium deposition in the cultured cells [4]. Also, osteogenic induced SHED has been reported to stimulate the upregulation of different bone markers such as ALP, bone sialoprotein, CBFA1 (Core-Binding Factor, Runt Domain Alpha Subunit 1), and MEPE (Matrix extracellular phosphoglycoprotein with ASARM motif) [5].

IL-17A is the member of IL-17 cytokines, consisting of IL-17A, IL-17B, IL-17C, IL-17D, IL-17E, and IL-17F, produced by Th17 cells [6]. IL-17A is the most studied subunit, particularly its pro-inflammatory activity, in which it actively promotes the production of pro-inflammatory factors in pathological conditions. IL-17A specifically binds to its receptor protein, IL-17RA. Any monoclonal antibodies directed against the receptor would eventually inhibit IL-17A-mediated activity, implying that binding is required to elicit IL-17A-specific biological responses [7].

Rapid advancements in microRNA studies in osteogenic differentiation have made this an interesting topic in which these microRNAs can help in the control of gene expression. [8]. Regulation occurs at post-transcriptional level by either translational suppression or mRNA degradation due to the action of the RNA-induces silencing complex (RISC) binding to the 3'UTR region of target sites with the assistance of microRNA [9].

In the present study, we predicted microRNA targeting IL-17RA using algorithmically programs, i.e. DIANA-micro T CDS, mirWalk v2.0, and TargetScan v7.1 and two microRNAs were selected. The hsa-miR-4524a-3p and hsa-miR-6761-5p were transfected into SHED which were pre-treated with IL-17A and the expressions of OPG and RANKL were evaluated by qPCR. To date, this is the first study to report on the effect of microRNAs targeting IL-17RA on the OPG and RANKL expressions in SHED. This study will pave the way for the possible use of microRNA targeting IL-17RA in regenerative medicine and bone diseases.

2 Materials and Methods

2.1 Cell Culture

SHED were purchased from AllCells, USA and were maintained in alpha minimum essential medium (Gibco, USA), completed with 10% fetal bovine serum (Gibco, USA), and 1% penicillin–streptomycin (Gibco, USA) at 37 °C and 5% CO_2 in humidified atmosphere. The medium was changed every 3 days.

2.2 Osteogenic Differentiation

Prior to transfection, SHED were maintained in osteogenic medium containing 50 μg/mL L-ascorbic (Wako, Germany), 10 mM β-glycerophosphate (Sigma, USA), and 10 nM dexamethasone (Sigma, USA) for 7 days. The cells were treated with 50 ng/mL of recombinant IL-17RA for 7 days before transfection and 24 h after the transfection.

2.3 microRNA Mimic Transient Transfection

The prediction of microRNAs targeting IL-17RA mRNA was performed via in silico study. List of potential microRNAs were shortlisted from three most recent algorithmically different programmes such as DIANA-microT CDS, mirWalk v2.0, and TargetScan v7.1 and were further analysed based on site features of mRNA-microRNA pairing. Selected microRNAs were transiently transfected using Lipofectamine® 3000 transfection reagent (Invitrogen, USA) diluted with 1X Opti-MEM® I reduced serum medium (Invitrogen, USA) onto SHED for 48 h. In this study, SHED were transiently transfected with 25, 50, and 100 nM microRNA concentrations (for optimisation) and 50 nM was selected for the actual study.

2.4 Quantitative Real Time-PCR

Total RNA was extracted using RNeasy® Mini Kit (Qiagen, Germany) as described by manufacturer. The purified RNA (2000 ng) was reverse transcribed to cDNA in 20uL reaction by using High Capacity cDNA Reverse Trancsription Kit (Applied Biosystem, USA). The expressions of IL-17RA, GAPDH, and osteogenic genes (OPG and RANKL) were quantified in triplicate by SYBR® Green expression assay on SYBR® Green PCR Master Mix (Applied Biosystems, USA) according to manufacturer's instruction. The expression of tested genes was normalized with internal control gene, reference gene ACTB. The relative gene expression level was calculated by using $2^{-\Delta\Delta CT}$ method [10]

2.5 *Statistical Analysis*

All experiments were carried out in three biological replicates and the quantitative data were reported as mean ± standard deviation. Independent t-tests and one-way analysis of variance (ANOVA) were used to determine significant differences between means, followed by post hoc multiple comparisons. The significance level for all statistical analyses was set at $p < 0.05$.

3 Results

3.1 *Prediction of microRNAS Targeting IL-17RA by in Silico Study*

Identification of microRNA recognition elements (MREs) which is 3' untranslated region (3'UTR) of IL-17RA gene were analysed by three algorithmically different programs (DIANA-micro T web server v5.0, TargetScan Release 7.1 and miRWalk 2.0). Application of these programs resulted in 36 non-repeating conserved microRNAs binding site at the 3'UTR of IL-17RA gene which were then analysed for their minimum free energy (MFE) by using RNAhybrid. Further analyses of microRNAs were evaluated for their most stable seed match which is 8-mer site type, resulting in 19 microRNAs being shortlisted. The best two potential microRNA mimics (hsa-miR-6761-5p and hsa-miR-4524a-3p) were selected based on the evaluation of their perfect Watson–Crick base pairing at the seed region, low minimal free energy (MFE) and have very good pairing to both 5' and 3' ends of the microRNA (5' dominant canonical), lack of G: U wobble pair and bulges at the seed region.

3.2 *Transfection Optimisation Efficiency Using microRNA Targeting GAPDH*

SHED were transfected with different concentrations of microRNA targeting GAPDH (25 nM, 50 nM, and 100 nM) to determine the most significant of GAPDH mRNA downregulation. After 48 h of transfection, the expression of GAPDH mRNA was measured. All the concentrations significantly downregulated the expression of GAPDH mRNA by 0.1237-fold at 25 nM ($p < 0.0001$), 0.0632-fold at 50 nM ($p < 0.0001$), and 0.0842-fold at 100 nM ($p < 0.0001$) as compared to controls (see

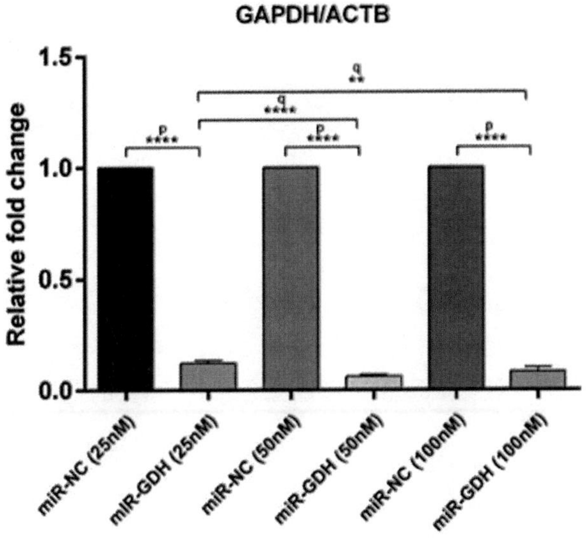

Fig. 1 Relative fold change of GAPDH mRNA level in SHED transfected with 25, 50 and 100 nM of microRNA-targeting GAPDH and non-targeting microRNA as negative control transfected for 48 h and normalized with *β-actin*. Error bars are standard deviation (SD) from three replicates. Asterisk (****) indicates $p < 0.0001$, (**) indicates $p < 0.01$. 'p' indicates compared to negative control and 'q' indicates comparison between microRNA-targeting GAPDH column

Fig. 1). Thus, 50 nM was selected as the optimal concentration of microRNA for downstream experiments.

3.3 Effects of the Predicted microRNAs Targeting IL-17RA on the Level of IL-17RA mRNA Transcript

The hsa-miR-4524a-3p and hsa-miR-6761-5p mimics were transfected into SHED respectively. The hsa-miR-4524a-3p mimic significantly downregulated IL-17RA mRNA expression by 0.195-fold ($p < 0.001$). The other predicted mimic, hsa-miR-6761-5p showed downregulation of IL-17RA mRNA expression by 0.6144-fold ($p < 0.001$). The results indicated that hsa-miR-4524a-3p mimic downregulated IL-17RA expression more effectively than hsa-miR-6761-5p mimic (see Fig. 2).

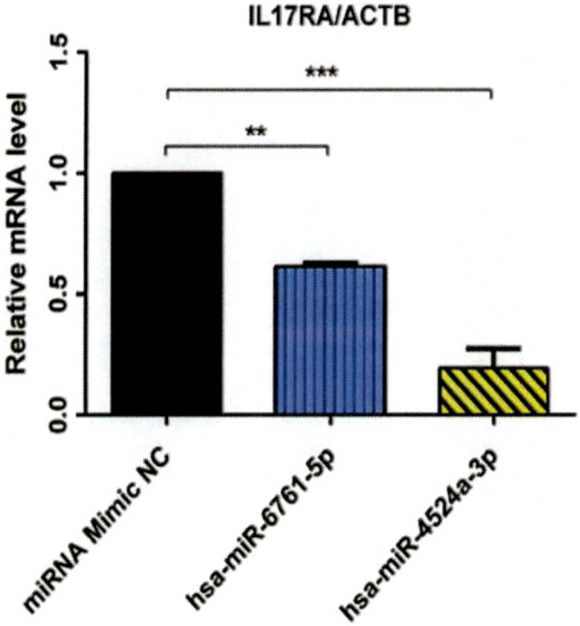

Fig. 2 Relative fold change of IL-17RA mRNA levels in SHED transfected with 50 nM of miR-6761-5p mimic, miR-4524a-3p mimic and non-targeting microRNA as negative control transfected for 48 h and normalized with *β-actin.* Error bars are standard deviation (SD) from two replicates. Asterisk (***) indicates $p < 0.001$ and (**) indicates $p < 0.01$ (One-way ANOVA)

3.4 Effect of microRNA Targeting IL-17RA on Osteogenic Marker Expression, OPG and RANKL by Quantitative Real-Time PCR

The effects of microRNA targeting IL-17RA, hsa-miR-4524a-3p and hsa-miR-6761-5p mimics were also evaluated on selected osteogenic markers expressions, OPG and RANKL. Both microRNAs group showed significant downregulation of OPG gene expression when compared to the control group; hsa-miR-6761-5p with 0.44-fold ($p < 0.01$) and hsa-miR-4524a-3p with 0.13-fold ($p < 0.001$). However, no significant reduction of RANKL gene expression in SHED treated with miR-6761-5p with 0.55-fold ($p > 0.05$) and miR-4524a-3p with 0.24-fold ($p > 0.05$) was observed compared to control (see Fig. 3a, b).

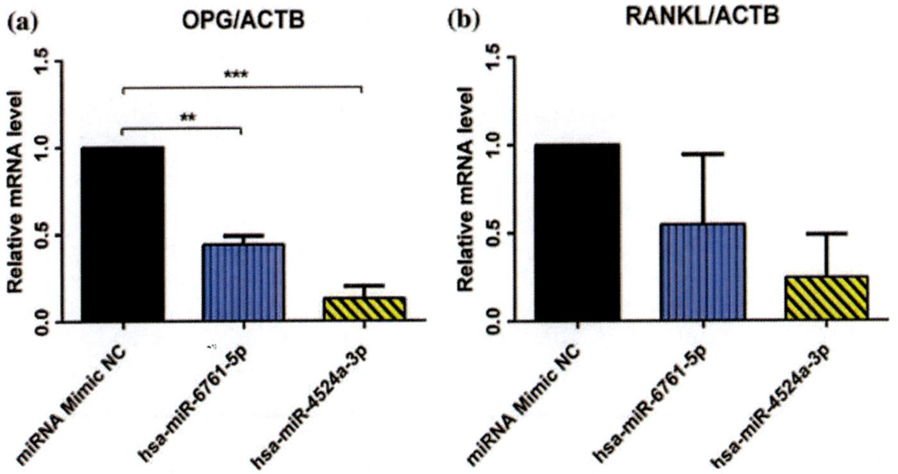

Fig. 3 Relative fold change of **a** OPG and **b** RANKL mRNA levels in SHED transfected with 50 nM of miR-6761-5p mimic, miR-4524a-3p mimic and non-targeting microRNA as negative control transfected for 48 h and normalized with *β-actin*. Error bars are standard deviation (SD) from two replicates. Asterisk (***) indicates $p < 0.001$ and (**) indicates $p < 0.01$ (One-way ANOVA)

4 Discussion and Conclusions

The current study was designed to figure out the effect of predicted microRNA that potentially binds to the 3'UTR of IL-17RA mRNA via in silico study. DIANA-micro T web server v5.0, TargetScan Release 7.1 and miRWalk 2.0 were the bioinformatics tools that have been used to manage the mounting flow of microRNA-related data. A total of 2825 predicted microRNAs were extracted from three algorithmically different program and only 36 non-repeating conserved microRNA were chosen from these programs. Only two shortlisted microRNAs were chosen for experimental validations which were hsa-miR-4524a-3p and hsa-miR-6761-5p. Hsa-miR-4524a-3p and hsa-miR-6761-5p have perfect WC match and microRNA target classification which is 8-mer and 5' dominant canonical. This finding is in agreement with Witkos et al., which stated the canonical with complete pairing within the seed region are the best choice of target for microRNA [11]. In addition, both microRNAs showed perfect number of match, low number of mismatch, absent in G-U wobble and bulges at seed position as well as more WC pairing at nucleotide 12–17 when compared to other predicted microRNAs. These features are important to enhance the effectiveness of microRNA-mRNA interactions which facilitate target prediction [12]

Optimizations for transfection are required to promote the success of genetic material into cells and optimise transfection efficiency. For optimal results, the efficiency of transfection should be reported as high as possible. It is important to conduct multiple transfections under different conditions to discover the ideal condition for maximal transfection effectiveness whenever working with a new cell line

[13]. In the present study, microRNA targeting GAPDH (positive control) significantly downregulate GAPDH gene expression at 25, 50, and 100 nM of mimic concentrations. In order to confirm that the mimic is efficiently knocking down the target, it is always important to include positive control microRNA, and it should be routinely transfected to maintain the optimal transfection condition in every experiment [14]. Furthermore, non-targeting mimics must be used as controls in experiments to demonstrate that the activity of the mimics is specific and not due to background influences [15].

Both predicted microRNAs (hsa-miR-4524a-3p and hsa-miR-6761-3p) targeting IL-17RA showed significant downregulation of IL-17RA mRNA transcript in SHED. Each microRNA might have different targets, leading to different roles and different responses according to the targets. In previous studies, predicted microRNAs have different important roles for instance, in a pilot study of microRNA transcriptome profiling in response to eCig (e-cigarettes), hsa-miR-6761-5p was expressed with eCig treatment [16]. Besides that, hsa-miR-4524a-3p, was discovered by a group of researchers by using next-generation sequencing expression analysis in breast cancer and showed that it has novel role in few subtypes of breast cancer [17]. These findings showed that both microRNAs have important roles in diseases. In contrast to our study, both predicted microRNAs also showed novel role in normal condition where these microRNAs significantly downregulated IL-17RA gene expression and demonstrated effects on osteogenic markers, OPG and RANKL.

IL-17A was previously demonstrated to have important roles in osteogenic differentiation of SHED, providing IL-17A-treated SHED a promising cell source for bone regeneration [18]. Furthermore, IL-17A also induced mineralization activity as well as altered OPG/RANKL ratio. In addition, IL-17A enhanced the proliferation and differentiation of MC3T3-E1 and hFOB and expected to be involved in mineralization via RANK signalling pathway [19]. The present study showed the IL-17A/IL-17RA interaction which affects the RANKL expression and suggested the role of RANKL-dependent IL-17RA expression in bone remodelling of SHED. Further work is required to validate the role of microRNA targeting IL-17RA whether directly or indirectly affects expression of RANKL.

In conclusion, this is the first study to describe the role of microRNA targeting IL-17RA in rIL-17A induced SHED and its effects on the osteogenic markers. These results are important to understand the potential molecular mechanism between IL-17A and IL-17RA in physiology of bone and provide insight into tissue engineering and other pathological research.

References

1. Boyce, B.F., Xing, L.: Functions of RANKL/RANK/OPG in bone modeling and remodeling. Arch. Biochem. Biophys. **473**(2), 139–146 (2008)
2. Walsh, M.C., Choi, Y.: Biology of the RANKL-RANK-OPG system in immunity, bone, and beyond. Front. Immunol. **5**(Oct), 1–11 (2014)

3. Weissman, I.L.: Stem cells: units of development, units of regeneration, and units in evolution. **100**, 157–168 (2000)
4. Miura, M., et al.: SHED: stem cells from human exfoliated deciduous teeth. **100**(10), 5807–5812 (2003)
5. Yasser, S., Nagy, N., Marei, M.K.: In vitro characterization of stem cells from human exfoliated. **5**(4), 389–396 (2012)
6. Moseley, T.A., Haudenschild, D.R., Rose, L., Reddi, A.H.: Interleukin-17 family and IL-17 receptors. **14**, 155–174 (2003)
7. Zhu, S., Qian, Y.: IL-17/IL-17 receptor system in autoimmune disease: mechanisms and therapeutic potential. Clin. Sci. **122**(11), 487–511 (2012)
8. Brennecke, J., Stark, A., Russell, R.B., Cohen, S.M.: Principles of microRNA-target recognition. PLoS Biol. **3**(3), 0404–0418 (2005)
9. Hofacker, I.L.: How microRNAs choose their targets. **39**(10), 1191–1192 (2007)
10. Livak, K.J., Schmittgen, T.D.: Analysis of relative gene expression data using real-time quantitative PCR and the 2–$\Delta\Delta$CT method. Methods **25**, 402–408 (2001)
11. Witkos, T.M., Koscianska, E., Krzyzosiak, W.J.: Practical aspects of microRNA target prediction. CMM., 93–109 (2011)
12. Wang, X.: Improving microRNA target prediction by modeling with unambiguously identified microRNA-target pairs from CLIP-ligation studies. **32**(Jan), 1316–1322 (2016)
13. Jackson, A.L., et al.: Expression profiling reveals off-target gene regulation by RNAi. Nat. Biotechnol. **21**(6), 635–638 (2003)
14. Taylor, P., Søkilde, R., Newie, I., Persson, H., Borg, Å., Rovira, C.: Passenger strand loading in overexpression experiments using microRNA mimics. RNA Biol. (June 2015), 37–41
15. Chang, F., Kai, J., Zhu, H., Cia, L., Wang, S.: Using artificial microRNA sponges to achieve microRNA loss-of-function in cancer cells. Adv. Drug Deliv. Rev. (2014)
16. Solleti, S.K., et al.: MicroRNA expression profiling defines the impact of electronic cigarettes on human airway epithelial cells. Sci. Rep. (Nov 2016), 1–10 (2017)
17. Persson, H., et al.: Identification of new MicroRNAs in paired normal and tumor breast tissue suggests a dual role for the ERBB2/Her2 gene. Cancer Res. **71**(1) (2011)
18. Sebastian, A.A., Kannan, T.P., Norazmi, M.N., Nurul, A.A.: Interleukin-17A promotes osteogenic differentiation by increasing OPG/RANKL ratio in stem cells from human exfoliated deciduous teeth (SHED). J. Tissue Eng. Regen. Med. **12**(8), 1856–1866 (2018)
19. Sritharan, S., Kannan, T.P., Norazmi, M.N., Nurul, A.A.: Interleukin 6 and Interleukin 17a enhance proliferation and differentiation of murine osteoblast and human foetal osteoblast cell lines. IMJM **13**(2), 35–40 (2014)

Synthesis of Polycaprolactone Using Novel Crude Lipase: Parameter Optimization

Paveethra Thegarathah, Muhamad Harith bin Amran, Jegalakshimi Jewaratnam, and Khanom Simarani

Abstract Polycaprolactone was synthesized using ring opening polymerization process by utilizing a novel lipase enzyme from *Aspergillus niger* sp. D-optimal design in DoE was used to optimize the reaction parameters for the synthesis of polycaprolactone. The variables selected were temperature (30–70 °C), time (30–150 min), mixing speed (100–500 rpm) and enzyme volume (5–9 mL). The response variable chosen is the number average molecular weight, Mn. Experimental results obtained was used to explain the interactions between parameters and responses were analyzed and validated. The result shows a good agreement with a minimum error between the actual and predicted values as the error is only 2.35%.

Keywords Polycaprolactone · Lipase · Polymerization

1 Introduction

Polycaprolactone (PCL) is an aliphatic polyester which is used in the biomedical industry. PCL has become popular in producing films, mats, drug delivery systems and scaffolds for various tissue engineering applications due to its biodegradability, biocompatibility, and adjustability. In addition, slow degradation of PCL and PCL-based materials make its preferable for bone substitute materials [1]. However, conventional method of synthesizing PCL using metal catalysts may causes harm to human body. It might leave traces of metal catalyst. Hence, there is a need for

P. Thegarathah · M. H. bin Amran · J. Jewaratnam (✉)
Department of Chemical Engineering, Faculty of Engineering, Universiti Malaya, 50603 Kuala Lumpur, Malaysia
e-mail: jegalaxmi24@um.edu.my

K. Simarani
Institute of Biological Sciences, Faculty of Sciences, Universiti Malaya, 50603 Kuala Lumpur, Malaysia

J. Jewaratnam
Faculty of Engineering, Center for Separation Science and Technology (CSST), Universiti Malaya, 50603 Kuala Lumpur, Malaysia

J. Usman et al. (eds.), *6th Kuala Lumpur International Conference on Biomedical Engineering 2021*, IFMBE Proceedings 86,
https://doi.org/10.1007/978-3-030-90724-2_61

a more sustainable method of PCL production to provide a better alternative while preventing the traces of metal catalyst.

The first reported synthesis of PCL is by using thermal treatment of its monomer, ε-caprolactone. Since then, PCL has been widely synthesized using ring-opening polymerization of ε-caprolactone metal catalyst. On the other hand, greener alternative uses lipase enzyme instead of metal catalysts, mainly due to its sustainability which requires milder reaction condition [2]. Therefore, constant stirring method has been utilised in the synthesis of PCL in this study because it is convenient to handle and inexpensive [3]. Eventually, the quality of the acquired PCL will be determined through its molecular weight distribution. The factors affecting the variety of results in the enzymatic polymerization are the enzyme activity of the enzyme, thermal properties of the enzyme, type of solvent used, pH values of the solvent, monomer-to-ratio solvent etc. *Candida Antarctica* lipase B (CALB) is one of the most promising biocatalysts in enzymatic polymerization of PCL. Nevertheless, there are still large amount of enzyme that has not been used in these are of studies.

In this study, a novel enzyme has been used. Lipase from *Aspergillus niger* sp. is produced in palm oil mill effluent (POME) and used in the enzymatic polymerization of PCL. The novel lipase best reacts at an optimal temperature of 40 °C. The reaction parameters for the synthesis of PCL were optimized by using response surface methodology (RSM) in design-of-experiment (DOE) software, called Statease. The parameters studied in this study are reaction temperature, reaction time, mixing speed and enzyme volume. Then, the responding parameter measured is the number of average molecular weight of the synthesized polymer. This study aims to determine the interaction between the reaction parameters and optimized conditions that will yield polymer with desired molecular weight.

2 Methodology

The lipase from *Aspergillus niger* sp. that was used in this enzymatic polymerization process was received from another study that was conducted along with this one. ε-Caprolactone, toluene, chloroform, and methanol of analytical grade were also obtained from Merck Sdn Bhd, Malaysia.

The preparation of PCL was conducted on a hot plate with constant magnetic stirring. Firstly, 10 ml of ε-caprolactone, 20 ml of toluene and a given volume of lipase enzyme were added into a conical flask with a magnetic stirrer. The reaction temperature, reaction time, mixing speed and enzyme volume were set according to the experimental runs given by DOE. After the desired period of constant stirring, cold chloroform was added to stop the reaction. After that, the solvent present and excess chloroform were removed through rotary evaporation. The acquired precipitate is dried overnight in an oven at 50 °C. Final sample obtained were sent for characterization study using nuclear magnetic resonance (NMR) spectroscopy.

Response surface methodology in DOE software was used to optimize the reaction parameters. The range of reaction parameters were chosen based on literature

Table 1 Reaction parameters chosen for optimization by D-optimal design of the research surface methodology

Reaction parameter	Annotation	Range	Interval	Units
Reaction temperature	A	30–70	10	°C
Reaction time	B	30–150	30	min
Mixing speed	C	100–500	100	RPM
Enzyme volume	D	5	9	mL

review. D-optimal design in RSM was used as it can thoroughly analyse the interaction between the reaction parameters (reaction temperature, reaction time, mixing speed and enzyme volume) and the responding parameter (number average molecular weight). Table 1 shows the reaction parameters and its range while Table 2 shows the experimental runs generated by the software.

3 Results and Discussion

The PCL obtained from this experiment is then characterized by nuclear magnetic resonance (NMR). Figure 1 shows the H1 NMR spectra for the product of the experiment. Peaks at 2.63 ppm, 4.16 ppm, 2.38 ppm, and 2.80 ppm indicate the presence of PCL, where each peaks represent methyl group end, hydroxyl group attached to methyl group, and overlapping hydroxyl methylene, respectively.

A total set of twenty-five experimental runs were generated by D-optimal factorial design with varying combinations of reaction parameters along with responding values are presented in Table 2. The results obtained were used to fit the observed data into polynomial equation (1) which displays the effect of parameters and their possible relations.

$$\text{Mn} = -258.68 * (\text{A}) + 168.22 * (\text{D}) + 1515.60 \quad (1)$$

From equation (1), it can be observed that the reaction temperature (A) and enzyme volume (D) are significant to the models and the reaction time (A) and mixing speed (C) is not very significant to the model. Table 3 shows the reduced quadratic model for the study. Table 3 shows that *P*-value less than 0.05 expresses that the model terms are significant. Factors A and D are found to be the significant terms (Table 4).

Predicted R^2 which is 0.2663 stays within reasonable agreement with the value of the Adjusted R^2 of 0.3715, where the difference is less than 0.2. Adequate Precision, which measures the signal to noise ratio, has a value of 7.4618. This implies that it is an adequate signal, where a ratio greater than 4 is much desired. This information can be used to navigate the design space of the model. DOE has successfully pinpointed the optimized values for each of the reaction parameters and is show in Table 5.

Table 2 Response values based on experimental runs

Run	Factor 1	Factor 2	Factor 3	Factor 4	Response 1
	A: temperature (°C)	B: time (min)	C: mixing speed (RPM)	D: enzyme volume (mL)	Mn
1	30	150	500	7	1667
2	30	150	100	5	1502
3	30	150	100	9	1348
4	30	30	500	5	2012
5	30	30	500	5	2241
6	70	30	500	7	1256
7	30	60	200	5	1733
8	70	150	100	7	1438
9	70	150	500	5	1885
10	50	150	300	7	1450
11	30	30	100	7	1724
12	70	30	200	9	1855
13	40	60	400	7	936
14	40	120	400	9	1392
15	60	30	100	5	2303
16	60	30	100	5	857
17	70	150	500	9	1237
18	30	30	500	9	1353
19	70	30	200	9	1895
20	50	90	100	9	2135
21	50	120	500	6	1426
22	30	150	500	7	1623
23	70	90	300	5	1201
24	30	60	200	9	731
25	70	150	500	9	1117

4 Conclusion

Optimization of enzymatic polymerization was obtained by conducting minimal number of runs generated by the D-optimal design. NMR analysis shows the presence of PCL in the sample obtained. The optimal conditions from the regression model were obtained at reaction temperature: 38 °C, reaction time: 90 min, mixing speed: 300 RPM and enzyme volume: 5 mL. The predicted and experimental values display a good agreement with a percentage error 2.35%. It can be concluded that the reaction temperature, mixing speed and enzyme volume are significant in the model.

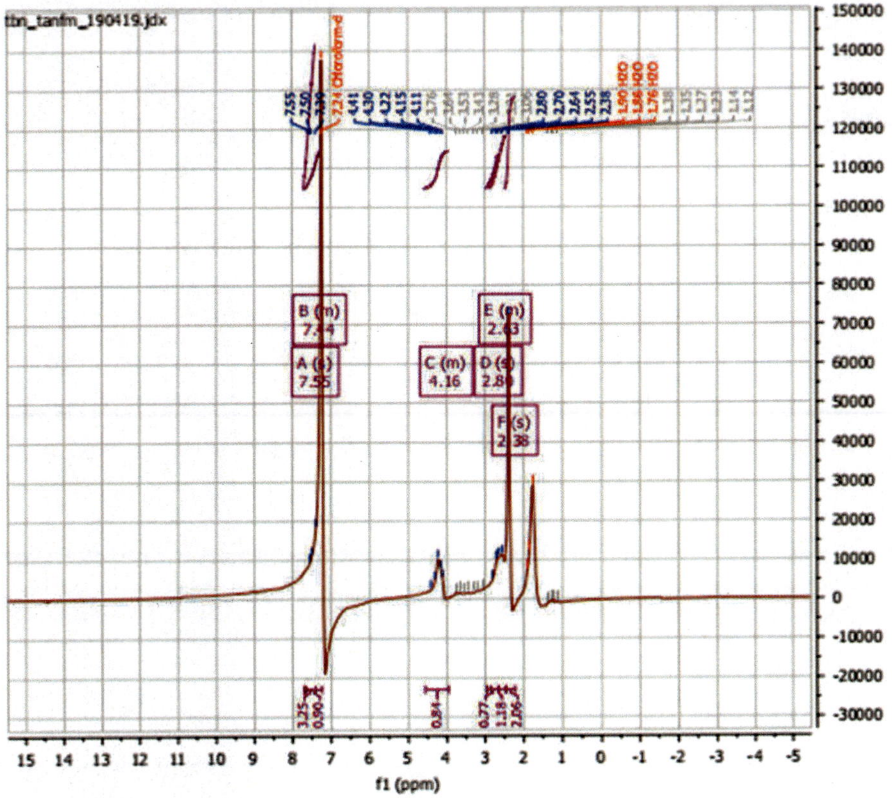

Fig. 1 H1 NMR spectra for polycaprolactone

Table 3 Reduced quadratic ANOVA model

Source	Sum of squares	df	Mean square	F-value	*P*-value	
Model	1.766E+06	2	8.829E+05	8.09	0.0023	Significant
A—Temperature	1.268E+06	1	1.268E+05	11.63	0.0025	
B—Enzyme volume	5.223E+05	1	5.223E+05	4.79	0.0396	
Residual	2.400E+06	22	1.091E+05			
Lack of fit	1.735E+06	17	1.021E+05	0.7669	0.6916	Not significant
Pure error	6.654E+05	5	1.331E+05			
Cor total	4.166E+06	24				

Table 4 Fit statistics for the regression model

Std. dev.	330.31	R^2	0.4239
Mean	1532.68	Adjusted R^2	0.3715
C.V. %	21.55	Predicted R^2	0.2663
		Adeq precision	7.4618

Table 5 Optimized values of the reaction parameters for the production of PCL

	Reaction temperature (°C)	Reaction time (min)	Mixing speed (RPM)	Enzyme volume (mL)	Mn
Predicted value	38.48	90	300	5.18	1511.94
Experimental value	38	90	300	5	1475.49
Percentage error (%)					2.35

Acknowledgements The research was financially supported by research university grant GPF030A-2019 from Faculty of Engineering, University of Malaya.

References

1. Malikmammadov, E., Tanir, T.E., Kiziltay, A., Hasirci, V., Hasirci, N.: PCL and PCL-based materials in biomedical applications. J. Biomater. Sci. Polym. Ed. 29(7–9), 863–893 (2018). https://doi.org/10.1080/09205063.2017.1394711
2. Albertsson, A.-C., Srivastava, R.K.: Recent developments in enzyme-catalyzed ring-opening polymerization. Adv. Drug Deliv. Rev. **60**(9), 1077–1093 (2008). https://doi.org/10.1016/j.addr.2008.02.007
3. Li, Q., Li, G., Yu, S., Zhang, Z., Ma, F., Feng, Y.: Ring-opening polymerization of ε-caprolactone catalyzed by a novel thermophilic lipase from Fervidobacterium nodosum. Process Biochem. **46** (2011). Bixler, A.: Family-Friendly Science: Increasing Family Engagement in STEM Education (2016)
4. dos Santos, J.C.S., Bonazza, H.L., de Matos, L.J.B.L., Carneiro, E.A., Barbosa, O., Fernandez-Lafuente, R., Gonçalves, L.R.B., de Sant' Ana, H.B., Santiago-Aguiar, R.S.: Immobilization of CALB on activated chitosan: application to enzymatic synthesis in supercritical and near-critical carbon dioxide. Biotechnol. Rep. 14:16–26 (2017). https://doi.org/10.1016/j.btre.2017.02.003
5. Foresti, M.L., Ferreira, M.L.: Synthesis of polycaprolactone using free/supported enzymatic and non-enzymatic catalysts. Macromol. Rapid Commun. **25**(24), 2025–2028 (2004). https://doi.org/10.1002/marc.200400392
6. Kumar, A., Gross, R.A.: Candida antartica Lipase B catalyzed polycaprolactone synthesis: effects of organic media and temperature. Biomacromol **1**(1), 133–138 (2000). https://doi.org/10.1021/bm990510p
7. Lam, C.X.F., Teoh, S.H., Hutmacher, D.W.: Comparison of the degradation of polycaprolactone and polycaprolactone–(β-tricalcium phosphate) scaffolds in alkaline medium. Polym. Int. **56**(6), 718–728 (2007). https://doi.org/10.1002/pi.2195

Experimental Study Between TPU Flex and Silicon Materials Mechanical Properties as an Alternatives in Development of the *CardioVASS* Heart Model

Nur Afikah Khairi Rosli, Mohd Azrul Hisham Mohd Adib, Mok Chik Ming, Nurul Natasha Mohd Sukri, Idris Mat Sahat, and Nur Hazreen Mohd Hasni

Abstract The development of a heart model for medical training purposes in the current market is still new. The mechanical properties and the selection of materials become the main elements in determining the type of materials used. This paper highlighted to study of the mechanical properties between TPU Flex and silicon to determine the suitability of the material for the development of the *CardioVASS* heart model. Both of the materials were assessed by utilizing the tensile, compression, and hardness test methods to prove the validity of the materials for the *CardioVASS* heart model. Results suggested that the TPU Flex was superior to the silicon materials in terms of strength and durability.

Keywords TPU · Polyurethane · Silicon · Polymer · Three-dimensional printing · Hardness test · *CardioVASS* device · Medical · Healthcare · Heart model

1 Introduction

The emergence of revolving technology nowadays had paved ways for the polymers group material to be explored in many sectors, including in the medical sectors. The flexible polyurethane thermoplastic (TPU) and silicon materials are the most

N. A. K. Rosli (✉) · M. A. H. M. Adib (✉) · M. C. Ming · N. N. M. Sukri
Medical Engineering and Health Intervention Team (MedEHiT), Department of Mechanical Engineering, College of Engineering, Universiti Malaysia Pahang, Lebuhraya Tun Abdul Razak, 26300 Kuantan, Pahang, Malaysia
e-mail: azrul@ump.edu.my

I. M. Sahat
Human Engineering Group (HEG), Faculty of Mechanical and Automotive Engineering Technology, Universiti Malaysia Pahang, 26600 Pekan, Pahang, Malaysia

N. H. M. Hasni
Family Health Unit, Pahang State Health Department, Jalan IM 4, Bandar Indera Mahkota, 25582 Kuantan, Pahang, Malaysia

J. Usman et al. (eds.), *6th Kuala Lumpur International Conference on Biomedical Engineering 2021*, IFMBE Proceedings 86,
https://doi.org/10.1007/978-3-030-90724-2_62

common materials of the polymers group that had marked their contribution especially in the current market [1–10]. However, some factors needed to be reviewed before implemented these elastomeric materials for further use; the mechanical properties factors. As the materials were known as soft, biocompatible, and flexural materials, therefore there were some concerns regarding the strength, durability, and endurance of the substance to be applied in long-term usage. Thus, this research was conducted to evaluate the following materials that include the experimental tensile test, compression test, and hardness test.

Silicon is one of the feasible materials that had been a preference for medical and healthcare applications. Poojari [11] in her research had suggested the encapsulation of the medical device implants by using silicone materials due to their excellent biocompatibility and mechanical properties. This material has excellent material properties, accompanied by high flexibility, low biological activity, ease of fabrication, chemical and thermal stability, biocompatibility, and hydrophobicity [11–13]. Rahaman et al. [14] had suggested the utilization of silicon nitride for ceramic implant materials, particularly in orthopedic surgery.

The TPU material commonly available as a rigid substance before extruded using the three-dimensional printer into the designated shapes. Most of the TPU usage revolved around the manufacturing and processing field that includes the footwear industry, cables, wires, and others [15]. Although the TPU Flex material was not as popular as silicone in the medical fields, however, this material can be applied for similar purposes as silicone and have outstanding mechanical properties compared to silicone. For instance, the TPU has good tensile strength, tear, and abrasion resistance compared to the silicone material [16, 17].

CardioVASS device or known as the cardiovascular simulator is a newly invented device that had been proposed to be utilized for the education and learning process. The history of this device started with the fabrication of an experimental heart-S apparatus [18, 19] that was evaluated into few models and now was known as the *CardioVASS* device. The research of this device was divided into three research modes; the physiology of blood circulation in the human heart [20], the observation of the heart's mechanism, and the comprehension of the pathophysiological state of the heart during the catheter insertion into the small arteries [21]. This research was also a continuation of the *CardioVASS* system study that focused on the fabrication of the heart model materials.

The objectives of this research are to study the mechanical properties of the TPU Flex and silicon materials to determine the suitability material characteristics to be fabricated as a heart model for the *CardioVASS* device.

2 Methodology

2.1 Fabrication of the Test Samples

The fabrication of the test samples started with designing the test samples using the Solidwork version 2016 software by referring to the ASTM D1621 for the compression test and ASTM D638 [22] specifications for the tensile test. The dog-bone specimens of the tensile test for TPU Flex materials were directly printed using the Ender 3 Pro printer by setting up the printer to be compatible with the material setting in Table 1. Figure 1a, b depicts the design and printing process during the experiment was carried out. Next, the compression test used a rectangular shape of specimens as shown in Fig. 2. The same method as the tensile test was applied while preparing for the compression test specimens. Since the silicon materials existed in the liquid form, the process of curing activities and mixture between silicon solution with the hardener solution were explained as in Fig. 3. Table 2 depicts the mechanical properties of the silicon materials.

The TPU Flex test samples were extruded from the TPU Flex filaments at room temperature to gain the specific test specimen as illustrated above. The TPU Flex

Table 1 Mechanical properties of the TPU Flex material [23]

Characteristics	Value
Durability	High
Strength	High
Flexibility	Very high
Chemical resistance	Medium–high
Abrasion resistance	High
Water resistance	Medium
Nozzle temperature	220–250 °C
Heated bed	Up to 60 °C

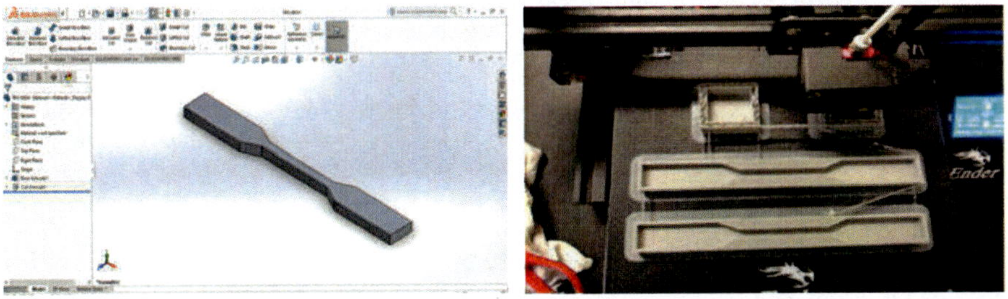

(a) (b)

Fig. 1 **a** Showed the designation of the test specimens for the TPU Flex tensile test. **b** Depicts the printing process for the molds of the tensile and compression test for the silicon materials

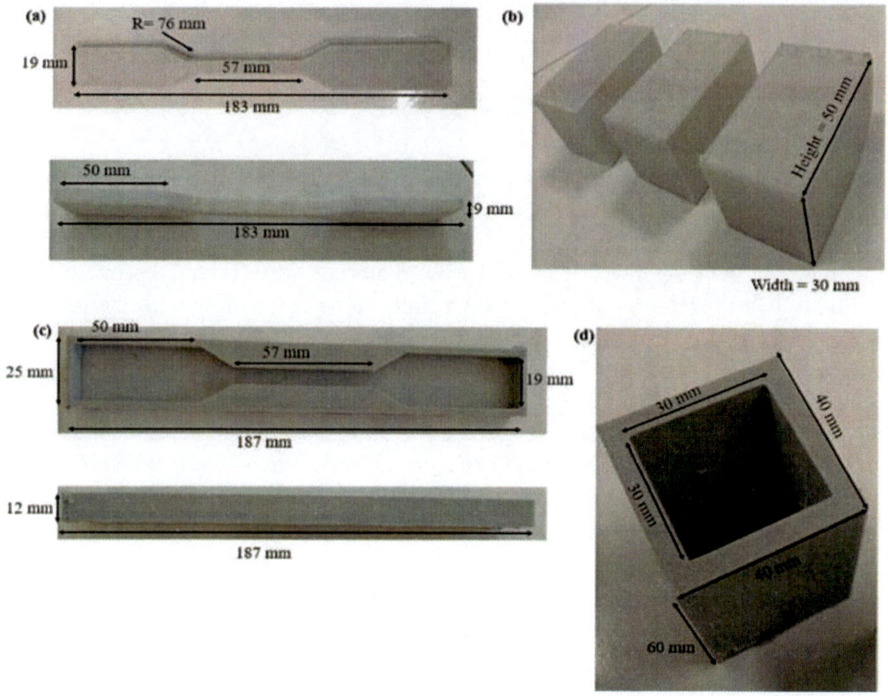

Fig. 2 **a** Depicts the specifications of the tensile test for the TPU Flex materials. **b** Showed the specifications of the compression test for the TPU Flex materials. **c, d** Depicts the molds for the silicon materials specifications

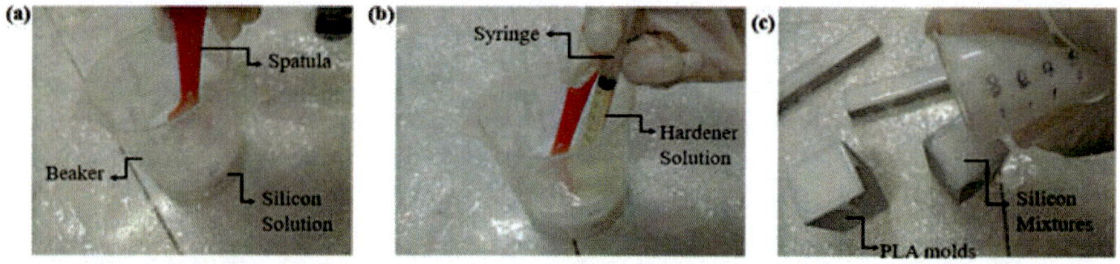

Fig. 3 **a** Shows the silicon solution was stirred completely before the mixing process to ensure the solution was even in viscosity. **b** Depicts the hardener solution that was poured into the beaker that contained the silicon solution based on the ratio of 3% of hardener to the total volume used for the silicon solution. The mixture was then stirred for about 5 min to blend them well. **b** Showed the silicon mixtures were poured into the molds to obtain the desired shapes for the test samples

samples utilized about 100 g approximately of TPU Flex filaments per test samples printed. The fabrication of the silicon samples used about 100 g of silicon mixtures per test specimens and cured at room temperature for 24 hours.

Table 2 Mechanical properties of the silicon materials

Characteristics	Value
Base viscosity	24,000 cP
Density	1.18 g/cc
Tear resistance	17/N mm
Hardness	After 72 h 21 ± 2 shA
Strength resistance	3/N mm^2
Elongation at break	400%

2.2 *Tensile and Compression Test*

The tensile and compression test were carried out by employing an Instron 300 K machines with a speed of 20 mm/min at the room temperature surroundings. The tensile samples were first marked with a marker to calibrate the tensile grips and the test specimen length. The samples were tested until achieved the breaking point (completely tear). Next, the compression test was conducted by applying for the parallel compression plates. The rectangular samples were then pressed until the maximum height of extension for the samples achieved. The data was then collected using the Instron software and tabulated as in Tables 3, 4, 5, and 6. Figure 4 depicts the tensile and compression test of the samples by using the Instron 300 K machines.

Table 3 The tensile test results of the TPU Flex specimens

	Tensile strain at maximum tensile extension (mm/mm)	Load at maximum tensile extension (N)	Modulus (automatic) (MPa)
Sample 1	2.29	2.22	3.29
Sample 2	1.67	68.20	8.23
Sample 3	2.26	−1.04	3.18

Table 4 The compression results for the TPU Flex material

	Minimum load (N)	Time at minimum load (s)	Energy at minimum load (J)	Extension at minimum load (mm)
Sample 1	−3532.19	134.22	8.43	−44.74
Sample 2	−10,592.03	137.00	17.48	−45.66
Sample 3	−12,776.37	106.71	18.73	−45.24

Table 5 The tensile test results for the silicon materials

	Tensile strain at maximum tensile extension (mm/mm)	Load at maximum tensile extension (N)	Modulus (automatic) (MPa)
Sample 1	1.37	−1.30	0.68
Sample 2	1.55	−0.91	0.68
Sample 3	1.35	−1.08	0.89

Table 6 The compression results for the silicon materials

	Minimum load (N)	Time at minimum load (s)	Energy at minimum load (J)	Extension at minimum load (mm)
Sample 1	−6464.43	135.91	34.60	−45.30
Sample 2	−6859.55	135.73	36.63	−45.24
Sample 3	−6029.81	135.98	33.01	−45.33

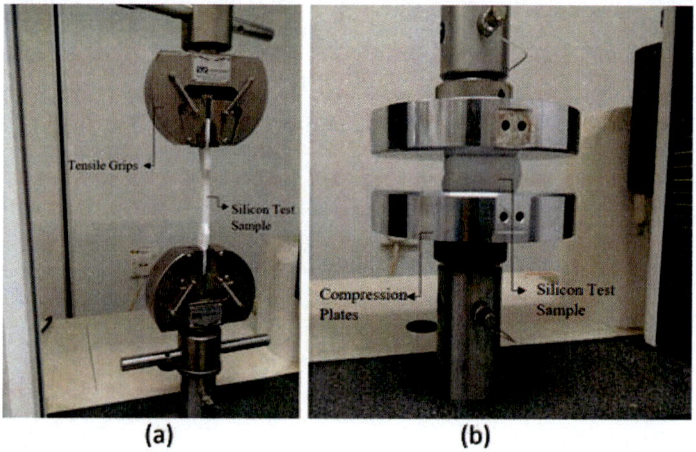

Fig. 4 **a** Showed the tensile load was exerted on the test samples. **b** Showed the compression load was applied on the silicon samples

2.3 Hardness Test

Hardness test is one of the methods that had been used in this experiment to measure the material's comprehensive performance reaction especially in the ability of the materials to withstand the resistance and to determine the elasticity of the materials. A digital shore durometer (type A) was utilized for measuring the hardness of the TPU Flex and silicon materials. The durometer type A instrument is suitable for medium hardness rubber such as plastic, rubber, leather, multi-grease, wax, and others. The range measured for the durometer instrument was varied from 0 to 100

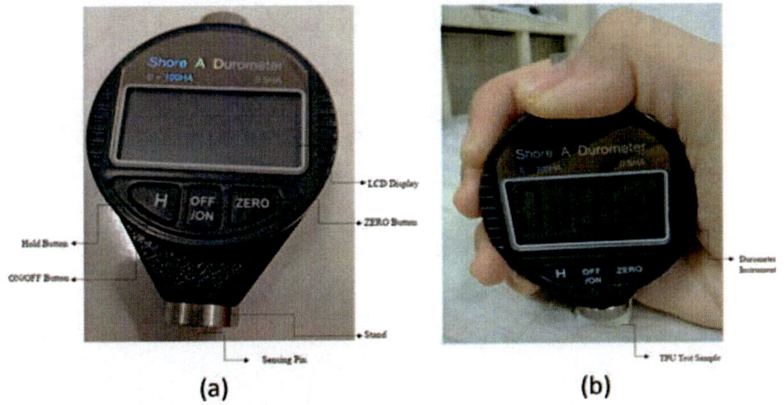

Fig. 5 **a** Shows the mechanism of the Durometer device. **b** Demonstrated the application of the Durometer device for measurement activities

HA. The higher the HA values, the higher the hardness of the material tested. By following the guidelines from ASTM D2240, a sample of the TPU Flex and silicon materials were prepared respectively before the experiments were conducted. The sensing pin that resembles needle-like stuff was penetrated the materials by a constant force and created resistance force from the samples that generated the hardness values for each of the samples [24] (Fig. 5).

3 Results and Discussions

3.1 Strength of Material

TPU Flex Material

The results of the tensile test for the TPU Flex materials were recorded and tabulated into the graph and Table 3. Three identical samples of the TPU Flex materials were analyzed and merged into the same graph to obtain a comparison of the graph trends during the experiments. In Fig. 6, the sample 1 and sample 3 achieved almost the same correlation values with the extension of the TPU Flex test samples achieved 400 mm respectively. The trends of both samples 1 and 3 were increasing significantly that demonstrated the elongation process occurred during the extension process of the samples before reaching the breaking point and dropped values that reached almost 400 N for both of the samples respectively. However, samples 2 displayed an odd shape of the graphs compared to samples 1 and 3. Sample 2 managed to achieved tensile extension at 170 mm approximately which is less than sample 1 and 3 results. Furthermore, sample 2 also conveyed 320 N of load approximately which showed a huge difference in the load values compared to samples 1 and 3. The irregular shapes at the end of the dropped values of the test samples 2 represented there was a

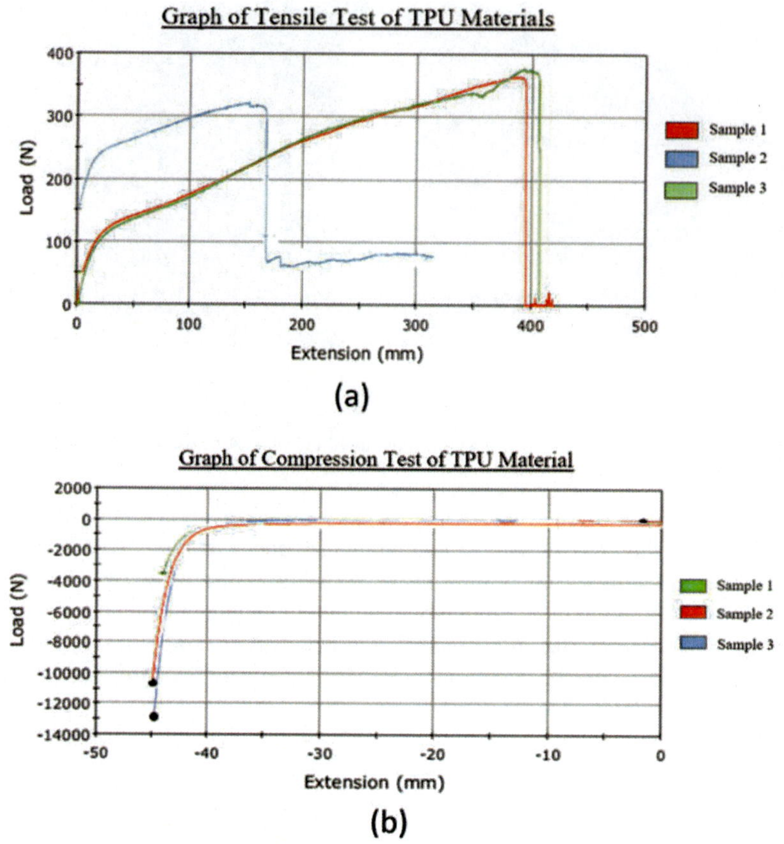

Fig. 6 **a** Showed the graphs of tensile load versus the tensile extension of the TPU Flex materials. **b** Depicts the compression load versus compression extension

continuous extension of the material even after the breaking point of the material was portrayed. These samples have different values and trends due to the different stress distribution for each of the specimens. Sample 1 and 3 were completely broken during the experimental process at the center point of the dog-bone specimens while sample 2 breaks at the end radius of the specimens. These situations may happen because of the distinct load from the tensile grips that were exerted on the specimens and the inconsistency of the filled volume of the TPU Flex specimens after the printing process that lead to the dissimilar stress distribution of the tensile specimens.

From the Fig. 6a, Hookean behavior were founded at the early stage of the tensile test. The linear elastic properties then changed to viscous behavior in the middle of the experiments with the additional load observed. In this phase, the stress and strain relationship were directly proportional. As the load exceeded the limitation of the TPU Flex material, the TPU Flex exhibit plastic behavior and finally break with permanent damage were recorded. Meanwhile, Fig. 6b form the viscoelastic behavior where the material return to their original shapes after the load was removed.

Silicon Material

The tensile test for the silicon material demonstrated similar increasing trends of extension due to the elastomeric properties of the silicon material before reached the breaking points where the tensile load values plummeted to zero values. The tensile strain at maximum tensile extension for samples 1, 2, and 3 were 1.37 mm/mm, 1.55 mm/mm, and 1.35 mm/mm respectively. The load at maximum tensile extension for sample 1 was −1.30 N, sample 2 was −0.91 N and sample 3 was −1.08 N. The automatic modulus analyzed were 0.68 MPa for both samples 1 and 2 while sample 3 showed slightly high values with 0.89 MPa.

The graphs in Fig. 7 illustrated the corresponding trends for all of the test samples where the compression extension results were decreased due to the force exerted on the specimens. Similar trends for the compression test as in the Fig. 6b were observed in the Fig. 7b where the silicon specimens underwent viscoelastic phase that enable the material to rebound back to the original length and shape with minimum exerted load recorded was 6000 N approximately and compressed until 90% of the height of the sample. Based in Table 6, the silicon material required less load compared to the TPU Flex material in Table 4 values with almost twice load values. However, the energy generated at minimum load of the silicon were twice of the TPU Flex material. Therefore, from these results we can deduce that the TPU Flex material have twice strength compared to the silicon material but at the other side, the silicon demonstrated twice elasticity than the TPU Flex material due to the ability of the silicon to absorb force from the applied load.

3.2 *Material Hardness*

The hardness of the materials can be measured through the hardness test by using the Durometer shore A device that utilizes the indentation method to calibrate the elasticity and the durability of the following materials. In Table 7, three distinct points of a single test specimen were used to determine the average values of the TPU Flex and silicon materials. The huge gaps between these two materials depicted that the TPU Flex materials were way too hard compared to the silicon materials. This relationship suggested that the increase the shore values, the harder the material hardness.

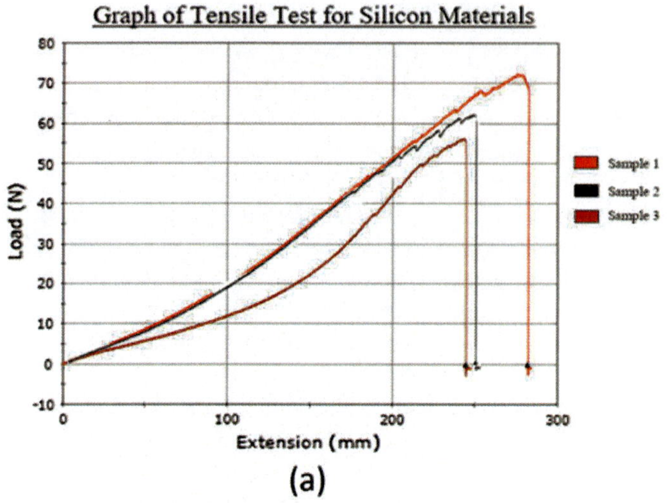

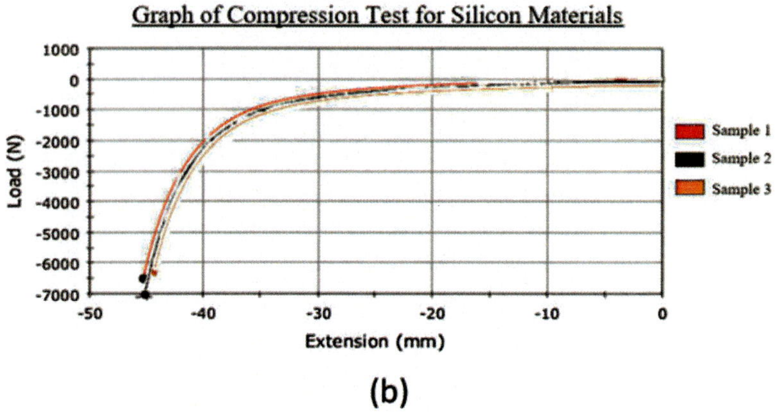

Fig. 7 **a** Showed the graph of tensile load versus tensile extension for silicon materials. **b** Depicts the compression load versus compression extension for the silicon materials

Table 7 Durometer hardness test for the TPU Flex and silicon materials

Material	1	2	3	Average (HA)
TPU Flex	76.5	73.5	77.5	75.8
Silicon	16.0	18.0	18.5	17.5

3.3 *The Suitability of the TPU Flex and Silicon Material in the Fabrication of the* CardioVASS *Heart Model*

In this research, we tried to highlight the suitability of the TPU Flex and silicon material for the fabrication of the *CardioVASS* heart model by studying the mechanical properties of the materials respectively. The research conducted by Adib et al. [21] and Khairul et al. [25] had implemented TPU Flex shore 85 A materials for the manufacturing of their heart model. Based on their research, they had successfully constructed a simple TPU Flex heart model but with multiple limitations confronted such as the difficulties in adjusting the strength and flexibilities of the model. Aiming to fabricate a functional heart model with good flexibilities and mimicking the actual heart, our *CardioVASS* project tried to solve the problems related to the heart models by studying the mechanical properties of the model to identify the strength and weaknesses of each of the material selected as in this paper. Previously, the TPU Flex shore 85 A was tested and compared with the soft epoxy resin material to identify the significance of the material with the fabricated heart model [15]. The results shown that the TPU Flex was able to demonstrate better elongation, flexibility and strength compared to the epoxy resin material. The maximum modulus gained for the TPU Flex shore 85 A was 13.78 MPa that almost multiple of the maximum modulus results for the TPU Flex shore 95 A with 8.23 MPa as in the Table 3. The values may vary due to the design implementation, infill, layer, thickness and temperature setting during the extrusion of the samples. The shore hardness of the TPU Flex material also may dropped during the extrusion process as represented in Table 7 where the average shore hardness dropped to 75.8 HA compared to the actual TPU Flex filament, 95 HA. Richard et al. [26] in his research mentioned that the polyurethanes was among the most feasible type of polymer for the heart valve applications that manage to achieve several hundred million cycles during the in vitro durability testing. Recent studies demonstrated by Hoashi et al. [27] had successfully constructed 20 custom made 3D printed heart model for preoperative surgical simulations to treat the congenital heart disease by utilizing the polyurethanes resins materials. The findings demonstrated that polyurethane resins can be recognized as having potential utility, particularly in understanding the relationship between intraventricular communications and great vessels, as well as in simulation for creating intracardiac pathways. Thus, we can deduce that the TPU Flex material was capable to be fabricated as heart model due to the excellent elastomeric properties. However, the application of the TPU Flex material for the fabrication of the heart model itself was not enough due to the insufficient strength and strain properties of the heart model prototypes and many researchers tried to solve the problems by mixing the polyurethanes materials with other polymer and materials to enhance their current properties [28, 29] (Table 8; Fig. 8).

Silicones material or known as siloxane was also one of the feasible types of polymer material that had used widely in manufacturing field, especially in the medical region. In this paper, the tensile and compression test had demonstrated that

Table 8 Mechanical properties for the TPU Flex [15]

	Modulus (automatic young's modulus) (MPa)	Tensile stress at tensile strength (MPa)	Tensile stress at break standard (MPa)	Force at tensile strength (kN)
Sample 4	13.78	2.31	0.02	0.31
Sample 5	11.57	2.32	0.01	0.31
Sample 6	12.07	2.34	0.01	0.31

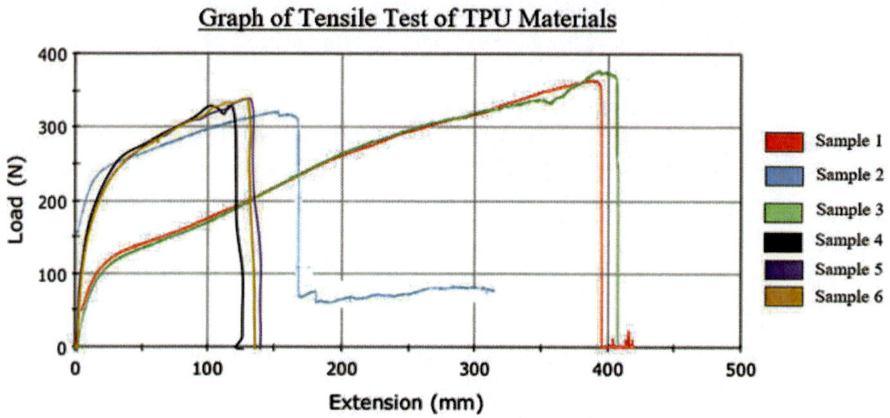

Fig. 8 Demonstrated a graph of tensile test versus extension for the TPU Flex material

the silicone material was twice weaker in strength compared to the TPU Flex material. However, the hardness test revealed that the silicone was four times weaker in terms of mechanical hardness shore. While hardness is dependent on ductility, elastic stiffness, plasticity, strain, strength toughness viscoelasticity and viscosity [30] of a material, it is understandable that there was some contradiction between the ratios as distinct mechanical test were conducted. On the contrary, because of the composition of silicon which allows free rotation along the chain, the silicone exhibits more elasticity than the TPU Flex as described earlier in Sect. 3.1, resulting in high polymer flexibility [31]. Nicholas [31] in his research had highlighted the application of the silicone elastomers for the fabrication of the artificial hearts agreed that the silicone elastomer was suitable for the soft artificial heart development because of the softness properties of the silicone itself. He also mentioned that the past artificial heart was commonly rigid due to the material properties constraint. The softness from the silicone was desirable as it can biomimicking the actual heart physiological blood flow and pumping.

In short, both TPU Flex and silicon material demonstrated high potential to be developed as heart model for the *CardioVASS* device. However, the materials still restricted to some weaknesses especially in strength, durability and elasticity compared to the actual heart. Improvement for both of the material were expected in the future for better heart model making.

3.4 Limitations

There were some limitations founded in this research. To begin with, the present work only represented a single type of polymer, silicone and TPU Flex shore 95 A only. By using a wide range of elastomeric polymer studies, we can make more strength and flexibilities comparison regarding the mechanical properties of the selected material. Next, the method that had been conducted to fabricate the samples were restricted to the FDM 3D printer only for the TPU Flex material and curing process method for the silicon. A better and compromise results expected when utilizing an advanced method in the fabrication process. For instance, using the stereolithography (SLA) and digital light projector (DLP) method that can produce a flexible and precise model sample with the complex geometries. Lastly, there was no addition of distinguished materials were presented in this work compared to the other research that known can establish the mechanical properties of the elastomeric materials especially. High scale of research must be done to study the most suitable material that can merge with the existing selected material that can improvise the mechanical properties of the material.

4 Conclusions and Recommendations

In conclusion, the tensile and compression test validate that the TPU Flex and silicon materials were able to demonstrate high strength and elasticity although have a soft structure of materials. Regardless, to achieve the actual heart strength, the TPU Flex and silicone strength were way too low in strength and durability. The results pointed out that the TPU Flex material was twice higher in strength compared to the silicon material. In contrast, the silicon material was twice elastic than the TPU Flex material. Here, we can conclude that both of the materials were capable to be fabricated as heart model for the *CardioVASS* device but the TPU Flex materials were preferred as the material have better strength, elongation, and durability compared to the silicon material. However, the softness properties from the silicone material was desirable for the development of the heart model due to the natural properties of silicon that biomimicking the actual heart. With the vast types of polymer, there still some room for the improvement for improvising the current mechanical properties of the material by merging different types of polymers or material and changing the method of material manufacturing by using advanced technological machine for 3D printing such as SLA printer. In the future, more research and development must be carried out to improvise the mechanical properties of the selected materials so that we can obtain an excellent heart model that can initiate the revolution of the local heart model in the market.

Acknowledgements The support from the Ministry of Higher Education (MOHE) under PRGS grant PRGS/1/2019/TK03/UMP/02/4, UMP under grant RDU190805 and PGRS2003198 and Medical Engineering and Health Intervention Team (MedEHiT) are gratefully acknowledged.

References

1. Su, S.H., Hua, Z.K., Zhang, J.H.: Design and mechanics simulation of bionic lubrication system of artificial joints. J. Bionic Eng. **3**, 155–160 (2006)
2. Bondurant, S., Ernster, V., Herdman, R., Implants, C.S.S.B., Medicine, I.: Safety of Silicone Breast Implants. National Academies Press, Washington, USA (2000)
3. Goudie, C., Gill, A., Shanahan, J., Furey, A., Dubrowski, A.: Development of an anatomical silicone model for simulation-based medical training of obstetric anal sphincter injury repair in Bangladesh. Cureus (2019). https://doi.org/10.7759/cureus.3991
4. Barton, A.: Medical adhesive-related skin injuries associated with vascular access: minimising risk with appeel sterile. Br. J. Nurs. **29**, S20–S27 (2020)
5. Swift, T., Westgate, G., Van Onselen, J., Lee, S.: Developments in silicone technology for use in stoma care. Br. J. Nurs. **29**, S6–S15 (2020)
6. Barboza, E.P., et al.: Evaluation of surgical gown textiles for resistance against aerosols: a preclinical double-blind study. Front. Dent. Med. **2** (2021)
7. Li, X., Koh, K.H., Farhan, M., Lai, K.W.C.: An ultraflexible polyurethane yarn-based wearable strain sensor with a polydimethylsiloxane infiltrated multilayer sheath for smart textiles. Nanoscale **12**, 4110–4118 (2020)
8. Chen, Q., et al.: Enhanced strain sensing performance of polymer/carbon nanotube-coated spandex fibers via noncovalent interactions. Macromol. Mater. Eng. **305** (2020)
9. Ashby, M.F.: Material profiles. In: Materials and the Environment (2013)
10. Curtis, J., Colas, A.: In: Ratner, B.D., Hoffman, A.S., Schoen, F.J. (eds.) Biomaterials Science: An Introduction to Materials in Medicine, pp. 80–86. Elsevier Academic Press, Amsterdam (2004)
11. Poojari, Y.: Silicones for encapsulation of medical device implants. Silicon **9**(5), 645–649 (2017). https://doi.org/10.1007/s12633-017-9603-4
12. Zhang, X., Brodus, D.S., Hollimon, V., Hu, H.: A brief review of recent developments in the designs that prevent bio-fouling on silicon and silicon-based materials. Chem. Cent. J. (2017). https://doi.org/10.1186/s13065-017-0246-8
13. Yeh, S.-B., Chen, C.-S., Chen, W.-Y., Huang, C.-J.: Modification of silicone elastomer with zwitterionic silane for durable antifouling properties. Langmuir **30**(38), 11386–11393 (2014)
14. Rahaman, M., Xiao, W.: Silicon nitride bioceramics in healthcare. Int. J. Appl. Ceram. Technol. **15**(4), 861–872 (2018). https://doi.org/10.1111/ijac.12836
15. Rosli, N.A.K., Adib, M.A.H.M., Sukri, N.N.M., Sahat, I.M., Hasni, N.H.M.: The Cardio-VASS heart model: comparison of biomaterials between TPU flex and soft epoxy resin for biomedical engineering application. In: 2020 IEEE-EMBS Conference on Biomedical Engineering and Sciences (IECBES), pp. 224–229 (2021). https://doi.org/10.1109/IECBES48179.2021.9398731
16. Chauvel-Lebret, D.J., Auroy, P., Bonnaure-Mallet, M.: Biocompatibility of elastomers. In: Dumitriu, S. (ed.) Polymeric Biomaterials, Revised and Expanded. Taylor & Francis, pp. 311–360 (2001)
17. Wasikiewicz, J.M., Roohpour, N., Vadgama, P.: Packaging and coating materials for implantable device. In: Inmann, A., Hodgins, D. (eds.) Implantable Sensor Systems for Medical Applications, pp. 68–107. Woodhead Publishing Limited, Oxford, UK (2013)

18. Adib, M.A.H.M., Hasni, N.H.M.: Study the heart valve elasticity and optimal of vortex formation for blood circulation measurement on the left ventricle using the heart simulator (Heart-S) apparatus. In: ACM International Conference Proceeding Series, pp. 58–62 (2017)
19. Liang, L.Q., Hui, K.Y., Hasni, N.H.M., Adib, M.A.H.M.: Development of heart simulator (heart-S) on the left ventricle for measuring the blood circulation during cardiac cycle. J. Biomimet. Biomater. Biomed. Eng. **36**, 78–83 (2018)
20. Rosli, N.A.K., Adib, M.A.H.M., Hasni, N.H.M., Abdullah, M.S.: Effect of hemodynamic parameters on physiological blood flow through cardiovascular disease (CVD)—the perspective review. J. Adv. Res. Fluid Mech. Therm. Sci. **74**, 19–34 (2020)
21. Adib, M.A.H.M., Yakof, K.S.A., Anuar, Z., Abdullah, N., Sahat, I.M., Hasni, N.H.M.: The cardio vascular simulator (CardioVASS) device on monitoring the physiology of blood flow circulation via angiographic image for medical trainee. J. Adv. Res. Fluid Mech. Therm. Sci. (2019)
22. E3-95: Standard practice for preparation of metallographic specimens. ASTM Int. **82**(C), 1–15 (2016)
23. Tractus3D: TPU material, Aug 2020 [Online]. Available: https://tractus3d.com/materials/tpu
24. Sharma, S., Jujhar, S., Harish, K., Abhinav, S., Vivek, A., Amoljit, S.G., Jayarambabu, J., Saraswathi, A., Rao, K.V.: Utilization of rapid prototyping technology for the fabrication of an orthopedic shoe inserts for foot pain reprieve using thermo-softening viscoelastic polymers: a novel experimental approach. Measur. Control **53**(3), 519–530 (2020)
25. Yakof, K.S.A., Zabudin, N.F., Sahat, I.M., Adib, M.A.H.M.: Development of 3D printed heart model for medical training. Lect. Notes Mech. Eng. **0**(9789811087875), 109–116 (2018)
26. Li, R.L., Russ, J., Poschalides, C., Ferrari, G., Waisman, H., Kysar, J.W., Kalfa, D.: Mechanical considerations for polymeric heart valve development: biomechanics, materials, design and manufacturing. J. Biomater. **225**, 119493 (2019)
27. Hoashi, T., Ichikawa, H., Nakata, T., Shimada, M., Ozawa, H., Higashida, A., Kurosaki, K., Kanzaki, S., Shirashi, I.: Utility of a super-flexible three-dimensional printed heart model in congenital heart surgery. In: 31st Annual Meeting of the European Association for Cardio-Thoracic Surgery, Vienna, Austria (2017)
28. Anna, K., Dominik, K., Michal, W., Elzbieta, J., Tomasz, C., Zbigniew, B.: Lab-on-a-chip system integrated with nanofiber mats used as a potential tool to study cardiovascular diseases (CVDs). Sens. Actuators B Chem. 330 (2021)
29. Ze-Wei, T., Siliang, W., Elizabeth, M.C.H., Jeffrey, G.J.: Evaluation of a polyurethane-reinforced hydrogel patch in a rat right ventricle wall replacement model. Acta Biomater. **101**, 206–218 (2020)
30. Geoff, B.: The Engineer's Guide to Plant Layout and Piping Design for the Oil and Gas Industries. Gulf Professional Publishing (2018)
31. Nicholas, H.C.: Silicone Elastomers for Artificial Hearts: 3D-Printing. Bioactive Glass and Potential. ETH Zurich, Germany (2018)

Assessment of the Cardiac Response to Sleep Arousal

Sobhan Salari Shahrbabaki and Mathias Baumert

Abstract Sleep arousal or transient unconscious wakefulness is a part of normal sleep. However, once its frequency increases, it may disturb the sleep and make it fragmented. The objective of this study is to assess the effect of sleep arousals on cardiovascular function. We investigated cardiac responses to sleep arousal in a large sample comprising 2656 older men. We quantified beat-to-beat QT and RR time intervals on ECG 15 s prior and following to arousal onset. Obtained results show that in more than three-quarters of the men, the average RR interval shortened during arousal compared to pre-and post-arousal intervals, while less than half of the men experienced average QT interval shortening during arousals. The QT and RR variability increased significantly during arousal, where RR variability changes were more prominent than QT variability changes. The QT variability index was weakly correlated with the apnea–hypopnea index and arousal index. In conclusion, arousal episodes trigger cardiovascular function, and their effect can be measured and quantified through cardiac QT and RR time intervals.

Keywords Sleep arousal · Heart rate · Cardiac time interval · Polysomnography · QT variability

1 Introduction

Sleep arousal is defined as transient unconscious wakefulness, can exert a strong effect on sympathetic activity such as heart rate, blood pressure and peripheral vasoconstriction [1, 2]. It occurs spontaneously or occurs as the body's response to potentially dangerous situations, such as noise or breathing becoming obstructed or any limb movements. Despite arousals are a part of normal sleep and do not often lead to complete awakening, an increase in the number of arousals may affect the sleep architecture and intensify the sleep fragmentation. As a consequence, it may cause excessive daytime sleepiness, poor executive functioning, fatigue and somnolence in

S. S. Shahrbabaki (✉) · M. Baumert
School of Electrical and Electronic Engineering, University of Adelaide, Adelaide, Australia
e-mail: sobhan.salarishahrbabaki@adelaide.edu.au

J. Usman et al. (eds.), *6th Kuala Lumpur International Conference on Biomedical Engineering 2021*, IFMBE Proceedings 86,
https://doi.org/10.1007/978-3-030-90724-2_63

following days [3]. Clinically, polysomnography (PSG) and manual scoring determine the rate and cause of arousal occurrence. Arousals often emerge as sudden shifts in the power of electroencephalogram (EEG) frequency to values >16 Hz with duration between 3 and 15 s [4]. The number of arousals per hour of sleep, arousal index (AI) is a marker of sleep fragmentation and quantifies sleep quality [5]. In addition, the duration of arousal episodes was demonstrated as an effective parameter in sleep fragmentation [2, 6]. Furthermore, the combination of duration and frequency of arousals known as arousal burden is associated with increased long-term cardiovascular mortality, particularly in women [7].

The influence of sleep arousal on the cardiovascular function can be measured through cardiovascular dynamics. Heart rate variability (HRV) has been assessed as a marker for the detection of sleep events and the prediction of different sleep breathing disorders [8, 9]. However, HRV does not perform as a relaible marker of potentially pro-arrhythmic changes that may occur in the cardiac or in the atrial or ventricular myocardium [10]. On the other hand, the QT interval is a marker of ventricular repolarization duration and can non-invasively assess the tonic sympathetic activity [11, 12].

Our main objective is to estimate QT and RR time interval variability before and after the occurrence of sleep arousals to quantify cardiac response to arousal activation and assess the influence of arousal episodes on heart function.

2 Methodology

2.1 Data Acquisition

The MrOS sleep study was conducted between December 2003 and March 2005 with 3155 community-dwelling men at six clinical centers in the United States. We had access to the PSG datasets of 2892 participants, where each dataset contained 22 biosignal recordings. Of those, 236 participants were excluded due to inadequate ECG recording or lack of manual scoring arousals. One channel electrocardiography (ECG) and one channel EEG (C1) of 2656 men were analysed. EEG was recorded at a sampling rate of 256 Hz while the sampling rate of ECG was 512 Hz. Sleep events like arousals and sleep disordered-breathing (SDB) episodes including obstructive sleep apnea, hypopnea, central apnea were manually scored by sleep technicians according to the American Academy of Sleep Medicine criteria. Apnea–hypopnea index (AHI) was computed based on the number of apneic events per hour of overnight sleep.

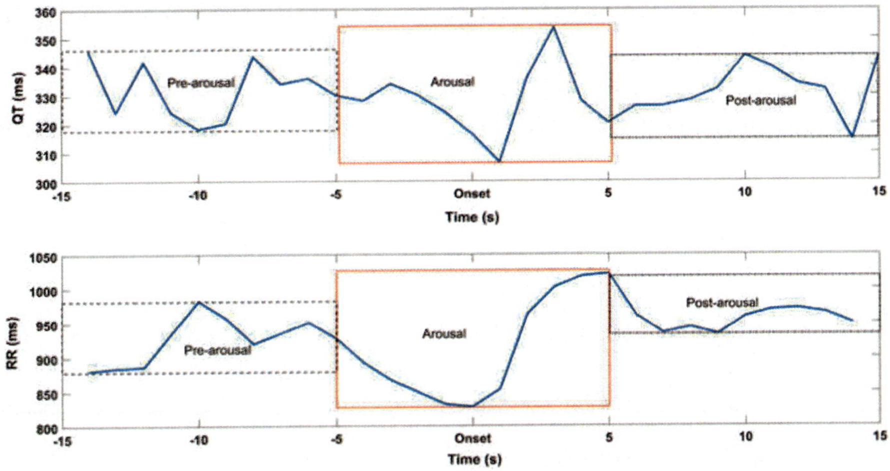

Fig. 1 An example of QT and RR time interval variability before, during and after arousal onset

2.2 *ECG Analysis*

To investigate the cardiac responses to arousal occurrence, the ECG time series around the onset was selected for every single arousal. The RR and QT time intervals were automatically computed using a 2-dimensional signal warping algorithm [13]. RR and QT time intervals were estiamted as the time interval taken between two consecutive R waves and the time delay between the start of the QRS complex to the T wave termination, respectively. Then, in each arousal episode, two time series for QT and RR were defined with considering arousal onset, (1) Pre-arousal for QT and RR intervals between 10 and 5 s prior to onset, (2) Arousal for QT and RR intervals from 5 s before to 5 s after arousal onset and (3) Post-arousal for QT and RR variation within 5 to 15 s after onset (Fig. 1). By this means, in each subject, six matrices were generated that each row represents 10 s QT or RR time series pre, during or post single arousal.

2.3 *Cardiac Interval Variability Measures and Statistical Analysis*

To evaluate QT/RR variability, we computed several statistical measures for intervals. MeanQT, MeanRR, SDQT and SDRR respectively represent the mean and standard deviation of QT and RR. Moreover, the QT variability index (QTVi) was also computed based on the equation proposed by Berger et al. [14].

To determine how measures vary before and after arousal and whether their changes were statistically significant, we applied Student's paired t-test. The

Pearson linear correlation coefficient also assessed any possible associations between computed parameters.

3 Results

In all 2656 participants, a total of 382,516 arousal episodes were scored (Mean ± SD: 144 ± 71.3 per subject). The arousal index in all men was 25.1 ± 12.5 h^{-1}.

As shown in Table 1, the average QT interval shortened during arousal in about 44% of men. In addition, in almost 38% of the men, the average post-arousal QT interval was more prolonged than after arousal onset. As shown in Fig. 2a, the difference between MeanQT before, during and after arousals is statistically significant but very small in absolute values.

The average RR time interval during arousal was significantly shorter than pre-arousal situations in more than 77% of men. On average, the RR interval shortened by about 20 ms during arousals (Fig. 2a). Measures of cardiac interval variability, SDQT and SDRR, significantely increased comparing to pre- and post-arousal. Arousal caused SDQT increased by 44% compared to pre-arousal, while arousal-related SDRR was 122% greater than pre-arousal SDRR. Thus, arousal-related RR interval variability seems to be almost three times stronger than QT variability.

As shown in Fig. 3, the correlation of MeanQT and MeanRR seems to be independent of arousal presence. On the other hand, the correlation between SDQT and SDRR during arousal was comparably lower than pre- and post-arousal ($\rho = 0.41$ vs. $\rho = 0.578$ and $\rho = 0.501$). That means that QT and RR changes caused by arousals are not necessarily in the same direction.

We also assessed the correlation of QTVi with two sleep metrics, AHI and AI (Fig. 4). Obtained results show that only arousal QTVi had a significant yet weak correlation with AHI and AI (AHI: $\rho = 0.044, p = 0.027$; AI: $\rho = 0.041, p = 0.044$).

Table 1 Men with average QT and RR interval shortening or lengthening caused by arousals

	Shortening (%)	Prolongation (%)	No change (%)
Pre-arousal versus arousal			
$QT_{pre} - QT_{aro}$	1164 (43.8)	1174 (44.2)	318 (12)
$RR_{pre} - RR_{aro}$	2051 (77.2)	591 (22.3)	14 (0.5)
Arousal versus post-arousal			
$QT_{post} - QT_{aro}$	1296 (48.8)	1007 (37.9)	353 (13.3)
$RR_{post} - RR_{aro}$	1240 (46.7)	1353 (51)	63 (3.3)

QT_{pre} and RR_{pre} Average QT and RR interval before arousal; *QT_{aro} and RR_{aro}* Average QT and RR intervals during arousals; *QT_{post} and RR_{post}* Average QT and RR interval after arousal

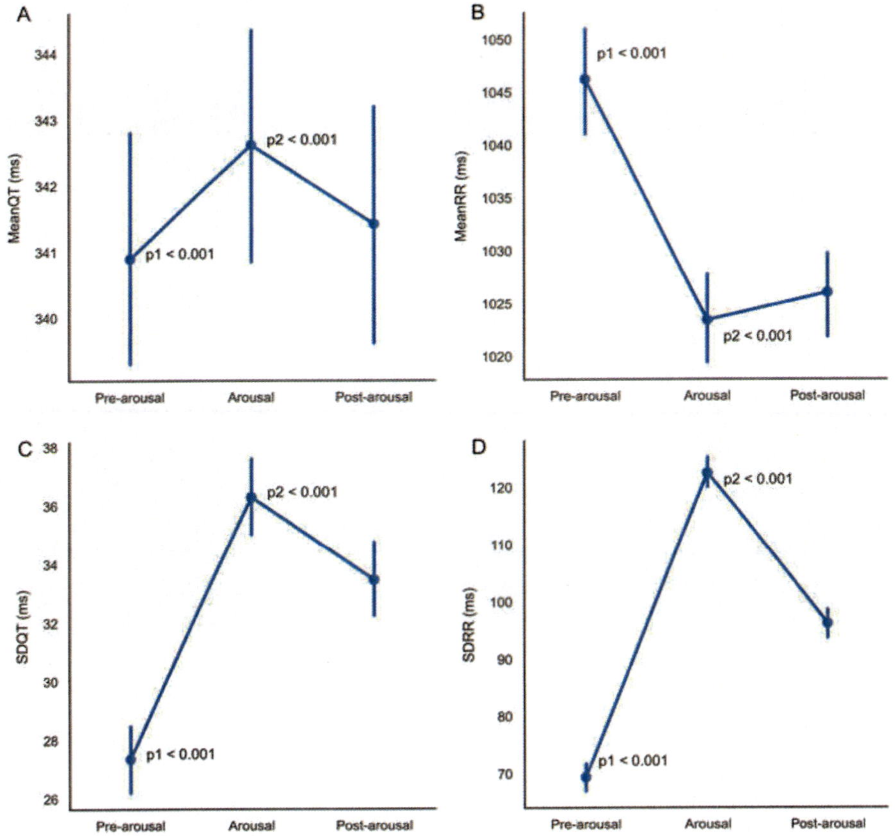

Fig. 2 Point-plots represent an estimate of the central tendency of cardiac time intervals measures before, during and after arousal onset. P1 values demonstrate the results of the Student's paired t-test for measures (MeanQT, MeanRR, SDQT and SDRR) before and during arousals. Similarly, P2 values represent paired t-test results for arousal and post-arousal onset measures

4 Discussion

This paper is the first to investigate the cardiovascular response to sleep arousals in a large cohort of older community-dwelling men. We extracted markers to quantify cardiac interval variability triggered by sleep arousals. Arousals not only intensify sleep fragmentation but also may increase the risk of cardiovascular mortality [7]. This manifests the importance of an investigation on the influence of sleep arousal on cardiac function.

The magnitude of QT variability can be considered as an indirect measure of the ventricular sympathetic control if it progressively increases as a function of the sympathetic drive, and this augmentation is accompanied by the rise of the amount of QT variability unrelated to RR changes and respiratory-related fluctuations [15,

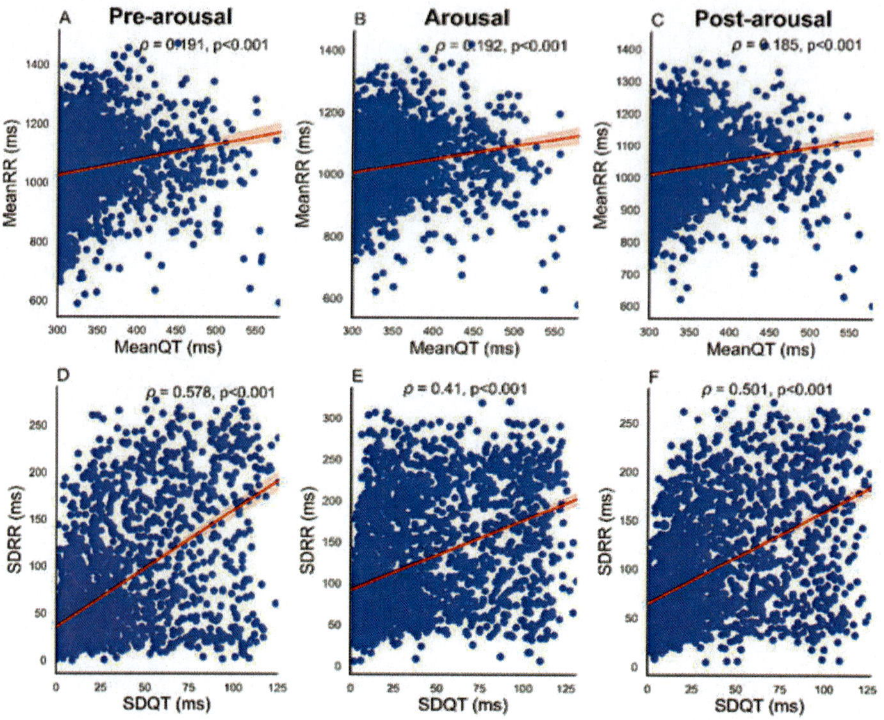

Fig. 3 Scatterplots show the correlation between QT and RR variability measures before, during and after arousal onset

16]. However, cardiac diseases may cause dissociation between QT and RR [17, 18]. Furthermore, ageing can lead to QT interval decoupling from the RR interval [19]. An arousal episode like a trigger causes a sympathetic surge which can be reflected as sudden alterations on QT modulation. QT variability has previously shown to be correlated with the severity of sleep apnea [20]. Our findings also indicate the correlation between QT beat-to-beat variability with AHI.

This study only focused on white older men.

5 Conclusion

The cardiovascular response to sleep arousal was quantified and assessed by cardiac time intervals variability markers. Sleep arousal leads to increased QT and RR intervals modulations where RR variability is more prominent than QT variability.

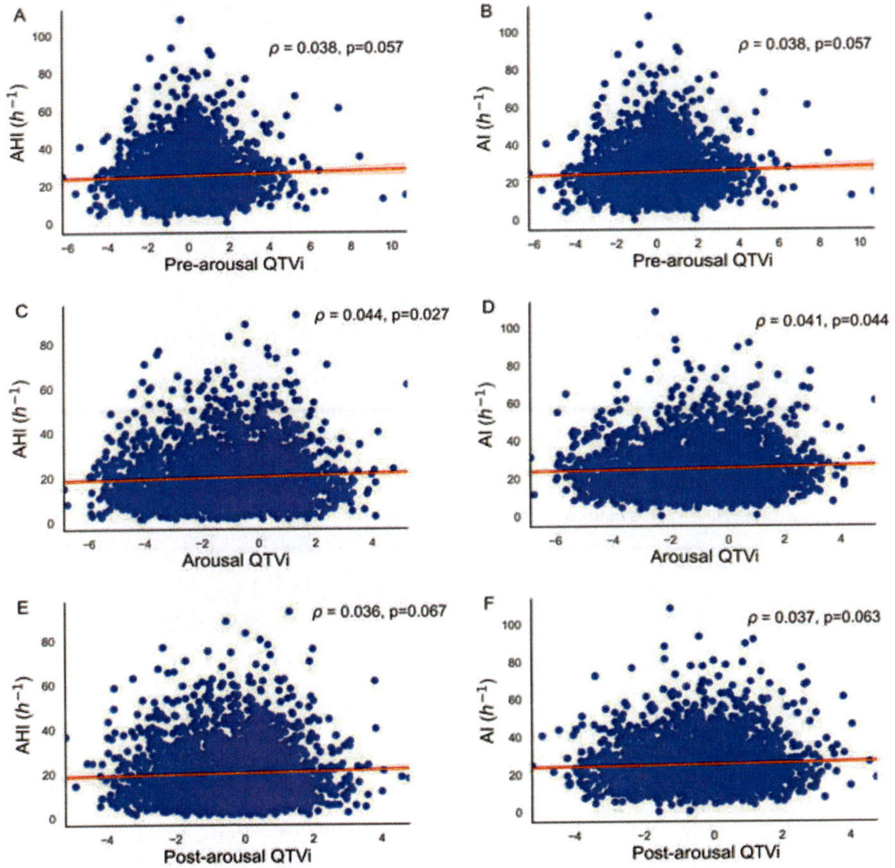

Fig. 4 Scatterplots show the correlation between QT variability index and arousal index (AI) and apnea/hypopnea index (AHI) before, during and after arousal onset

References

1. Morgan, B.J., Crabtree, D.C., Puleo, D.S., Badr, M.F., Toiber, F., Skatrud, J.B.: Neurocirculatory consequences of abrupt change in sleep state in humans. J. Appl. Physiol. **80**(5), 1627–1636 (1996)
2. Trinder, J.A., Allen, N.B., Kleiman, J., Kralevski, V., Kleverlaan, D., Anson, K., Young, K.: On the nature of cardiovascular activation at an arousal from sleep. Sleep **26**(5), 543–551 (2003)
3. Martin, S.E., Engleman, H.M., Deary, I.J., Douglas, N.J.: The effect of sleep fragmentation on daytime function. Am. J. Respir. Crit. Care Med. **153**(4), 1328–1332 (1996)
4. Iber, C., Ancoli-Israel, A., Chesson, A., Quan, S.F.: *The AASM Manual for the Scoring of Sleep and Associated Events: Rules, Terminology and Technical Specifications*. American Academy of Sleep Medicine, Westchester, Illinois, USA (2007)
5. Smurra, M.V., Dury, M., Aubert, G., Rodenstein, D.O., Liistro, G.: Sleep fragmentation: comparison of two definition of short arousals during sleep in OSAS patients. Eur. Respir. J. **17**, 723–727 (2001)

6. Nigro, C., Rhodius, E.: Variation in the duration of sleep arousal in obstructive sleep apnea. Med. Sci. Monit. **11**(4), CR188–192 (2005)
7. Shahrbabaki, S.S., Linz, D., Hartmann, S., Redline, S., Baumert, M.: Sleep arousal burden is associated with long-term all-cause and cardiovascular mortality in 8001 community-dwelling older men and women. Eur. Heart J. **42**(21), 2088–2099 (2021)
8. Fornasa, E., De Felice, A., D'Addio, G., Insaiaco, G., Balzano, G., Accardo, A.: HRV analysis in obstructive sleep apnea syndrome by means of LF/HF ratio and fractal dimension. Eur. Respir. J. **44**(58) (2014)
9. Smith, J.H., Baumert, M., Nalivaiko, E., McEvoy, R.D., Catcheside, P.G.: Arousal in obstructive sleep apnoea patients is associated with ECG RR and QT interval shortening and PR interval lengthening. J. Sleep Res. **18**(2), 188–195 (2008)
10. Nalivaiko, E., Catcheside, P.G., Adams, A., Jordan, A.S., Eckert, D.J., McEvoy, RD.: Cardiac changes during arousals from non-REM sleep in healthy volunteers. Am. J. Physiol. Regul. Integr. Comp. Physiol. **292**(3) (2007)
11. Baumert, M., Porta, A., Vos, M.A., Malik, M., Couderc, J.P., Laguna, P., Piccirillo, G., Smith, G.L., Tereshchenko, L.G., Volders, P.G.: QT interval variability in body surface ECG: measurement, physiological basis, and clinical value: position statement and consensus guidance endorsed by the European heart rhythm association jointly with the ESC working group on cardiac cellular electrophysiology. Europace **18**(6), 925–944 (2016)
12. Baumert, M., Schlaich, M.P., Nalivaiko, E., Lambert, E., Sari, C.I., Kaye, D.M., Elser, M.D., Sanders, P., Lambert, G.: Relation between QT interval variability and cardiac sympathetic activity in hypertension. Am. J. Physiol. Heart Circ. Physiol. **300**(4), H1412-1417 (2011)
13. Schmidt, M., Baumert, M., Porta, A., Malberg, H., Zaunseder, S.: Two-dimensional warping for one-dimensional signals—conceptual framework and application to ECG processing. IEEE Trans. Signal Process. **62**(21), 5577–5588 (2014)
14. Berger, R.D., Kasper, E.K., Baughman, K.L., Marban, E., Calkins, H., Tomaselli, G.F.: Beat-to-beat QT interval variability: novel evidence for repolarization lability in ischemic and nonischemic dilated cardiomyopathy. Circulation **96**(5), 1557–1565 (1997)
15. Porta, A., Tobaldini, E., Gnecchi-Ruscone, T., Montano, N.: RT variability unrelated to heart period and respiration progressively increases during graded head-up tilt. Am. J. Physiol. Heart Circ. Physiol. **298**(5), H1406–H1414 (2010)
16. El-Hamad, F., Lambert, E., Abbott, D., Baumert, M.: Relation between QT interval variability and muscle sympathetic nerve activity in normal subjects. Am. J. Physiol. Heart Circ. Physiol. **309**(7), H1218-1224 (2015)
17. Nayyar, S., Roberts-Thomson, K.C., Hasan, M.A., Sullivan, T., Harrington, J., Sanders, P., Baumert, M.: Autonomic modulation of repolarization instability in patients with heart failure prone to ventricular tachycardia. Am. J. Physiol. Heart Circ. Physiol. **305**(8), H1181–H1188 (2013)
18. El-Hamad, F.J., Bonabi, S.Y., Müller, A., Steger, A., Schmidt, G., Baumert, M.: Augmented oscillations in QT interval duration predict mortality post myocardial infarction independent of heart rate. Front. Physiol. **11**, 578173 (2020)
19. Baumert, M., Czippelova, B., Porta, A., Javorka, M.: Decoupling of QT interval variability from heart rate variability with ageing. Physiol. Meas. **34**(11), 1435–1448 (2013)
20. Baumert, M., Smith, J., Catcheside, P., McEvoy, R.D., Abbott, D., Sanders, P., Nalivaiko, E.: Variability of QT interval duration in obstructive sleep apnea: an indicator of disease severity. Sleep **31**(7), 959–966 (2008)

Achieving Carbon-Balanced Ecosystem: Case Study of Carbon Sequestration Analysis in Universiti Malaya

Nurshafira Hazim Chan, Ayman Khallel Ibrahim Al-Ani, Nahrizul Adib Kadri, Sarah Abdul Razak, Hanee Farzana Hizaddin, Mohd Istajib Mokhtar, Muhammad Mokhzaini Azizan, Khin Wee Lai, and Khairunnisa Hasikin

Abstract As part of promoting an eco-campus facility in University of Malaya, this project has developed an automated carbon sequestration monitoring system using few sensor modules and analysis of tree growth. The tree growths (i.e., diameter and height) has been monitored to quantify carbon sequestration. The calculated carbon sequestration is also compared with the data collected from the proposed sensor. The study area was conducted at Rimba Ilmu, UM and the prediction of the carbon sequestration for the next 10 years is also presented in this paper. The analysis presented in this paper has added new insight on achieving carbon balanced ecosystem in the campus through the tracking and quantification of the carbon stored in the tree.

Keywords Sustainability · Carbon-balanced · Carbon sequestration · Tree growth

N. H. Chan · A. K. I. Al-Ani · N. A. Kadri · K. W. Lai · K. Hasikin (✉)
Department of Biomedical Engineering, Faculty of Engineering, Universiti Malaya, Lembah Pantai, 50603 Kuala Lumpur, Malaysia
e-mail: khairunnisa@um.edu.my

S. A. Razak
Faculty of Science, Institute of Biological Science, Universiti Malaya, Lembah Pantai, 50603 Kuala Lumpur, Malaysia

H. F. Hizaddin
Department of Chemical Engineering, Faculty of Engineering, Universiti Malaya, Lembah Pantai, 50603 Kuala Lumpur, Malaysia

M. I. Mokhtar
Department of Science and Technology Studies, Faculty of Science, Universiti Malaya, Lembah Pantai, 50603 Kuala Lumpur, Malaysia

M. M. Azizan
Department of Electrical and Electronic Engineering, Faculty of Engineering and Built Environment, Universiti Sains Islam Malaysia, Bandar Baru Nilai, 71800 Nilai, Negeri Sembilan, Malaysia

J. Usman et al. (eds.), *6th Kuala Lumpur International Conference on Biomedical Engineering 2021*, IFMBE Proceedings 86,
https://doi.org/10.1007/978-3-030-90724-2_64

1 Introduction

As part of promoting an eco-campus facility in the University of Malaya (UM), the first step the university has taken, is quantifying the carbon storage in the campus. UM has a unique campus, with over 1600 species that occupies an area of 80 ha. Prior to this project, there is no proper and real time monitoring system on carbon sequestration in the campus.

Carbon sequestration is a process that removes carbon dioxide which trapping heat in the atmosphere. As a result, the heat builds up and warms up the atmosphere and the Earth. This phenomenon can induce climate change and rise in global warming issues. Plantation of trees can make way for lesser carbon dioxide in our surroundings, thus reduces the trapped heat as whole. With the capability of storing large amount of carbon through their woods, trees add carbon stock as they grow. Generally, major carbon storage reservoir generated from faster growing trees which contributed to higher annual sequestration rates.

Since UM has pledged to be ecofriendly campus, continuous efforts on maintaining carbon storage reservoir have been great interest to the campus community. UM is also subjected to an increase scrutiny of their sustainability practices since it participated in green matric ranking among other universities in the world.

A tool of real time monitoring system on carbon sequestration of the planted trees in the campus will provide a great insight on pertaining a carbon balanced ecosystem could be achieved in the campus. This can be done by proper carbon management through quantification of carbon sequestered in trees on campus [1]. Therefore, this paper presents an analysis on carbon sequestration rate of campus trees located at our in-house tropical forest, namely Rimba Ilmu.

2 Climate Change and Low Carbon Cities Assessment System

Since July 2019, Malaysia government has taken conscious initiatives in addressing the impact of global warming by launching National Green Technology Policy (NGTP). This remark as breakthrough in the country's history in addressing sustainable development issues. Besides NGTP, the government has initiated Low Carbon Cities Framework (LCCF) as part of their serious efforts in reducing carbon emission to achieve sustainable development. As stated in LCCF, landscaping and regular maintenance f the trees both have significant impact on the amount of carbon that they can sequestered. Realizing this scenario, a tool to quantify the carbon sequestration and tree growth will provide valuable information for proper landscape planning for sustainable living.

Alarming concern over greenhouse gas emission and its impact towards climate change renews anxiety on whether existing efforts on global term is suffice [2]. It is known to many that most strategies center onto reducing greenhouse gas emission to a much lower level, it is equally important that sinking of carbon is made complementary to existing mitigation methods [3]. In this agenda, sinking of carbon requires extensive carbon storage agents, which naturally are the trees [4]. Through their natural processes, trees absorb carbon dioxide into their woods and convert it to biomass, while at the same time produces oxygen through its leaves. Reducing carbon in the atmosphere pave the ways for heat to be removed and therefore creating cooler surroundings [5].

Considerable effort is undergoing to conduct this natural carbon storage on smaller scale, as at the level of local region such as businesses and institutions. Trees play major role in carbon cycle due to their capability in sequestering and storing carbon. During photosynthesis process, the carbon dioxide will be converted to sugars and stored as biomass [6]. It is estimated that the terrestrial forests able to sequester 3 billion tons of anthropogenic carbon per year, which covers almost 30% of fossil fuel- and deforestation-related CO_2 emissions globally [3].

During carbon sequestration process, individual trees are carbon sinks due to their capabilities in locking CO_2 in their tissue and can only released to the atmosphere when the trees are decomposed. It is reported in [7] that larger trees have larger foliage biomass which are likely to sequester more carbon per year. However, if trees exceed the growth rate, their capability as carbon sources significantly reduced and could increase deforestation chances. Therefore, proper management and tracking of these carbon stores are important to be maintained.

Carbon sequestration capacity of small groups of trees regardless of the species can be beneficial within the context of the smaller community. This is the whole idea of localized or regionalized mitigation of carbon emission. The reasoning behind localized or regionalized mitigation method is that the control over carbon storage practice is easier and immediate, thus enabling faster decision making by the stakeholders. Information collected over smaller groups of trees absorbing carbon can be integrated into existing platform for analytics for decision making on management and mitigation.

This project focuses on characterizing carbon sequestration by individual trees in a localized or regionalized environment, which in specific for this research is university campus. To date, there is no proper monitoring system on carbon sequestration implemented by any party in UM, only logged data on general population of trees are recorded. Therefore. This project has developed a tool to monitor carbon sequestration in relation to tree growth in our campus.

3 Tree Growth and Carbon Sequestration in University of Malaya

Carbon sequestration depends on number of factors, including climate region, primary productivity of the area, tree species, age, tree growth rate, and diameter of the tree. There are many different approaches can be used to estimate the carbon sequestration, however, most models estimate the carbon sequestration based on the age of the tree, diameter, height of the tree, tree species and location of the tree. The carbon sequestration estimation relies on the wood density which depends on the tree species. Different tree species will have different capability in absorbing carbon and thus will provide different carbon sequestration rate.

This study looked at the important of urban forest in our campus and their sequestration as well as carbon offset potential. It provides equations to estimate the amount of carbon stored and sequestered in Rimba Ilmu. We cover up to 50 species of trees in Rimba Ilmu, where initial data of tree growth was collected at the beginning of the project (i.e. in November 2018). The tree growth data is collected once again after 6 months of the project to monitor the rate of growth (i.e., in April 2019). We also monitor the surrounding parameters which include temperature, humidity and concentration of carbon dioxide throughout this span.

Correlation between tree growth and surrounding parameters will be used to estimate the sequestration rate of the trees at Rimba Ilmu. We also estimate expected carbon sequestration rate based on the growth rates of the trees. We hope that this data could be compared with the annual carbon emissions at the campus, in order to attain carbon-balanced ecosystem.

In this study, we have developed a tool to quantify the sequestration rate and correlation with its surrounding environment. The outline of the proposed system is presented in Fig. 1. The amount of biomass and carbon dioxide (CO_2) in standing

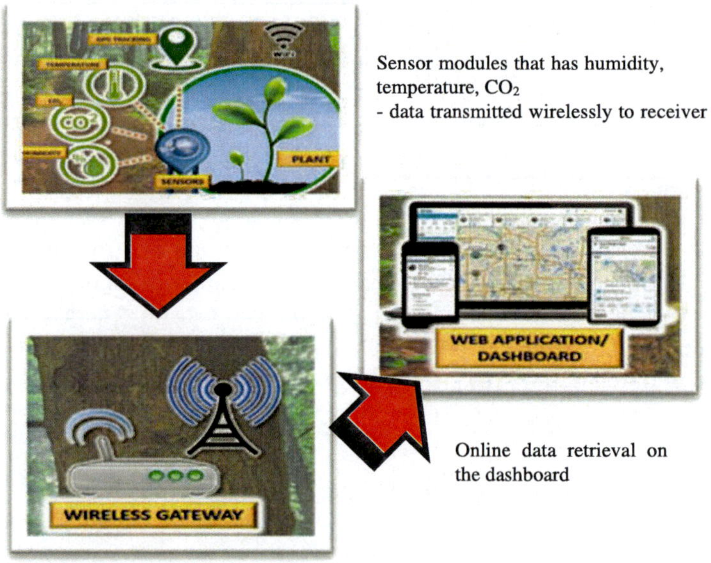

Fig. 1 The outline of the proposed system that consists of sensor modules and receiver as well as live dashboard

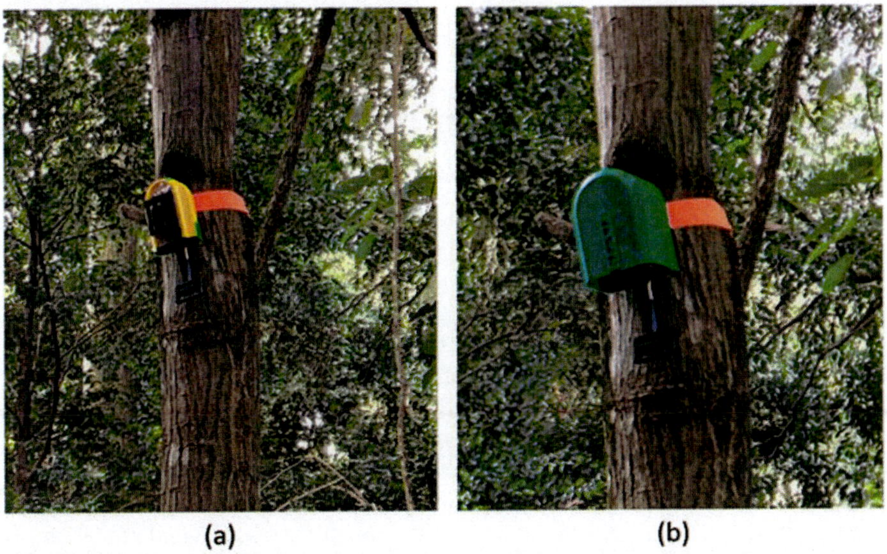

Fig. 2 The sensor modules that were installed on *Mangifera foetida* (Anacardiaceae); **a** sensor without weatherproof casing **b** sensor with weatherproof casing

woody biomass of selective few tree species was calculated and presented in this paper. The analytical data that we obtained from the calculation is then compared with the data that we attained directly from the sensor. The sensor was setup to attain live data of CO_2 concentration for few days at Rimba Ilmu as shown in Fig. 2. The sensor measured the CO_2 concentration within 50 m radius of the study area and was mounted to the higher tree (more than 2 m height).

To estimate biomass of different trees, non-destructive method was used. The biomass of tree was estimated on the basis of diameter at breast height (DBH) and tree height. The above ground biomass (AGB) of tree includes the whole shoot, branches, leaves, flowers and fruits. The AGB is calculated using:

$$AGB\left(\frac{\text{kg}}{tree}\right) = Volume\,of\,tree\,\left(\text{m}^3\right) \times wood\,density\,\frac{\text{kg}}{\text{m}^3} \tag{1}$$

where

V = volume of the cylindrical shaped tree in m^3
R = radius of the tree (m)
H = height of the tree (m).

Equation (2) shows the below ground biomass (BGB) which is calculated by estimating the root shoot ratio. The BGB is correlated with AGB by 0.26 factor as shown in the equation below.

$$BGB = AGB\left(\frac{kg}{tree}\right) \times 0.26 \quad (2)$$

Once the AGB and BGB are calculated, total biomass of the tree can be estimated by taking the sum between the two, TGB = AGB + BGB (kg/tree). For any plant species, it is estimated 50% of its biomass is considered as carbon (Biomass × 50%).

Table 1 tabulates the GPS location, carbon sequestered by the single tree of five different species from Rimba Ilmu. CS is analytically calculated using the above equations while CS^+ is the carbon sequestered by the tree as recorded by the sensor. The discrepancy between two data is approximately 6.8% for all types of the tree. We select these five species to be discussed in this book chapter since these species aged more than 30 years and able to sequester high carbon. The correlation between the CO_2 sequestered recorded by the sensor and temperature for a daily reading with an average humidity of 65.63% is shown in Fig. 3. It can be concluded that the carbon sequestration is higher at night as the photosynthesis is majorly done during night.

We also calculated the prediction of total weight of CO_2 to be sequestered by the five species in Fig. 4a–e for the next ten years. Analyses in Fig. 4a–e are made based on the assumption that the incremental diameter was estimated at 0.4 cm per year and the incremental height is at 0.6 m per year for trees that are less than ten years of age. Meanwhile, diameters of trees aged 11–40 years were estimated to be incremented at 0.38 cm per year with the height increment at 1 m per year. As for.

Trees that aged more than 40 years old, the diameter and height remained constant [7].

In this paper, we presented the amount of CO_2 that will have been sequestered for five species in the next ten-years. As a result, the tress that aged less than 40 years

Table 1 Carbon sequestrated by single tree of different species in Rimba Ilmu (5 samples)

Name of the tree	GPS	DBH (m)	H (m)	TB (kg/tree)	CS (kg/tree)	CS^+ (kg/tree)
Koompassia malaccensis (Caesalpiniaceae)	3° 7′ 47″ N 101° 39′ 27″ E	0.46	8.79	1422.44	2607.54	2785.133
Anisoptera scaphula (dipterocarpaceae)	3° 7′ 47″ N 101° 39′ 27″ E	0.08	1.59	6.39	11.72	12.5145
Dipterocarpus verrucosus (Dipterocarpaceae)	3° 7′ 47″ N 101° 39′ 26″ E	0.24	11.25	427.37	783.45	418.4024
Streblus elongatus (Moraceae)	3° 7′ 47″ ’N 101° 39′ 26″ E	0.47	5.85	1181.40	2165.68	2313.179
Lepisanthes senegalensis (Sapindaceae)	3°7′ 43″ N 101° 39′ 23″ E	0.15	3.13	45.23	82.91	88.55621

GPS global positioning system
DBH diameter at breast height
H height of the tree
TB total biomass
CS carbon sequestered per tree
CS^+ carbon sequestered data extracted from sensor (the data of carbon sequestered is per 10,000 volume (m^3)

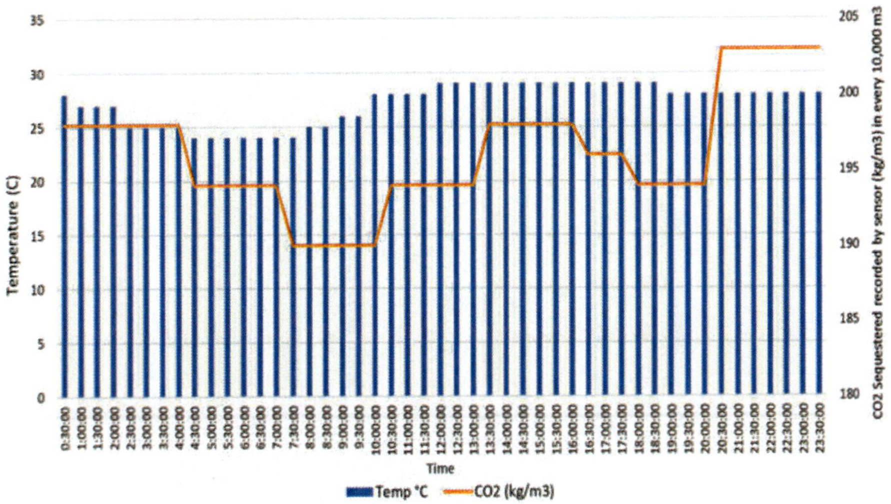

Fig. 3 Average weight of CO_2 sequestered in trees in one day per 10,000 kg m^{-3} in correlation with daily temperature (average humidity of 65.63%)

show an increment more than 50% in their capability to store carbon. However, the capability of trees at UM to store additional carbon will start to reduce if the trees are aged more than 40 years,

4 Conclusion

This study calculated the carbon sequestered in five species of trees at Rimba Ilmu, UM and estimated the annual expected sequestration over the next ten years. It also estimated that the tree growth for the tree aged less than 40 years will increase exponentially in the next 10 years. However, it is observed that the diameter and height remain constant for the tree that aged more than 40 years. This has resulted in constant carbon sequestration rate throughout the campus. UM has a relatively large campus, allowing for many trees. If the carbon emission in the campus can be quantified and known, proper practice and policy implications to provide carbon balanced ecosystem could be achieved. Increasing the potential of carbon mitigation in campus could be achieved by offsetting the carbon emission with the carbon sequestration in trees.

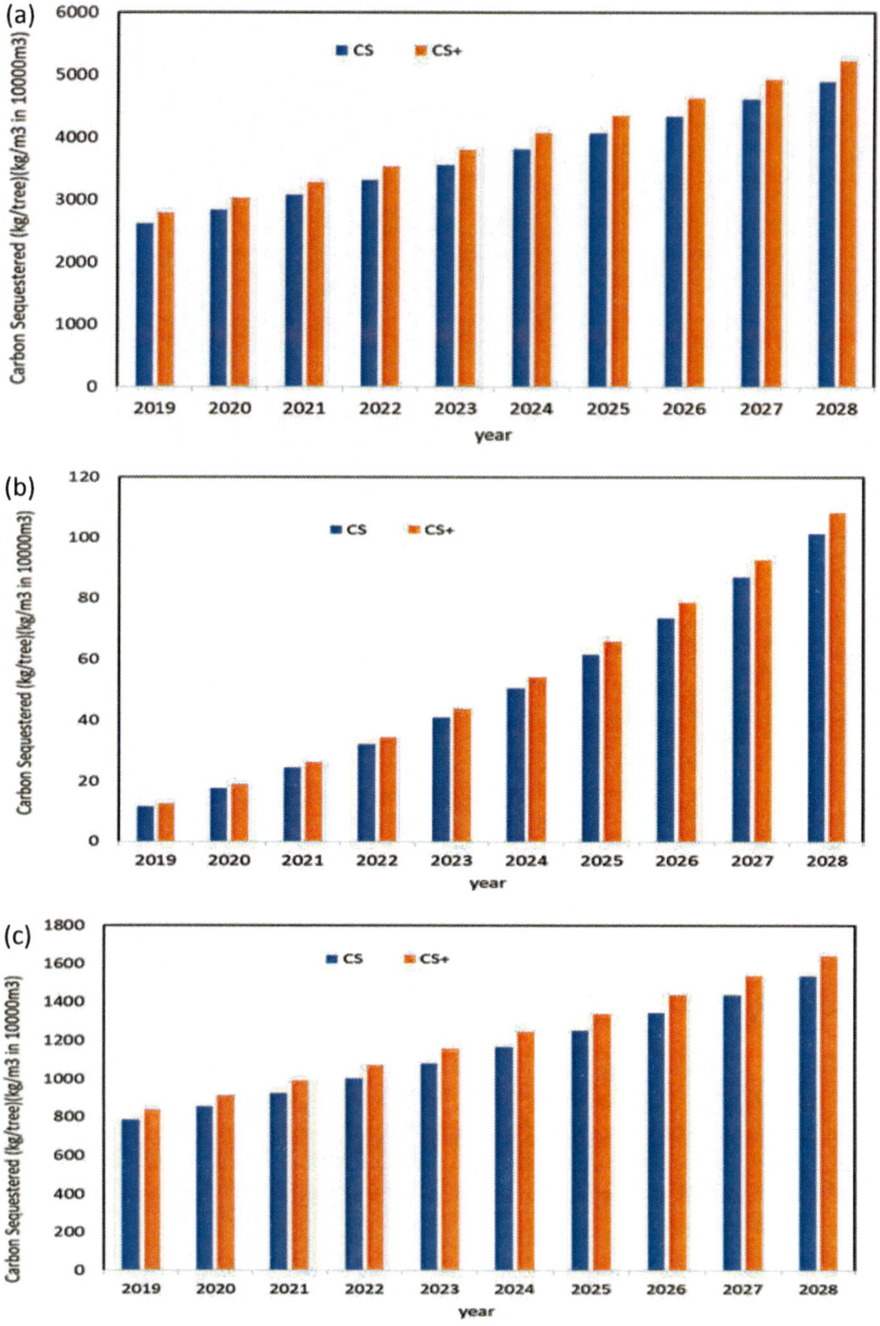

Fig. 4 Prediction of total weight of CO_2 to be sequestered in trees in the next ten years for 5 species. **a** *Koompassia malaccensis* (Caesalpiniaceae). **b** *Anisoptera scaphula* (dipterocarpaceae). **c** *Dipterocarpus verrucosus* (Dipterocarpaceae). **d** *Streblus elongatus* (Moraceae) and **e** *Lepisanthes senegalensis* (Sapindaceae)

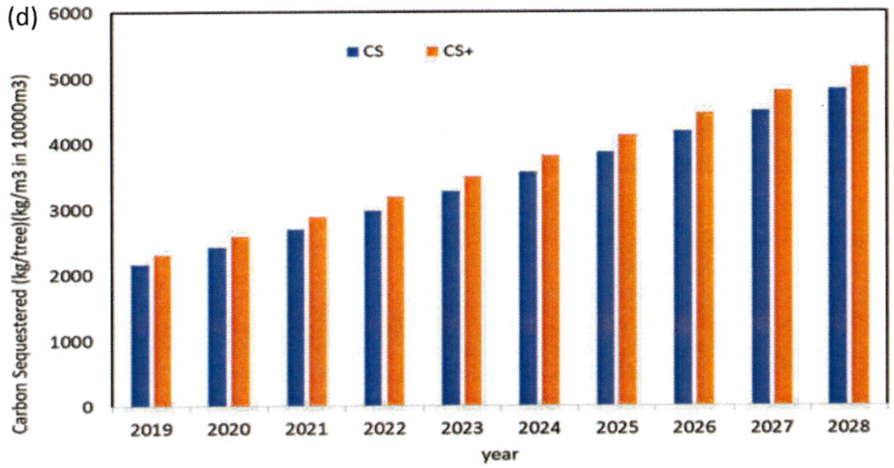

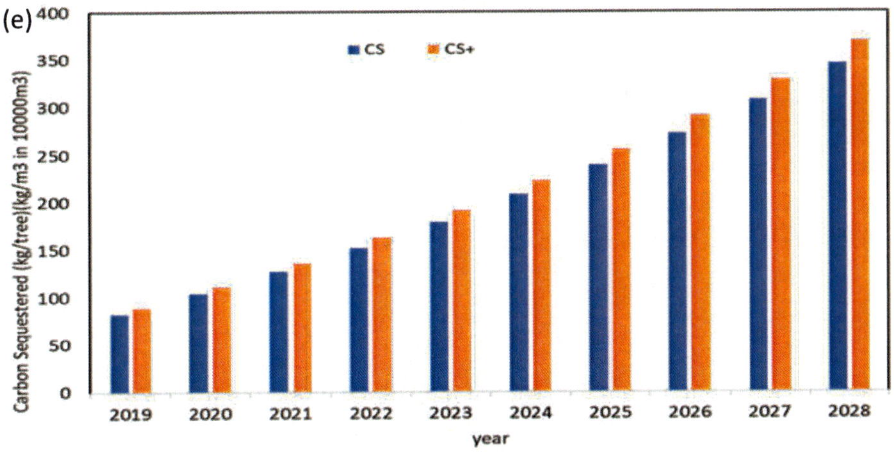

Fig. 4 (continued)

Acknowledgements The authors would like to thank Universiti Malaya for the continuous support and the UM Living Lab research funding LL037-18SUS granted by UM Eco-Campus Secretariat and Ministry of Higher Education on MYRGS grant MR001-2019. Special appreciation goes to the Rimba Ilmu specifically to Dr. Sugumaran A/L Manickam and Dr. Yong Kien Thai for helping our team during installation of the sensor at Rimba Ilmu.

References

1. Xu, B., Mitchell, N.: Carbon Sequestration by Trees on the City Campus. The University of Auckland, Auckland (2011)
2. United Nations: The Paris Agreement, Paris (2015)
3. Tang, K.H.D.: Climate change in Malaysia: trends, contributors, impacts, mitigation and adaptations. Sci. Total Environ. **650**, 1858–1871 (2019). https://doi.org/10.1016/j.scitotenv.2018.09.316
4. McLaughlin, C., Elamer, A.A., Glen, T., AlHares, A., Gaber, H.R.: Accounting society's acceptability of carbon taxes: expectations and reality. Energy Policy **131**, 302–311 (2019). https://doi.org/10.1016/j.enpol.2019.05.008.
5. Rötzer, T., Rahman, M.A., Moser-Reischl, A., Pauleit, S., Pretzsch, H.: Process based simulation of tree growth and ecosystem services of urban trees under present and future climate conditions. Sci. Total Environ. **676**, 651–664 (2019). https://doi.org/10.1016/j.scitotenv.2019.04.235
6. Nowak, D.J., Crane, D.E.: Carbon storage and sequestration by urban trees in the USA. Environ. Pollut. **116**(3), 381–389 (2002). https://doi.org/10.1016/S0269-7491(01)00214-7
7. Kavehei, E., Jenkins, G.A., Adame, M.F., Lemckert, C.: Carbon sequestration potential for mitigating the carbon footprint of green stormwater infrastructure. Renew. Sustain. Energy Rev. **94**, 1179–1191 (2018). https://doi.org/10.1016/j.rser.2018.07.002

Surface Water Quality Assessment: A Case Study of Merbok River, Kuala Muda, Kedah

Wen Yee Wong, Ayman Khallel Ibrahim Al-Ani, Sarah Abdul Razak, Hanee Farzana Hizaddin, Mohd Istajib Mokhtar, Muhammad Mokhzaini Azizan, and Khairunnisa Hasikin

Abstract This paper presents a case study on surface water quality assessment at Merbok river, Kuala Muda, Kedah. The study provides an insight on the feasibility of environmental pollution monitoring through in-situ water quality measurement. The study was conducted in the span of five months from November 2020 to March 2021 where the water quality samples were taken twice daily using water quality system and turbidity probes of EUTECH CyberScan PCD650 and EUTECH-TN100 respectively. The measured water quality parameters are pH, dissolved oxygen, conductivity, total dissolved solids, salinity, resistivity, and turbidity. Results from the sampling analysis have shown that water quality parameters of Merbok River are categorized as Class III according to the National Water Quality Standards (NWQS). The study identified a spike in pH (8.9) and dissolved oxygen in February possibly caused from dumping of industrial waste. Turbidity shows an increase during monsoon season followed by an increase in conductivity, resistivity and salinity in the dry season which implies surface runoff from industrial discharges. The state of Merbok

W. Y. Wong · A. K. I. Al-Ani · K. Hasikin (✉)
Department of Biomedical Engineering, Faculty of Engineering, Universiti Malaya, Lembah Pantai, 50603 Kuala Lumpur, Malaysia
e-mail: khairunnisa@um.edu.my

S. A. Razak
Faculty of Science, Institute of Biological Science, Universiti Malaya, Lembah Pantai, 50603 Kuala Lumpur, Malaysia

H. F. Hizaddin
Department of Chemical Engineering, Faculty of Engineering, Universiti Malaya, Lembah Pantai, 50603 Kuala Lumpur, Malaysia

M. I. Mokhtar
Department of Science and Technology Studies, Faculty of Science, Universiti Malaya, Lembah Pantai, 50603 Kuala Lumpur, Malaysia

M. M. Azizan
Department of Electrical and Electronic Engineering, Faculty of Engineering and Built Environment, Universiti Sains Islam Malaysia, Bandar Baru Nilai, 71800 Nilai, Negeri Sembilan, Malaysia

J. Usman et al. (eds.), *6th Kuala Lumpur International Conference on Biomedical Engineering 2021*, IFMBE Proceedings 86,
https://doi.org/10.1007/978-3-030-90724-2_65

River requires necessary attention from authorities and policy makers, to prevent future contamination that degrades the diverse ecosystem.

Keywords Sustainability · Mangrove estuarine · Environmental pollution · Water pollution

1 Introduction

Surface water quality is sensitive to land use changes that has been ongoing since the era of industrialization and urbanization. It is evident that human activities are the cause of the increase in pollution and nutrients in rivers, groundwater, and estuaries [1, 2]. The contaminated water is prone to spread water-borne diseases from the disposal of manure, garbage, industrial wastes and runoff [3]. These discharge contains nutrients such as nitrogen, and phosphorus were an excess in nutrients could host problems in estuarine and fresh water systems, leading to a hypoxia condition from low dissolved oxygen concentration [4].

Estuaries are complicated in terms of biological, chemical, and physical characteristics as it is a mix of freshwater and saltwater of different density and water masses. The estuarine ecosystem acts as a shelter of various flora and fauna, and as a source of food, transportation, and development sites for humans. It is vital to monitor the ecosystem continuously to detect changes in water quality and take immediate action to prevent future damage.

The change and status of water quality can be reflected through long term monitoring of substantial water quality parameters. Dissolved oxygen (DO) is the amount of oxygen present in the water. Dissolved oxygen is essential for aquatic organisms to survive. It is the most important measure of water quality as it indicates the water bodies' ability to sustain aquatic life. Another crucial parameter is the power of hydrogen (pH) that defines the acidity or alkalinity of water. In rivers, pH sets as the foundation of support for the availability of nutrients.

In addition, to understand the amount of impurities present in water, salinity (SAL) quantifies the dissolved salt content in water and total dissolved solid (TDS) derives the amount of organic matter in the water solution. Since dissolved salts and other organic chemicals can conduct electric current, thus conductivity correlates with TDS and increases with salinity. Electrical conductivity (EC) measures the ability of water to pass an electrical current. Both conductivity and TDS are water quality parameters used as the salinity indicator. The two parameters are not only affected by salinity, but also material contents which can be expressed as $TDS = k\,EC$ (25 °C), given that the value k is characterized with the concentration of ions in water [5]. Subsequent water quality variables are resistivity (RES), which is the opposite of conductivity; it signifies the ability of water to resist an electric current. Water of higher concentration of dissolved salts will have lower resistivity.

Turbidity (TUR) is the water quality parameter used to describe the clarity and haziness of water. A high turbidity contains a high intensity of clay, slit and organic matter. The level of turbidity affects light transmission in water which affects photosynthesis rate of aquatic plants in water, hence consequently affecting dissolved oxygen levels [6].

In the present study, sampling analysis and daily observation was carried out in Merbok River, Kuala Muda, Kedah to assess the variation of water quality parameters. The water quality parameters as described above shall be used as variables for the assessment of this study as these water quality parameters could easily reveal the condition of water bodies. This study is helpful to understand the environment impacts and evaluate the water quality status in understanding possible threats to the ecosystem.

2 Materials and Methods

2.1 Study Area

This study was conducted at Merbok River situated between latitudes 5° 39 N and 541° N and longitudes 100° 20 E to 100° 24 E in the northwest of Peninsular Malaysia of Kuala Muda District, Kedah (Fig. 1). There are two sampling sites in this study, namely Site A (Fig. 2) at Laguna Jetty Point and Site B (Fig. 3) 1.0 km from Site A. The river is about 35 km long, 2.5 km wide and approximately 3–15 m deep. Merbok River is tidally influenced, with most of the river being a mangrove estuarine. The main sources of the river are from Bongkok River and Puntar River, Gurun.

The climate characteristics of Merbok River is dry and wet twice per year. Dry seasons occurs during December, January and February while rainfall is highest

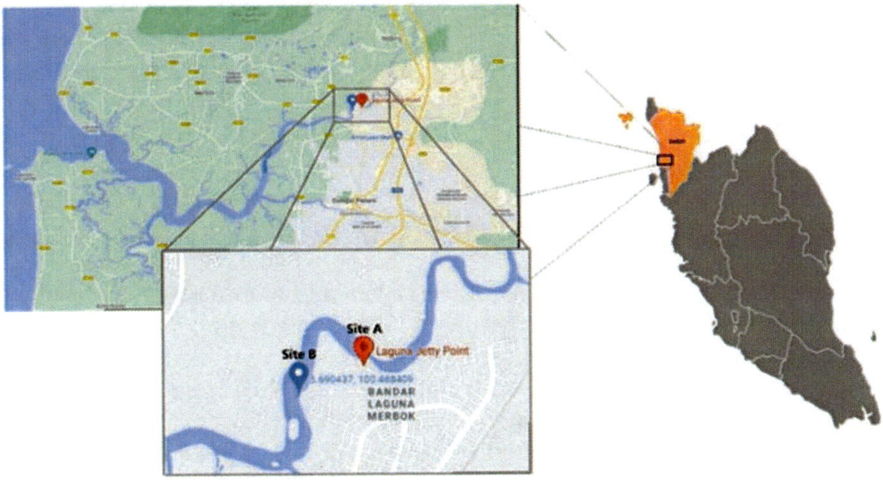

Fig. 1 Location of study area at Merbok River, Kuala Muda District, Kedah

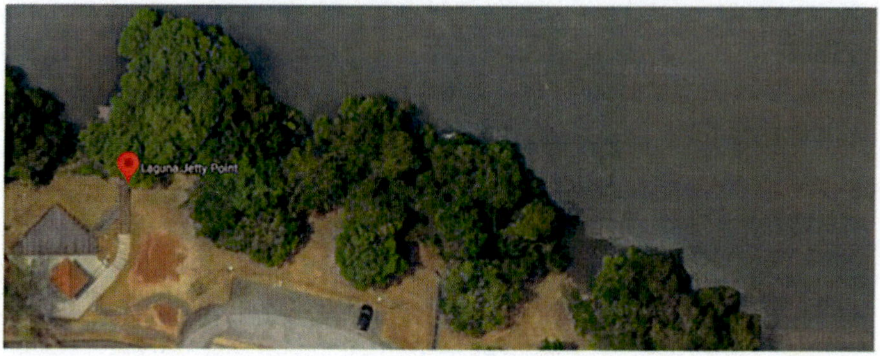

Fig. 2 Aerial view of the location of site A, Laguna Jetty Point

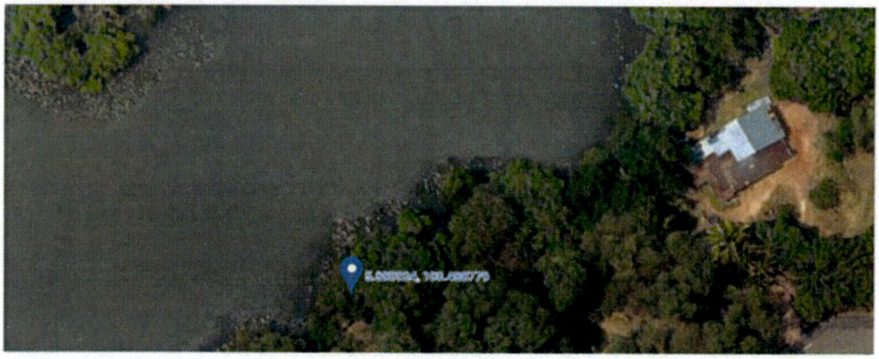

Fig. 3 Aerial view of site B (5° 41.4 N; 100° 29.28 E)

during November in the north east monsoon and May in the south west monsoon [7]. The annual rainfall varies between 200 and 250 cm with average daily temperature ranges between 22 and 32 °C and average humidity in the range of 80–90%. Tidal range of Merbok River has a mean of 1.7 m with mean neap tide of 0.8 m and mean spring tide of 2.3 m [8].

The Merbok river catchment was chosen in this study due to its increase in land use activities over the years. Major activities around the catchment are oil palm and rubber plantations in the upper and middle catchment. Whereas the middle and lower catchment is saturated with residential areas and urbanization. The lower catchment is then distributed with swamp and mangroves. The tributaries are currently suffering from point source pollutions originating from household sullage, wastewater treatment plant and industrial runoffs. Other polluting sources are coming from restaurants, development areas, disposal sites, and aquacultural activities [9]. The increase in economic and population growth has taken a toll on the ecosystem balance of Merbok basin, particular on the surrounding mangrove habitat.

Table 1 National water quality standards for Malaysia (INWQS) [11]

Parameter	Unit	Class					
		I	IIA	IIB	III	IV	V
pH	–	6.5–8.5	6–9	6–9	5–9	5–9	–
DO	mg/l	7	5–7	5–7	3–5	<3	<1
EC	μS/cm	1000	1000	–	–	6000	–
TDS	mg/l	500	1000	–	–	4000	–
SAL	mg/l	0.5	1	–	–	2	–
TUR	NTU	5	50	50	–	–	–
TEMP	°C	–	Normal + °C	–	Normal + °C	–	–

2.2 *Sampling Protocol*

Two points were designated around Laguna Jetty Point (5° 41.63 N, 100° 26.60 E) for daily water sample collection. The water samples were collected at depths 0.5 m from water surface, and at riverbanks between 07:00 and 10:00 AM in the morning and 06:00 and 09:00 PM in the evening from November 2020 to March 2021.

In-situ water quality parameters that are pH, temperature (TEMP), dissolved oxygen (DO), conductivity (COND), total dissolved solids (TDS), and salinity (SAL) were measured using the EUTECH CyberScan PCD650 multiparameter meter, while turbidity (TUR) is analyzed using the EUTECH-TN100 turbidity meter. Calibration is performed every three days according to the standards of pH buffer 4,7 and 10, saturation of dissolved oxygen at 80–100% at sea level, 12,880 μS/cm conductivity standard, and turbidity calibrated to 0.2 NTU, 20 NTU, 100 NTU, 1000 NTU to ensure equipment accuracy.

Water quality analysis is a fundamental assessment of the level of pollution of the water body. The Malaysian Department of Environment (DOE) has categorized water quality into 5 groups (Table 1) that have different purposes. Class I is classified as unpolluted and safe for drinking; Class II is fit for recreational use yet require conventional treatment; Class III is considered as polluted water supply hence requires extensive treatment; Class IV is only for irrigation or domestic use whereas Class IV cannot be utilized for any purposes [10].

3 Results and Discussion

3.1 *Temperature, pH and Dissolved Oxygen*

Throughout the sampling period from November to March, wet season occurred from November 2020 to January 2021 while the dry season happened during February and March. The average water temperature of samples is shown in Fig. 4, ranging

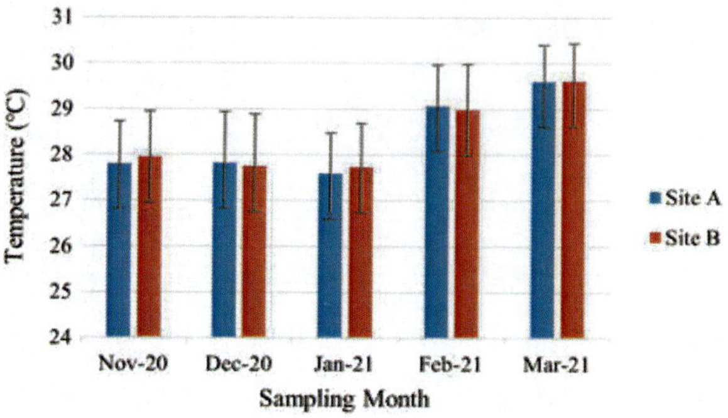

Fig. 4 The mean value of daily water temperature from sampling points

between 27.0 and 31.0 °C. Temperature is lower during the wet season where rainfall is regular.

The measured values of pH, DO, TDS, salinity, and turbidity are tabulated in Table 2 with their respective mean value and standard deviation. It can be deduced that the water quality in Merbok River is semi-polluted. Based on daily observations, the surface of the water is only cloudy or hazy during monsoon seasons and relatively calm throughout the dry season. Litter and garbage were seen occasionally flooding the area specifically after rainfall. Most of the time, the riverbank area is filled with lively aquatic life such as prawns and school of fishes; jellyfish was sighted twice during the end of February. Laguna Merbok Jetty Point (Site A) is a recreational spot that is usually crowded with jogging residents, whereas Site B is a common fish netting spot for fishermen.

The range of pH value of Merbok River along the study period is 6.5–8.9 pH, with an average of 7.08. The average pH value is within the neutral range as per the NWQS and ideal for biological productivity that is between pH 7.0–8.5 [12]. Nevertheless, it was observed that there is a significant spike in pH during February followed by a spike in saturated dissolved oxygen. The high value of pH is likely due to point source pollution from agricultural or wastewater runoff. High pH values can also be associated with a high photosynthesis rate from dense phytoplankton blooms. However, the increase in pH levels was then lowered in the following month. Minor changes in pH levels could have long term effects on nutrient solubility. The minor increase of pH could also form an oligotrophic state that is high in dissolved oxygen, this could cause the water to become eutrophic when the demand of dissolved oxygens increases with the growth of algae [13] (Fig. 5).

Table 2 The average and standard deviation (average ± standard deviation) of measured pH, DO, TDS, salinity, and turbidity in Merbok River

Sampling site	pH	DO (mg/l)	TDS (mg/l)	Salinity (mg/l)	TUR (NTU)
Site A	7.04 ± 0.27	3.57 ± 1.74	14.50 ± 10.21	18.76 ± 14.11	31.49 ± 65.63
Site B	7.13 ± 0.35	3.94 ± 2.24	18.23 ± 10.32	23.99 ± 14.59	25.29 ± 50.08
Classification	I	III	–	–	II

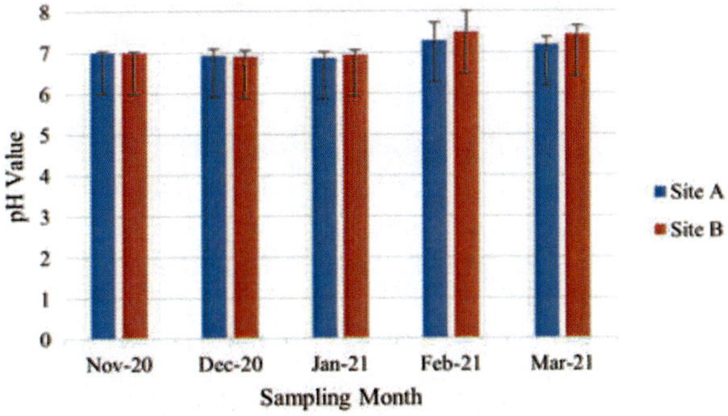

Fig. 5 The mean value of daily pH from sampling points

Figure 6 shows the average range of DO values at Merbok River that is between (1.40 and 13.35 mg/l) with an average of 3.71 mg/l. Similar DO results were recorded by Fatema et al. [14] in 2011. During the study period, the highest DO value was recorded in February which corresponded with the increase of pH value. Overall, throughout the study period the DO levels are classified in Class III, hence suggesting the semi-polluted condition of Merbok River. Along the duration of study, an occurrence of fishes crowding to the water surface in November was observed. Fishes ventilate at the top layer of water for respiration where the surface contains higher concentration of dissolved oxygen. The event signifies the hypoxic water condition from low levels of oxygen in water. The low DO level in water bodies is associated to the increase of oxygen demand caused from the increased concentration of anaerobic bacteria and organic matter in water [15]. Prolonged conditions of low dissolved oxygen saturation could impair river ecology, prompting serious hypoxia events [16].

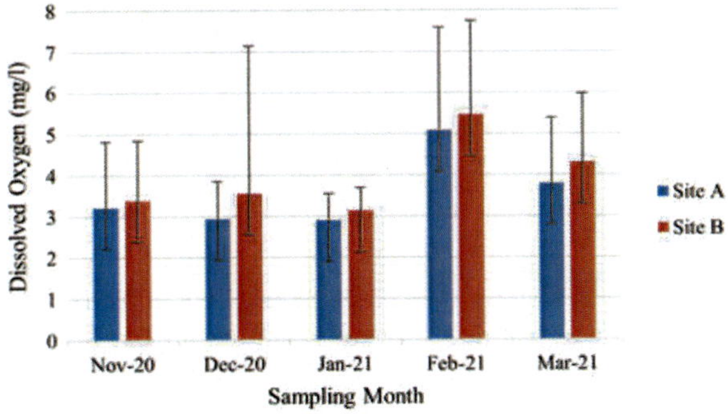

Fig. 6 The mean value of daily dissolved oxygen from sampling points

3.2 *Conductivity, Total Dissolved Solids, Salinity and Resistivity*

Figures 7, 8, 9 and 10 measures the conductivity value, total dissolved solids, salinity (NaCl) and resistivity in Merbok River from November 2020 to March 2021. It is observed that the trend of conductivity, TDS and salinity are similar. The three water quality parameters peaked during March and have similar range of mean values.

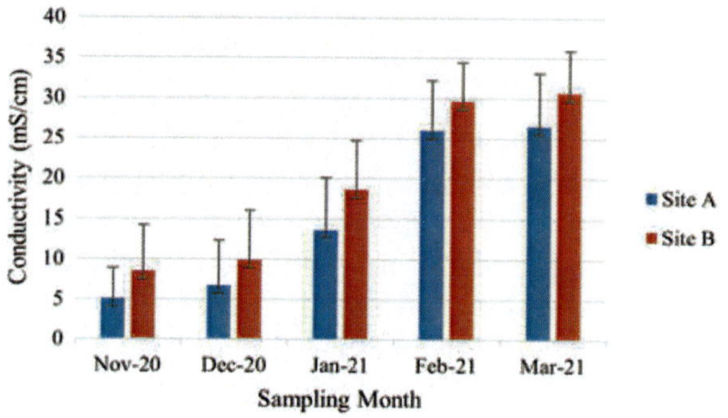

Fig. 7 The mean value of daily conductivity from sampling points

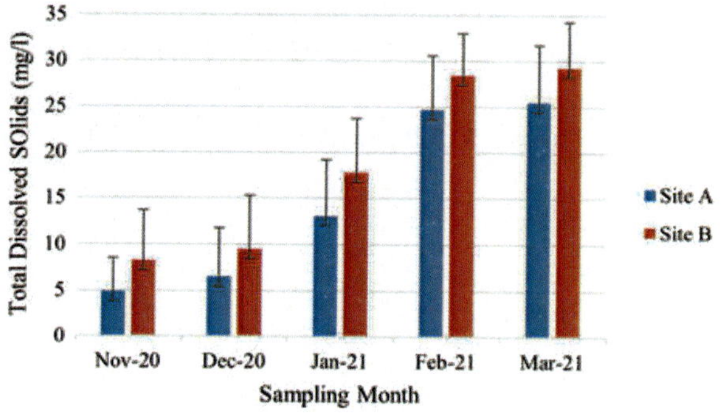

Fig. 8 The mean value of daily total dissolved solids from sampling points

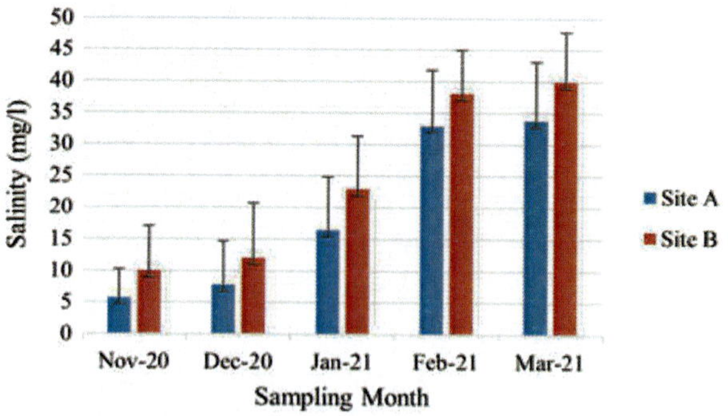

Fig. 9 The mean value of daily salinity from sampling points

Fig. 10 The mean value of daily resistivity from sampling points

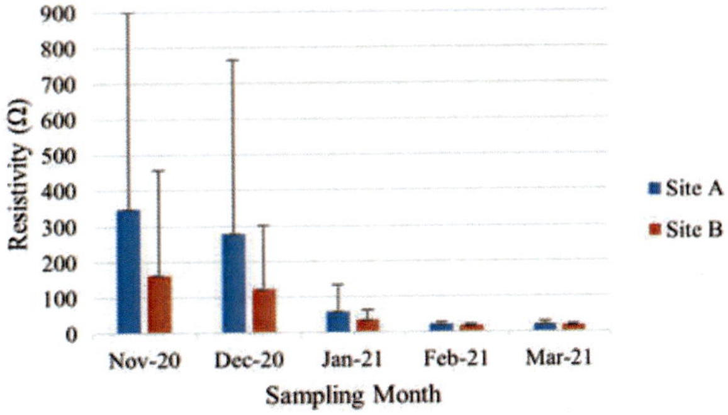

Significant changes in conductivity indicates that there are impurities coming from pollution source or discharge present in the water. This is due to the additional increase of chloride, phosphate and nitrate ions from sewage leakage or agricultural waste [17]. Moreover, higher temperature could also lead to higher conductivity. The increase in temperature increases the mobility of ions in water. In this study, during February and March the dry season, temperature has increased by 2 °C, therefore an increase in conductivity is observed.

Salinity analysis from Fig. 9 shows that the value of salinity in ppt (mg/l) is between 0.188 and 59.22 ppt with an average of 21.38 ppt. Generally, the range of salinity for estuaries is between 0.5 and 35 ppt. The average value of salinity is still within threshold limit. However, the rise in salinity was observed during March where there is little rainfall in the dry season. Findings from our study correlates with the results by Manikannan et al. [18] where salinity levels are maximum during summer (dry season) and lowest in the monsoon season. Rising level of salinity is reflected from the increase in evaporation and precipitation rate [19]. High level of salinity could decrease the performance and survival of organisms [20].

In this study, it is evident that the relation between resistivity and salinity is inversely proportional. Resistivity was the lowest during January, February and March, while salinity and conductivity was the highest during that time. After a heavy rainfall, the values of conductivity, total dissolved solids and salinity are the lowest. It is concluded that during the monsoon season where rainfall is peak, conductivity is decreased since the salinity of water is diluted [17].

3.3 *Turbidity*

Continued in this section is the measure of turbidity throughout the study period. As depicted in Fig. 11, turbidity could range from as low as 1.13 NTU to 555 NTU. Low turbidity was observed during the dry season, starting from January. High turbidity is common during the monsoon season where rainfall is the heaviest in November.

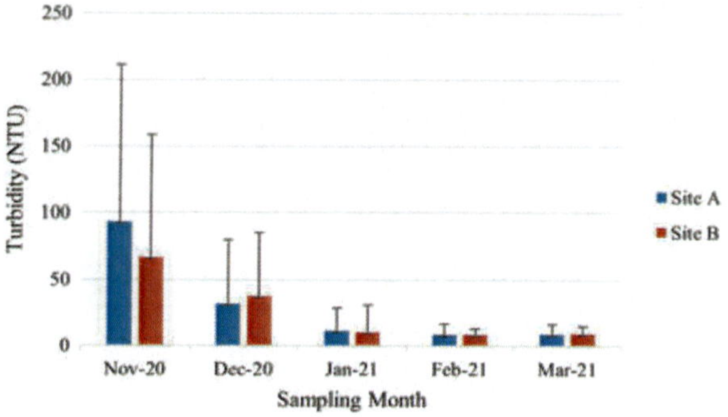

Fig. 11 The mean value of daily turbidity from sampling points

The average turbidity of Merbok River throughout the study period is 28.39 NTU falling into Class II as per the NWQS.

The observed results matches the research conclusion by Ismail et al. [21] during 2018, where suspended sediment concentration and suspended sediment load increases significantly during the wet season compared to the dry season, hence increases the turbidity. Surface runoffs are a major contributing factor to the elevated levels of sediment and turbidity. These runoff are due to industrial discharges into the river [22]. The extreme rise in turbidity poses risk to underwater organism, high level of turbidity shades sunlight from penetrating into the water, which encourages the smothering of benthic habitats such as mollusks and polychaetes. Moreover, the disturbance of sediments in water tend to absorb heat, causing an increase in water temperature that would reduce the dissolving rate of oxygen. The high concentration of particulate matter affects ecological productivity, and reducing the resiliency of aquatic life [23].

4 Conclusion

From the five month in-situ sampling at Merbok River, daily observations and values of pH, water temperature, dissolved oxygen, conductivity, total dissolved solids, salinity, resistivity and turbidity, the river is categorized as semi-polluted (Class III). Water quality between Site A and Site B are similar in average, yet aquatic life were found to be more dominant at Site B since dissolved oxygen levels were higher and hence fishery activities were more common at Site B. The predominant fluctuating factor of the river are pH, dissolved oxygen and turbidity which are heavily influenced by weather and seasonal factors coupled with underlying point source pollution from industrial activities.

The occasional peak in pH and dissolved oxygen from an undetected source poses a long-term risk on the aquatic life in Merbok River, as this phenomenon encourages the growth of algae and increases the demand for dissolved oxygen. When the supply of oxygen gets depleted, yet the demand remains high, this might create an imbalance where the ecosystem could become eutrophic. Moreover, the high level of turbidity specifically during the wet season could affect the future coastal and estuarine fisheries. With ongoing urbanization and industrialization taking place surrounding the area, water quality might deteriorate further.

Forth coming work such as soil sampling analysis of the sediments and collection of nitrogen or phosphate concentration could be carried out to understand heavy metal concentration and nutrient levels within the Merbok estuary. Future research and strategies to improve the coastal ecosystem should be implemented to preserve the dynamic ecosystem at Merbok River, where mangroves and aquatic life are dominant in the area.

Acknowledgements The authors would like to thank Ministry of Higher Education on Malaysian Young Researchers Grant (MYRGS), MR001-2019 and Universiti Malaya for the continuous support through UM Living Lab research funding LL037-18SUS granted by Universiti Malaya Community and Sustainability Centre.

References

1. Gburek, W., Folmar, G.: Flow and chemical contributions to streamflow in an upland watershed: a baseflow survey. J. Hydrol. **217**(1–2), 1–18 (1999)
2. Jickells, T.: Nutrient biogeochemistry of the coastal zone. Science **281**(5374), 217–222 (1998)
3. Nollet, L.M., De Gelder, L.S.: Handbook of Water Analysis. CRC Press (2000)
4. Rabalais, N.N., Turner, R.E., Wiseman, W.J., Jr.: Hypoxia in the Gulf of Mexico. J. Environ. Qual. **30**(2), 320–329 (2001)
5. Rusydi, A.F.: Correlation between conductivity and total dissolved solid in various type of water: a review. In: IOP Conference Series: Earth and Environmental Science, vol. 118, no. 1, p. 012019. IOP Publishing (2018)
6. Berry, W., Rubinstein, N., Melzian, B., Hill, B.: The biological effects of suspended and bedded sediment (SABS) in aquatic systems: a review. U.S. Environ. Protect. Agency Duluth **32**(1), 54–55 (2003)
7. Ismail, W.R., Ibrahim, M.N.: An assessment of sediment and nitrogen input into the upper Merbok estuary, Kedah, Malaysia. Water Qual. Expo. Health **7**(1), 79–88 (2015)
8. Khuzaimah, Z., Ismail, M.H., Mansor, S.: Mangrove changes analysis by remote sensing and evaluation of ecosystem service value in Sungai Merbok's mangrove forest reserve, Peninsular Malaysia. In: International Conference on Computational Science and Its Applications, pp. 611–622. Springer (2013)
9. Kamrudzamana, A.N., Nordina, A.M.A., Aziza, R.A., Ab Jalilb, M.F.: Mapping status for river water quality index of Sungai Merbok, Kedah, Malaysia. Int. J. **3**(1) (2012)
10. Othman, F., et al.: Efficient river water quality index prediction considering minimal number of inputs variables. Eng. Appl. Comput. Fluid Mech. **14**(1), 751–763 (2020)
11. DOE: Environmental Quality Report (EQR) 2006. Department of Environment, Ministry of Natural Resources and Environment Malaysia, Kuala Lumpur (2006)
12. Abowei, J.: Salinity, dissolved oxygen, pH and surface water temperature conditions in Nkoro River, Niger Delta, Nigeria. Adv. J. Food Sci. Technol. **2**(1), 36–40 (2010)
13. Fondriest Environmental, Inc.: pH of water. Fundamentals of Environmental Measurements [Online]. Available: https://www.fondriest.com/environmental-measurements/parameters/water-quality/ph/

14. Fatema, K., Maznah, W.W., Isa, M.M.: Spatial and temporal variation of physico-chemical parameters in the Merbok Estuary, Kedah, Malaysia. Trop. Life Sci. Res. **25**(2), 1 (2014)
15. Cooper, C.: Biological effects of agriculturally derived surface water pollutants on aquatic systems—a review. J. Environ. Qual. **22**(3), 402–408 (1993)
16. Jassby, A., Van Nieuwenhuyse, E.E.: Low dissolved oxygen in an estuarine channel (San Joaquin River, California): mechanisms and models based on long-term time series. San Francisco Estuary Watershed Sci. **3**(2) (2005)
17. Fondriest Environmental, Inc.: Conductivity, salinity and total dissolved solids. In: Fundamentals of Environmental Measurements [Online]. Available: https://www.fondriest.com/environmental-measurements/parameters/water-quality/conductivity-salinity-tds/
18. Manikannan, R., Asokan, S., Ali, A.H.M.S.: Seasonal variations of physico-chemical properties of the Great Vedaranyam Swamp, Point Calimere Wildlife Sanctuary, South-east coast of India. Afr. J. Environ. Sci. Technol. **5**(9), 673–681 (2011)
19. Ridd, P.V., Stieglitz, T.: Dry season salinity changes in arid estuaries fringed by mangroves and saltflats. Estuar. Coast. Shelf Sci. **54**(6), 1039–1049 (2002). https://doi.org/10.1006/ecss.2001.0876
20. Velasco, J., et al.: Effects of salinity changes on aquatic organisms in a multiple stressor context. Philos. Trans. R. Soc. B **374**(1764), 20180011 (2019)
21. Ismail, W., Ibrahim, M., Najib, S.: Longitudinal changes in suspended sediment loading and sediment budget of Merbok River catchment, Kedah, Malaysia. Pertanika J. Sci. Technol. **26**(4), 1899–1911 (2018)
22. Ateshan, H.M., Misnan, R., Sinang, S.C., Koki, I.B.: Evaluation of water pollution and source identification in Merbok River Kedah, Northwest Malaysia (2020)
23. Paul, S.: Turbidity: description, impact on water quality, sources, measures—a general overview. Descr. Impact Water Qual. Sources Measur. **3**, 2–4 (2008)